CONCEPTS
OF
BIOCHEMISTRY

W0235528

CONCEPTS OF BIOCHEMISTRY
(For Physiotherapy / Pharmacy)

S.P. Singh

Ph.D, FACBI, Former WHO Fellow-
Texas A & M University, Texas, U.S.A.
Nominated by Government of India for Commonwealth Medical Fellowship- 1983
Professor and Head, Department of Biochemistry,
MLB Medical College, Jhansi- 284128, U.P.
and
Chief Consultant in Biochemistry,
MLB Medical College Associated Hospital, Jhansi

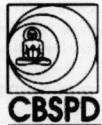

CBS Publishers & Distributors Pvt Ltd

New Delhi • Bengaluru • Chennai • Kochi • Kolkata • Lucknow • Mumbai
Hyderabad • Jharkhand • Nagpur • Patna • Pune • Uttarakhand

Disclaimer

Science and technology are constantly changing fields. New research and experience broaden the scope of information and knowledge. The author has tried his best in giving information available to him while preparing the material for this book. Although all efforts has been made to ensure optimum accuracy of the material, yet it is quite possible some errors might have been left uncorrected. The publisher, the printer and the author will not be held responsible for any inadvertent errors, omissions or inaccuracies.

Concepts of Biochemistry for Physiotherapy and Pharmacy

ISBN: 978-81-239-1391-9

Copyright © Author & Publisher

First Edition: 2006
Reprint: 2007, 2009, 2014, 2019, 2023

All rights reserved. No part of this book may be reproduced or transmitted in any form or by any means, electronic or mechanical, including photocopying, recording, or any information storage and retrieval system without permission, in writing, from the author and the publisher.

Published by **Satish Kumar Jain** and produced by **Varun Jain** for

CBS Publishers & Distributors Pvt Ltd

4819/XI Prahlad Street, 24 Ansari Road, Daryaganj, New Delhi 110 002, India.
Ph: 011-23289259, 23266861, 23266867   Website: www.cbspd.com
Fax: 011-23243014   e-mail: delhi@cbspd.com;

Corporate Office: 204 FIE, Industrial Area, Patparganj, Delhi 110 092
Ph: 011-4934 4934   Fax: 011-4934 4935   e-mail: publishing@cbspd.com;
                                                                             publicity@cbspd.com

Branches

- **Bengaluru:** Seema House 2975, 17th Cross, KR Road, Banasankari 2nd Stage, Bengaluru 560 070, Karnataka, India
  Ph: +91-80-26771678/79   Fax: +91-80-26771680   e-mail: bangalore@cbspd.com
- **Chennai:** 7, Subbaraya Street, Shenoy Nagar, Chennai 600 030, Tamil Nadu, India
  Ph: +91-44-26680620, 26681266   Fax: +91-44-42032115   e-mail: chennai@cbspd.com
- **Kochi:** 42/1325, 1326, Power House Road, Opp KSEB, Power House, Ernakulum Kochi 682 018, Kerala, India
  Ph: +91-484-4059061-65,67   Fax: +91-484-4059065   e-mail: kochi@cbspd.com
- **Kolkata:** 147, Hind Ceramics Compound, 1st Floor, Nilgunj Road, Belghoria, Kolkata-700056, West Bengal, India
  Ph: +033-25633055, 033-25633056   e-mail: kolkata@cbspd.com
- **Lucknow:** Basement, Khushnuma Complex, 7 Meerabai Marg (Behind Jawahar Bhawan),Lucknow-226001, UP, India
  Ph: +0522-4000032   e-mail: tiwari.lucknow@cbspd.com
- **Mumbai:** PWD Shed, Gala no 25/26, Ramchandra Bhatt Marg, Next to JJ Hospital Gate no. 2, Opp. Union Bank of India,
  Noorbaug, Mumbai-400009, Maharashtra, India
  Ph: 022-66661880/89   e-mail: mumbai@cbspd.com

Representatives

- Hyderabad   0-9885175004   • Jharkhand   0-9811541605   • Nagpur   0-9421945513
- Patna   0-9334159340   • Pune   0-9923910676   • Uttarakhand 0-9716462459

Printed at   SRK Graphic, Shadara, Delhi

PREFACE TO THE FIRST EDITION

Occasional visits to the departments of **Physiotherapy** and **Pharmacy** as an examiner to various universities of our country fed me an idea to write one cozy book for the students pursuing such courses as I found them consulting large size voluminous books of 'Biochemistry'.

I have written this book after consulting syllabi of various Indian Universities of both the courses. I am sure this book shall serve the purpose of such courses. If any short coming (s), I am sure the valuable readers (students and the learned teachers) shall bring it to my notice for further improvement and oblige.

15th August '2006   - S.P. Singh

(Independence Day of India)

ACKNOWLEDGEMENT

First of all, I express my deep gratitude to my family members i.e., **wife Dr. (Smt) Manju Singh, Reader, History Department, Bundelkhand Postgraduate College, Jhansi; sons Er. Vikrant Singh and Er. Vijyant Singh, daughter-in-law Smt. Charu Singh, pets Pasha, Gini and Laina who all always not only inspired me but also encouraged me from time to time for this gigantic work as writing of a book paralyses one's social and family life.**

I shall fail in my duties if I do not express my gratitude to my well wishers i.e.; Lt. Colonel (Retd) A.R.N. Setalvad, Secretary, Medical Council of India (a thorough gentleman who speaks little and says everything from eyes); Dr. Narendra Kumar Jain, Vice Chancellor, Rajasthan University, Jaipur (inspirer for me for writing work); Dr. R.K. Srivastava, Director - General, Ministry of Health and Family Welfare, Govt of India, New Delhi (who acts as a **'lamp'** for me), Dr. A.K. Gupta, Principal & Dean, M.L.B. Medical College, Jhansi, Professor (Smt) Mridula Kapur, Professor R.K. Gandhi, Prof R.P. Srivastava, Professor Bhakt Prakash Mathur, Dr. K.P. Singh, Prof. V.N. Pandey, Principal, Bundelkhand Postgraduate College, Jhansi; Sri M.P. Gupta, Senior Advocate, Jhansi; Prof. R.K. Bhatia, History Department, BKD College, Jhansi; Er. S.S. Chaturvedi, Er. V.N. Pathak, Sri K.V. Srivastava, Sri Bishan Lal, (Librarian), Sri S.A. Siddiqui, Sri S.S. Shukla, Sri Ashok Kumar Srivastava, Sri Chintamani, Sri Khalak Singh, Sri Vinod Kumar - all of M.L.B. Medical College, Jhansi.

I am also indebted to my well wishers i.e., Sri Satish Kumar Jain, Sri Vinod Kumar Jain, Sri Sonu Jain, Sri B.M. Singh, Sri B.M. Sharma, Sri Dharam Veer, Sri Nayar- all of M/s CBS Publishers, New Delhi; Dr. D.P. Singh Maurya (Meerut) and Sri Sudhir Arora, M/s English Book Depot, Sadar Bazar, Jhansi who all always guided me for creative works from time to time.

I am also really indebted to **Mr. Prakash Sahu**, Compositor, 390, Sadar Bazar, Jhansi and **Mr. Sunil Sharma,** Artist, Nagra, Jhansi for preparing beautiful figures of this book in such a short period.

15th August '2006   - S.P. Singh
(Independence Day of India)

By
the grace and kind blessings
of
Lord Sri Ram Raja Sarkar ji, ORCHHA
(Tikamgarh, Madhya Pradesh)

Dedicated
To
The Primary School
Ratti Ka Nangla (Across Railway Loco Shed)
TUNDLA JUNCTION (AGRA)
Where I took my primary education

AND

My Late respected laborious mother **Smt MUKANDI DEVI ji,**
who taught me upto standard 3rd after all odds

AND

My Late respected intelligent, diligent and honest father **Sri Devi Prasad Singh ji,**
B.A., L.L.B., Station Master/ Yard Master, **Tundla Junction (Northern Railway)**, who taught me
upto 12th standard after enormous tiring, stressful and exhausted duties of Railways.

AND

My dear Brothers and Sister **Sri C.P. Singh ji,** Retired Jt Director, Cement Research Institute,
Ballabhagarh (Haryana), **Sri I.P. Singh ji,** Retired Works Manager, N. Rly Workshop,
KALKA (Haryana), **Sri. V.P. Singh,** Civil Defence Officer, Mathura (U.P.), **Sri. A.P. Singh,**
Assistant Office Supdt., D.R,M. Office, N.Rly, Moradabad (U.P.), **Smt. Shakuntala Devi,** Jai
Narain Vyas Colony, Bikaner (Rajasthan)

BIOCHEMICAL ABBREVIATIONS

Ac	:	Acetate
Ac CoA	:	Acyl coenzyme A
A	:	Adenine
ACD bottle	:	Acid citrate dextrose bottle
ALD	:	Aldolase
AIDS	:	Acquired immune deficiency syndrome
AMP	:	Adenosine monophosphate (adenylic acid)
ADP	:	Adenosine diphosphate
ACE	:	Angiotensin converting enzyme
ACP	:	Acid phosphatase
ALT	:	Alanine transaminase (previously GPT)
AST	:	Aspartate transaminase (previously GOT)
ATP	:	Adenosine triphosphate
ADPR	:	Adenosine diphosphate ribose
ATPase	:	Adenosine triphosphatase
AT-10	:	Dehydrotachysterol (antitetany compound-10)
AZT	:	Azidothymidine the only drug effective against AIDs, this is going to be marketed in India by 'Cipla' under the name of 'Zidovir'
BCG	:	Bacillus Calmette and Guerin
BMR	:	Basal metabolic rate
CF	:	Citrovorum factor (folinic acid)
CoA	:	Coenzyme A
CoA SH	:	Coenzyme A reduced
C	:	Cytosine
CMP	:	Cytosine monophosphate (cytidylic acid)
CDP	:	Cytosine diphosphate
cDNA	:	Complementary DNA
CT	:	Computed tomography
CTP	:	Cytosine triphosphate
cTnT	:	Cardiac troponin T
Cal	:	Calorie, large (kilocalorie)
ChE	:	Choline esterase
CPK	:	Creatine phosphokinase
DAP	:	Dihydroxyacetone phosphate
DFP	:	Diisopropyl fluorophosphate
1,25 DHCC	:	1,25 dihydroxy cholecalciferol
DMD	:	Duchenne muscular dystrophy
DNP	:	2, 4 - dinitrophenol
DPN^+	:	Diphosphopyridine nucleotide, oxidized
$DPNH_2$	:	Diphosphopyridine nucleotide, reduced

DNA	:	Deoxyribonucleic acid
DOC	:	Deoxycorticosterone
DOPA	:	Dioxyphenylalanine or Dihydroxyphenylalanine
EDTA	:	Ethylene diamine tetra acetic acid
EAA	:	Essential amino acids
EFA	:	Essential fatty acids
FA	:	Folic Acid
FAD	:	Flavin adenine dinucleotide
FDP	:	Fructose 1, 6-diphosphate
FH_2	:	Dihydro folic acid
FH_4	:	Tetrahydro folic acid
FMN	:	Flavin mono nucleotide
FAO	:	Food and Agriculture Organization
GC-MS	:	Gas Chromatograph-Mass spectrometer
GA	:	Glyceraldehyde
GPx	:	Glutathione peroxidase
GSH	:	Glutathione (reduced form)
GSSG	:	Glutathione (oxidized form)
γ-GT	:	γ- glutamyl transferase
G	:	Guanine
GMP	:	Guanosine monophosphate (guanylic acid)
GDP	:	Guanosine diphosphate
GTP	:	Guanosine triphosphate
GDH	:	Glucose dehydrogenase
GLDH	:	Glutamate dehydrogenase
GnRH	:	Gonadotropin- releasing hormone
HbCO	:	Carboxy(Carbon monoxy) hemoglobin
HBsAG	:	Hepatitis B surface antigen i.e., Australia antigen
HBV	:	Hepatitis B virus
HPLC	:	High performance liquid chromatography
HIV	:	Human immuno-deficiency virus
IAA	:	Iodoacetate
I	:	Inosine
ICD	:	Isocitrate dehydrogenase
IMP	:	Inosine monophosphate (Inosinic Acid)
IDP	:	Inosine diphosphate
ITP	:	Inosine triphosphate
KG	:	α- Ketoglutarate
LTs	:	Leukotrienes
Mb	:	Myoglobin

MB	:	Methylene blue
MRI	:	Magnetic resonance imaging
NMN	:	Nicotinamide mononucleotide
NAD^+	:	Nicotinamide adenine dinucleotide (older name is DPN^+, also known as Co I)
$NADP^+$	:	Nicotinamide adenine dinucleotide phosphate (older name is TPN^+, also known as Co II)
NPN	:	Non protein nitrogen
OAA	:	Oxaloacetate
OD	:	Optical density
PABA	:	Para amino benzoic acid
PBI	:	Protein bound iodine
PEP	:	Phosphoenolpyruvate
3-PGA	:	3- Phosphoglyceric acid
PGE_2	:	Prostaglandin E_2
Pi	:	Inorganic phosphate
PP	:	Pyrophosphate
PKU	:	Phenylketonuria
POMC	:	Pro-opio melanocortin
PSA	:	Prostate specific antigen (semenogelase)
RNA	:	Ribonucleic acid
RNAse	:	Ribonuclease
R-5-P	:	Ribose-5-Phosphate
R.Q.	:	Respiratory Quotient
SOD	:	Superoxide dismutase
SRP	:	Signal recognition particle
STH	:	Somatotropic hormone
TCA	:	Trichloroacetic acid
THAM	:	Tris (hydroxymethyl) aminoethane
TPP	:	Thiamine pyrophosphate
TPN^+	:	Triphosphopyridine nucleotide (oxidized form)
$TPNH_2$	:	Triphosphopyridine nucleotide (reduced form)
U	:	Uracil residue
UMP	:	Uridine monophosphate (uridylic acid)
UDP	:	Uridine diphosphate
UTP	:	Uridine triphosphate
UDPG	:	Uridine diphosphoglucose
UDPGal	:	Uridine diphosphogalactose
USP	:	United States Pharmacopoeia
WHO	:	World Health Organization
XMP	:	Xanthosine monophosphate
Xyl	:	Xylose
Xul	:	Xylulose

AMINO ACIDS

Ala	:	Alanine
Arg	:	Arginine
Val	:	Valine
His	:	Histidine
Leu	:	Leucine
Ile	:	Isoleucine
Met	:	Methionine
Pro	:	Proline
Phe	:	Phenylalanine
Trp	:	Tryptophan
Asp	:	Aspartic acid
Asn	:	Asparagine
Gln	:	Glutamine
Glu	:	Glutamic acid
Gly	:	Glycine
Ser	:	Serine
Thr	:	Threonine
Thx	:	Thyroxine
Tyr	:	Tyrosine
Cys-SH	:	Cysteine
Cys-S-	:	1/2 Cystine
Lys	:	Lysine

HORMONES

ACTH	:	Adrenocorticotrophic hormone
FSH	:	Follicle stimulating hormone
GH	:	Growth hormone
HCG	:	Human chorionic gonadotropin
ICSH	:	Interistitial cell stimulating hormone
LH	:	Luteinizing hormone
LTH	:	Leuteotrophic hormone
MSH	:	Melanocyte stimulating hormone
PTH	:	Parathyroid hormone
TSH	:	Thyroid stimulating hormone
T_3	:	Triiodothyronine
T_4	:	Tetraiodothyronine (thyroxine)

MISCELLANEOUS

AHG	:	Antihemophilic globulin
BAL	:	British anti- lewisite
IR	:	Infrared
PRPP	:	Phosphoribosyl pyrophosphate
UV	:	Ultraviolet
VDM	:	Vasodepressor material
HRP	:	Horseradish peroxidase

Biochemical Abbreviations

TMB	: Tetra methyl benzidine	EGF	: Epidermal Growth Factor
Eukaryotes	: Mammalian cells	Enz	: Enzyme (Also E)
Prokaryotes	: Bacteria	Figlu	: Formiminoglutamic acid
NEPH	: Nephelometry	GIP	: Gastric inhibitory polypeptide
REP	: Radio electrophoresis	HAL	: Hepatic acylglycerol lipase
RU	: Radio uptake	HMG-CoA	: β-Hydroxy-β-methylglutaryl-CoA
CC	: Column Chromatography	HMM	: Heavy meromyosin
CDFD	: Centre for DNA finger printing & diagnostics (Hyderabad)	HSL	: Hormone-sensitive lipase
		I	: Isoproterenol
RIA	: Radio-immunoassay	IGF	: Insulin-like growth factor
CLIA	: Chemiluminescence immunoassay	IL	: Interleukin
ELISA	: Enzyme linked Immunosorbent assay	kat	: Katal
HAA	: Haem agglutination assay	kJ	: Kilojoule
ABP	: Androgen- binding protein	LATS	: Long- acting thyroid stimulator
ACAT	: Acyl-CoA: cholesterol acyltransferase	LMM	: Light meromyosin
ADH	: Alcohol dehydrogenase	LPH	: Lipotropic hormone
ADH	: Antidiuretic hormone, vasopressin	LPL	: Lipoprotein lipase
AFP	: α_1-Fetoprotein	MCR	: Metabolic clearance rate
AIP	: Aldosterone-induced protein	MDR	: Minimum daily requirement
ALA	: Aminolevulinic acid	MIT	: Monoiodotyrosine
BDGF	: Bone-derived growth factor	MJ	: Megajoule
BMP	: Bone morphogenic protein	NE	: Norepinephrine
CaBP	: Calcium- binding protein	NGF	: Nerve growth factor
CBG	: Corticosteroid- binding globulin	NSN	: Nicotine-sensitive neurophysin
CCK	: Cholecystokinin	PAF	: Platelet-activating factor
COMT	: Catechol-O-methyltransferase	PAPS	: Phosphoadenosine-phosphosulfate
CRBP	: Cellular retinol-binding protein	PGI	: Prostacyclin
CRH	: Corticotropin-releasing hormone	RDA	: Recommended daily (dietary) allowance
D	: Dopamine receptor		
DA	: Dopamine	SAM	: S - Adenosylmethionine
DES	: Diethylstilbestrol	SC	: Secretory component
DHEA	: Dehydroepiandrosterone	SDS	: Sodium dodecyl sulfate
DHT	: Dihydrotestosterone	SMP	: Submitochondrial particle
DIT	: Diiodotyrosine	TG	: Thyroglobulin
DPG	: Diphosphoglycerate	TMP	: Thiamine monophosphate
dsRNA	: Double-stranded RNA	TPA	: Tissue plasminogen activator
E	: Epinephrine	VIP	: Vasoactive intestinal polypeptide
		VMA	: Vanillylmandelic acid

CONTENTS

CHAPTER 1

BIOCHEMISTRY - THE 'YOGA' AND THE HEALTH

Do some 'Yoga' daily atleast half an hour and advise others also for the same after the age of 20 years atleast as the body's biochemistry starts deteriorating very gradually. Increase its time after the age of 40 years to atleast one hour. It will keep the body's biochemistry fit and in order and will keep you away from a doctor.

'Yoga' is a complete science of Ancient Indian system of Medicine which is more than 5,000 years old whereas the present more prevalent system of allopathic medicine is nearly 200 years old only.

Plus points of allopathic system of Medicine are that it is of great value in completely curing diseases caused due to bacteria/microorganisms; in surgical/accidental (traumatic)/emergency cases, whereas the 'yoga' system of medicine has got the capability to cure incurable diseases permanently. If 'yoga' and ancient system of medicine i.e., Ayurvedic are used simultaneously for curing a disease then the results are quicker but it's not always advisable to take Ayurvedic pills. 'Yoga' alone is a very good system of medicine which to a greater extent can cure innumerable diseases/ disorders of human beings permanently whereas there is no such permanent cure of such diseases in allopathic system. To name such incurable diseases, following are the

few examples:

1. Blood pressure (Hypertension)
2. Hypercholesterolaemia/ hypertriglycerid-aemia
3. Obesity (reduction in weight)
4. Parkinson's disease
5. Polio
6. Alzheimer's disease
7. Heart- aliments
8. Psoriasis
9. Asthma
10. Hyperacidity
11. Piles
12. Joint problems like ankylosis, prolapse disc, lumbago (pain in the lumbar region), cervical and lumbar spondylosis, osteo-arthritis, rheumatoid arthritis, gout, arthralgia (pain in joints), frozen shoulders, sprains, etc.
13. Bronchitis
14. Atherosclerosis

15. SLE (partially)
16. Tumours
17. Cancers (to some extent, Ist stage only)
18. Anaemia
19. Mysthenia gravis
20. Diabetes mellitus
21. Hyperthyroidism
22. Baldness
23. Greyish of hairs
24. Varicose veins
25. Fibroids in the uterus
26. Deafness
27. Muscular dystrophy
28. For gain in body weight
29. Neurological disorders
30. Depression
31. Epilepsy
32. Scleroderma
33. Leucoderma
34. Eye sight
35. Glaucoma
36. Osteoporosis
37. Constipation
38. Ulcers in the gastrointestinal tract
39. Spinal problems
40. Renal problems
41. Psychic problems
42. Sharpness of the wisdom
43. Paralysis
44. Insomnia
45. Vitality
46. Respiratory problems, etc.

- **The science of 'Yoga' demands regularity, sincerity, dedication and time.**
- Duration of time in performing 'Yoga' has got more meaning.
- By the application of 'Yoga', one can lead a long smooth life, may be hundred years or more as there are examples of Indian Rishis and Munis having longevity as much as 150 years or so. What 'Yoga' does to the biochemistry of human beings?

- It brings out proper synchronisation and balance of various hormones **(endocrine system)** and enzymes of our system which play innumerable vital role in thousands of biochemical reactions of our body.
- It reactivates and re-energises cells of our system.
- It regenerates cells.
- It checks degeneration process which is mainly associated with the advancing age.
- It reactivates various organs like pancreas, lungs, etc.
- It brings out inhalation of proper quantity of oxygen.
- It keeps the biochemistry of the body fit and in order which one can realise and come across the consequences in one's own life.

Credit for revolution in 'Yoga' in the present era goes to the untiring efforts of **Param Pujya yogi swami Ram Dev Ji Maharaj of Haridwar of Uttranchal state whose dream is first to see every Indian healthy and then the human race round the globe.**

Although, this science of 'Yoga' is not the new one but 'Yogi ji' is solely responsible for bringing awareness in the masses.

He deserves 'Bharat Ratna' while alive. Govt. of India must confer upon him this prestigious award. He has awaken all of us. We were really sleeping for more than fifty years like 'Kumkhkaran' (brother of Rawan) of 'Ramayana Age'. **He emphasizes mainly on three 'yogic exercises', namely :**

(i) Anulom - Vilom,

(ii) Kapalbhati, and

(iii) Bhastrika

CHAPTER 2

BIOCHEMISTRY : IMPORTANCE AND APPLICATIONS

Biochemistry, these days is treated to be the most important subject of life-sciences whether medical sciences or plant-sciences. Nearly 70 years ago, this subject was in infancy but now it is deep rooted and possesses an unique position because it is said to be the foundation of the modern medicine on which it is erected.

> **The word 'Biochemistry' is very broad in its meaning which may be defined as the study of different chemical processes going on in the body at molecular level, no matter it's a plant or animal body.**
>
> Besides, it also deals with the nature of the chemical constituents of the living organisms; the functions and transformations of such chemical entities in the biological systems and also with the chemical and energetic changes associated with such transformations during the course of activity.
>
> Day by day, its applicability in the field of life sciences is going on increasing and it is being utilized for the benefit of mankind and plant kingdom as well.

The history of biochemistry as it is in the present form is not very old. Most of the work in the field of biochemistry has been carried out in the last half-century. In this period of development, it is being increasingly recognized as an essential discipline among the life-sciences. In some of the advanced Western countries, there are full fledged independent institutes of biochemistry but unfortunately there is even not a single separate full fledged independent institute of Biochemistry in India because of the want of which our country is lagging behind as far as *biochemical sciences* are concerned. Unfortunately our country has neither got a separate *'Institute* of *Biochemistry'* nor *'Biochemical Engineering';* whereas now the time is fully mature to establish such an independent institute in India, so that we could keep pace with the Western world. Although, we have some good institutes of Science and Technology like **Central Drug Research Institute at Lucknow; Industrial Toxicology Research Centre at Lucknow; National Institute of Immunology at New Delhi; National Institute of Nutrition at Hyderabad; Centre for Food & Technological Research Institute at Mysore; Indian Institute of Science at Bangalore; Centre for Biochemical Technology at New Delhi; National Chemical Laboratory at Pune; Indian Institute of Chemical Technology at**

Hyderabad; Bhabha Atomic Research Centre at Trombay (Mumbai); Tata Institute of Fundamental Research at Mumbai; All India Institute of Medical Sciences at New Delhi; Centre for Cellular and Molecular Biology at Hyderabad, Centre for DNA Finger Printing & Diagnostics at Hyderabad; National Brain Research Centre at Manesar (Haryana); Institute of Genomics & Integrative Biology at New Delhi; International Centre for Genetic Engineering & Biotechnology at New Delhi etc, which have got very good well equipped biochemistry sections. Scientists and doctors are working whole heartedly round the clock at these centres to make 'science' more approachable and meaningful to the mankind. We have some eminent biochemists in India like *Prof G.P. Talwar, Padam Shree (Ex-Professor & HOD, Department of Biochemistry, AIIMS, New Delhi & ex-*Director, National Institute of Immunology, New Delhi), and at present Director, Talwar Research Foundation, New Delhi, whose team has so far been able to publish wonderful research papers in the field of 'Immunology' in world class journals and still working on several projects like "developing peptide based vaccine for **Plasmodium vivax malaria**" etc; **Dr. Lalji Singh, Director, Centre for Cellular and Molecular Biology, Hyderabad;** whose team is working on several projects related to

CBT	: New Delhi
CDRI	: Lucknow
CFTRI	: Mysore
CCMB	: Hyderabad
ITRC	: Lucknow
ICGEB	: New Delhi
IGIB	: New Delhi
I.I.Sc	: Bangalore
IICT	: Hyderabad
NCL	: Pune
NII	: New Delhi
NIN	: Hyderabad
TIFR	: Mumbai
CDFD	: Hyderabad
NBRC	: Manesar (Haryana)

DNA finger printing technology, uses of various biochemical techniques/ applications in forensic sciences, etc., for e.g., in establishing **parentage problems/issues,** etc. *Prof D.P. Burma,* Ex-Professor and Head of the Department of Biochemistry, Institute of Medical Sciences, B.H.U., Varanasi, now a days settled at Calcutta is a worker on *Nucleic Acids (Ribosomologist); Prof P.P. Singh,* Ex-Head of the Department of Biochemistry, R.N.T. Medical College, Udaipur is a worker on *Urolithiasis; Prof T.N. Pattabiraman,* Ex-Head of the Department of Biochemistry, Kasturba Medical College, Manipal, is an *Enzymologist; Prof. B.C. Harinath, Ex-* Head of the Department of Biochemistry, Mahatma Gandhi Institute of Medical Sciences, Sevagram (Wardha, Maharastra), is an *Immunologist* of repute and high profile. **Dr. P.M. Bhargava,** Ex- Director, CCMB, Hyderabad is a Biochemist of repute who is working with his team on several projects of National interest.; **Dr. G.K. Khullar,** Professor & Head, Biochemistry Department, P.G.I., Chandigarh is a Biochemist of repute working on **'designing polymer based novel drug carriers for Experimental Tuberculosis; Professor Balaram,** Chairman, Division of Biological Sciences, Indian Institute of Science, Bangalore is a Biochemist of repute working on several projects of human interest; **Dr. K. Taranath Shetty,** Professor and Head Department of Biochemistry, NIMHANS, Bangalore, is a Biochemist of repute working on several projects related to **neurobiochemistry; Dr. V. S. Chauhan,** Director, International Centre for Genetic Engineering & Biotechnology, New Delhi whose team is working on hereditary and allied disorders; **Dr. Samir Brahmachari,** Director, Institute of Genomics & Integrative Biology, New Delhi whose team is working on **'Genome Project'** and allied topics; **Dr. Sandeep Basu,** Director, National Institute of Immunology, New Delhi whose team is working in developing vaccines for various disorders; **Dr. P. N. Tandon,** Director, National Brain Research Centre whose team is working on several projects of brain chemistry and **Dr. Seyed E Hasnain,** Director, Centre for DNA Finger Printing & Diagnostics, Hyderabad whose team is working on several topics of human interest.

We are having **National Institute of Nutrition at Hyderabad,** an institute of its type in whole of Asia which is dedicated towards the inventions of cheaper sources of proteins, vitamins, etc. and also trying to evolve cheaper vegetable/plant substitutes of animal proteins for the vegetarians as in our country quite a sizable population is vegetarian and in the Western world too quite a good number of people conscious to health and obesity are now a days turning to vegetarianism. This institute also attracts young doctors having aptitude for research in medicine; institute is also dedicated in quality research work in bringing out solution of the diseases being caused due to the deficiency of vitamins and hormones, also involved in the search of good cheaper easily available sources of calories so that the poorer around the world may be benefited. Besides, **institute is also doing work as to how sufferers of certain diseases like diabetes mellitus, kwashiorkor, marasmus, protein energy malnutrition (PEM),etc. may get rid of such fierceful diseases/ states.** Institute is also looking after various interests of pregnant and lactating women with special reference to poverty.

CFTRI (Mysore), is also looking after the interest of the good health of the people of the globe with special reference to pure drinking water, beverages, adulterations (trend of adulteration is on increase day by day in some countries like India where the punishment for the adulterators, if at all existing is either of mild nature or nil) etc. Adulteration in edibles/ beverages like sweets, oils, spices, condiments, milk, medicines, flour, and a number of variety of preparations which are used in daily routine by the human beings and the animals has become a common thing now-a-days. **Adulteration is the mother of so many diseases and a perfect sound 'Nation' can not be footed so long the adulterators are alive.** Therefore, the Governments should be very strict in dealing with such adulterators.

C.D.R.I. (Lucknow) is also dedicated towards the search of newer, safer, potent drugs having no or lesser toxicity.

I.T.R.C. (Lucknow) is likewise dedicated in studying various aspects of toxicity to mankind with special reference to pollutants, gases, adulteration of toxic substances like lead, cadmium, cobalt etc. i.e., non-permitted (banned) colours etc, to the edibles. They are also working to see the effect of poisonous gases/ materials etc. on the health of factory/industry workers.

NII (New Delhi) is dedicated towards the synthesis of newer vaccines of certain diseases. They are also doing work towards the synthesis of *'birth control vaccine';* it shall be the most revolutionary day in the history of science. It shall be a laurel not only to the Indian Scientists but to the entire scientific community of the world. *Prof. G.P. Talwar,* Ex-Head of the Department of Biochemistry, All India Institute of Medical Sciences, New Delhi and at present working in NII as an emeritus scientist is engaged for more than last two decades towards the synthesis of birth control vaccine. One such group from Mumbai, besides some groups from the Western world are also engaged for the same cause. These days, control of the explosion of the population is the ever biggest challenge before the entire scientific community of the world.

A lot of work is being done both on basic and applied fields of biochemistry in order to make it more useful and viable for the benefit of mankind and understanding the secrets of life. The discipline has so far established an unique position in the field of medicine because of the fact that it is forming a **major tool in explaining the development of disorders and diseases in the body;** that is why, one finds sophisticated latest update biochemical instruments like **PCR, gas liquid chromatography, atomic absorption spectrophotometer, autoanalysers, radioisotope laboratory, tissue culture laboratory, etc.** in the well established good departments/sections/units of biochemistry. The knowledge of biochemistry has been able to pinpoint the exact site of the disorder and to give a clue towards the line of treatment in most of the diseases. **The new offshoot of biochemistry i.e. genetic engineering is flourishing like anything in the Western advanced countries like U.S.A., U.K., Germany, France, Japan, etc. which may bring solution of several disorders like those of hereditary disorders and other incurable diseases, the treatment of which is not possible at the moment. Scientists and doctors are working day and night in these countries to synthesize genes responsible for various genetic defects but unfortunately in our own country, this science is still lagging behind. It is a cause of serious concern to the Government of India.**

Hereditary diseases, which are considered to be incurable at present might be easily controlled or treated satisfactorily in the near future by simply changing the nature of the particular gene(s) responsible for the causation of such disease(s). **Attempts are being made to synthesize genes biochemically. Success in this field is bound to bring revolutionary, miraculous changes in the world of life-sciences.** Genes are the carriers of hereditary characters. After the synthesis of newer genes, it might be quite possible to produce off-springs of ones own choice. Suppose, then, if someone wishes a wrestler, or an athlete or a gymnast or a tall fellow, or a very intellectual one, it would

be quite possible to have it. This also means that the usage of genes for the betterment of mankind may also be misused by someone, hence, care must be taken for its 'use' and not 'misuse'; therefore the Governments must enact some law(s) in future for the use of **'genes'** and the power of its usage should never be vested in a single hand (single doctor), rather in a board comprising of atleast 5-7 highly qualified specialists of that field.

Dr Har Gobind Khorana, India born Chemist, turned into a Biochemist, now-a-days settled in U.S.A. (a permanent citizen of U.S.A at present) is working for more than a quarter century on DNA and the synthesis of genes for which he was awarded the most prestigious award i.e. *"Nobel Prize"* in the year 1968.

The knowledge of biochemistry is also being extensively used in the field of diagnosis of diseases. Estimations of the levels of biogenic compounds and enzymes in the circulating blood/urine have been proved to be of valuable guidance to the Physicians/Surgeons in making the diagnosis of diseases, for instance, blood sugar level gets elevated in diabetes mellitus, blood urea and creatinine levels get raised in nephritis, serum calcium level gets elevated in hyperthyroidism and gets decreased in infantile tetany, serum inorganic phosphorus gets decreased in rickets, serum cholesterol level gets elevated in nephrosis, diabetes mellitus, obstructive jaundice, myxoedema and xanthomatosis and may be decreased in *hyperthyroidism,* level of enzyme acid phosphatase gets increased in the carcinoma of prostate glands, serum glutamic oxaloacetic transaminase (GOT) and creatine phosphokinase (CPK or CK) levels get elevated in myocardial infarction, and so on.

Certain qualitative tests in urine, e.g. for the detection of sugar, protein, bile pigments, bile salts, blood, chyle, etc. are of great importance to the Physicians/Surgeons in making proper diagnosis. Besides qualitative tests, certain quantitative tests in urine like that of the estimation of total proteins in a 24 hrs urine sample is of diagnostic value in cases of nephritic syndrome.

Estimations of hormones in serum are of equally great diagnostic value, e.g. the estimations of T_3 and T_4 are most reliable means of confirming the diagnosis of hyperthyroidism or hypothyroidism. Highly specific and sensitive radioimmunoassays are used to measure serum T_3 and T_4 concentrations. In thyrotoxic states, serum TSH concentration is almost always low or undetectable. This is of little diagnostic value, since most assays can not distinguish between

NORMAL RANGE		
T_4	:	4 -12 µg/dl
T_3	:	80-100 ng/dl
TSH	:	Less than 5 µU/ml

normal and subnormal values. Measurement of serum TSH is the best means of distinguishing between untreated hypothyroidism of thyroid origin, in which the values are invariably increased, and pituitary or hypothalamic hypothyroidism, in which the values are usually undetectable or within the normal range.

Certain diseases are merely controlled by using specific enzyme inhibitors or activators. Recent studies have proved that the medicines mostly act by influencing certain enzyme or enzyme systems. The same also holds true for hormones. Structure activity relationships have been established in most of the cases. Such studies are covered in the field of *biochemical pharmacology*. After ascertaining the site of action and the structure responsible for a particular activity, it has now become possible to synthesize newer medicines having lesser toxicity and greater beneficial effects.

Radioisotopes are of great use in certain types of diseases like malignancies (cancers) of different origin of various organs/tissues. Isotopes of cobalt, iodine, etc. are used satisfactorily with very good results in different types of early diagnosed cancers by the radiophysicists under the guidance/consultation of Physicians/Surgeons treating such patients. In our country, establishment of radioisotope laboratory requires clearance by the *Bhabha Atomic Research Centre (BARC), Trombay as* one must take all kinds of precautions in the handling of radioisotopes. All staff members connected with such a laboratory must be well versed with the *"Radiation Hazards",* which are otherwise very fatal and injurious to the humans, many times more fatal than the X-Rays.

Disposal of the used radioactive material is also a cause of great concern. This material must be disposed as per the guidelines and instructions laid down by BARC, Trombay. All kinds of wares i.e: plasticwares/glasswares etc. being used for the estimation purposes or therapy purposes or otherwise should not be used for routine work, hitherto must be disposed safely. **Radioactive material, if handled casually, may otherwise kill the normal healthy cells, may also cause 'mutation' which may even persist in the off-springs (1-2-3 generations).**

Biochemistry plays an important role for 'Physiotherapists' and 'Pharmacists'; unless the students pursuring such courses are not well versed with the topics, such as: (i) Carbohydrates, (ii) Lipids (Fats), (iii) Proteins (immunoglobulins), (iv) Nucleic acids, (v) Enzymes and isoenzymes, (iv) pH, buffers, acids, bases, (vii) Vitamins, (viii) Nutritional biochemistry, (ix) Detoxification, (x) Muscle physiology and biochemistry, (xi) Biochemistry of nervous tissue, (xii) Hormonal biochemistry, (xiii) Metabolism, (xiv) Biophysical chemistry, etc, it shall not be possible for them to correlate properly the diseases, understand their causes, means to cure them by dietary habitat, etc. Therefore, to understand the **'human biochemistry'** for them is very essential and to the point.

CHAPTER 3

THE CELL

What is a cell?

Cells are the fundamental functional and structural biological units, which are capable of performing all the functions of living matter. They may be defined as the smallest organised unit of element or atom of life, which are capable of independent existence and maintaining and propagating themselves in any suitable environment other than the interior of the cell. This definition includes not only the animal and plants, but also all the single celled animals (Protozoa: Goldfuss, 1817), single celled plants (Protophyta) and other micro-organisms. The distinguishing feature between a protozoa and a protophyta is that the nutrition in former is holozoic and in latter holophytic, though there are holophytic protozoans also. Hence a clear cut and absolute distinction of the two groups is not possible. Such organisms were placed in a single group 'Protista' by the scientist Haeckel.

A cell is strictly a bounded system. It is bounded by a thin plasma-membrane about 100 Å thick (Å-1 angstrom is $10^{-4}\mu$ or 10^{-8} cm), which is comprised of a few layers of protein and lipid molecules. **The main constituent of a cell is the living matter called protoplasm.**

Claude Albert (Belgium) a Cytologist; de Duve, Christian (Belgium) a Biochemical Cytologist and Palade, George E. (Rumania/USA) a Molecular Biologist were together awarded Nobel Prize in Medicine in 1974 for their discoveries concerning the structure and functional organisation of the cell.

Protoplasm

Since almost all the methods of chemical analysis lead to the death of the living material i.e., protoplasm, its exact chemical composition is not very accurately known, but it is clear that it's an aqueous medium of organic compounds like carbohydrates, proteins, lipids, nucleic acids, and other molecules. These constituents are themselves not alive and it is only when these molecules become organised in a precise way that the phenomenon of life appears. **The minimum unit of this living matter that can live is called the cell.**

As microscopes improved, evidence for cell theory accumulated, as more and more structures could be distinguished within the jelly-like substance of the cell. **Jan Evangelista Purkinje,** an outstanding Czech Anatomist who had a religious training, called the jelly of the cell as **'protoplasm'** after the theological term 'protoplast', which means the first formed being.

The protoplasm was at first thought to be just liquid, and late to be a colloid, like paste or clay but eventually particles and fibrils could be distinguished within it. The protoplasm has since proved to be composed of an enormous variety of remarkable structures. Many of these structures have been extensively studied under the light microscope, but it has taken the resolving power of the electron microscope to reveal the organisation of the cell in significant detail.

Protoplasm is a translucent, greyish, slimy and viscous substance, which is capable of flowing.

Protoplasm is composed of both organic and inorganic substances. The most important of inorganic substances is water, which is about 50-90 per cent of the aqueous medium. It is an essential medium for the existence of life itself. **Water is an electrolyte and has a remarkable dissolving power.** It not only dissociates itself but has high dissociative power and can dissociate most solutes. **Water also has high tension power and a low viscosity. Finally, it has great capacity of absorbing heat. This last quality is very important as it enables protoplasm to protest itself against abnormal variation of temperature.**

The other important characteristic of protoplasm is its high content of potassium ions and its low content of sodium and chloride ions. It is the most striking feature in the sense that the **World is very rich in sodium ions,** but poor in potassium ions and this becomes a limiting factor in the environmental tolerance of the organisms. This proportion of energy is required for osmotic work.

Other inorganic constituents that compose the living matter are certain cations and anions. The cations are magnesium, calcium and ammonium. The other two cations i.e., potassium and sodium have already been mentioned above. The anions are bicarbonate, carbonate, nitrate, chloride, sulphate and phosphate, etc.

The principal organic constituents of the protoplasm are the following, i.e.,

(i) Proteins,

(ii) Carbohydrates,

(iii) Lipids, and

(iv) Nucleic acids

Professor E. Ruska built the first electron microscope in the year 1933. Since then these instruments have been steadily improved and can now magnify one million times or even more.

The great disadvantage of the electron microscope is that it cannot be used to observe living material, because the specimen has to be held dry in a vacuum to avoid disturbing the electron beam. For this reason it is not possible to understand how the cell really works simply by looking at it-even if one uses an electron microscope.

It is the test tube, rather than the microscope, which has made the cell understandable in terms of the atoms and the molecules of which it is composed. Nineteenth century chemists analysed and synthesised organic compounds and found that they were made from the same chemical elements as inorganic compounds. They isolated and identified many of the most important chemical constituents of the living cells including haemoglobin, the red pigment of the blood; and chlorophyl, the green pigment in plants. They also studied the role of the enzymes in the process of digestion.

Shortly after the turn of the century the

approaches of biochemists and the cell biologists began to converge; though it has only been during the last two decades, with the growth of molecular biology, that cell biology has really flourished. **The usual approach of the biochemist is to break open cells by grinding them up with sand,** or by homogenizing them by some mechanical means. He then studies the chemistry of the parts of the cell. Once the biochemist has ground up his cells, he usually proceeds to separate out different parts of the cell by some process of purification. The method most frequently used is to spin test tubes full of homogenized cells in a centrifuge for varying lengths of time; heaviest parts of the cell are soon thrown to the bottom of the tube and the lighter particles are thrown down progressively until there remains only the cell sap, which contains all the soluble substances of the cell including the enzymes.

The cell nucleus, containing the cell's quota of DNA, is the first part of the broken cell to sediment when centrifuged. Next come the various cell organelles like mitochondria, etc. All these organelles can be separated from one another and purified by using powerful centrifuges.

The first high-speed centrifuges, invented by Swede, Theodore Svedberg, in 1925 were able to generate a force hundreds of thousands of times as great as that of gravity, and attain speeds of more than a million revolutions per minute. The introduction of these high-powered instruments to biochemistry in increasing numbers since the Second World War has brought about a technical revolution perhaps even greater than the electron microscope.

Science proceeds by gathering information in whatever way it can and then by putting this information together to get an overall perspective. The studies of the light microscopists, electron microscopists and biochemist thus complement each other to give a composite picture of the cell and its parts. This picture has been put together piece by piece, rather like the pieces of a jigsaw puzzle, and although there may still be some pieces missing we can now see the general plan.

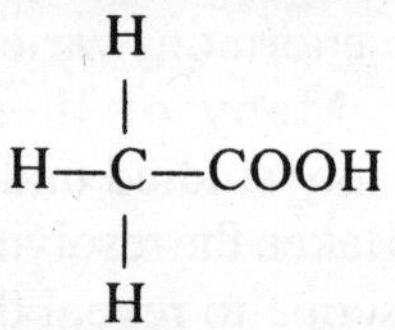

$$
\begin{array}{cc}
\text{H} & \text{NH}_2 \\
| & | \\
\text{H—C—COOH} & \text{H—C—COOH} \\
| & | \\
\text{H} & \text{H} \\
\text{acetic} & \text{glycine} \\
\text{acid} & \text{(amino acetic acid)}
\end{array}
$$

(i) Proteins:

These are complex nitrogenous compounds of carbon, hydrogen, oxygen and nitrogen. Sometimes, they may also contain other elements like sulphur, phosphorus, iron, etc. They have high molecular weight and on hydrolysis, i.e., decomposition on reaction with water, they form amino acids. An amino acid, is an organic compound which contains amino group (NH_2) and on hydrolysis yields glycine (aminoacetic acid). **Now, 20 different amino acids have been isolated from different proteins.**

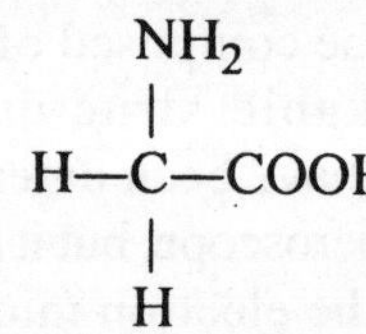

(ii) Carbohydrates

These are the compounds of carbon, hydrogen and oxygen. On hydrolysis, these yield simple sugars, Sugars are aldehyde or ketone derivatives of poly hydric alcohols, i.e., of glycerol (—OH = alcohol group), glyceric aldehyde (—CHO = aldehyde group), or dihydroxyacetone (—CO = ketone group). Monosaccharide, disaccharide and polysaccharide are all carbohydrates but the most important carbohydrate in nature is dextrose (glucose). All carbohydrates are converted into it before oxidation in tissues.

H	O	H
|	||	|
H—C—OH	C—H	H—C—OH
|	|	|
H—C—OH	H—C—OH	C=O
|	|	|
H—C—OH	H—C—OH	H—C=OH
|	|	|
H	H	H
glycerol	glyceric-aldehyde	dihydroxy-acetone

(iii) Lipids

These are natural fats, oils and waxes and like carbohydrates are the compounds of carbon, hydrogen and oxygen. They occur in plant and animal tissues and are insoluble in water but are soluble in organic solvents like chloroform, benzene, ether, alcohol, etc.

(iv) Nucleic acids

These are the largest and most fascinating molecules found in living matter. These are the carriers and mediators of genetic information from one generation to another and exert primary control over the basic life processes in all organisms. **Like proteins, nucleic acids are also polymers.**

CELL STRUCTURE (Fig 3.1)

Shape and Size

Cells vary greatly in shape and size. Usually they are microscopic, but some of them are also visible to the naked eyes. They range from 0.2 to 0.5 micron in diameter (one micron is 1/1000 mm). Eggs are also single cells. Ostrich egg, single called plants such as Acetabularia and nerve cells may be 10 cm or more in length.

Cells can be of any conceivable shape. Their shape usually reflects the functions it carries out in an organism, e.g., nerve cells which have to transmit impulses to long distances are long; muscle cells are elongated. Cells may be flat, spindle shaped, cuboidal and of other shapes as well.

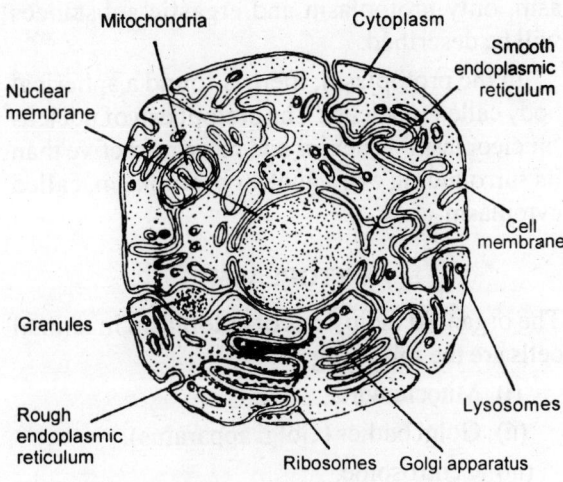

Fig. 3.1: Cellular components

All cells have certain common features. Presence of nucleus in cells is one such main feature (Brown, 1883). Nucleus in cells is the controlling centre. In Gloeocaspa (A blue-green algae), nucleus is not visible though it contains chromatin and chlorophyll and performs all the functions of a living cell. Bacteria and viruses are other variations. Both are devoid of a typical nucleus. Viruses have no recognisable structure of a generalised cell. They are so small that usually they are not visible without the help of an electron microscope. They do not have cytoplasm, however, they are crystals of nucleoprotein.

CELL PARTS

Meyer has divided the morphological structure of cells into the following three parts:

(i)   the active living part **'protoplasm'**
(ii) partially active part **'alloplasm'**, and

(iii) the passive and lifeless inclusions called **'ergastic substances'**.

In cells, the ergastic substances are the products of cellular metabolism. As it is not easy to differentiate between protoplasm and alloplasm, only protoplasm and ergastic substances will be described.

In the protoplasm, there is found a spherical body called 'nucleus'. The protoplasm of nucleus 'nucleoplasm' is denser and more refractive than its surrounding extra nuclear protoplasm, called cytoplasm.

CYTOPLASM

The organoid inclusions of cytoplasm in animal cells are the following:

  (i) Mitochondria,

  (ii) Golgi bodies (Golgi apparatus),

  (iii) Centrosome,

  (iv) Fibrilla, and

  (v) Chromidial substances.

(i) Mitochondria :

The mitochondria (Fig. 3.2) are granular and filamentous or spherical or rod-shaped bodies. They vary in diameter from 0.5-1.0 micron and may be upto about 7 microns long. They are microscopic and are not easily visible. They require special techniques to make them microscopically visible. They vary in number in each cell. In active cells like those of liver they may be over a thousand per cell.

When seen under an electron microscope, the mitochondria appear to be hollow structures bounded by a double membrane. This membrane is made up of lipoprotein. The inner membrane is convoluted or folded internally to form mitochondria cristae. The surface of the mitochondria cristae is studded with small spheres which are most probably associated with electron transport activity. The interior of mitochondria is filled with a fluid, which is very rich in enzymes. Mitochondria can expand and contract like cell membrane.

Mitochondria contain cytochromes, dehydrogenase enzymes, respiratory pigment flavin and some other enzymes that participate in lipid metabolism and the Krebs Cycle. In Krebs cycle, the products are exposed to successive dehydrogenation. Cytochrome provides a mechanism whereby the electrons resulting from the oxidation of hydrogen are transported to oxygen functioning as acceptor for hydrogen ions to form water. Mitochondria act as high energy storage centre taking active part in metabolism.

The mitochondria convert the potential energy of different food materials into a kind of energy that can be used to carry out different activities of cell like re-absorption, growth, reproduction, respiration etc. In view of this, they usually congregate in the most active regions of the cell. They usually occur in large number in nerve cells, muscle cells and secretory cells. **Thus, mitochondria are actually the power-houses or batteries of a cell and therefore, of the organism as a whole.**

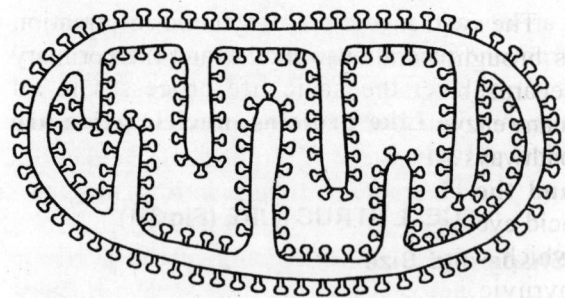

Fig. 3.2 : Diagrammatic section through a mitochondrion showing how the cristae arise as infoldings of the inner membrane.

There may be anything from one to more than a thousand mitochondria in a single cell. In the mitochondria, pyruvic acid (derived from sugar) is burned releasing energy for use by the cell. This energy is used to synthesise molecules of adenosine triphosphate (ATP) which diffuse out of the mitochondria to all parts of the cell. ATP, often called high-energy phosphate, releases its energy in serving the needs of the cell and is destroyed in the process. All biochemical reactions are reversible, but a reaction may be, and often is, much slower in one direction than the other. ATP speeds up reactions by supplying energy so that they occur in the direction and at a rate which is useful to the cell.

The mitochondrion is a highly organised double walled sac. The outer membranous wall is smooth, but the inner membrane is full of convolution and deformations which stretch right across the interior of the organelle. These deformations, called cristae, stick out from all sides of the inner membrane. Although under the electron microscope, both these membranes appear similar to other cell membranes, in fact they differ a great deal biochemically. They are made up of a mixture of protein and fatty material held together by what are called hydrophobic bonds—chemical bonds which are not water-soluble. The protein part of the membrane consists of some proteins which have a structural function and others have an enzymic function.

The synthesis of ATP by the mitochondrion is brought about by the conjugation of two separate biochemical pathways, each involving many enzymes. These two separate biochemical pathways are called the **Krebs citric-acid cycle and the electron-transfer chain.** The citric acid cycle is a collection of about 10 enzymes which work together to remove energy from pyruvic acid molecules in a series of easy stages. This might be thought of as a process of slow and controlled burning in which the heat energy is trapped in ATP molecules. Actually, the energy is liberated in the form of energy carrying hydrogen and electron which are then passed along the electron transfer chain so that ultimately hydrogen combines with oxygen to form water and the electrons give up their energy to assist in the synthesis of ATP. This type of **energy release** is called aerobic energy release:

that is, it uses oxygen from the air. Anaerobic (without air) energy release is effected by some organisms, such as yeast, by means of alcoholic fermentation, which is carried out by enzymes in the cytoplasm, outside the mitochondria.

Citric-acid cycle enzymes are believed to occur in solution in the centre of the mitochondrion between the cristae. The 'enzymes of the ETC (electron transfer chain) remain located in the membranes of the cristae themselves. High-power electron microscope pictures of the cristae exhibit structures shaped like a knob on the end of a stick studded all over the inner surface of the cristae. These are the molecules of the enzyme adenosine triphosphatase which catalyses the final synthesis of ATP from AMP and inorganic phosphate.

Now since DNA has been discovered in mitochondria, therefore, it has become clear that mitochondria normally arise by the division of other mitochondria.

The quantity of DNA in mitochondria is in fact quite small-probably just enough to code for three or four average sized proteins. It is the amount of DNA which might be found in a rather small virus. The mitochondria DNA is circular, like the DNA of many viruses and bacteria. It is not known which proteins of the mitochondria are coded by the mitochondria DNA. However, since there are found more than 5 different proteins in the mitochondrion, the majority of these mitochondria proteins must be coded for in the nucleus and synthesised in the cytoplasm, before migrating to the mitochondrion.

The mitochondrion appears to have a system of protein synthesis which is different from that of the cell-a system sensitive to inhibition by certain antibiotics which do not affect the normal protein synthesis in the endoplasmic reticulum.

(ii) Golgi body (Golgi apparatus)

In 1898 an Italian scientist Camillo Golgi made preparation of the nerve cells of the

barn owl and the cat, which he stained with silver salts and osmium tetroxide. He saw a dark staining part of the cytoplasm of the cell quite distinct from the nucleus. This structure, called after him the Golgi apparatus, is a system of membranes similar to the smooth membranes of the endoplasmic reticulum. For a long time its existence remained disputed by biologists—partly because of its variable appearance in cells—but now electron microscope studies have establi-shed its existence without any doubt. ·

Recently the Golgi apparatus has been shown to play a most important role in preparing and packaging proteins secreted by cells. Such proteins are made on the ribosomes in the normal way and then accumulate in the Golgi apparatus. The Golgi apparatus then adds some carbohydrate molecules to the protein molecule and wraps together a large number of the molecules in a single membrane. This package may then pass to the edge of the cell and release its contents outside: the mucus part of the saliva is made in this way in the cells of the salivary glands and the digestive enzymes of the gut are also put into packets by the Golgi apparatus before being liberated into the intestine. However, this apparatus is also responsible for packing certain enzymes into parcels—called **lysosomes**—which remain within the cell.

Membranes: The membranes (Fig. 3.3) of the cell—the nuclear membrane, the cell's outer membrane and the endoplasmic reticulum-are all very similar. The membranes of the mitochondria are also of the same general type as is found in the rest of the cell. For this reason there is considered to be one basic type of cell membrane, called the unit membrane. Under the electron microscope, these membrane appear as a double line of dense material with a space of transparent material in between. The dense material on the outside is thought to be protein

and the light material in the centre of the sandwich to be fat. Membranes from different parts of the cell do, however, vary in thickness from about 0.007-0.01 micron.

About one third of the membrane by weight is fatty material and most of the rest is protein. There is no general agreement at present about the way in which the protein and fat are organised in the membrane. Fat soluble substances readily penetrate the cell membrane, but so do water soluble substances. There are also some quite simple molecules which cannot penetrate the cell. Some substances are taken into the cell actively and reach much higher concentrations within it than in the surrounding liquid. This process, called active transport, is performed by enzymes called permeases and is an energy-requiring process, There may be holes in the membrane which allow some substances to pass through and not other. Alternatively, the membrane has been considered to be a mosaic of protein and fat with areas where fatty substances can dissolve through the membrane and other areas where water soluble substances can dissolve through it. Both the protein and the fat are necessary for the integrity of the cell membrane, since if agents which dissolve fats or denature proteins are applied to the membrane, it is destroyed.

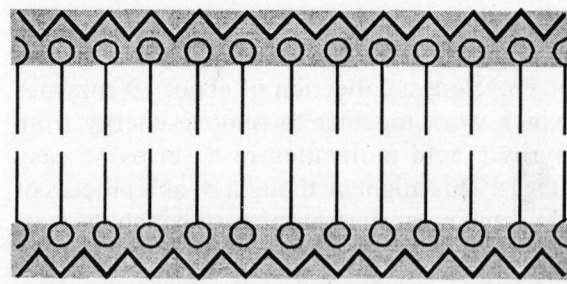

Fig. 3.3 : All cell membranes appear to have the same basic structure - two one - molecule thick layers of proteins enclosing a two - molecule - thick layer of fat. The shaded areas in the diagram indicate how this, the unit membrane, acquires its distinctive 'double' appearance in electron microscope pictures.

Lysosomes — the 'Suicide Bags'

In 1949, scientist Christian de Duve, while studying enzymes extracted from rat liver in his laboratory in Louvain, Belgium, was unable to explain why the quantity of one enzyme varied in apparently identical experiments. Then he noticed that when he homogenised the rat liver cells gently, he obtained much less of this enzyme than when he homogenised the same cells vigorously. This was the first clue to the existence of a new cellular particle—the **lysome** (Fig. 3.4). The particles were given this name; because they contain highly active enzymes able to destroy, or lyse the cell.

Lysosomes are little membranous sacs which contain a battery of enzymes. These sacs are easily broken when the cell is homogenised. Their diameter is from 0.25-0.8 microns and contain enzymes capable of digesting proteins, carbohydrates, RNA and DNA. The enzymes contained in the lysosomes cannot damage the cell unless the lysosome membrane is intact but as soon as the cells are broken down by grinding them, these lysosomes may also be broken down releasing enzymes which damage other parts of the cell unless great care is taken.

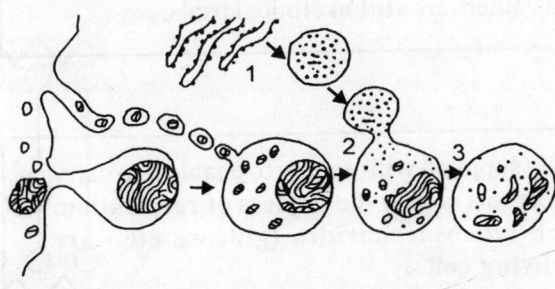

Fig. 3.4 : Cell digestion. Ribosomes (1) associated with the endoplasmic reticulum form a lysosome, which fuses (2) with a food vacuole. In the digestive vacuole so formed (3) lysosomal enzymes break down the trapped food particles and digestive products are absorbed through the surrounding membrane, until finally the vacuole's residual contents are expelled.

One of the main functions of the lysosomes is to digest pieces of food taken in by the cell. This is done in special food vacuoles. The white cells of the blood (phagocytes), for example, have an important function as scavengers. They engulf pieces of dead tissue or perhaps whole bacteria; and destroy them with the assistance of lysosomes which release their digestive enzymes into the vacuole, or space, in the cytoplasm, surrounding the engulfed material. The membrane round the vacuole prevents the digestive enzymes from damaging the cell itself.

Protozoa such as **Amoeba** and **Paramecium** also digest food by the liberation of lysosomes into vacuoles containing food particles.

Worn out parts of the cell, too are digested in similar vacuoles and the molecules of these worn out parts are put back into circulation once more as food. In an old cell the lysosomes may dissolve and result in the cell's complete breakdown-for which reason they are sometimes called **"suicide bags"**. The lysosomes play an important part in the death of the cells in the course of embryonic development. When a tadpole develops into a frog, its tail is "reabsorbed"-a result of the action of lysosomes in the tail cells which literally digest away the tail from within. Cell death brought about by lysosomes is now known to be a normal part of the processes by which tissues and organs are remodelled during embryonic development.

Besides, the lysosomes may play an important part in some disease processes as well as in disease resistance. **Silicolosis,** a disease very common in miners, caused by the inhalation of silica dust, may result from an accumulation of these silica particles in the lysosomes in the lung cells, and therefore cause corrosive enzymes to leak out of the lysosomes. Excessive quantities of other substances, such as vitamin A, are also known to cause the lysosome membranes to become unstable. Whereas, other substances such as cortisone and hydrocortisone stabilise the lysosome membrane, and this may account for the well known anti-inflammatory properties of these substances.

(iii) Centrosome:

There is found a body near the nucleus which is called as 'centrosome'. The centrosome actually consists of two separate bodies about a fifth of a micron in diameter, which are called as centrioles. When the cell divides, the centrioles move to opposite ends of the cell and appear to play an important part in the formation of the spindle on which the chromosomes are arranged during cell division. Electron microscope pictures reveal that usually each centriole is a paired structure, rather like two cylinders at right angles to each other.

Topoisomerase I Inhibitors

A variety of antibiotics and antineoplastic drugs exert their therapeutic effects by interaction with topoisomerase I and disruption of DNA synthesis during phase of dividing cells. Topoisomerase I is essential for DNA replication and cell growth. The enzyme relieves torsional stress in DNA by inducing reversible single- strand breaks. The interaction of topoisomerase I and certain drugs produces double strand breaks in DNA that are irreversible and can lead to cell death.

A variety of antibiotics and antineoplastic drugs function as topoisomerase I inhibitors; these include the quinoline antibiotics, anthracyclines (doxorubicin), epipodophylotoxins (etoposide), and the **camptothecins**, which are active in treating lung, ovarian, and colorectal cancers. The camptothecins also are used in the treatment of myelomonocytic syndromes, **chronic myelomonocytic leukemia (CMML),** acute leukemia, and **multiple myeloma.** A variety of synthetic analogues of natural camptothecins are being tested clinically for efficacy and safety in the treatment of these aggressive cancers. The camptothecins were discovered in extracts from the **Chinese tree Camptotheca acuminata.** Initial studies showed that camptothecins had antitumor activity, but clinical trials demonstrated severe side effects and toxicity. Numerous camptothecin analogues have been synthesised; several have received FDA approval (irinotecan and topotecan), whereas others are still in clinical trials.

To maintain the living state, a cell must be constantly supplied with energy to enable it to carry out its vital functions. This energy is made available to a cell by the process of **respiration. Respiration is a continuous process in which monosaccharides (glucose etc.) are oxidised to carbon dioxide and water by the living cell.**

$$C_6H_{12}O_6 + 6O_2 \longrightarrow 6CO_2 + 6H_2O + Energy$$

ATP is a complex compound. It is present in the living matter of each cell. It was first discovered by **Fritz Lipmann** (1941), who pointed out the importance of ATP as a reservoir and source of supply of energy. He was awarded the **'Nobel Prize'** for this work.

CHAPTER **4**

CELL BIOLOGY (HISTORY etc.)

Prokaryotic and Eukaryotic Cells (Table 4.1)

Prokaryotes include all types of bacteria, divided into two separated categories i.e., **eubacteria** and **archaebacteria**. Most bacteria studied in laboratories are eubacteria. The eubacteria include the photosynthetic organisms formerly known as blue-green algae but these days better known as **cyanobacteria.**

Less is known about the archaebacteria, which grow in unusual environments. The methanogens live only in oxygen-free milieus such as swamps. These bacteria produce methane (CH_4), also known as **"swam gas"** 'by the reduction of CO_2, Other archaebacteria include the **halophiles** which require high concentrations of salt to survive, and the **thermoacidophiles, which grow in hot ($80^{\circ}c$) sulphur springs, where a pH of less than 2 is common.**

Eukaryotes include all member of the protist, fungus, animal and plant kingdoms that is to say from the most primitive form to the most complex flowering plants, and from amoebas and simple sponges to insects and mammals. The variety of organisms classified as eukaryotes is very large but they all share certain structural features.

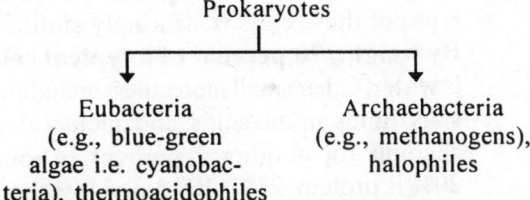

Eukaryotes: Examples are all members of the animal and plant kingdoms.

Living Matter

If a living material such as green wood is burned in a fire, after it is burned away, only ash will be left. This ash is the mineral or inorganic residue of the wood, which is all that remains after burning. While the wood gets burnt, carbon dioxide and water are given off as gas and vapour. Molecules of water consist of one atom of oxygen and two atoms of hydrogen. Molecules of CO_2 consist of one atom of carbon and two atoms of oxygen. The organic material of wood and other living substances consist of mineral ash, carbon, hydrogen and oxygen. Other elements such as nitrogen, sulphur and phosphorus, which may be contained in the mineral ash are given off as gases are also important. These elements are the inorganic

Table 4.1 : Difference between prokaryotic and eukaryotic cells

Prokaryotic cells	Eukaryotic cells
1. They have a relatively simple structure.	1. These have relatively a very complicated structure.
2. In prokaryotes, in general, only one type of membrane called as the plasma membrane from the boundary of the cell proper. This membrane is permeable to certain gases, such as O_2 and CO_2 and to water and impermeable to most molecules that the cell must obtain from its environment such as sugars, amino acids and inorganic ions.	2. . Eukaryotic cells also remain surrounded by a plasma membrane but they contain extensive internal membrane that enclose specific regions, separating them from the rest of the cytoplasm, the region of the cell lying out side the nucleus. These membranes define a collection of subcellular structures called organelles.
3. Prokaryotes and Eukaryotes contain similar macromolecules. The volume of a typical animal or plant cell is several hundred times that of a typical bacterial cell yet the chemical composition of both types of these cells is strikingly similar. **By weight, 70 percent of a typical cell is water.** Other small molecules, including salts, lipids amino acids, and nucleotides account for another 7 percent. About 20% is protein, 2% is RNA and less than 1% is DNA, the genetic material.	3. Prokaryotes and Eukaryotes contain similar macromolecules. The volume of a typical animal or plant cell is several hundred times that of a typical bacterial cell yet the chemical composition of both types of these cells is strikingly similar. **By weight, 70 percent of a typical cell is water.** Other small molecules, including salts, lipids amino acids, and nucleotides account for another 7 percent. About 20% is protein, 2% is RNA and less than 1% is DNA, the genetic material.
4. They contain less DNA than the eukaryotic cells.	4. They contain more DNA.
5. In prokaryotic cells, nucleus is never membrane bound.	5. Here, the nucleus is always membrane bound.
6. In all prokaryotes studied to date, most or all cellular DNA remains in the form of a single circular molecule.	6. The number and size of individual chromosomes vary widely among different eukaryotes. Yeast for e.g., possess 12-18 chromosomes. **Human cells contain 2 sets of 23 chromosomes.**
7. The cell is said to have a single chromosome.	7. Each eukaryotic chromosome is believed to contain a single, linear double-stranded DNA molecule.
8. Despite their many differences, prokaryotic and eukaryotic cells have many biochemical pathways in common and in most aspects the translation of m-RNA into proteins is similar in all cells. Hence prokaryotes and eukaryotes are believed to be descended from the same primitive cell. Their divergence must have occurred before the separation of plant and animal cells.	8. Despite their many differences, prokaryotic and eukaryotic cells have many biochemical pathways in common and in most aspects the translation of m-RNA into proteins is similar in all cells. Hence prokaryotes and eukaryotes are believed to be descended from the same primitive cell. Their divergence must have occurred before the separation of plant and animal cells.

building blocks of the cells. The are joined together in various ways to form a vast inventory of organic molecules.

What is Cell Biology?

Cell Biology is that branch of biology that more or less directly deals with the structural and functional organisation of protoplasm and its relation to the phenomena of metabolism, growth, differentiation, heredity and evolution.

History

The term "cell" was first of all given by an Englishman **Robert Hooke** but the credit must go to this Dutch counterpart, Antony Van Leeuwenhoek (1632-1723), discovered microscope. Cells are so minute that they cannot be seen by naked eyes and it is doubtful that without the discovery of microscope they would have never been discovered. In the year 1665 Robert Hooke studied at thin piece of cork cut by a sharp knife under a microscope. He found that it was all perforated and porous like a honey-comb. Though this perforation was not regular, yet it wall as not unlike honey-comb. He called these minute pores surrounded by a firm was "cell". In the seventeenth century two other scientists namely **Grew and Malpighi,** made the same observations, but called the pores **'utricles'** or **"vesicles"**. It was only in 19th century that important discoveries were made. In 1801 a French surgeon-cum-anatomist named as M.F.X. Bichat (1771-1802), observed that various organs of animal were composed of aggregates of structural elements. He called these aggregates of structural elements by the name of 'tissues'. In 1824 Rene Dutrochet found that when plant material was boiled in nitric acid, it got split into tiny box-like 'units' very similar to those described by Hooke. He reported that plants are composed entirely of 'cells' and of organs that are obviously derived from cells. **The same also holds good for animals**. Other

scientists also confirmed the fact that plants were composed of cells. In 1833 **Robert Brown** described **'nucleus'** as a central feature of cells.

The Cell Theory

By now, many scientists began to take keen interest in the cellular organisation of living organisms and more information began to accumulate. In the first decade of 19th century, a new concept began to take form —could it be that all living things were composed of 'cells', **Rene Dutrochet** had already stated that plants are composed of cells. Other scientists also confirmed this finding. Previously, another German biologist, **K.W.F. Wolff,** had stated that both the plants and the animals were composed of cells. Many other scientists came to the same conclusion, yet a definite answer was only possible in the years 1838-39. In 1838, a German Botanist, **Matthias Jakob Schleidon** (1804-1881), and in 1839 his Zoologist co-worker, **Theodore Schwann** (1810-1882) made the greatest contribution. The former held that "cells" are morphological units in plants and the latter after having studied many animal tissues in detail applied the same thesis to animals. This generalisation is called the **'Cell Theory'** and marks an important landmark in 'Cell Biology'. The theory states that the bodies of all plants and animals are composed of minute units or structures called as 'cell'. The cell is the fundamental, morphological and physiological unit.

Citing the work of Schleiden, Schwann states that **'Cell was functional Biological Unit'**.

In short the cell theory may be summarised in three main ideas:

(i) Cell is the unit of structure of living organisms.

(ii) Cell is the unit of function in living organisms with a constant exchange of energy and matter within the cell in the process of living.

(iii) All cells come from the division of pre-existing cells. A multicellular animal begins life as a single cell which undergoes repeated division to form its body.

Difficulties in Cell Theory

Today, there is an increasing opinion that 'all' living things are not **cellular** and that some organisms are '**acellular**', i.e., without cell. A cell is defined as having a single distinct nucleus, but this description does not hold true to all cells. Some fungi, for example rhizopus are made up of an undivided mass of protoplasm, which has numerous nuclei scattered about in it. Distinct nucleus bounded by a membrane is also not found in the cells of **blue-green algae**, however regions containing DNA are present in them. Bacteria are also like blue-green algae and are devoid of nucleus. **Viruses** are also exceptions to cell theory. They are organisms having nucleic acids but exhibit none of the attributes of life, however, they cause drastic changes in the pattern of cell's living when introduced in other cells. These may be considered as exceptions and should not be treated as barriers in the study of cell structure and function.

Protoplasm

In the beginning, the cell theory emphasised the cell wall more and the contents less. **The cell contents were named as 'protoplasm' by the scientist Purkinje in the year 1840.** Dujardin made extensive studies of Protozoan protoplasm and named it '**Sarcode**' in 1835. Later on a German biologist, Max Schultz (1825-1874), in 1861 established the similarity between 'Sarcode' and 'Protoplasm' of animal and plant cells and declared- '**A cell is a lump of protoplasm inside which lies a nucleus**'. Thus, he offered a theory which was called "**Protoplasm Theory**" by the scientist O. Hertwig in the year 1892 which states-"**The cell is an accumulation of a living substance 'protoplasma' possessing a nucleus and a cell membrane.** Both the constituents are equally important and the disappearance of one or the other destroys the cell concept."

THE ORIGIN OF CELLS

With the establishment of the fact that all animals and plants were made up of minute units called '**cells**', the next question that immediately arose was "where do cells come from"? Schwann believed that new cells were formed spontaneously out of the living substance, but other biologists noticed that one cell seemed to divide into two. The German scientist, Rudolf Virchow (1821-1902), agreed with this view and wrote 'Omnis', '**cellulae cellula**', which means '**all cells from cells**'.

There were, of course, other scientists who believed in spontaneous generation, but today all biologists accept the cell theory of Schleiden and Schwann and Virchow's hypothesis that all cells come from pre-existing cells. It is true that some animals and plants are unicellular or single-celled where cell and organism are one, but the ones with which we are most familiar (multi-cellular animals) are made up of many kinds of cells which perform a variety of functions. The cells are integrated for proper functioning.

Ultimately, in the twentieth century great advancement has been made in this field and the development of '**electron microscope**' has recently added more information about the structure of the cell. **Now, the cell is defined as a highly organised unit.**

Nucleus is not only the control-centre of the physiological activities, it is also very important for cell- division. A denucleated cell can neither grow nor reproduce. It has been reliably established that the `gene', which are the actual determiners of hereditary characters lie is nuclear chromosome.

CHAPTER 5

CARBOHYDRATES

We are very important for the human beings as we are the driving force (petrol) for them. We are polyhydroxy aldehydes or ketones or their derivatives. To achieve us is very easy and we are inexpensive but teeth should take care of us, especially the infants and the children. When you eat us like other things and do not brush, we get accumulated in the interspaces of teeth, thus invite bacteria to grow which results in caries, a fierceful disease. We have storehouses in the body like liver, muscles, etc.

INTRODUCTION

The class of substances known as carbohydrates is comprised of a large number of relatively heterogenous compounds. They are especially prominent constituents of plants, but also do occur and serve important functions in animals.

Carbohydrates serve as the chief source of energy in the food of humans and many other animals. As is evident from the name itself, these are generally the compounds of carbon, hydrogen and oxygen but the higher carbohydrates have also been found to possess nitrogen and sulphur in their structures.

Carbohydrates may be defined as polyhydroxy-aldehydes or polyhydroxy-ketones or their derivatives. Their molecular weight ranges from less than 100 to well over 1 million and in general are, white solids, sparingly soluble in organic solvents but soluble in water except some high molecular weight carbohydrates.

Carbohydrates

‖

carbon + hydrogen + oxygen

or

carbon + hydrogen + oxygen +

nitrogen + sulphur

They are found in abundance in plant kingdom in the form of cellulose and starch; besides are also found in abundance in animal kingdom as well in the form of glucose or glycogen or chondroitin sulphates, etc.

Classification (Table 5.1)

For convenience, carbohydrates may be classified into three major groups namely :

(a) Monosaccharides or simple sugars (mono = single or one; saccharide = sugar moiety i.e. unit).

(b) Oligosaccharides (oligo = a few)

(c) Polysaccharides (poly = many)

(d) Derived carbohydrates; these include :

    (i) Oxidation products (ascorbic acid, uronic acids, aldonic acids, saccharic acids, etc.)

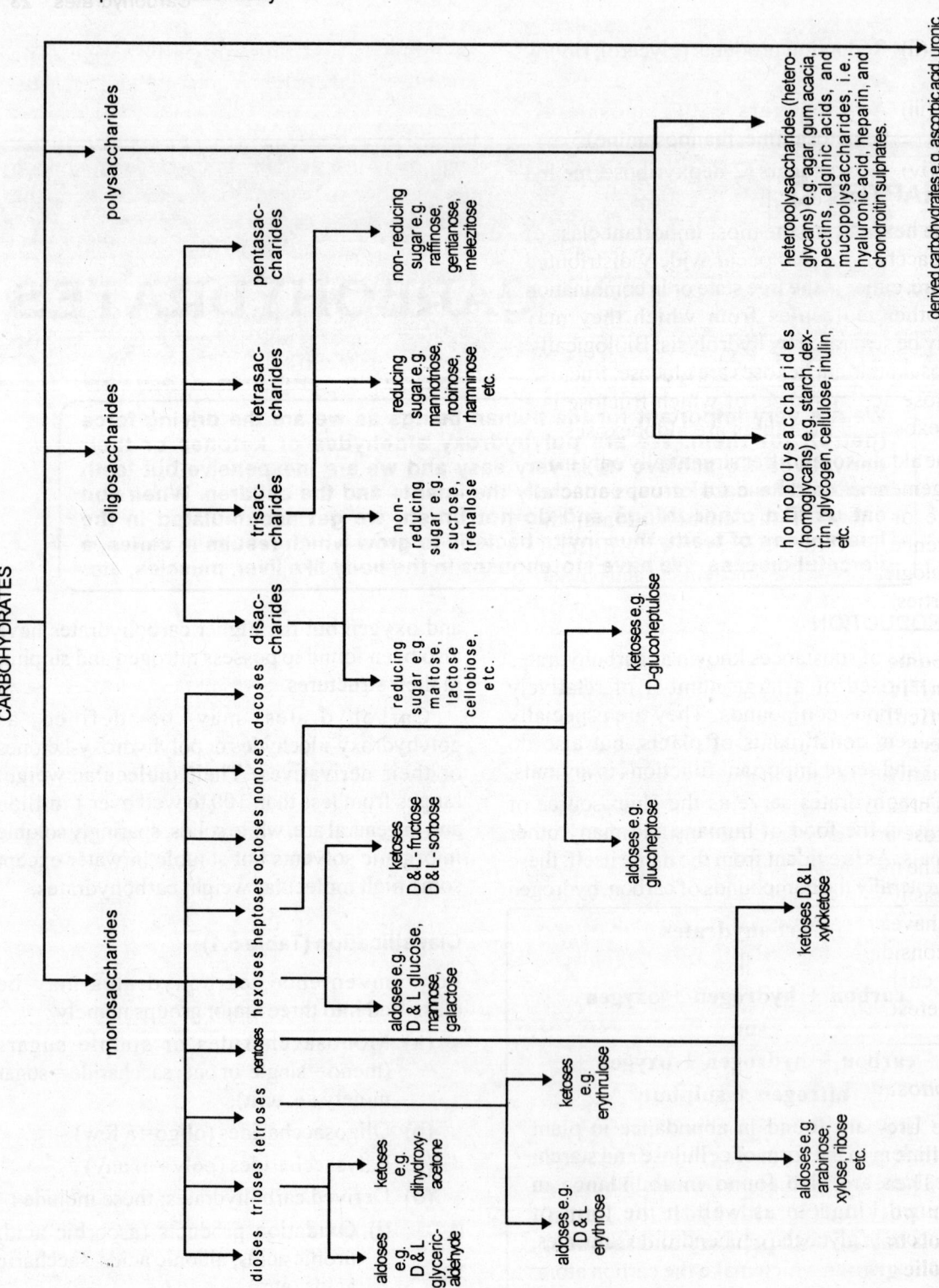

Table 5.1 : Classification of Carbohydrates

(ii) Reduction products (glycerol, ribitol, inositol).

(iii) Aminosugars (glucosamine, galactosamine, mannosamine).

(iv) Deoxysugars (2-deoxyribose, methyl pentoses).

The hexoses are the most important class of monosaccharides and occur widely distributed in nature, either in the free state or in combination with other molecules from which they may usually be separated by hydrolysis. Biologically, the most important hexoses are glucose, fructose, galactose and mannose, of which fructose is a ketohexose and the others are aldohexoses.

The aldohexoses differ structurally only in the arrangement of the H and OH groups attached to one or more of the carbon atoms; this difference may result in markedly different physiological, as well as in chemical and physical properties.

Some of the aldopentoses also are of significant biological importance, particularly ribose and deoxyribose. Others, such as arabinose and xylose, are primarily important in the plant kingdom.

Three disaccharides, maltose lactose and sucrose are important in nature.

The monosaccharides and disaccharides are easily soluble in water, are optically active and have a sweet taste. Glucose, which may be considered to be the most important of the carbohydrates, is also one of the sweetest.

(a) Monosaccharides

These are simple sugars, colourless and crystalline substances having more or less sweet taste. These are soluble in water. **These are either polyhydric aldehydic or ketonic alcohols having both primary and secondary alcoholic groups** which make the carbon atoms asymmetric and thus optically active. The presence of aldehyde or ketone groups i.e. aldose sugars (aldoses) and ketone sugars (ketoses); the suffix- ose can be taken to mean that a compound is a carbohydrate. Depending upon the number of carbon atoms present in the molecule, these are named as 'dioses', 'trioses', 'tetroses', 'pentoses', 'hexoses' etc. (Table 5.2). The simplest carbohydrate is glycolaldehyde.

In the nature mostly 'D' (dextrorotatory) form occurs. Sugars may show mostly cyclic structures. They form either α or β rings. The 6 membered ring is known as "pyranose" ring in which one of the members is oxygen atom, whereas the 5 membered ring is known as "furanose" ring. Again one member of the furanose ring is oxygen atom. The sugars, by virtue of their alcoholic group can form esters with acids, all the free hydroxy groups being replaceable. In the biological systems, the alcoholic groups at position "6" or "1" are found to be most reactive.

Being aldehydes or ketones, they can readily reduce copper*, bismuth** or silver solutions. They can condense with hydroxylamine or phenylhydrazine forming oximes and osazones.

The important sugars belonging to monosaccharides are **glucose (dextrose), fructose (levulose),** mannose, galactose, ribose, ribulose, xylose, xylulose, erythrose, sedoheptulose, glyceraldehyde, dihydroxyacetone etc.

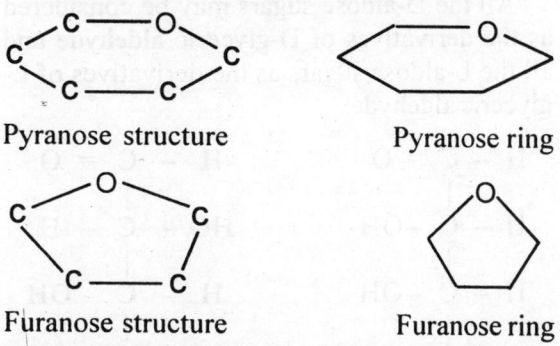

| Pyranose structure | Pyranose ring |

| Furanose structure | Furanose ring |

---

* *Basis of Fehling's test, Barfoed's test and Benedict's test*
** *Basis of Nylander's test*

Table 5.2 : Classification of monosaccharides

General formula $C_n(H_2O)_n$	Aldoses	Ketoses
Dioses, $C_2H_4O_2$	glycolaldehyde	
Trioses, $C_3H_6O_3$	D-&L*-glycerose or glyceric aldehyde	dihydroxyacetone
Tetroses, $C_4H_8O_4$	D-&L-erythrose	erythrulose
	D-&L-threose	
Pentoses, $C_5H_{10}O_5$	D-&L-ribose	D-&L-xyloketose
	D-&L-arabinose	
	D-&L-xylose	
Hexoses, $C_6H_{12}O_6$	D-&L-glucose	D-&L-fructose
	D-&L-mannose	D-&L-sorbose
	D-&L-galactose	
	D-&L-gulose	
Heptoses, $C_7H_{14}O_7$	glucoheptose	D-glucoheptulose
	mannoheptose	L-glucoheptulose

* *Levorotatory*

If the primary alcoholic group of the monosaccharides is oxidized to -COOH; the acid formed is known as "uronic acid" such as glucose forms glucuronic acid, galactose forms galacturonic acid etc. Such uronic acids are found in mucoproteins.

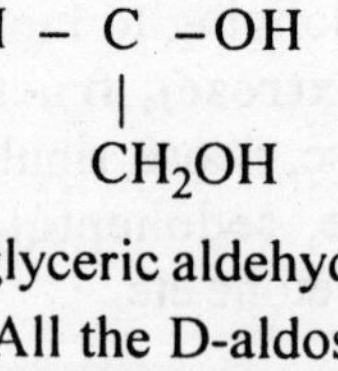

D-glyceric aldehyde 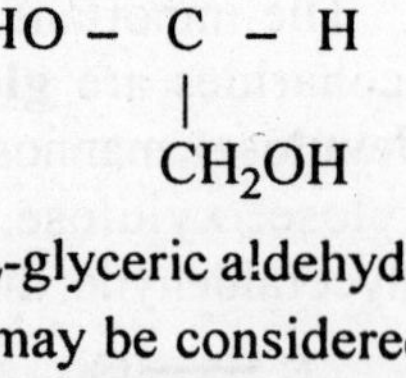   L-glyceric aldehyde

All the D-aldose sugars may be considered as the derivatives of D-glyceric aldehyde and all the L-aldose sugars as the derivatives of L-glyceric aldehyde.

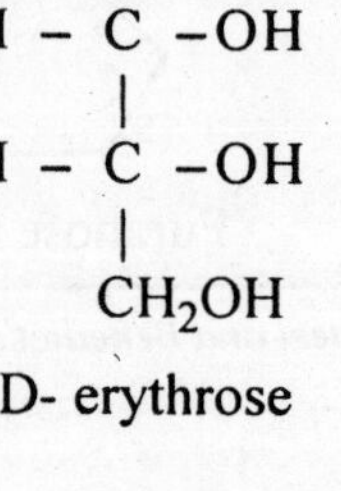

D- erythrose 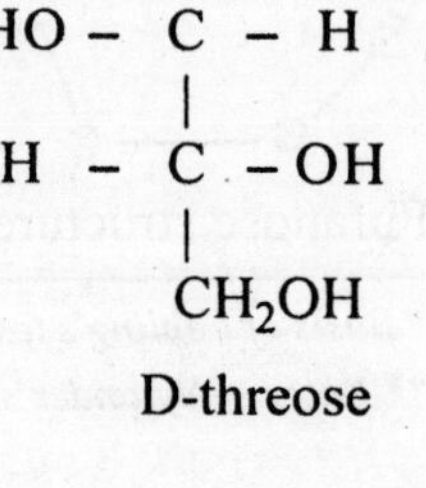   D-threose

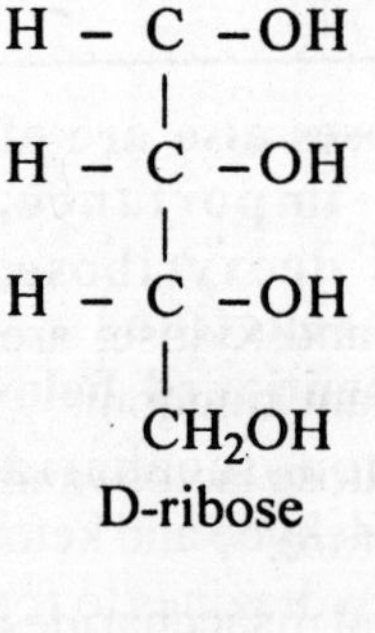

D-ribose 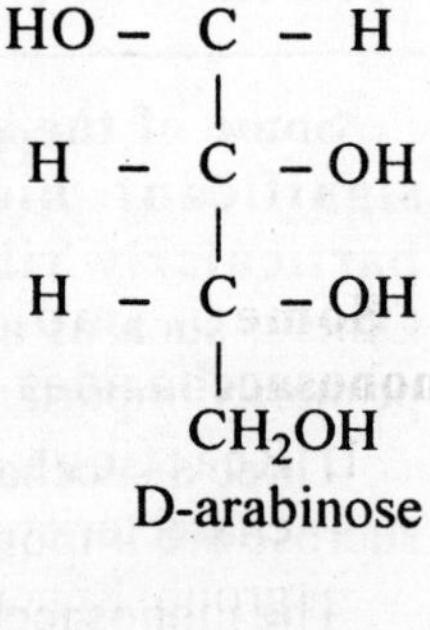   D-arabinose

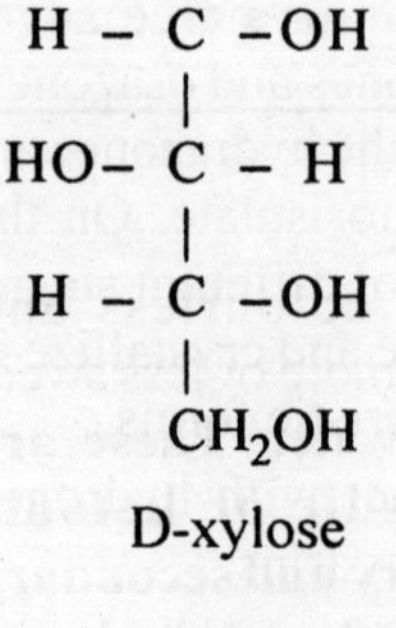

D-xylose 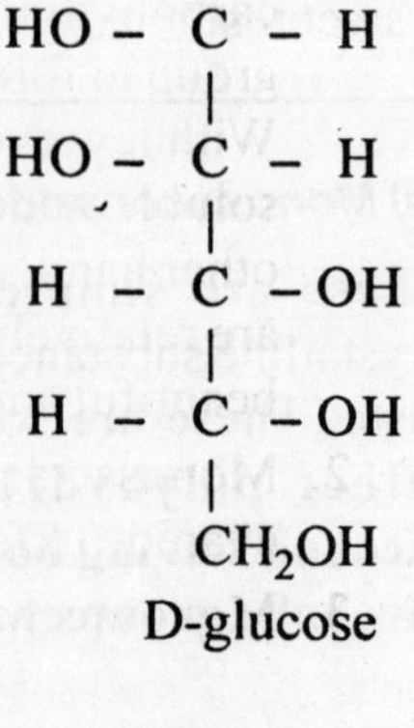   D-glucose

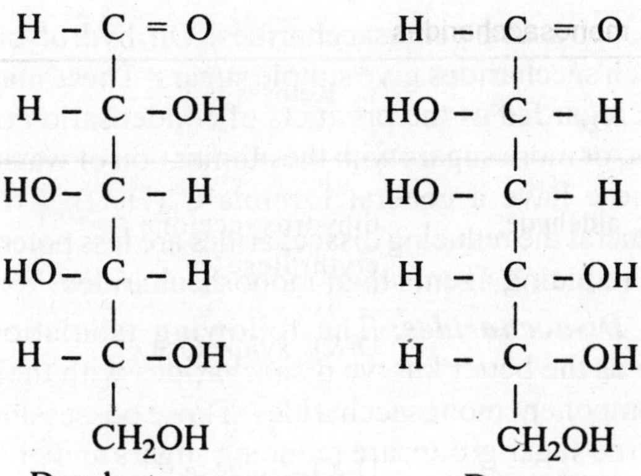

```
   H – C = O              H – C = O
       |                      |
   H – C –OH             HO – C – H
       |                      |
  HO– C – H             HO – C – H
       |                      |
  HO– C – H              H – C – OH
       |                      |
   H – C –OH              H – C – OH
       |                      |
      CH₂OH                  CH₂OH
   D-galactose            D-mannose
```

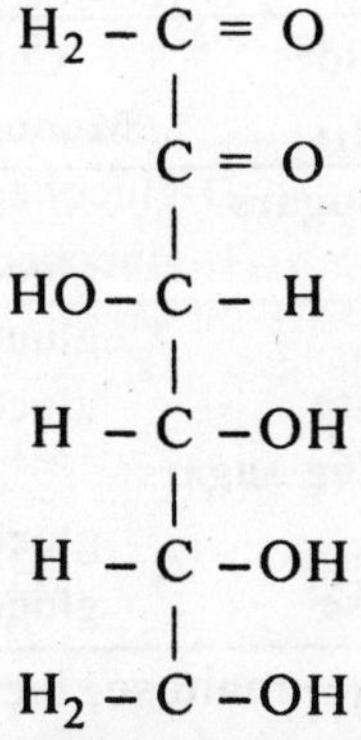

```
         H₂ – C = O
              |
              C = O
              |
         HO – C – H
              |
          H – C –OH
              |
          H – C –OH
              |
         H₂ – C –OH
         D-fructose
```

Some important reactions of monosaccharides are as mentioned below:

1. Reactions of monosaccharides characteristic of the aldehyde and ketone group. Reaction with hydrazines to form hydrazones and osazones:

   Phenylhydrazine and substituted hydrazones react with the monosaccharides and other carbohydrates containing a free sugar group to form hydrazones and osazones. With few exceptions, the hydrazones are soluble and difficult to isolate. On the other hand, osazones of different sugars are relatively insoluble and crystallize in beautiful and characteristic forms.

2. Monosaccharides react with hydrogen cyanide to form cyanhydrins.

3. Monosaccharides react with hydroxy-lamine to form oximes.

4. Reduction to form sugar alcohols: Both aldoses and ketoses may be reduced to the corresponding polyhydroxy alcohols. This may be accomplished with sodium amalgam, or better, electrolytically or by hydrogen under high pressure in the presence of a catalyst. Thus, the alcohols formed from glucose, mannose and fructose are as follows :

   D- glucose $\longrightarrow$ D - sorbitol
   D-mannose $\longrightarrow$ D - mannitol
   D-fructose $\longrightarrow$ D-mannitol, D-sorbitol

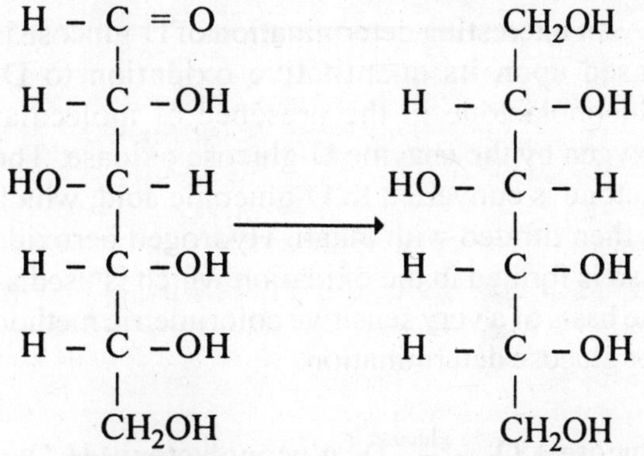

```
   H – C = O                      CH₂OH
       |                            |
   H – C –OH                    H – C – OH
       |                            |
  HO – C – H      ───────▶    HO – C – H
       |                            |
   H – C –OH                    H – C – OH
       |                            |
   H – C –OH                    H – C – OH
       |                            |
      CH₂OH                        CH₂OH
   D-glucose                     D-sorbitol
```

5. Monosaccharides get oxidized to form sugar acids, for example:

   D-glucose $\xrightarrow{\text{bromine water}}$ D-gluconic acid

6. Reducing action of sugars in alkaline solution:

Determination of sugars

All the sugars that contain free sugar group undergo enolization and various other changes when placed under alkaline solution. The enediol forms of the sugars are highly reactive and are easily oxidized by oxygen and other oxidizing agents. This means that these sugars in alkaline solution are very powerful reducing agents. They readily reduce oxidising ions such as Ag^+, Hg^{++},

Bi^{+++}, Cu^{++} and $Fe(CN)_6^{---}$ and the sugars are odixized to complex mixture of acids. This reducing action of sugars in alkaline solution is utilized for both the qualitative and quantitative determination of sugars. Reagents containing Cu^{++} ions are most commonly used. These are generally alkaline solutions of cupric sulphate containing sodium potassium tartarate (Rochelle salt) or sodium citrate. Sodium or potassium hydroxide is used as the alkali in the older reagents such as Fehling's solution; but weaker alkalies such as Na_2CO_3 and $NaHCO_3$ are used in the more recent reagents, such as those of Benedict, Folin and Shaffer and Hartmann.

An interesting determination of D-glucose is based upon its quantitative oxidation to D-gluconolactone in the presence of molecular oxygen by the enzyme D-glucose oxidase. The lactone is converted to D-gluconic acid, which is then titrated with alkali. Hydrogen peroxide also is formed in the oxidation which is used as the basis of a very sensitive colorimetric method for glucose determination.

$$glucose + O_2 \xrightarrow[\text{oxidase}]{\text{glucose}} gluconolactone + H_2O_2$$

$$+ H_2O$$

$$\downarrow$$

D- gluconic acid

$$H_2O_2 + o - dianisidine$$

$$\downarrow$$

peroxidase

yellow compound

(b) Oligosaccharides

The term 'oligosaccharide' is used for compounds made up by the condensation of 2-10 molecules of simple sugars. The important carbohydrates of this group are sucrose, maltose, lactose and raffinose. These are distinguished from each other by nomenclature such as disaccharides,

tri, tetra and pentasaccharides. On hydrolysis such saccharides give simple sugars. These may be regarded as the products of condensation of two or more sugars with the elimination of water. These have a general formula $C_n(H_2O)_{n-1}$. In general the reducing disaccharides are less potent as reducing agents than monosaccharides.

Disaccharides: The following tabulation gives the better known disaccharides with their component monosaccharides. Those possessing a free sugar group, are reducing sugars and give reactions characteristic of monosaccharides.

Disaccharides $C_{12}H_{22}O_{11}$	Constituent Monosaccharides
I **Reducing sugars**	
(a) Maltose	glucose+glucose
(b) Lactose	glucose+galactose
(c) Cellobiose	glucose+glucose
II **Non-reducing sugars**	
(a) Sucrose	glucose+fructose
(b) Trehalose	glucose+glucose

Of the above, maltose, lactose and sucrose are the most important examples of disaccharides.

Maltose: It is composed of two glucose units (Fig. 5.1) and is formed when the enzyme amylase or diastase hydrolyzes starch. It is a product of the action of salivary amylase (ptyalin) and pancreatic amylase (amylopsin) upon starch during the process of digestion. It is also formed as an intermediate product in the acid hydrolysis of starch and is an important constituent of corn syrups, which are prepared by partial hydrolysis

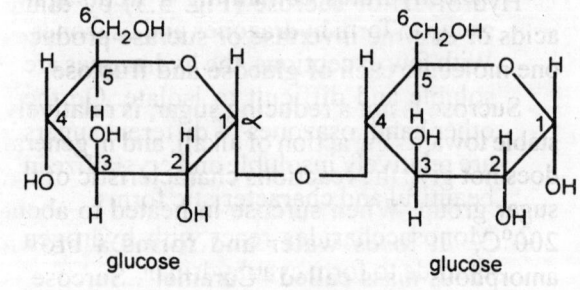

Fig 5.1 : Maltose

of starch with dilute acids. Enzyme maltase hydrolyzes it to glucose.

Lactose : It is formed by the secretory cells of the mammary glands during lactation and occurs to the extent of about 2 - 6 percent in the milk. It is prepared commercially from milk whey. It is hydrolyzed by acids and the **specific enzyme lactase** into its constituent monosaccharides, glucose and galactose. It is a reducing sugar, forms osazones, a cyanhydrin, and an oxime, and is decomposed by alkali. It accordingly contains a free sugar group in its structure (Fig 5.2).

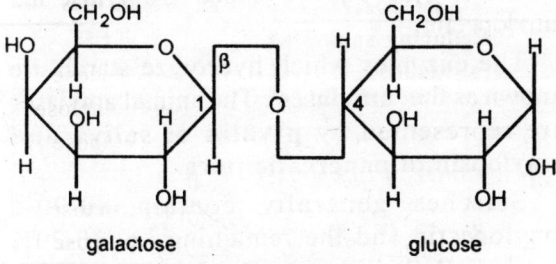

Fig 5.2 : Lactose

It is of interest to know that the human milk differs from cow's milk in containing, in addition to regular lactose, **other oligosaccharides, such as L-fucosyl lactose.**

Sucrose: It occurs especially in the juices of plants such as sugar beets, sugar cane, sorghum, sugar maple and pineapple and in smaller quantities in the juices of many other plants. Ripe fruits are rich in sucrose. It is by far the most abundantly distributed of the sugars.

Hydrolysis of sucrose (Fig. 5.3) by dilute acids or enzyme invertase or sucrase produces one molecule each of glucose and fructose.

Sucrose is not a reducing sugar, is relatively stable towards the action of alkali, and in general does not give the reactions characteristic of the sugar group. When surcose in heated to about 200°C, it loses water and forms a brown amorphous mass called "Caramel". Surcose is readily fermented by yeast. It is first split into

glucose and fructose by invertase, and the monosaccharides are then fermented by the zymase system of enzymes.

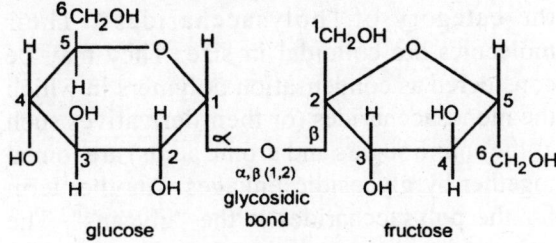

Fig. 5.3 : Surcose

Trisaccharides. Several oligosaccharides containing three monosaccharide units occur in nature. These are given in the following tabulation (Table 5.3) :

Amongst the trisaccharides, the most important of them is raffinose which occurs in sugar beets and is concentrated in sugar beet molasses. Cottonseed meal contains about 7 percent of raffinose. It is also frequently found in higher plants and fungi. It is hydrolyzed by enzymes of the gastrointestinal bacteria of herbivorous animals and serves as food for these animals whereas it is not well utilized as food by the human beings. Raffinose is fermented by yeast.

Table 5.3 : Classification of trisaccharides

Trisaccharides	Constituent monosaccharides with order of linkage
I **Reducing sugars**	
(a) Mannotriose	galactose, galactose, glucose
(b) Robinose	galactose, rhamnose, rhamnose
(c) Rhamninose	galactose, rhamnose, rhamnose
II **Non-reducing sugars**	
(a) Raffinose	fructose, glucose, galactose
(b) Gentianose	fructose, glucose, glucose
(c) Melezitose	glucose, fructose, glucose

(c) Polysaccharides

Carbohydrates composed of ten or more monosaccharide units are generally classified in the category of "polysaccharides". Their molecules are colloidal in size. They may be considered as condensation polymers in which the monosaccharides (or their derivatives such as the amino sugars and uronic acids) are joined together by glycosidic linkages. Another term for the polysaccharides is the "glycans". The polysaccharides such as starches, glycogen and cellulose, which are made up of a single kind of monosaccharide, are called "homoglycans" i.e. homopolysaccharides and the polysaccharides composed of two or more kinds of monosaccharides (or their derivatives), such as the **mucopolysaccharides,** are called as **"heteroglycans"** i.e. heteropolysaccharides made up of mannose and xylose are called as **"mannans"** and **"xylans"** respectively etc.

Some polysaccharides contain units that are derivatives of the monosaccharides, for example, chitin is made up of the amino sugar glucosamine and hyaluronic acid is composed of glucuronic acid and glucosamine.

Since the monosaccharide units of polysaccharides are joined together by glycosidic linkage, the polysaccharides are readily hydrolyzed by mineral acids but are resistant to alkaline hydrolysis.

The polysaccharides are hydrolyzed by the group or enzymes called "polysaccharidases". Important examples of polysaccharides include starch, glycogen, cellulose, dextrins, inulin etc. their molecules are so large that they can't be obtained in the form of true solution. **They give colloidal solutions except cellulose, which is insoluble.** Determination of their molecular weight reveals that a particular type of compound may have different molecular weights and shapes. Polysaccharides such as cellulose, starch, glycogen and dextrins are made up of many D-glucose units. They can be readily hydrolyzed to glucose by boiling with dilute acids except cellulose which is hydrolyzed by strong acids only. The polysaccharide **inulin is a compound made up of fructose units exclusively.**

HOMOPOLYSACCHARIDES

Starches

These occur widespread as reserve carbohydrate in tubers such as potatoes, in grains and seeds, in many fruits and in the rhizomes and pith of plants. Native starches are a mixture of two types of compounds that are separable from each other and are named as amylose and amylopectin.

The enzymes which hydrolyze starch are known as the **'amylases'.** The animal amylases are represented by **ptyalin of saliva and amylopsin of pancreatic juice.**

Starches generally contain 80-90% amylopectin and the remaining i.e. 10-20% amylose. Both the amylose and amylopectin are hydrolyzed by acid to D-glucose. Partial acid hydrolysis gives complex mixtures of dextrins, maltose and glucose.

Amylose

Molecule of amylose consists of many glucose units joined together through α-glycosidic linkage, chiefly as found in maltose. The glucose units of amylose are linked in the unbranched chain. The amylose structure (Fig.5.4) may be considered as an expanded maltose structure with a free sugar group on one end.

Amylose may be easily hydrolyzed by acids

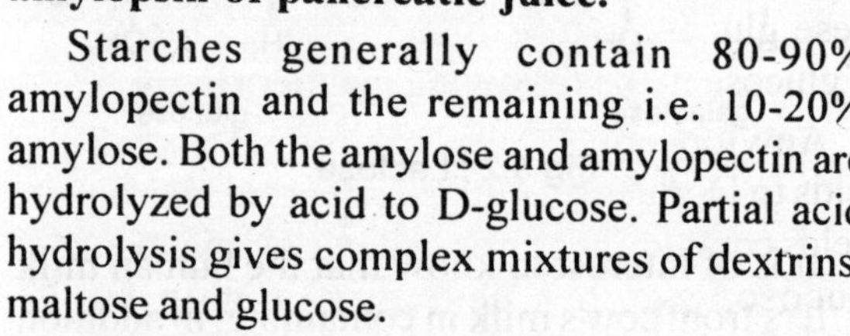

Fig 5.4 : Amylose

to D-glucose. Partial acid hydrolysis gives complex mixtures of dextrins, maltose and glucose. Starches generally contain 10-20 percent amylose, though in a few instances the amylose content is higher. The amylose extracted from starch grains is a mixture of molecules of different sizes. Amylose fractions with molecular weights from 4,000 to 4,00,000 have been obtained. It gives a characteristic colour reaction with iodine. **It produces a blueblack colour with iodine solution.** The colour disappears upon heating the solution and reappears upon cooling.

Amylopectin

Like that of amylose molecule, it too consists of many glucose units joined together through α-glycosidic linkage, chiefly as found in maltose. Its molecule also contains chains of glucose units like that of amylose and also has branches of these glucose chains linked through the 6-OH of glucose in the following manner:(Fig. 5.5).

Amylopectin is also easily hydrolyzed by acids to D-glucose units. Partial acid hydrolysis yields complex mixtures of dextrins, maltose and glucose. Starches generally contain 80-90 percent amylopectin. Its molecules differ from amylose molecules not only in possessing many branched chains, but also in being larger. The molecular weight of amylopectins apparently vary from 50,000 to about 1000,000. **It gives a characteristic violet to red-violet colour with iodine solution. As with amylose, the colour disappears upon heating the solution and reappears upon cooling.**

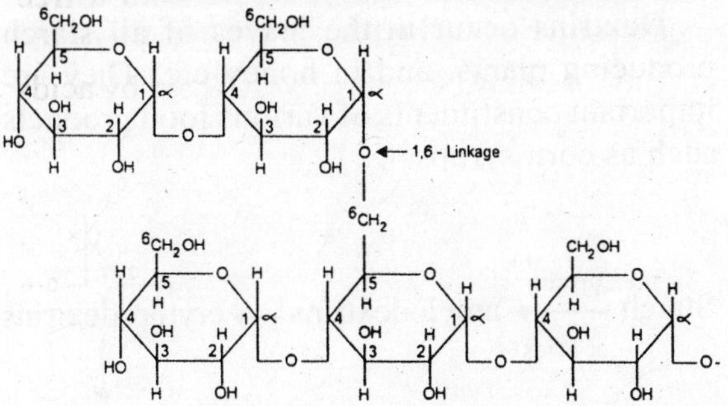

Glycogen

It is the carbohydrate reserve of animals. It is stored chiefly in the liver and muscles. It is also found in the plants which have no chlorophyll content such as fungi and yeast. Its structure is similar to that of amylopectin in that it is a branched molecule. It has been found to have 7 to 12 glucose residues per non- reducing end group and hence it is even more highly branched. Molecular weights ranging from 270,000 to 100 million have been reported. It is readily soluble, **its solution is opalescent and gives a red-brown or red colour with iodine solution.** It yields D-glucose upon complete hydrolysis. Its structure may be represented as shown below (Fig. 5.6), where each head of chain represents a glucose molecule.

Biochemically, glycogen is one of the most important substances in the body. Liver glycogen is broken down to glucose and passed into the blood stream for use by the tissues. **Muscle glycogen is a source of energy for muscle contraction. Mollusks such as oysters and clams are usually rich in glycogen.**

Amylo- 1-6-glucosidase is involved in the

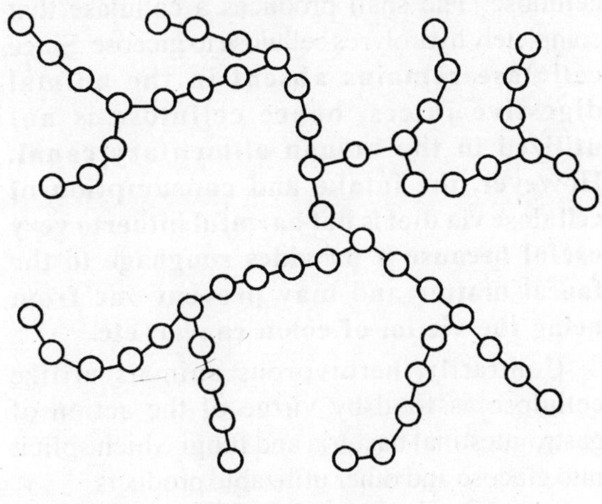

Fig. 5.5 : Amylopectin

Fig. 5.6 : Model of a glycogen molecule

specific cleavage, by hydrolysis, of the 1,6-branching linkage of glycogen, releasing free glucose. The combined action of the phosphorylase and the amylo 1,6-glucosidase results in the liberation of glucose- 1-phosphate and glucose. Indeed, the ratio of these two defines the extent of branching in a glycogen (or amylopectin) molecule.

Cellulose

Cellulose is the chief constituent of the fibrous parts of the plants and consequently **is the most abundant organic material in nature.** The cellulose content of flax, ramie and cotton amounts **from 97 to 99 percent,** while the content in wood varies from 41 to 53 percent. Cereal straws contain from 30 to 43 percent cellulose. Thus, it is the most abundant **structural polysaccharide of plant kingdom. It does not occur in animal body.**

Although usually considered to be only a plant product, **cellulose (tunicin) is also found in certain marine animals.**

Cellulose yields D-glucose as the final product of hydrolysis. It is resistant to hydrolysis and requires the action of strong acids. Various bacteria and other lower forms possess enzymes **called cellulases,** capable of hydrolyzing cellulose. The snail produces a cellulase that completely hydrolyzes cellulose to glucose. **Since cellulase remains absent in the animal digestive juices, hence cellulose is not utilized in the human alimentary canal. However, the intake and consumption of cellulose via diet is not harmful hitherto very useful because it provides roughage to the faecal matter and may prevent one from being the victim of colon cancer, etc.**

Contrarily, herbivorous animals utilize cellulose as food by virtue of the action of gastrointestinal bacteria and fungi which split it into glucose and other utilizable products.

Partial hydrolysis of cellulose by acids yields a mixture of cellodextrins, various oligosaccharides, cellobiose and glucose.

Studies seem to indicate that cellulose is a linear polysaccharide consisting of β-1,4 linked glucose units. The M.W. of cellulose samples vary from 200,000 to 2,000,000. It is insoluble in water. It does not give characteristic colour with iodine solution.

Cellulose may be nitrated to form nitrocellulose which is of much importance in the manufacture of explosive celluloid and other substances. Cellulose acetates are used in making photographic films, rayon and various plastic materials.

Dextrins

Partial hydrolysis of starch by acids, or α-and β- amylases, produces substances known as "dextrins". These substances consist of a very complex mixture of molecules of different sizes and structures and are known as amylodextrins, erythrodextrins and achrodextrins. **Amylodextrin** gives **blue colour** with iodine, **erythrodextrin** gives **reddish- brown colour** whereas **achrodextrin does not give any colour.** Their reducing property is feeble and they have got faint sweet taste. **They are generally soluble in water and produce sticky solutions and hence are used as adhesives and binders.** All dextrins have free sugar groups and accordingly reduce alkaline copper solutions and give other sugar reactions.

Dextrins occur in the leaves of all starch producing plants, and in honey etc. They are important constituents of various food products such as corn syrups.

$$\text{Starch} \xrightarrow[\text{or acids}]{\text{ptyalin}} \text{amylodextrins} \longrightarrow \text{erythrodextrins} \longrightarrow \text{achrodextrins}$$

Inulin

It is a polysaccharide which exclusively contains **D-fructose units.** It occurs as the reserve carbohydrate in the tubers of chicory, Jerusalem artichoke, dahlia and in the bulbs of onion and garlic. It is a white, more or less crystalline powder. It is very easily hydrolyzed by acids. It is not hydrolyzed by amylase **but is split by inulinase.**

Inulin is used as a source of commercial fructose. It is also administered to animals in the studies of glomerular membrane filtration rates. It is not hydrolyzed by any of the enzymes of the gastrointestinal tract and is not utilized as food.

HETEROPOLYSACCHARIDES (HETEROGLYCANS)

Agar

Agar is a vegetable mucilage obtained from seaweeds. It is a sulfuric acid ester of a complex galactose polysaccharide. It is odourless and tasteless. It swells strongly in cold water but does not dissolve. It gets dissolved in hot water to form a sol which upon cooling sets into a gel. A 1 percent agar gel is fairly rigid, and a 2 percent gel is very rigid. Agar is non-digestible and at times is given to provide bulk to the faeces in the treatment of constipation.

Gum Acacia or Gum Arabic

The vegetable gums are carbohydrate materials containing hexoses or pentoses or both in glycosidic union and a carbohydrate acid group. It is one of the most important and best- known gums. Gum arabic appears to be the salt of a high polymer of arabic acid which upon complete hydrolysis yields galactose, arabinose, rhamnose and glucuronic acid.

Gum arabic is used in the preparation of pharmaceuticals, in confections, and as an adhesive.

Pectins

"Pectin" is the term used to represent the substance or substances which in the presence of sugar and the proper acid concentration causes the formation of jellies. **It occurs in abundance in nature and is found especially in the pulp of citrus fruits, apples, carrots, beets, etc.** Commercial pectin is generally prepared from lemons or apples. When soluble, pectin is boiled with dilute acid, it is slowly hydrolyzed to pectic acid and methyl alcohol.

Large amounts of pectin are used in the fruit conserving industry and for other purposes.

"Pectin" is a group term and a number of different pectins are known today, some of which are insoluble and useless for gelation.

Alginic Acids

Alginic acids consist chiefly of linear polymers of D-mannuronic acid units. Its molecular weights range from 50,000 to 1,85,000. These are found in many marine algae and in giant kelp, which is a commercial source. Large amounts are used as emulsifier and smoothening agents in food industries.

Mucopolysaccharides (Glycosaminoglycans)

These are referred to as the substances which are composed of amino sugar and uronic acid units as the principal components, though some are chiefly made up of amino sugar and monosaccharide unit without the presence of uronic acid. The hexosamine present is generally acetylated.

Mucopolysaccharides are essential components of tissues. **They may be combined with proteins as mucoproteins or mucoids.** Important examples of mucopolysaccharides include hyaluronic acid, heparin and the chondroitin sulphates.

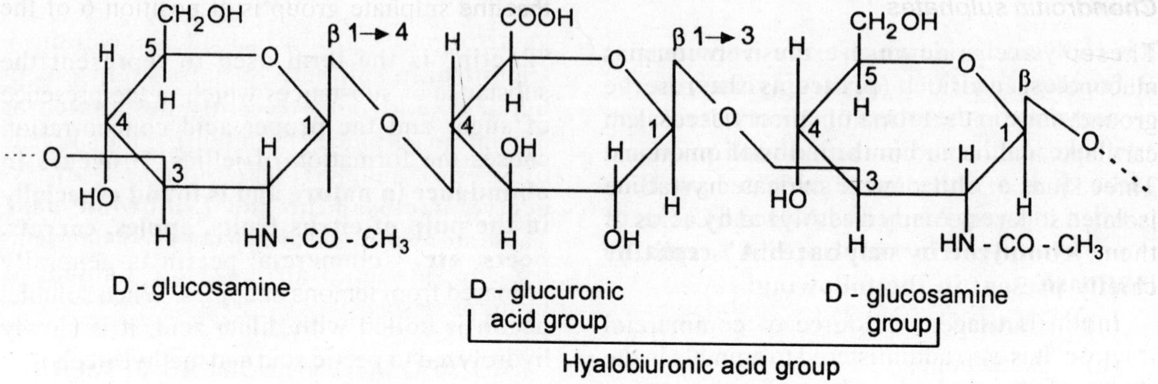

Fig. 5.7 : Repeating units in hyaluronic acid structure

Hyaluronic acid

It is found in vitreous humour, synovial fluid, skin, umbilical cord and other sources. It appears to serve as an integral part of the gel-like ground substance of connective and other tissues and as lubricant and shock absorbent in joints. It acts as an intercellular cement. It is a viscous, high molecular weight (several million) polysaccharide consisting of chains of N-acetylglucosamine and glucuronic acid residues. **Hyaluronidase** is a the enzyme which hydrolyzes it into its constituents, This enzyme is widely distributed in microorganisms and mammalian tissues (Fig 5.7).

Heparin

It is a blood anticoagulant which is found in liver, lung, thymus, spleen and blood. It is a polymer of **D-glucosamine and D-glucuronic acid.** The amino groups and some of the hydroxyl groups remain combined with sulphuric acid. The molecular weight of heparin appears to be in the range of 17,000 to 20,000. **It is strongly acidic due to the presence of sulphuric acid group and readily forms salts. It inhibits the transformation of prothrombin to thrombin, preventing the conversion of fibrinogen to fibrin, which is catalyzed by thrombin. The probable repeating units are as follows (Fig. 5.8).**

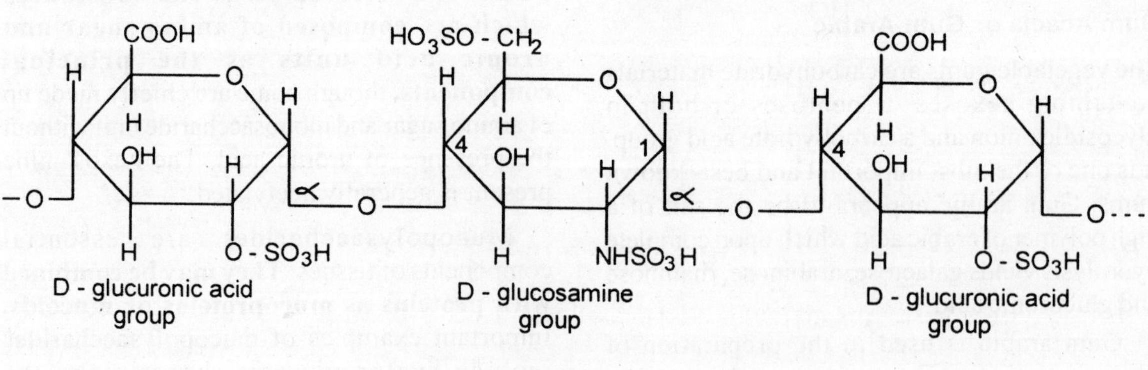

Fig. 5.8 : Repeating units in heparin

Chondroitin sulphates

These are among the principal mucopolysaccharides **(proteoglycans)** in the ground substance of mammalian tissues and cartilage, and occur **combined with proteins**. Three kinds of chondroitin sulphate have been isolated so far and named as A, B and C. Out of them, **chondroitin sulphate 'A' remains chiefly present in the following:**

(a) Cartilage,

(b) Adult bone,

(c) Cornea, etc.

Chondroitin sulphate 'B' remains chiefly present in:

(a) Skin

(b) Heart valves

(c) Tendons, etc.

Chondroitin sulphate 'C' remains chiefly present in:

(a) Cartilage

(b) Tendons, etc.

The basic structure of chondroitin sulphate 'A' consists of repeating unit of **N-acetyl galactosamine** and **glucuronic acid** with esterified sulphate at position 4 of galactosamine. The structure of chondroitin sulphate 'C' is the same as that of chondroitin sulphate 'A' except

that the sulphate group is at position 6 of the galactosamine group instead of position 4. **Chondroitin sulphate `B', also known as β-heparin, and more recently designated as dermatan sulphate** (from skin), is the sulphate of a polysaccharide composed of **N-acetylgalactosamine and L-iduronic acid.** These are hydrolyzed to their corresponding units by the mammalian enzyme named as hyaluronidase.

MUTAROTATION, ANOMERS, EPIMERS

The α-and β-forms of glucose spontaneously undergo interconversion (mutarotation) in water (Fig. 5.9). α-D-glucose and β- D- glucose differ only in the conformation of the hydroxyl group on carbon atom number 1. **These and other pairs of sugar molecules that differ only in**

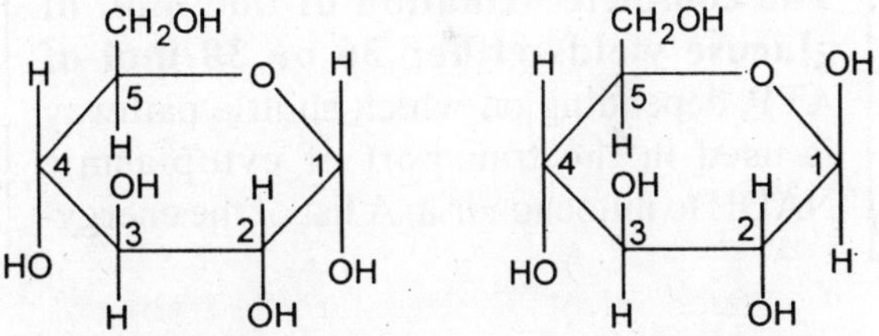

Fig. 5.9 : Two conformations of D-glucose

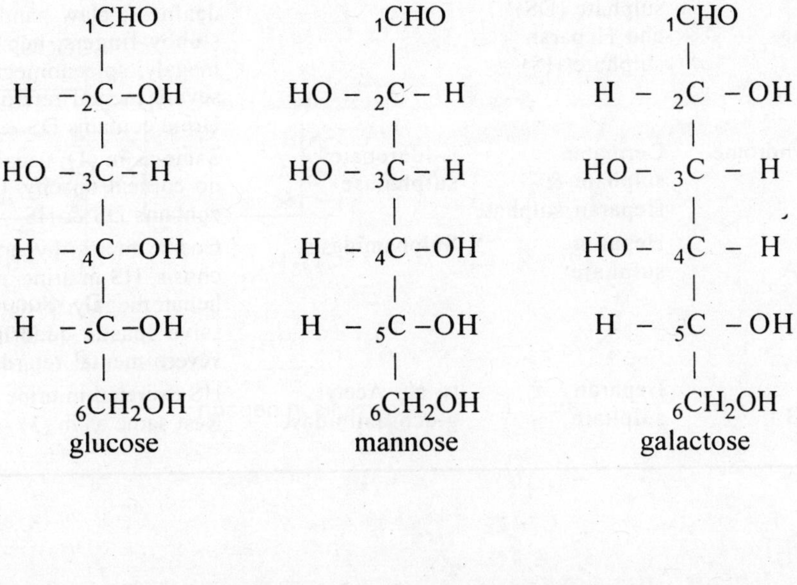

glucose

mannose

galactose

this respect are termed as anomers.

Such isomers which differ only in the configuration of a single carbon atom are termed as "epimers". Examples of epimeric pairs include those of glucose-mannose and glucose-galactose. Glucose and mannose are epimers with respect to carbon atom 2; whereas glucose and galactose are epimers with respect to carbon atom 4.

Mucopolysaccharidoses (Table 5.4) are the hereditary disorders caused due to the absence/deficiency of certain enzymes of the metabolism of mucopolysaccharides leading to the accumulation of certain mucopolysaccharide(s) in one or the other tissue(s) of the body; there are atleast seven types of such disorders out of which two are of paramount importance, **namely Hurler's syndrome** and **Hunter's syndrome.**

> **The complete oxidation of one mol. of glucose yields either 36 or 38 mol of ATP,** depending on which shuttle pathway is used in the transport of cytoplasmic NADH to mitochondria. A list of the energy-

yielding reactions of glucose oxidation is as shown below:

Energy yielding reactions in the complete oxidation of Glucose:

Reaction	Net moles of ATP generated per mole of glucose
Glycolysis	
(phosphoglycerate kinase, pyruvate kinase; 4 ATPs are formed whereas 2 are utilized)	2
NADH shuttle	
glycerol-phosphate shuttle (or malate-aspartate shuttle)	4 (6)
Pyruvate dehydrogenase (NADH)	6
Succinyl CoA synthetase	
(GTP is equivalent to ATP)	2
Succinate dehydrogenase	
(succinate $\longrightarrow$ fumarate + FADH$_2$)	4
Other TCA cycle reactions	
(isocitrate $\longrightarrow$ α-ketoglutarate, α-ketoglutarate $\longrightarrow$ succinyl CoA, malate $\longrightarrow$ oxaloacetate; total of 3NADH generated)	18
Total	36 (38)

Table 5.4 : Different types of Mucopolysaccharidoses

Sl. No.	Name of disorder	Affected compound (s)	Enzyme defect	Clinical manifestations	Age of onset
1.	Hurler's syndrome (Mucopolysaccharidose -I)	Dermatan sulphate (DS) and Heparan sulphate(HS)	α-L-Iduronidase	Corneal opacity, deafness, claw hands, stubby fingers, hepatomegaly, spleenomegaly, severe mental retardation. Urine contains DS & HS.	1 year
2.	Hunter's syndrome (MPS-II)	Dermatan sulphate & Heparan sulphate	L-Iduronate sulphatase	Same as in (1); usually no corneal opacity. Urine contains DS & HS	1 year
3.	MPS-III A Sanfilippo A syndrome	Heparan sulphate	Sulphamidase	Coarse facies, hypertrichosis, HS in urine, mild hepatomegaly, progressive spastic quadriparesis, severe mental retardation	2 - 3 years
4.	MPS-III B Sanfilippo B syndrome	Heparan sulphate	α- N - Acetyl glucosaminidase	HS excreted in urine Rest same as in (3)	2 - 3 years

CHAPTER 6

LIPIDS

> We do not have affinity with water but have with organic solvents. We make the food palatable and delicious. We are some what costly. We are found in many food oils/ seeds/ pulses and other innumerable eatables. In excess, we make you run to the doctor, hence use us with full precautions. We have store houses in the body like subcutaneous tissue, omentum, adipose tissue, etc. We can disfigure your body if consumed in excess.

Lipids are the organic compounds that are poorly soluble in water but quite soluble in organic solvents such as the structural components of cell membranes, as storage forms of energy, as metabolic fuel and as emulsifying agents. Surprisingly, four of the vitamins (A, D, E and K) are lipids. In addition, the prostaglandins, substances that stimulate smooth muscle contractions and function in intracellular regulatory processes, are lipid derivatives. The transport of lipids through the blood plasma is an extremely important subject from the standpoint of health, because the abnormalities in these processes are thought to be a major factor in the development of coronary artery diseases which are on the increase throughout the globe. **Obesity results from the storage of excessive amounts of lipids in the body. Such common diseases like diabetes mellitus, obstructive jaundice, pancreatitis, and hypothyroidism have associated plasma lipid transport abnormalities. In addition,** there are a number of rare inherited diseases, known as the lipid storage diseases or lipidoses. For instance, Tay-Sach's disease, Niemann-Pick disease, Gaucher's disease, Fabry's disease, Farber's disease, etc.

To summarize, lipid is a term used to describe a group of fats and fat like substances that constitute a major portion of tissue components and a major foodstuff.

Isolation of lipids from tissue

The chloroform- methanol (2:1) solvent introduced by Folch for lipid extraction has largely replaced the older well-known ethanol- ether (3:1) solvent introduced by Bloor..

Classification of lipids

There is no single internationally accepted system of classification for the lipids. However, generally accepted classification is given in Table 6.1.

Table 6.1 : Classification of lipids

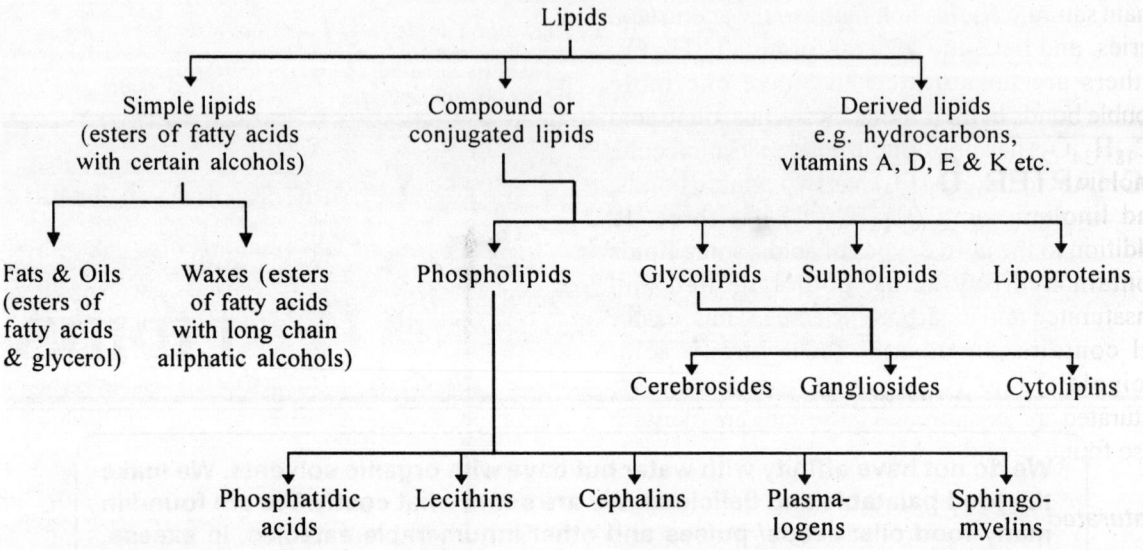

Functions of lipids

There are numerous functions of lipids in the animal body. They play vital functions in the body which may be remembered as given in Table 6.2.

Table 6.2 : Functions of lipids

Sl. No.	Lipid	Function(s)
1.	Fatty acids	Metabolic fuel, building blocks for other lipids
2.	Prostaglandins	Intracellular modulators
3.	Glyceryl esters	
(a)	Acylglycerols	Fatty acid storage, metabolic intermediates
(b)	Phospho-glycerides	Membrane structure
4.	Sphingolipids	
(a)	Sphingomyelin	Membrane structure
(b)	Glycosphingo-lipids	Membranes, surface antigens
5.	Sterol derivatives	
(a)	Cholesterol	Membrane and lipoprotein structure
(b)	Cholesterol esters	Storage and transport
(c)	Bile acids	Lipid digestion and absorption

Sl. No.	Lipid	Function(s)
(d)	Steroid hormones	Metabolic regulation
(e)	Vitamin D	Calcium and Phosphorus metabolism
6.	Terpenes	
(a)	Vitamin A	Vision, epithelial integrity
(b)	Vitamin E	Lipid antioxidant
(c)	Vitamin K	Blood coagulation

Simple lipids

These are the esters of fatty acids with certain alcohols. They are usually further classified according to the nature of the alcohols, as follows:

Fats and Oils

These are the esters of fatty acids and glycerol. If they are solid at room temperature, then they are known as fats and if liquid at room temperature, then they are termed as oils.

Fatty acids. Fatty acids found in fats and other lipids are of various types. Some of them, like palmitic acid ($CH_3(CH_2)_{14}.COOH$) and stearic acid ($CH_3(CH_2)_{16}.COOH$) are straight-chain saturated acids belonging to the acetic acid series, and have the general formula $C_nH_{2n}O_2$. Others are unsaturated and have one more double bonds in their molecules. Thus, oleic acid ($C_{18}H_{34}O_2$) has one double bond in its molecule, linoleic acid ($C_{18}H_{32}O_2$) has two double bonds, and linolenic acid ($C_{18}H_{30}O_2$) has three. In addition to the above types of acids, some lipids contain hydroxy acids, both saturated and unsaturated and dicarboxylic acids. Thus, castor oil contains an unsaturated hydroxy acid, ricinoleic acid ($C_{18}H_{32}O_3$). Certain cyclic saturated and unsaturated fatty acids are likewise also found in nature (Table 6.3).

Saturated fatty acids

They are generally represented by the general formula $C_nH_{2n}O_2$ or $C_nH_{2n+1}COOH$. Physical properties of the saturated fatty acids depend upon their molecular weights. Whereas those fatty acids that contain ten carbon atoms or fewer in their molecules are liquids at room temperature, the remainder are solids whose melting points rise with increasing molecular weight. The liquid acids are also known as **volatile fatty acids,** since they may be distilled with steam, whereas the others, the **nonvolatile acids,** are carried over by steam distillation only in traces or not at all. Fatty acids with four carbon atoms or fewer are miscible with water in all proportions. As the length of the carbon chain increases beyond this, the solubility rapidly decreases to zero. The important examples of straight chain **saturated fatty acids** found in nature as constituents of lipid molecules include **butyric, caproic, caprylic, capric, lauric, myristic, palmitic, stearic** etc. (Table 6.3).

Unsaturated fatty acids

These are characterized by the presence of one or more double bonds in the molecule.

Table 6.3 : Classification of the fatty acids

Common name	Formula	Occurrence
1. Saturated acids, $C_nH_{2n+1}COOH$, unbranched chain		
(a) Acetic (2)*	CH_3COOH	Vinegar
(b) Butyric (4)	C_3H_7COOH	Butter fat
(c) Caproic (6)	$C_5H_{11}COOH$	Butter fat, coconut oil
(d) Caprylic (8)	$C_7H_{15}COOH$	Butter fat, coconut oil
(e) Capric (10)	$C_9H_{19}COOH$	Butter fat, coconut oil
(f) Lauric (12)	$C_{11}H_{23}COOH$	Laurel kernel oil, butter fat, coconut oil
(g) Myristic (14)	$C_{13}H_{27}COOH$	Nutmeg fat, butter, vegetable fats
(h) Palmitic (16)	$C_{15}H_{31}COOH$	Most vegetable & animal fats
(i) Stearic (18)	$C_{17}H_{35}COOH$	Most vegetable & animal fats
(j) Arachidic acid (20)	$C_{19}H_{39}COOH$	Peanut oil
(k) Behenic acid (22)	$C_{21}H_{43}COOH$	Rapeseed oil, peanut oil
(l) Lignoceric acid (24)	$C_{23}H_{47}COOH$	Cerebrosides, sphingomyelin, peanut oil

II, Unsaturated fatty acids

A. **Monoethenic**, $C_nH_{2n-1}COOH$, one double bond (Monounsaturated)

(a) **Paimitoleic**, Δ^9 (16)	$C_{15}H_{29}COOH$	⎫
(b) **Oleic acid**, Δ^9 (18)	$C_{17}H_{33}COOH$	Animal and vegetable fats
(c) **Erucic acid** Δ^{13} (22)	$C_{21}H_{41}COOH$	
(d) **Nervonic acid** Δ^{15} (24)	$C_{23}H_{45}COOH$	⎭

B. **Dienoic**, $C_nH_{2n-3}COOH$, two double bonds (Diunsaturated)

*number of carbon atoms in the fatty acid molecule

Linoleic acid, $\Delta^{9,12}(18)$ $C_{17}H_{31}COOH$ Linseed oil, animal & plant fats, corn oil, soyabean oil, peanut oil etc.

C. Trienoic, $C_nH_{2n-5}COOH$, three double bonds (Triunsaturated)

Linolenic acid, $\Delta^{9,12,15}(18)$ $C_{17}H_{29}COOH$ Linseed oil, rapeseed oil soyabean oil, liver oil etc.

D. Polyenoic, $C_nH_{2n-7}COOH$, more than three double bonds. (Many unsaturations)

Arachidonic acid, $\Delta^{5,8,11,14}(20)$ $C_{19}H_{31}COOH$ Fats, phospholipids etc.

III. Branched-chain acids

(a) Isobutyric acid (4) C_3H_7COOH Waxes

(b) Tuberculo-stearic acid (19) $C_{18}H_{37}COOH$ Wax of tubercle bacillus

IV. Hydroxy acids

(a) Cerebronic acid (24) $C_{23}H_{46}(OH)COOH$

(b) Ricinoleic acid (18) $C_{17}H_{32}(OH)COOH$ Animal and vegetable fats

(c) Hydroxy-nervonic Acids (24) $C_{23}H_{44}(OH)COOH$

V. Cyclic acids

(a) Chaulmoogric acid   *R-$(CH_2)_{12}$-COOH   seed oils

(b) Hydnocarpic acid   *R-$(CH_2)_{10}$-COOH   seed oils

* Where R is

$$CH=CH \atop | \quad\quad\quad \searrow C- \atop CH_2-CH_2 \nearrow \quad\; H$$

They have been classified in accordance with the number of double bonds and named by reference to the parent hydrocarbon, the position of the double bond or bonds in the chain being indicated by a number referred to the carboxyl carbon atom as number one.

Nomenclature of fatty acids

Carbon atoms are numbered from the carboxyl carbon (carbon No. 1). The carbon atom adjacent to the carboxyl carbon (No.2) is also known as α- carbon. Carbon atom No.3 is the β-carbon, and the end methyl carbon is known as a ω-carbon or n- carbon. Various conventions are in use for indicating the number and position of the double bonds; for e.g., Δ^9 indicates a double bond between carbon atoms 9 and 10 of the fatty acid. The ω- 9 indicates a double bond on the 9th carbon counting from the ω-carbon atom. Widely used conventions to indicate the number of carbon atoms, the number of the double bonds, and the positions of the double bonds are prevalent. To cite an example, see the structure of oleic acid.

Oleic (C'_{18}) $C_{18}H_{34}O_2$

$$18:1;9 \text{ or } \Delta^9 \; 18:1$$

$$\overset{18}{C}H_3-\overset{17}{C}H_2-\overset{16}{C}H_2-\overset{15}{C}H_2-\overset{14}{C}H_2-\overset{13}{C}H_2-\overset{12}{C}H_2-\overset{11}{C}H_2-\overset{10}{C}H$$

$$=\overset{9}{C}H\overset{1}{(CH_2)_7} COOH$$

OR

$$\overset{\omega}{C}H_3-\overset{2}{C}H_2-\overset{3}{C}H_2-\overset{4}{C}H_2-\overset{5}{C}H_2-\overset{6}{C}H_2-\overset{7}{C}H_2-\overset{8}{C}H_2-\overset{9}{C}H_2$$
n

$$\overset{10}{=CH}\overset{18}{(CH_2)_7} COOH$$

In animals, additional double bonds are introduced only between the existing double bonds e.g., $\omega9$, $\omega6$, or $\omega3$ and the carboxyl carbon, leading to three series of fatty acids known as the $\omega9$, $\omega6$ and $\omega3$ families, respectively.

Some unsaturated fatty acids of physiologic and nutritional importance are as given below:

Number of carbon atoms and position of double bonds	Series	Common name
Monoenoic acids (one double bond)		
16:1;9	$\omega 7$	Palmitoleic
18:1;9	$\omega 9$	Oleic
22:1;13	$\omega 9$	Erucic

Dienoic acids (2 double bonds)

18 : 2 ; 9, 12   ω 6   Linoleic

Trienoic acids (3 double bonds)

18 : 3; 6, 9, 12   ω 6   γ - Linolenic

18 : 3; 9, 12, 15   ω 3   α - Linolenic

Tetraenoic acids (4 double bonds)

20 : 4; 5, 8, 11, 14   ω 6   Arachidonic

Triglycerides (Neutral fats)

The neutral fats (triglycerides) are important because the bulk (as much as 90 per cent) of the lipid material stored in the adipose tissue of the body is **neutral fat** and represents a concentrated form of energy stored until required for metabolic purposes.

Glycerol reacts with one molecule of fatty acid to form a **monoglyceride,** with two molecules to form a **diglyceride** and with three to form a **triglyceride** as shown below:

$$
\begin{array}{ccccc}
CH_2OH & & HO.OC.C_3H_7 & & CH_2.O.CO.C_3H_7 \\
| & & & & | \\
CHOH & + & HO.OC.C_3H_7 & \longrightarrow & CH.O.CO.C_3H_7 \quad + \quad 3H_2O \\
| & & & & | \\
CH_2OH & & HO.OC.C_3H_7 & & CH_2.O.CO.C_3H_7 \\
\text{glycerol} & & \text{butyric acid} & & \text{tributyrin} \\
& & \text{(3 moles)} & & \text{(a triglyceride)}
\end{array}
$$

General formula for a fat is

$$
\begin{array}{c}
CH_2.O.CO.R_1 \\
| \\
CH.O.CO.R_2 \\
| \\
CH_2.O.CO.R_3
\end{array}
$$

where R_1, R_2 and R_3 may be derived form the same or different fatty acids.

Compound or conjugated lipids

These are the esters of fatty acids which, upon hydrolysis, yield other substances in addition to the fatty acids and an alcohol. Some important members of this group are:

1. Phospholipids (Phosphatides)

Lipids which upon hydrolysis, yield fatty acids, phosphoric acid, sometimes, but not always, glycerol and a nitrogenous base. These are subdivided into the following groups:

(A) Phosphatidic acids: Lipids which when hydrolyzed yield one molecule each of glycerol and phosphoric acid and two molecules of fatty acids of which one is probably saturated and the other unsaturated.

(B) Lecithins: These are the lipids containing fatty acids, phosphoric acid, glycerol, and the nitrogenous base choline.

The saturated fatty acids present in lecithin molecules include palmitic and stearic acids while the unsaturated fatty acids present include oleic, linoleic, linolenic and arachidonic acids. Lecithins are widely distributed in animal tissues for instance brain, liver, blood, cardiac muscles etc., they are also found in vegetable sources e.g. plant seeds etc.

Lecithins when purified are waxy white substances but soon become brownish when exposed to air and light, owing to autoxidation and decomposition. They are soluble in ordinary

$$^1CH_2 - O - CO - R$$
$$|\qquad\qquad \text{(saturated fatty acid)}$$
$$R-CO-O-^2CH\qquad O$$
(unsaturated
fatty acid)
$$^3CH_2-O-P-O-\overline{CH_2-CH_2-N}\equiv (CH_3)_3$$
$$|\qquad\qquad\qquad +$$
$$OH\qquad\qquad OH$$

choline

α - Lecithin

fat solvents like ethanol, ether etc. but not in acetone. **Large quantities of soyabean lecithins are used these days as emulsifying and smoothening agents in the food industry.**

Lecithins are hydrolyzed by boiling with alkalies and dilute mineral acids and also by the corresponding enzymes i.e. **lecithinases (phospholipases).** The nature of hydrolysis depends upon the kind of phospholipase acting. Scientist **'Hanahan' has shown that lecithinase A (phospholipase A) found in certain snake venoms (cobra, cotton mouth moccasin, vipers), poisons of scorpions and bees, and various mammalian tissues, specifically hydrolyzes off the fatty acid (unsaturated) present at C_2 of α- lecithin molecule to form lysolecithins. The lysolecithins so formed are very powerful haemolytic agents which rapidly haemolyze blood erythrocytes, and are considered to be responsible for harmful physiological effects of venoms containing phospholipase A.**

$$H_2{}^1C - O - CO - R$$
$$|$$
$$HO -^2C - H$$
$$|\qquad\qquad O$$
$$\qquad\qquad\quad ||$$
$$H_2{}^3C - O - P - O - CH_2.CH_2.N \equiv (CH_3)_3$$
$$|\qquad\qquad\qquad\qquad +$$
$$O\qquad\qquad\qquad OH$$

L-α-Lysolecithin

Four kinds of lecithinases i.e. A, B, C and D are known today which are very specific in nature. These are found in different vegetables, mammalian tissues and microorganisms.

(C) Cephalins. Lipids which upon hydrolysis yield fatty acids, glycerol, phosphoric acid, and either the nitrogenous base ethanolamine (colamine) or the amino acid serine. Lipids of uncertain structures which contain inositol, fatty acids, phosphoric acid, ethanolamine, and possibly galactose and tartaric acid have also been included in this class.

$$^1CH_2 - O - CO - R$$
$$|$$
$$R-CO-O-^2CH$$
$$|\qquad\qquad O$$
$$\qquad\qquad\quad ||$$
$$^3CH_2 - O - P - O - \overline{-CH_2.CH_2.NH_2}$$
$$|$$
$$OH\qquad \text{ethanolamine}$$

α-Cephalin (L-α-Phosphatidyl ethanolamine)

Cephalins contain the saturated fatty acid called stearic acid and the unsaturated fatty acids, **oleic, linoleic** and **arachidonic acids.** They are found in various animal tissues e.g. brain, liver, egg yolk, erythrocytes and cardiac muscles and are also found to be present in various plant sources i.e. plant seeds etc. Cephalins, like lecithins, are hygroscopic solids and are decomposed on exposure to air. These are insoluble in alcohol and acetone, but soluble in ether.

The cephalins are hydrolyzed by boiling with alkalies and dilute mineral acids. Lecithinase A from snake venom hydrolyzes cephalins to form lysocephalins which are similar to the lysolecithins formed from lecithins.

(D) Plasmalogens. These on hydrolysis yield one molecule each of aliphatic aldehyde, fatty acid, glycerol, phosphoric acid, and a nitrogen containing base (ethanolamine or choline). These

contribute to an appreciable proportion (about 10 percent) of the phospholipids of muscles and brain. Cardiac muscles and erythrocytes also contain plasmalogens.

(E) Sphingomyelins. These on hydrolysis yield a nitrogenous base sphingosine, a single fatty acid molecule, phosphoric acid, and choline, but no glycerol. These are soluble in hot ethanol, but not in ether, acetone or cold ethanol. They are found in brain, liver, blood, cardiac muscles etc.

2. Glycolipids

As the name indicates, these are the complex lipids containing carbohydrate in combination with long chain aliphatic acids or alcohols.

(A) Cerebrosides. Lipids which contain carbohydrate (galactose or glucose), one fatty acid, and sphingosine, but no phosphoric acid or glycerol. The fatty acids of the cerebrosides chiefly are lignoceric, behenic, and palmitic acids.

$$CH_3(CH_2)_{12} - CH = CH - CH - CH - CH_2 - O - C$$

sphingosine group

Cerebroside

Various cerebrosides have been obtained from brain and nerves which are differentiated from each other by the presence of other fatty acids they possess. Such fatty acids are cerebronic acid, lignoceric acid, nervonic acid, and oxynervonic acid.

These are found in large amounts in the white matter of brain and in the myelin sheaths of nerves. In smaller quantities, they appear to be very widely distributed in animal tissues. **Large**

amounts of the cerebrosides accumulate in the liver and spleen in Gaucher's disease- a rare hereditary disease of lipid metabolism. This disease was for the first time noticed by the scientist Gaucher in a patient in whom the splenic pulp was replaced entirely by large pale cells, which now are known after his name as "Gaucher Cells". These cells are found particularly in spleen, brain, and bone marrow.

(B) Gangliosides. These arc related to the cerebrosides and contain sphingosine, long-chain fatty acids, hexoses (usually galactose or glucose) and neuraminic acid (sialic acid). These are rich in carbohydrates. Brain gangliosides are known to be complex one.

Gangliosides have been isolated from nerve cells, spleen and red blood cell stroma. Large amounts of it are found in the brain in cases of Tay-Sachs disease and Niemann-Pick disease (diseases of lipid metabolism).

(C) Cytolipins. These lipids contain fatty acids, sphingosine, glucose and galactose.

3. Sulpholipids

Lipid material containing sulphur has long been known to be present in the tissues, examples being liver, kidney, brain, salivary glands, testicles, tumours etc. It's most abundantly found to be present in the white matter of the brain. In composition, these are similar to the cerebrosides except for the fact that sulphuric acid is present as cerebronic acid ester.

4. Lipoproteins

These compounds found in mammalian plasma are composed of lipid material bound to the proteins. The lipid moiety consists mainly of cholesterol esters and phospholipids containing principally stearic, palmitic and oleic acids although palmitoleic, linoleic and arachidonic acids have also been identified.

A number of proteins in serum are called lipoproteins because their function is to transport lipids; without them, the lipids could not exist in a dissolved state in the blood. The four major classes of lipoproteins are chylomicrons, pre-beta lipoproteins, beta lipoproteins and alpha lipoproteins. This classification is based on paper electrophoresis, which separates the lipoproteins into these four groups. They can also be separated by ultracentrifugation, and, although basically same groups are observed, different names are applied. These alternate names as well as the lipid content of the lipoprotein fractions are summarised in the following Table 6.4 (Also consult chapter on lipid metabolism).

Table 6.4: Lipoproteins

Category based on paper electrophoresis	Category based on ultracentrifugation	Major lipid component
Chylomicrons	Chylomicrons	Triglycerides
Pre-beta lipo-proteins	Very low density lipoproteins (VLDL)	Triglycerides
Beta lipoproteins	Low density lipoproteins (LDL)	Cholesterol
Alpha lipoproteins	High density lipoproteins (HDL)	Phospholipid

Lipoproteins not only are named but also measured in terms of the separation provided by electrophoresis or ultracentrifugation. These measurements are carried out principally in cases of increased concentrations of blood lipids (hyperlipidemia), which, of course, mean that the lipoprotein concentrations also must be increased (hyperlipoproteinemia) since they involve the same lipids. Various combinations of lipoproteins can be increased in these disorders; correlation of hyperlipidemia; hyperlipoproteinemia and clinical disorders is under intensive study these days, but no universally acceptable explanation is available so far.

Hyperlipidemia currently is receiving considerable attention of the scientists because it has been positively correlated with atherosclerotic cardiovascular disease, which has a high mortality and morbidity rate.

Derived lipids

Derived lipids are substances formed during the hydrolysis of simple or compound lipids which still retain the properties of this class of compound.

1. **Fatty Acids:** Saturated and unsaturated acids

2. **Alcohols:** Compounds of high molecular weight but not glycerol. These may be classified as follows:

   (A) **Aliphatic alcohols** such as cetyl, stearyl and myricyl alcohols.

   (B) **Sterols** which contain the phenanthrene nucleus (cholesterol, ergosterol, sitosterol and stigmasterol).

Steroids

A large number of compounds found in nature belong to the class of compounds known as steroids. These have the parent nucleus named as perhydrocyclopentanophenanthrene, which consists of three six-membered rings (A, B and C) and a five membered ring (D) which is known as a cyclopentane ring. These rings are joined together as shown in Fig. 6.1 with a total of 17 carbon atoms.

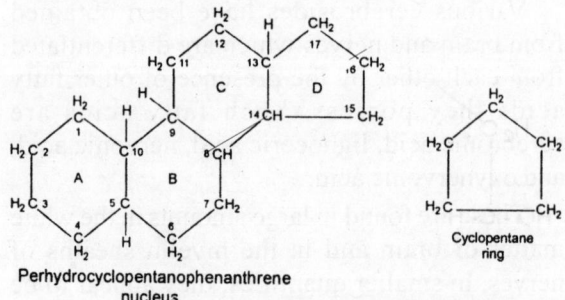

Perhydrocyclopentanophenanthrene nucleus

Cyclopentane ring

Fig. 6.1 : Structures of perhydrocyclopentanophenanthrene and cyclopentane ring

Steroids may be classified in the following categories:

(a) Sterols

(b) Bile acids

(c) Male sex hormones

(d) Female sex hormones

(e) Adrenal corticosteroids

(f) Vitamins D

(g) Saponins

(h) Cardiac glycosides

Sterols

The best known of the sterols is cholesterol. In the animal kingdom, the most abundant steroid is the sterol called as cholesterol. It remains present in all animal cells and is particularly abundant in nervous tissue. It is not found in vegetables and plant tissues. Because of its abundance, its historical interest, structure and clinical importance to man will be considered in some detail over here.

As early as 1815, **Chevreul** gave the name cholesterine to a white waxy material that could be isolated **from gallstones.** It was later identified as an alcohol stable to boiling with strong alkali. Fatty acid esters of the alcohol were also isolated from certain tissues.

Cholesterol, literally means bile solid-alcohol; derives its name from the fact that it was first isolated from human gallstones, of which it is generally the chief component. The amount of cholesterol in animal tissues varies widely. It is particularly abundant in brain, nerve tissue, adrenal glands and egg yolk. Dry white matter of brain contains about 14 per cent of cholesterol, and spinal cord 10-15 per cent. Scientist Bloor, an authority on lipids gives the percentage values (Table 6.5) for the average cholesterol content of dry tissues.

Cholesterol is usually accompanied by dihydrocholesterol and 7-dehydrocholesterol. It has the structure as shown in Fig. 6.2.

Cholesterol generally crystallizes as white, shining rhombic plates. It melts at 149°-150°C. It is tasteless and odourless. It is insoluble in water, acids and alkalies, somewhat soluble in soap solutions and much more soluble in the solution of bile salts. It is readily soluble in ether, benzene, chloroform, petroleum ether, carbon bisulfide and acetone. It is also readily soluble in hot alcohol, but only slightly soluble in cold alcohol. It dissolves readily in oleic acid and liquid

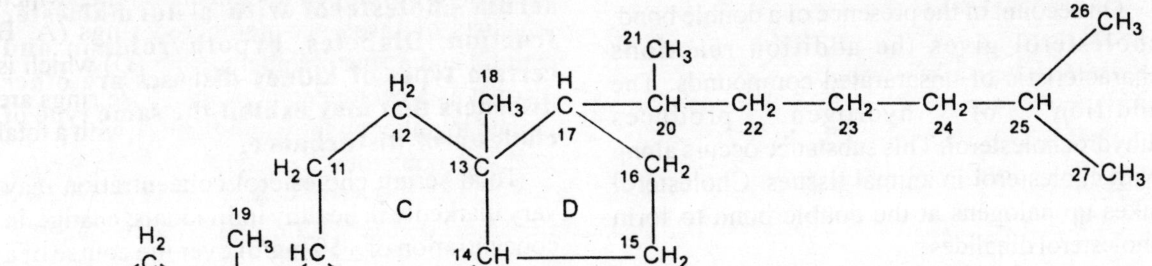

$$C_{27}H_{45}OH$$

Fig. 6.2 : Structure of cholesterol

Table 6.5 : Percentage of cholesterol in dry tissues

Sl.No.	Tissue	%
1.	White matter of brain	14.00
2.	Gray matter of brain	6.00
3.	Kidney	1.60
4.	Spleen	1.50
5.	Skin	1.30
6.	Liver	0.93
7.	Mammary glands	0.70
8.	Whole blood	0.65
9.	Smooth muscle	0.55
10.	Diaphragm	0.35
11.	Skeletal muscle	0.25

fats. It is commercially produced from the spinal cords of the cattle. It may be readily prepared in the laboratory by extraction from gallstones or brain tissue with the help of organic solvents.

Since cholesterol is a poor conductor of electricity and has a high dielectric value, it's a good insulator against electric discharge. Possibly, as an abundant constituent of brain, nerves and spinal cord, it functions as an insulating covering of impulse generating and transmitting structures. It is well established that brain and nerve impulses are electrical in character.

On account of the presence of a double bond, cholesterol gives the addition reactions characteristic of unsaturated compounds. The addition of hydrogen produces dihydrocholesterol. This substance occurs along with cholesterol in animal tissues. Cholesterol takes up halogens at the double bond to form cholesterol dihalides.

Upon oxidation, it gives various ketones, hydroxy compounds and acids, the products depending upon the oxidizing agents and conditions used.

Cholesterol is the best known and most widely determined lipid and is an important intermediate in the synthesis of steroid hormones. In the blood it occurs both in the free and esterified forms. The latter form is a mixture of many cholesterol esters, each of which has a different fatty acid bound in ester linkage to cholesterol at the OH group. Usually, only the total cholesterol concentration is of clinical interest but occasionally separate estimation of the free and esterified forms is of value to the clinicians. The normal range of cholesterol esters is between 70 and 75% of the total with free cholesterol making up the remaining 25 to 30%. **The normal range of the concentration of cholesterol in the serum is from 150 to 200 mg/dl. In normal infants and children lower values of cholesterol are found in the serum whereas higher values are found in normal older persons. The concentration of total cholesterol gets elevated in several diseases like nephrosis, diabetes mellitus, and hypothyroidism. Low values may be found in hyperthyroidism, malnutrition, Gaucher's disease and acute hepatitis.** However, the increase usually is not clinically diagnostic of these diseases. In some diseases, total cholesterol concentration is affected, while in others only the ester fraction is disturbed. **Jaundice of obstructive type usually is accompanied by an elevated level of total serum cholesterol with a normal ester fraction. Diabetes, hypothyroidism and certain types of kidney diseases are other disorders that may exhibit the same type of cholesterol disturbance.**

Total serum cholesterol concentration may vary markedly in healthy individuals; change in concentration of ± 50 mg/dl over the course of a few hours have been noted.

Since, the liver cells esterify cholesterol, infectious hepatitis cirrhosis and most types of liver damage are accompanied by a decreased percentage of cholesterol esters. Only the ester percentage is significant, not the absolute ester concentration.

In the recent years, interest in lipid metabolism has increased tremendously, primarily as a result of possible relationship between lipid metabolism and atherosclerosis.

Other Animal Sterols: A number of sterols closely related to cholesterol are found in various tissues. 7-dehydrocholesterol is a precursor of vitamin D_3. **Skin is a good source of both Δ^7- cholesterol (lathosterol) and 7 - dehydrocholesterol.** Desmosterol (24-dehydrocholesterol) and several methyl derivatives such as lanosterol and agnosterol have been isolated from skin lipids and are recognised as intermediates in cholesterol biosynthesis. Lanosterol and agnosterol are also present in wool lipids. Their structures are as given over here:

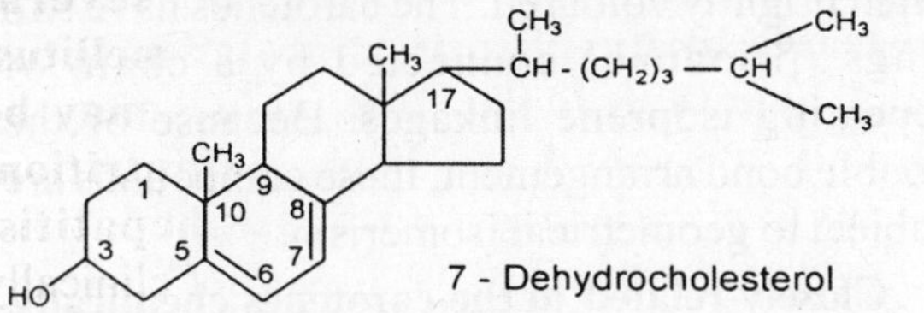

7 - Dehydrocholesterol

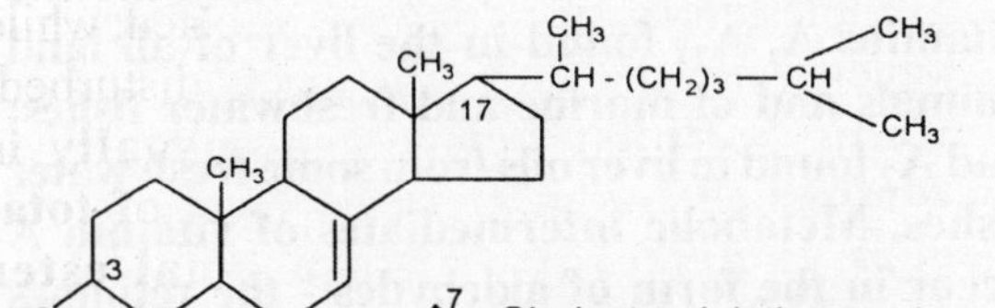

Δ^7 - Cholesterol, lathosterol

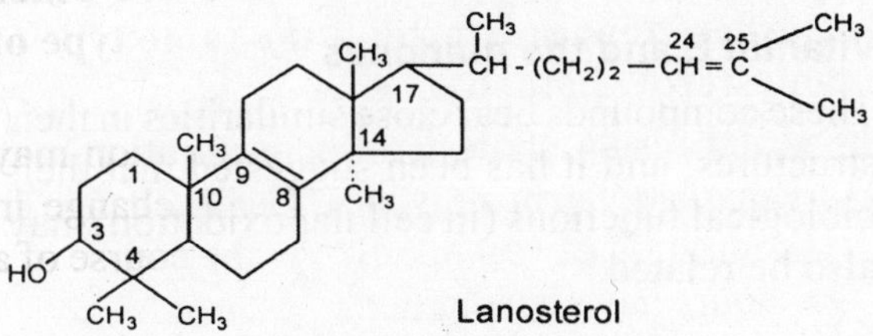

Lanosterol

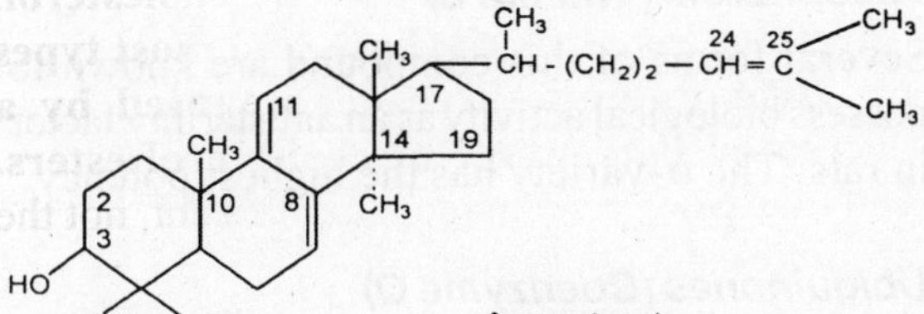

Agnosterol

Bile Acids

Human bile contains three different bile acids cholic, deoxycholic, and chenodeoxycholic acids.

Deoxycholic acid is microbial in origin and is absorbed from intestinal contents. The bile acids are present largely as derivatives of glycine and taurine. The bile acids differ from the sterols because of the *trans* relationship of its OH group at the 3- carbon to the angular CH_3 group. Structures of some of the bile acids are as given in Fig. 6.3.

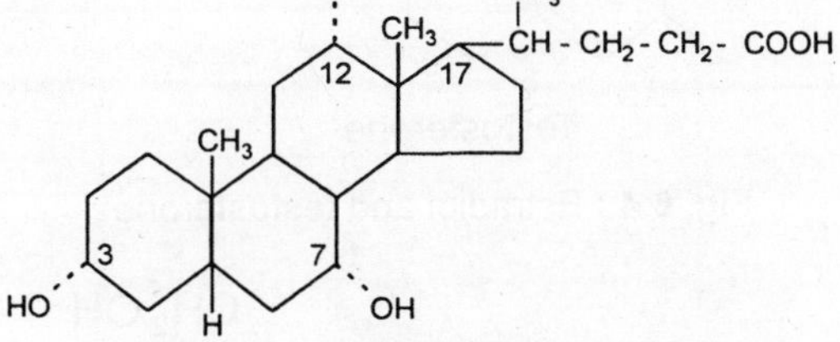

Cholic acid
3,7,12 - Trihydroxycholanic acid

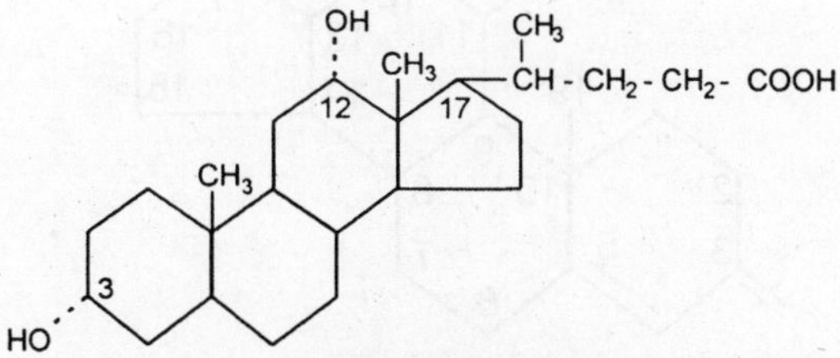

Deoxycholic acid
3,12 - Dihydroxycholanic acid

Fig. 6.3 : Cholic and deoxycholic acids

Sex hormones

The principal hormone of the ovary is estradiol and that of the testis is testosterone. Their structures are as shown in Fig 6.4.

Adrenal corticosteroids

The adrenal cortex synthesizes a number of steroids of metabolic importance. One of the very important of these is corticosterone (Fig 6.5).

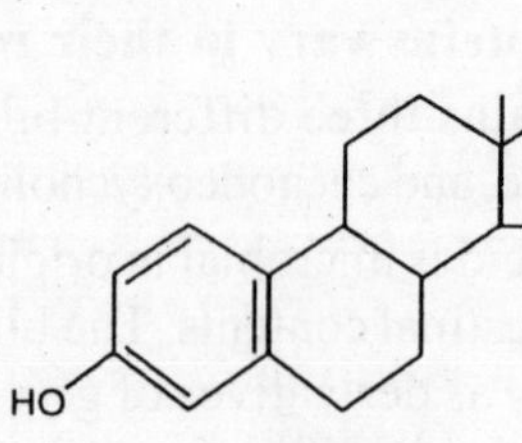

Estradiol

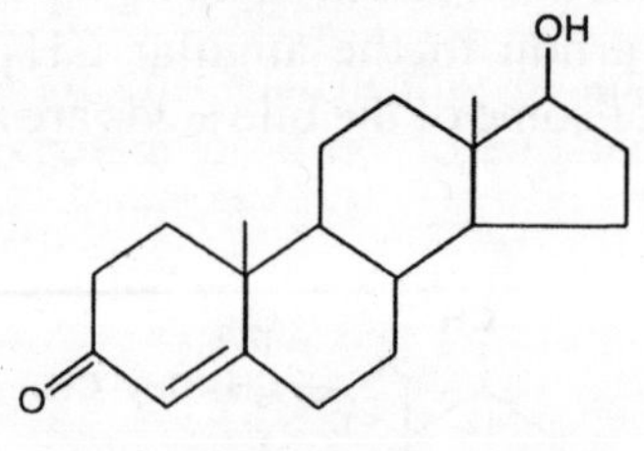

Testosterone

Fig. 6.4 : Estradiol and testosterone

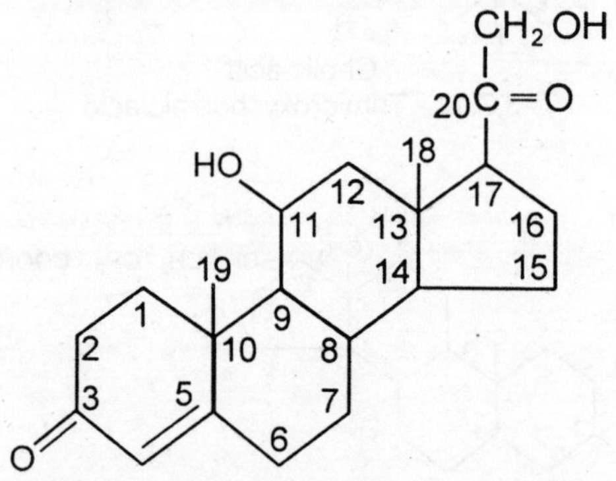

Fig. 6.5 : Structure of corticosterone

Vitamin D

Irradiation with ultraviolet light converts a number of sterols to compounds with vitamin D activity.

Saponins

Digitonin (Fig. 6.6) is a plant glycoside of a steroid-digitogenin in which the sugar residues are attached to the OH group at the 3-carbon. Digitonin (Fig. 6.6) forms insoluble addition compounds with sterols such as cholesterol.

Cardiac glycosides

These compounds have therapeutic applications.

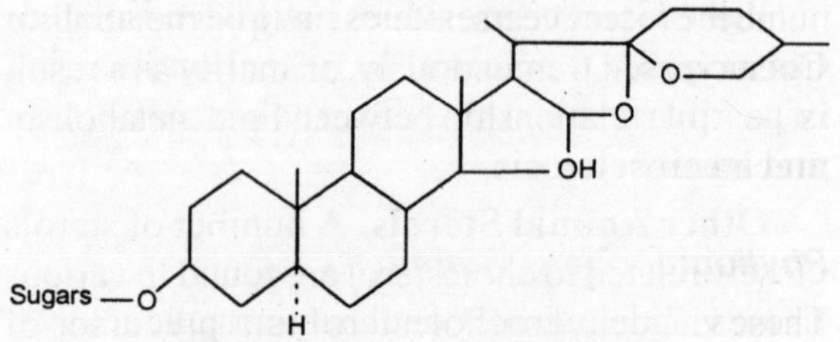

Fig. 6.6 : Structure of digitonin

Strophanthin is a glycoside of the steroid strophanthidin.

Carotenoids and Vitamin A

Carotenoids are isoprenoid hydrocarbons of plant origin containing 40 carbon atoms. Because carotenoids have a system of conjugated double bonds, they show strong light absorption and are often brightly coloured. The carotenes have two rings (β-ionone) connected by a chain of repeating isoprene linkages. Because of the double bond arrangement, these compounds are subject to geometrical isomerism.

Closely related to the carotenes chemically, and derived from them biochemically, are the vitamins A, A_1, found in the liver of all land animals and of marine and freshwater fishes; and A_2 found in liver oils from some fresh water fishes. Metabolic intermediates of vitamin A occur in the form of aldehydes - the retinines (for details, consult chapter on vitamins).

Vitamin E and the quinones

These compounds bear close similarities in their structures, and it has been suggested that their biological functions (in cellular oxidation) may also be related.

Tocopherols (Vitamin E)

Several forms of this compound are known to possess biological activity as an antisterility factor in rats. The α-variety has the highest potency.

Ubiquinones (Coenzyme Q)

A group of related quinones with variable

number of isoprene residues have been isolated. **Coenzyme 'Q' is found in mitochondria and is a part of the electron transport mechanism.**

Phylloquinones (Vitamin K)

These vitamins display antihaemorrhagic activity.

Plastoquinone

This quinone is found in the chloroplasts and is not found in the animal kingdom.

Lipoproteins

As is evident from the name itself, lipoproteins are the mixtures of lipids and proteins (lipoproteins = lipids + proteins). They are complex molecules and are found in blood.

Lipoproteins may be said as the large assemblies of lipid and protein. Different classes of lipoproteins vary in their relative content of lipid. They also have a wide range of density. They possess different size. They can be separated from each other either by electrophoresis or centrifugation in solutions of appropriate density which is the basis of their classification (Table 6.6) as shown over here :

An important enzyme in plasma is *lipoprotein lipase,* which hydrolyzes triacylglycerols and has the effect of reducing chylomicrons and VLDL to smaller fragments i.e fatty acids and glycerol. This enzyme is called as a *'clearing factor'* as after a fatty meal it has a tendency to clear the milky appearance of plasma that is due to the large quantities of chylomicrons being absorbed from the intestine.

Lipoprotein lipase is activated by apoprotein C_{11}.

Table 6.6 : Classification of lipoproteins

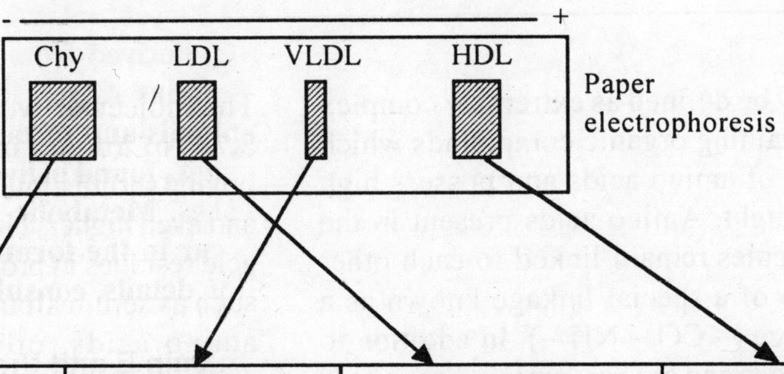

Name	Chylomicrons	Very low density lipoprotein (VLDL) or Pre-β-lipoprotein	Low density lipoprotein (LDL) or β-lipoprotein	High density lipoprotein (HDL) or α-lipoprotein
Site of synthesis	Intestine	Intestine and liver	In blood (and liver)* from VLDL	Liver
Size	Very large (1000-10,000 Å)	Large (300- 700 Å)	Smaller (150 - 250 Å)	Smallest (75 - 100 Å)
Density	0.94 g/ml	0.94-1.006 g/ml	1.006-1.063 g/ml	1.063-1.21 g/ml
Composition	Wt%			
(a) Protein	1	10	20	50
(b) Phospholipid	4	19	24	30
(c) Cholesterol	6	19	45	18
(d) Triglyceride	90	50	10	5

* It is not yet clear whether all β-lipoprotein is formed from VLDL in blood or whether some may be directly synthesized in the liver.

represise Theme mitochondrial Terminal
enzyme C is found in most eukaryotic
is a part of the electron transport
mechanism

CHAPTER **7**

CHEMISTRY OF AMINO ACIDS, PROTEINS AND IMMUNOGLOBULINS

We are very complex substances having large molecular weights and are expensive of all the foodstuffs and found in innumerable eatables. We have the wonderful unimaginable properties like involvement in (i) blood clotting (ii) hereditary transmission (iii) transport of O_2 and CO_2 (iv) defence (antibodies) mechanisms (v) enzymes (vi) cementing substances (vii) buffers and many more.

There will come no end in our inventions and our contribution in various physiological/ biochemical/ metabolic processes is everlasting.

Proteins may be defined as extremely complex nitrogen containing organic compounds which are polymers of amino acids and possess high molecular weight. Amino acids present in the protein molecules remain linked to each other with the help of a special linkage known as a peptide linkage (– CO – NH –). In addition to carbon, hydrogen and oxygen, proteins invariably contain nitrogen and generally sulphur also. **Besides, proteins have also been found to contain phosphorus, iron, copper, iodine, manganese, zinc and other elements.**

Consequently, there is a great variety and range of proteins according to their composition, size and shape. They are of utmost importance in biological processes; although some have a purely structural function; however the majority not only plays a static role in living tissues but a very dynamic role. Such proteins include the **enzymes.**

The molecular weight of proteins ranges from **5,734 of human insulin** through the 60, 000 of bovine serum albumin to the 6,00,000 of myosin and even higher. The proportion of various amino acid residues in proteins vary considerably; some such as serum albumin contains all the common amino acids, others for e.g. insulin lacks methionine, tryptophan and cysteine. **Collagen,** the protein of connective tissue contains 33% glycine residues and 12% each of alanine and proline with very low proportion of the other amino acids.

Proteins may be highly insoluble, such as **keratins** of hair and nails or highly soluble such as albumins of the blood plasma.

Chemistry of amino acids

Normally occurring amino acids are those amino acids which contain (i) amino group and (ii) carboxyl group in the carbon atom and are represented by the following general formula:

$$\begin{array}{c} COOH \\ |\alpha \\ R - C - NH_2 \\ | \\ H \end{array}$$

α - amino acid

All amino acids (structures as given ahead) found in living systems i.e. plant and animal proteins are L -α - amino acids (derived from L-glyceraldehyde). In nature, glycine is the only amino acid which is optically inactive and cannot be resolved into D - or L - form because of symmetry on the α - carbon atom. Rest amino acids are optically active.

The configuration of L - α - amino acid is as follows :

$$\begin{array}{c} COOH \\ |\alpha \\ NH_2 - C - H \\ | \\ R \end{array}$$

L- amino acid

Classification of the amino acids

Amino acids have been classified in many ways. They can either be classified according to the presence of (a) acidic, basic, or neutral groups or due to the presence of (b) polar groups, non-polar groups, sulphur containing groups, aromatic groups, heterocyclic ring, branched chain, etc. in their structures.

It is as metioned ahead in Table 7.1

1. Aliphatic amino acids.

Table 7.1 : Classification of amino acids

Amino acids
- Aliphatic amino acids
  - Neutral
    - Hydrocarbon side chain, e.g. glycine, valine, alanine, leucine, and isoleucine
    - Sulphur containing amino acids e.g. cysteine, and methionine
    - Hydroxyl containing, e.g., serine, and threonine
  - Acidic, e.g. aspartic acid, and glutamic acid
  - Basic, e.g. arginine, and lysine
- Aromatic amino acids, e.g. phenylalanine, and tyrosine
- Heterocyclic amino acids, e.g. proline, hydroxy-proline, histidine, and tryptophan

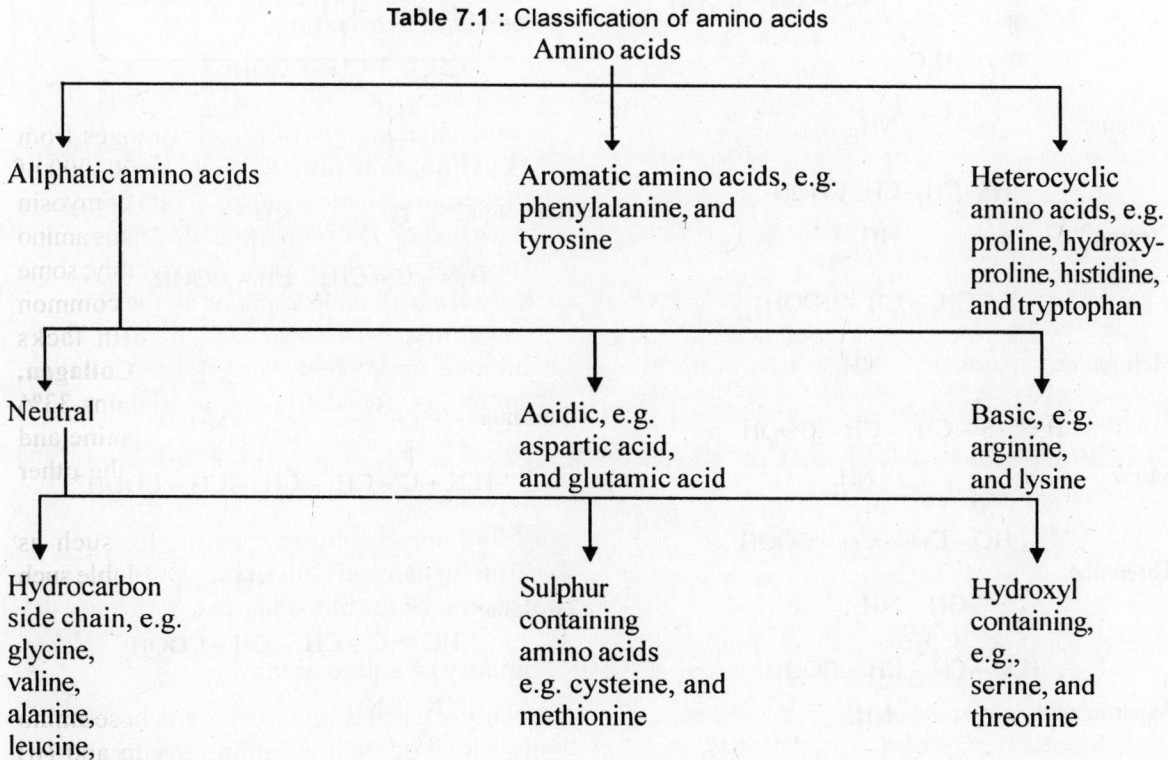

Glycine

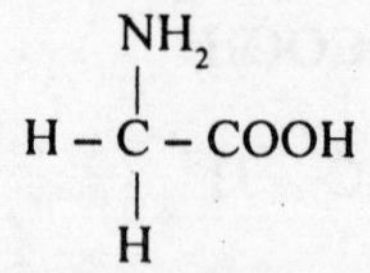

$$H - \underset{\underset{H}{|}}{\overset{\overset{NH_2}{|}}{C}} - COOH$$

Alanine

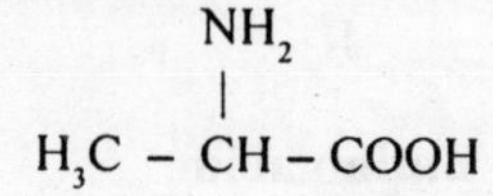

$$H_3C - \underset{\underset{}{|}}{\overset{\overset{NH_2}{|}}{CH}} - COOH$$

Valine

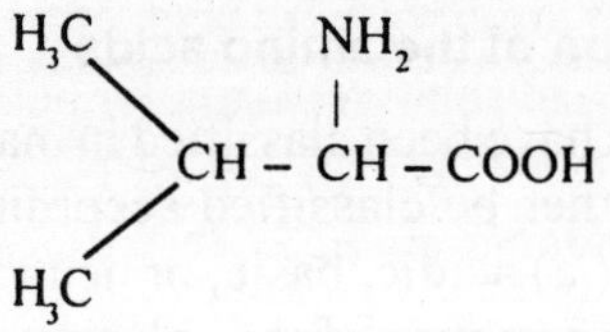

$$\underset{H_3C}{\overset{H_3C}{>}} CH - \underset{}{\overset{\overset{NH_2}{|}}{CH}} - COOH$$

Leucine

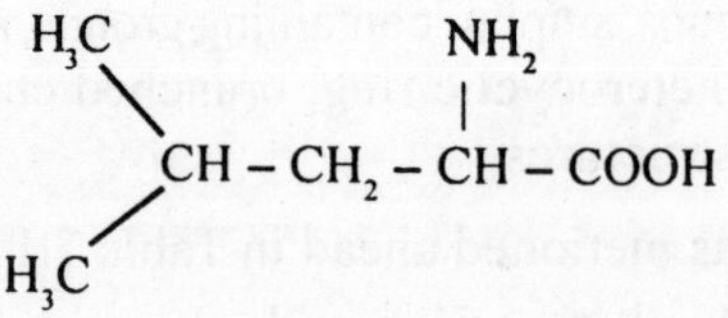

$$\underset{H_3C}{\overset{H_3C}{>}} CH - CH_2 - \overset{\overset{NH_2}{|}}{CH} - COOH$$

Isoleucine

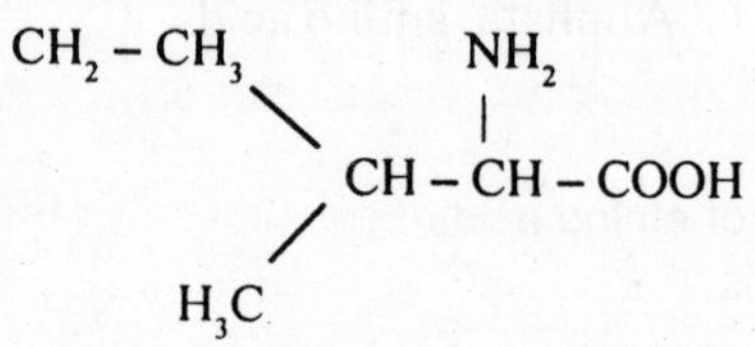

$$\underset{H_3C}{\overset{CH_2 - CH_3}{>}} CH - \overset{\overset{NH_2}{|}}{CH} - COOH$$

Cysteine

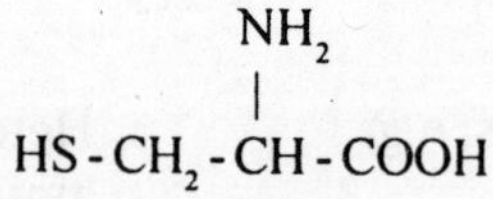

$$HS - CH_2 - \overset{\overset{NH_2}{|}}{CH} - COOH$$

Cystine

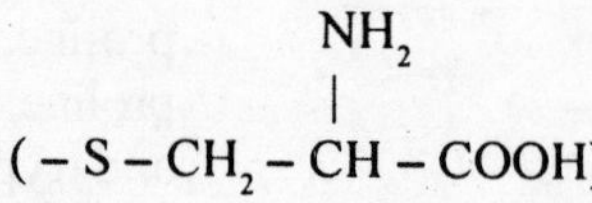

$$(- S - CH_2 - \overset{\overset{NH_2}{|}}{CH} - COOH)_2$$

Methionine

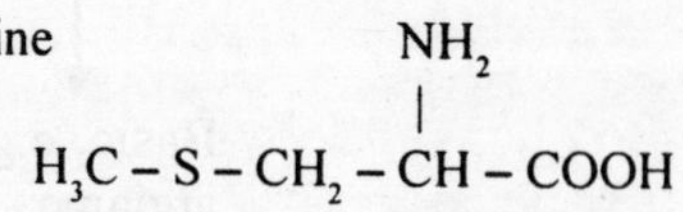

$$H_3C - S - CH_2 - \overset{\overset{NH_2}{|}}{CH} - COOH$$

Serine

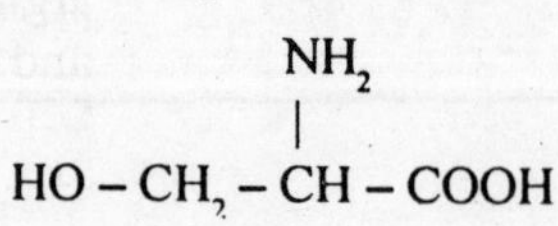

$$HO - CH_2 - \overset{\overset{NH_2}{|}}{CH} - COOH$$

Threonine

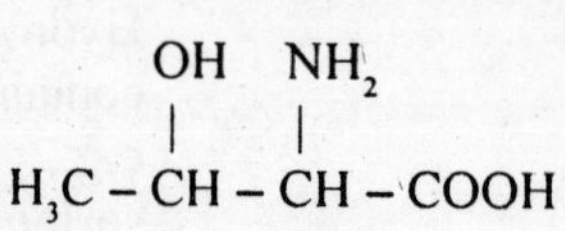

$$H_3C - \overset{\overset{OH}{|}}{CH} - \overset{\overset{NH_2}{|}}{CH} - COOH$$

Aspartic acid

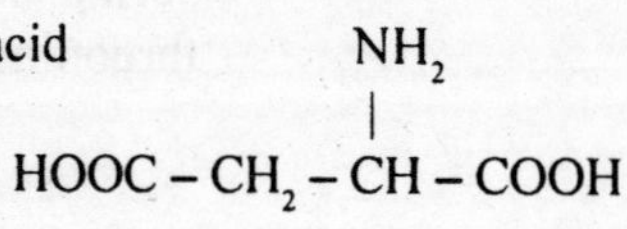

$$HOOC - CH_2 - \overset{\overset{NH_2}{|}}{CH} - COOH$$

Glutamic acid

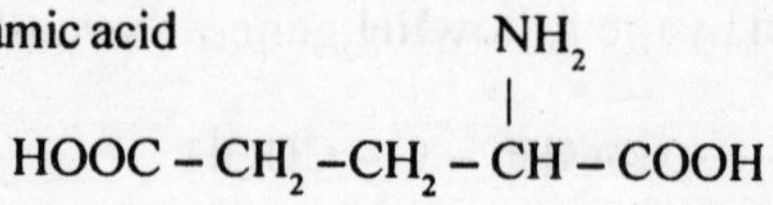

$$HOOC - CH_2 - CH_2 - \overset{\overset{NH_2}{|}}{CH} - COOH$$

Arginine

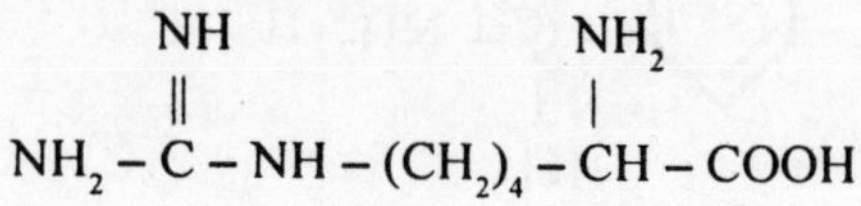

$$NH_2 - \overset{\overset{NH}{||}}{C} - NH - (CH_2)_4 - \overset{\overset{NH_2}{|}}{CH} - COOH$$

Lysine

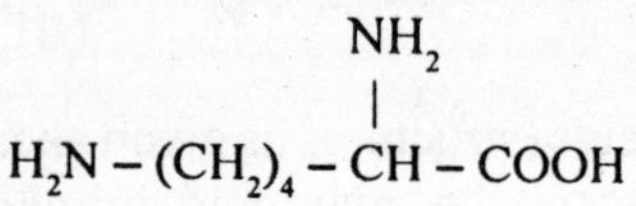

$$H_2N - (CH_2)_4 - \overset{\overset{NH_2}{|}}{CH} - COOH$$

Phenylalanine

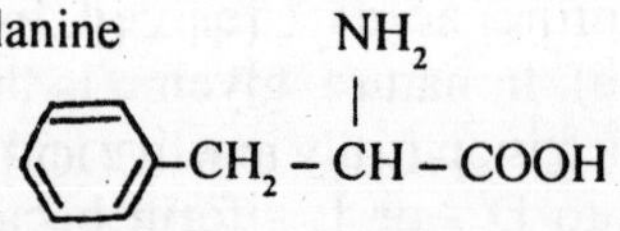

$$\bigcirc - CH_2 - \overset{\overset{NH_2}{|}}{CH} - COOH$$

Tyrosine

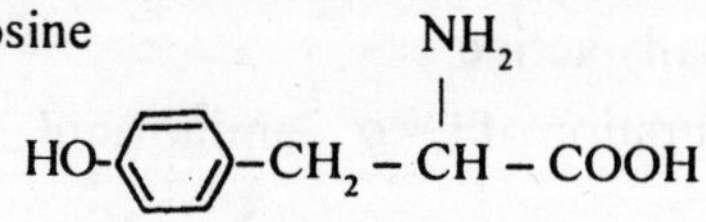

$$HO - \bigcirc - CH_2 - \overset{\overset{NH_2}{|}}{CH} - COOH$$

Proline

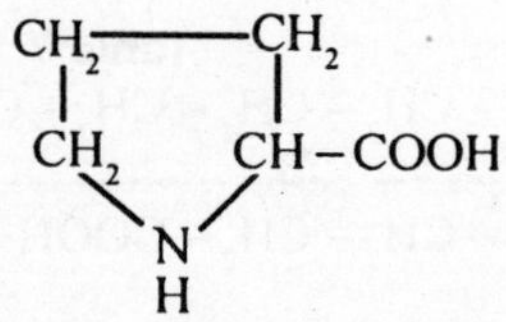

$$\begin{array}{c} CH_2 - CH_2 \\ | \quad\quad | \\ CH_2 \quad CH - COOH \\ \backslash \quad / \\ N \\ | \\ H \end{array}$$

Asparagine

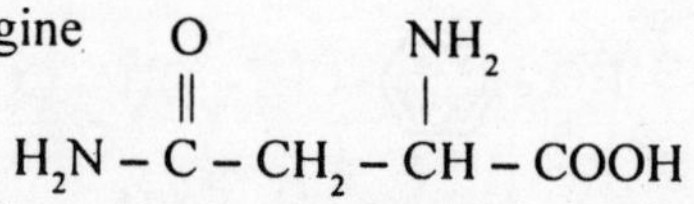

$$H_2N - \overset{\overset{O}{||}}{C} - CH_2 - \overset{\overset{NH_2}{|}}{CH} - COOH$$

Glutamine

$$H_2N - \overset{\overset{O}{||}}{C} - CH_2 - CH_2 - \overset{\overset{NH_2}{||}}{CH} - COOH$$

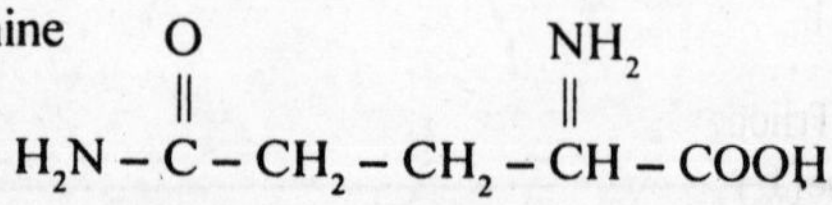

Histidine

$$\begin{array}{c} \quad\quad\quad NH_2 \\ \quad\quad\quad | \\ HC = C - CH_2 - CH - COOH \\ |\quad\quad | \\ N \quad NH \\ \backslash \quad / \\ C \\ | \\ H \end{array}$$

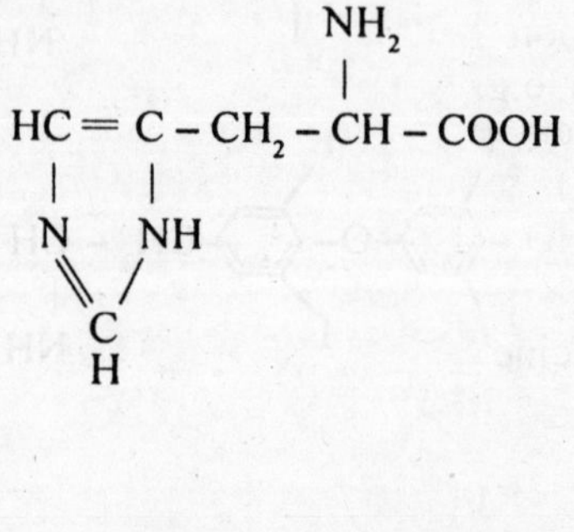

Tryptophan

$$\text{Ar} - C - CH_2 - \underset{H}{\overset{NH_2}{C}} - COOH$$

$$\underset{\underset{N}{|}}{\overset{||}{CH}}$$
$$\underset{H}{}$$

Ornithine

$$H_2N - CH_2 - CH_2 - CH - H - COOH$$
$$\overset{NH_2}{\underset{|}{C}}$$

Cirtulline

$$CH_2 - CH_2 - CH_2 - CH - COOH$$
$$\underset{NH}{|} \qquad \underset{NH_2}{|}$$
$$\underset{C=O}{|}$$
$$\underset{NH_2}{|}$$

γ - Amino butyric acid (GABA)

$$H_2N - CH_2 - CH_2 - CH_2 - COOH$$

β - Alanine

$$H_2N - CH_2 - CH_2 - COOH$$

3-Monoiodotyrosine

$$HO - \overset{3\ 2}{\underset{5\ \gamma}{\bigcirc}} - CH_2 - \underset{|}{\overset{NH_2}{CH}} - COOH$$

3,5-Diiodotyrosine

$$HO - \overset{3}{\underset{5}{\bigcirc}} - CH_2 - \underset{|}{\overset{NH_2}{CH}} - COOH$$

3,5, 3'- Triiodo-thyronine (T$_3$)

$$HO - \overset{3}{\underset{5}{\bigcirc}} - O - \overset{3'}{\underset{5'\ \gamma}{\bigcirc}} - CH_2 - \underset{|}{CH} - COOH$$
$$\underset{NH_2}{}$$

3,5,3',5'- Tetraiodo-thyronine (T$_4$)

$$HO - \overset{3}{\underset{5}{\bigcirc}} - O - \overset{3'}{\underset{5'}{\bigcirc}} - CH_2 - \underset{|}{CH} - COOH$$
$$\underset{NH_2}{}$$

2. Aromatic amino acids
3. Heterocyclic amino acids

Besides the regular 20 amino acids, there are number of special amino acids which are found in free or combined form but do not occur in protein molecules, these include triiodothyronine (T_3), tetraiodothyronine (T_4), ornithine, citrulline, β-alanine, γ- aminobutyric acid, etc.

Examples of relatively smaller peptides that possess biological activity include:

(i) glutathione,
(ii) oxytocin, and
(iii) vasopressin, etc.

Out of the above **glutathione is a tripeptide** which consists of glutamic acid, cystine and glycine in its structure and is found in RBCs. **Oxytocin and vasopressin are *octapeptides*** and are secreted by the posterior part of the pituitary gland, each is made up of 8 amino acids. *Oxytocin* **causes contraction of smooth muscles and is used in obstetrics to initiate labour whereas vasopressin increases blood pressure and reduces the formation of urine.**

Functions of of amino acids

Amino acids play very important role in human system and serve as :

(1) **Building blocks of proteins, and**
(2) **As precursors of:**
   (a) **hormones,**
   (b) **purines,**
   (c) **pyrimidines,**
   (d) **porphyrins,**
   (e) **vitamins, etc.**

Essential amino acids (EAA)

EAA are those amino acids which are not synthesized in the body and hence have to be provided in the diet. They are also termed as *indispensable* amino acids and are eight in number. To remember them, there is a formula known as M $\boxed{A}$ TTVIL Ph Ly in which A is silent; these are as follows:

(i) Leucine,

(ii) Isoleucine,

(iii) Valine

(iv) Methionine

(v) Tryptophan

(vi) Phenylalanine

(vii) Lysine, and

(viii) Threonine

Histidine is treated under the category of 'Essential' in case of infants, otherwise semiessential.

Sufficient amounts of EAA are required to maintain the proper nitrogen balance. Deficiency of one or more EAA in the diet affects the synthesis of proteins resulting failure in the growth of the child, negative nitrogen balance in the adults and fall in the levels of plasma proteins and haemoglobin.

Semiessential amino acids: Are those amino acids which are required half-heartedly by the body for proper growth and development, these include:

(i) Arginine

(ii) Tyrosine

(iii) Cystine

(iv) Glycine

(v) Serine and

(vi) Histidine

Non-essential Amino Acids

These are not required by the body but are synthesized by the body and include aspartic acid, glutamic acid, proline, hydroxyproline, etc. These are derived from the carbon skeletons of carbohydrates and lipids metabolism or from the transformation of essential amino acids.

Nitrogen Balance

The ratio of:

$\dfrac{\text{Intake of N}}{\text{Output of N}}$ = 1, i.e., nitrogen equilibrium. Normal adults are in nitrogen equilibrium.

> 1, i.e., Positive Nitrogen Balance, e.g., p r e g n a n c y, convulsions and growth.

< 1, i.e., Negative Nitrogen Balance, e.g., malnutrition and certain wasting diseases where there is tissue breakdown.

Ionic properties of Amino Acids:

The amphoteric (property of behaviour either as an acid or a base) properties of amino acids account for their separation of electrophoresis on paper at pH 6.0 (Fig. 7.1).

The amphoteric nature of α - amino acids determines that, in the absence of other acids or bases, the carboxyl and amino groups are both

```
COO⁻           CH₃            NH₃⁺
 |              |              |
CH₂            CH.NH₃⁺        (CH₂)₄
 |              |              |
CH.NH₃⁺        COO⁻           CH.NH₃⁺
 |             Alanine         |
COO⁻                          COO⁻
Aspartic                      Lysine
acid
```

$$
\begin{array}{ccc}
COO^- & CH_3 & NH_3^+ \\
| & | & | \\
CH_2 & CH.NH_3^+ & (CH_2)_4 \\
| & | & | \\
CH.NH_3^+ & COO^- & CH.NH_3^+ \\
| & \text{Alanine} & | \\
COO^- & & COO^- \\
\text{Aspartic acid} & & \text{Lysine}
\end{array}
$$

negatively charged   isoionic   positively charged

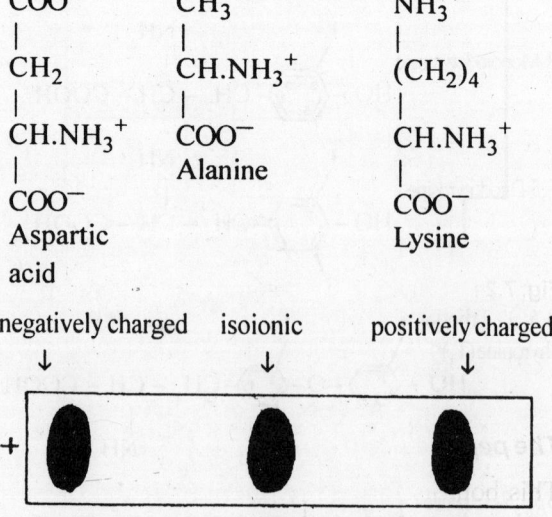

point of application of the mixture

Fig. 7.1 : To show pattern of electrophoresis

ionized fully to give rise to the term zwitterion (German zwitter = hybrid or hermaphrodite). This kind of nature may be understood as follows:

Separation of Amino acids by Ion-Exchange Chromatography (Fig 7.2)

In addition to permitting the separation of amino acids by electrophoresis, their ionic properties also permit their separation by ion-exchange chromatography. Ion-exchange is performed using a resin to which positively charged groups (anion-exchange resin) or negatively charged groups (cation-exchange resin) are covalently bound and thus immobilized. Ions passed down a column of such a resin bind competitively to the charged groups. Principle of ion-exchange chromatography has been shown as in (Fig. 7.2):

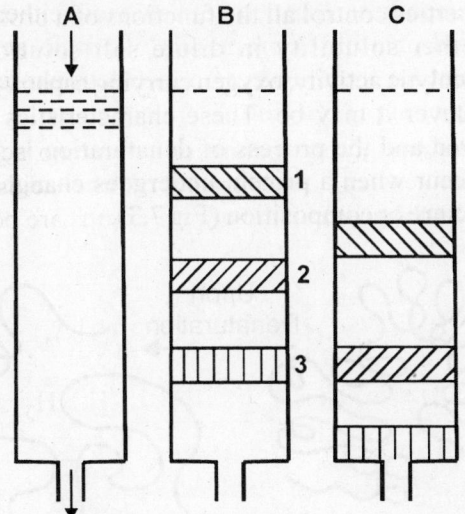

Fig. 7.2 : Principle of column chromatography. Material applied at top of column (A) gets separated into three components (B and C)

The peptide bond

This bond is formed by the interaction of two amino acids with the elimination of water between the NH_2 and COOH groups as shown below.

$$\left(\begin{array}{c} O \quad H \\ \parallel \quad | \\ -C-N- \end{array} \right)$$

The Biuret Reaction

Biuret has the formula $NH_2CONHCONH_2$, and is a simple substance containing a peptide bond. **When *Biuret* is treated with $CuSO_4$ in alkaline solution, a purple colour is produced. This is known as the *Biuret Reaction*. All proteins give a positive reaction.**

Isoelectric point

The isoelctric point is that pH at which the protein carries a net charge of zero because at this pH the sum of positive charge is equal to the sum of negative charge. That is why proteins do not migrate in an electric field. At this pH, amino acids (constituents of a protein molecule) exist in the zwitterion form. According to the isoelectric point, proteins are described as basic, neutral or acidic depending or whether their overall charge at physiological pH is positive, approximately zero, or negative. Isoelectric points of some common proteins are as follows:

Protein	Isoelectric point
Serum albumin	4.7
α_1, - Globulin	2.0
γ_2, - Globulin	5.8
Fibrinogen	5.8
Hemoglobin	7.2
Pepsin	1.0
Insulin	5.4
Cytochrome	9.8
Lysozyme	11.1

High Performance Liquid Chromatography (HPLC)

This is the most latest kind of chromatography

in which an instrument named as Bio-Rad protein Chromatography system is used. **By this technique, separation of a variety of peptides may be done, for example:**

   (i) Oxytocin

   (ii) Met-Enkephalin

   (iii) TRH

   (iv) α - Endorphin

   (v) α - MSH

   (vi) β - Endorphin

   (vii) Angiotensin II

   (viii) Substance P

   (ix) LHRH

   (x) Neurotensin, etc.

The technique depends upon the use of microfine column matrixes to give high resolution rapidly.

α_1 Antitrypsin (AT) and its role in Emphysema

The predominant component of the α_1 - globulin band consists of a protein named as α_1-antitrypsin (AT). It has been wrongly named because it is active against elastase rather than trypsin and is a member of a group of **Serine Proteinase Inhibitors or, Serpins.**

In normal young, the destructive power of enzyme elastase released from the neutrophils in checked by AT. **Cigarette smoking increases the number and activity of lung neutrophils and consequently the amount of enzyme elastase.** Moreover, oxidation reduces the protection afforded by a given amount of circulating AT.

α_1- antitrypsin is less active after oxidation; elastase then causes tissue breakdown and loss of elasticity in the lungs vis-a-vis emphysema. **It means that smoking leads to a tendency of emphysema.**

Proteins

Proteins may be defined as extremely complex nitrogen containing organic compounds which are polymers of amino acids and possess high molecular weight. Amino acids present in the protein molecules remain linked to each other with the help of a special linkage known as a peptide linkage $(- CO - NH -)$. In addition to carbon, hydrogen and oxygen, proteins invariably contain nitrogen and generally sulphur also.

Proteins have also been found to contain phosphorus, iron, copper, iodine, manganese, zinc and other elements.

Denaturation

A protein is said to be a native protein if its amino acid composition and stereochemical structures remain unchanged from the natural state. These properties control all the functions of a protein, whether solubility in dilute salt solutions, proteolytic activity, oxygen carrying capacity, or whatever it may be. These characteristics are altered and the process of denaturation is said to occur when a protein undergoes changes in structure or composition (Fig 7.3).

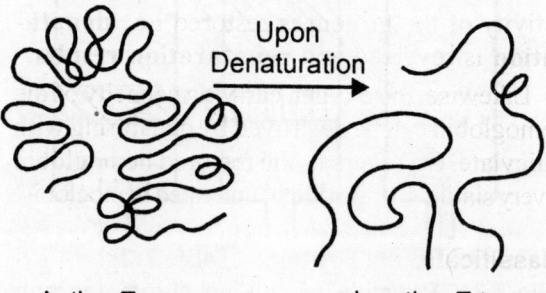

Active Enzyme   Inactive Enzyme

Fig. 7.3 : Representation of denaturation of protein

Chemical and physical agents that cause these changes are called denaturing agents. Their action involves the splitting of some or all the protein cross linkages with their possible reformation, in some cases, to cause a rearrangement of the peptide chains.

Denaturation may be caused by the following:

1. Heat
2. Mineral acids and alkalies
3. Shaking or stirring
4. Grinding
5. Ultraviolet radiations
6. Ultrasonic waves
7. Neutral Chemical agents, etc.

Renaturation

Denatured proteins may, however, under certain conditions, be restored to proteins with many of the properties of the original protein. This process is known as 'renaturation'. It appears, however, that renaturation seldom results in the complete restoration of the denatured protein to its original state.

Pepsin can be denatured and so loses its proteolytic properties if it is warmed to the proper temperature.

When the solution is cooled, the proteolytic activity of the protein is restored i.e., **denaturation** is reversed and **renaturation results.**

Likewise, the oxygen carrying capacity of the hemoglobin can be destroyed by denaturing with salicylate. On reversal, the restored hemoglobin is very similar to the original untreated hemoglobin.

Classification of Proteins (Table 7.2) :

Proteins have been classified on the basis of their composition as follows:

I Simple proteins

Simple proteins are made up of amino acids only and upon hydrolysis yield a mixture of amino acids only.

Examples

(A) **Fibrous (insoluble) proteins**	: Also called as **scleroproteins.** They impart a supporting or protective function in the animal. These are insoluble in water.
(a) Collagens	: Principal supporting proteins of skin, tendons and bones. They possess very large amount of hydroxyproline. They are **resistant to peptic and tryptic digestion.**
(b) Elastins	: Found in elastic tissues like tendons and arteries. **Readily digested by trypsin and pepsin.** It contains smaller amount of hydroxyproline.
(c) Keratins	: Found in animal skin, nails, horns, hoofs, hair, feathers, etc. They possess high cystine content.
(B) **Globular (soluble) proteins**	: Are soluble proteins with definite molecular weights. Each molecule contains one or more peptide chains, held in a coiled configuration by disulfide bridges and other bonds.
(a) Albumins	: Include ovalbumin from egg white, serum albumin from blood serum, and lactalbumin from milk. They are coagulable by heat

and soluble in pure water. They are precipitated from solution by **full saturation of ammonium sulphate.**

(b) Globulins : Include serum globulins, lactoglobulin from milk, thyroglobulin from thyroid gland. Also found in many plant seeds, e.g. edestin from hempseed. Are soluble in dilute salt solutions and are precipitated from solution by **half saturation of ammonium sulphate.** Coagulated by heat.

(c) Plant proteins (glutenins, prolamins) : Cereal proteins such as glutelins of wheat, orygenin of rice and zein of maize. Soluble in very weak acids or alkalies but insoluble in all neutral solvents.

(d) Protamines : They are simpler polypeptides. Uncoagulable by heat and possess strong basic properties. Rich in arginine. **Example is salmine from salmon sperms.**

(e) Histones : Are soluble in water but insoluble in dilute ammonia. Rich in arginine and lysine and possess strong

basic properties. Example scombrone from mackerel sperms.

(C) Denatured Proteins

When proteins are subjected to certain physical and chemical agents, they get denatured. In fact, they undergo intramolecular changes which cause changes in solubility and other properties. Soluble proteins for example albumins and globulins are converted by heat, ultraviolet light, mechanical agitation or long contact with alcohol, etc. into insoluble materials known as coagulated proteins. Such coagulated proteins are denatured one.

II Conjugated Proteins

Are those proteins which consist of protein combined with some non protein substance (the prosthetic group). They are classified according to the nature of the prosthetic group, as indicated below:

III Derived Proteins

Include those substances formed from simple and conjugated proteins. It is the least well defined of the protein groups. These are subdivided into primary derived proteins and secondary derived proteins.

1. Primary derived proteins : Slight change with little or no hydrolytic cleavage of peptide bonds.

(a) Proteans : Insoluble products, example fibrin from fibrinogen

(b) Metaproteins : Generally soluble in very dilute acids and alkalies but insoluble in neutral solvents. Examples are acid and alkali albumin-ates.

(c) Coagulated : Insoluble products formed by the action of heat or alcohol upon natural proteins. Examples are cooked egg albumin, cooked meat, etc.

2. Secondary derived: proteins

These are formed in the progressive hydrolytic cleavage of the peptide unions of proteins. They represent very complex molecules of different size and amino acid composition. They are roughly grouped into following three categories :

(a) **Proteoses**

(b) **Peptones**

(c) **Peptides**

Structure of Proteins

Proteins exhibit four levels of organization

1. **Primary structure**
2. **Secondary structure**
3. **Tertiary structure**
4. **Quaternary structure**

Primary Structure: It refers to the sequence of individual amino acids in the polypeptide chain or chains that comprise the protein and the location of disulfide bonds, if any.

– Ala – Gly – Gly – His – Leu –

Secondary Structure: It refers to the conformation of polypeptide chains. The term *conformation* refers to the relative positions of each of the constituent atoms of a molecule in the space (Fig. 7.4).

Globular proteins (example insulin) indicate a coiled structure in which peptide bonds are folded in a regular manner. The foldings are the results of linking of the carboxyl and amino groups of the peptide chains by means of hydrogen bonds and disulfide bonds. Such foldings are referred to as the secondary structure of the protein (Fig. 7.4).

Conjugated Protein = Protein part + prosthetic group

		Prosthetic group	*Example*
1.	Nucleoproteins	= Nucleic acid	Virus proteins
2.	Glycoproteins and Mucoproteins	= Carbohydrate or a derivative of carbohydrate	Mucin of saliva
3.	Phosphoproteins	= Phosphoric acid	Casein of milk, ovovitellin of egg yolk
4.	Chromoproteins	= Metalloporphyrin or some similar substance which absorbs visible light	Haemoglobin
5.	Metalloproteins	= Metals(copper, Mn, Mg, Zn, Mo, etc.)	Tyrosinase, arginase,anhydrase, xanthine oxidase, etc.
6.	Lipoproteins	= Lipids (cholesterol, phospholipids triglycerides, etc.)	Serum lipoproteins, lipoproteins of egg yolk

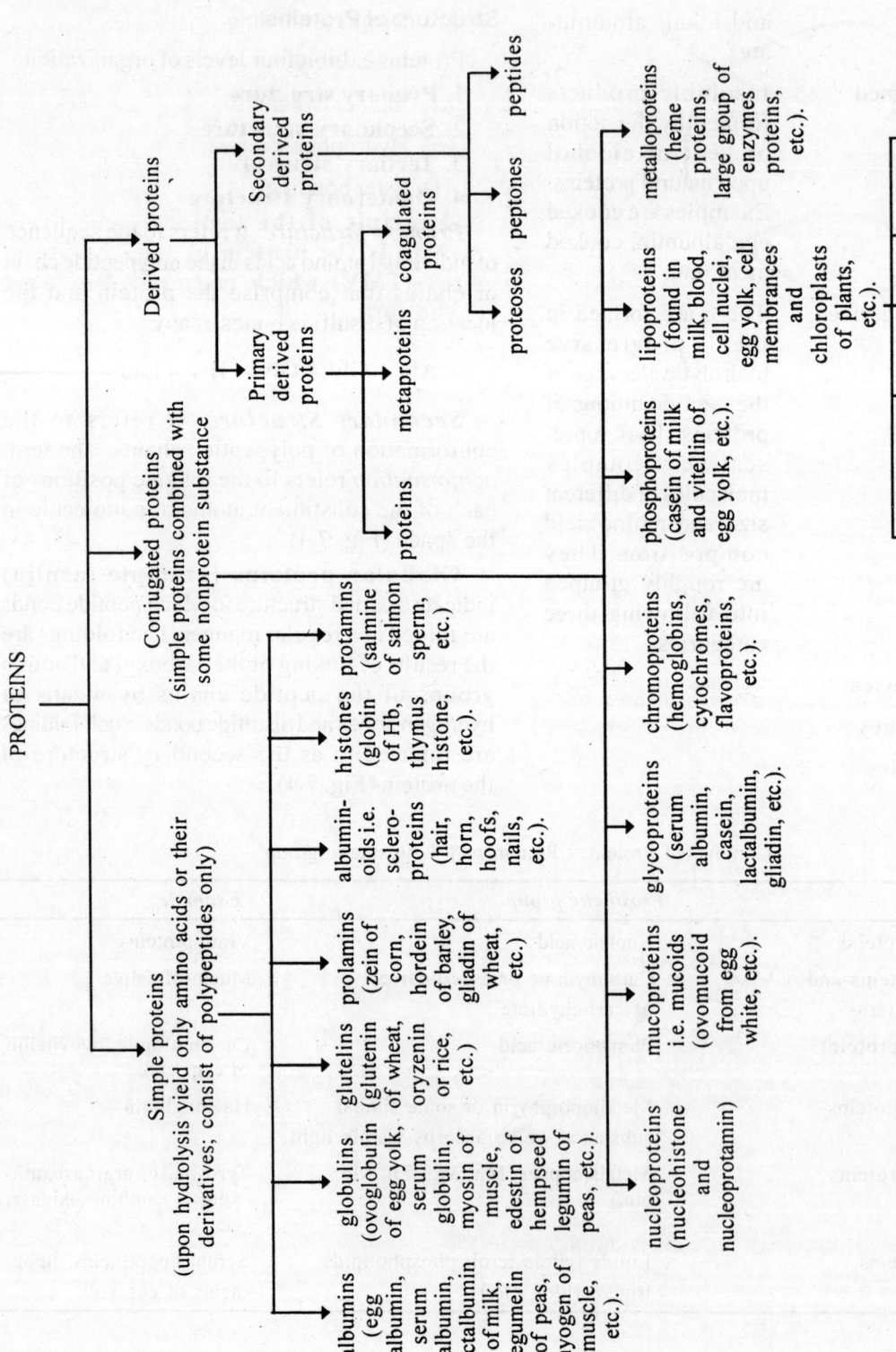

Table 7.2 : Classification of proteins

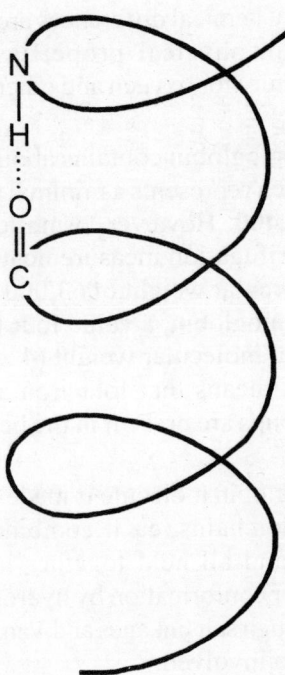

Fig. 7.4 : Secondary structure

Tertiary Structure: It refers to the coiling of several helical portions of single helix into a three dimensional structure (Fig. 7.5).

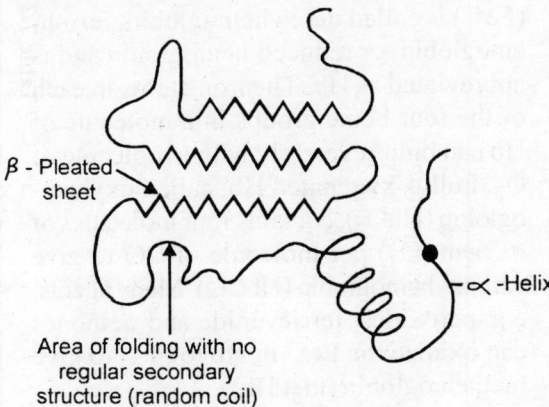

Fig 7.5 : Tertiary structure

The tertiary structure of proteins is stabilised and maintained by :

   (a) Hydrogen bonding

   (b) Disulfide bonding

   (c) Ionic interactions

   (d) Vander Waal's forces

   (e) Hydrophobic interactions

   (f) Ester bonding

Example of the tertiary structure of protein is the protein of tobacco mosaic virus (TMV) which resembles the kernel of the corn.

Quaternary Structure

Proteins containing more than one polypeptide chain display fourth level of structural organization called **quaternary structure**. In this type, the individual polypeptide chain is arranged in relation to each other so as to give a simple three dimensional structure on the overall protein molecule. Each polypeptide chain in such a protein is called a subunit. Depending upon the number of subunits present, such proteins are called as dimers, trimers, tetramers or polymers, etc. **Examples are haemoglobin, ferritin, etc.**

Biochemical functions/roles or biological importance of proteins

They play very important roles in the human body and are very essential substances. They play following important roles in the human body.

   1. Proteins may be said as the essence of life processes.

   2. All enzymes are made up of proteins.

   3. Many of the hormones are proteïnous in nature for example **insulin, glucagon, oxytocin, vasopressin, etc.**

   4. They serve as building block units for subcellular, cellular and organic structures.

   5. They act as defence against infections by way of protein antibodies.

   6. They are involved in blood clotting through

thrombin, fibrinogen and other protein factors.

7. Cementing substances and the reticulum which bind the cells as tissues/organs are partly made up of proteins.

8. They perform hereditary transmission by way of nucleoproteins found in the cell nucleus.

9. They act as buffers.

10. They help in the transport of oxygen and CO_2 by way of haemoglobin and certain special enzymes which are found in red blood cells.

Hemoglobins

The red colour of blood is caused by the hemoglobin content of the erythrocytes. There is about 12 to 17g hemoglobin/dl blood, depending upon the age and sex of the individual. Under normal conditions, all the hemoglobin of the blood remains present inside the erythrocytes. Hemoglobin is made in immature erythrocytes in the bone marrow and not during the 120 to 135 days life span of the erythrocyte in the circulation.

Centrifugation of a blood sample causes the cells to pack at the bottom of the centrifuge tube. These cells occupy about 40 to 47% of the blood volume; the percentage value of packed cells is called the *hematocrit*. Since the vast majority of these cells are erythrocytes, the hematocrit is a measure of the amount of erythro-cyte hemoglobin to the first approximation.

Hemoglobins are the respiratory proteins of vertebrate erythrocytes. These are formed by the conjugation of basic proteins globins with ferroheme (ferroprotoporphyrin).

The hemoglobins of the various species are different as shown by differences in crystal form. These differences are due to variations in the amino acids of the globin part of the molecule since the heme component is the same in all

hemoglobins. Chemical differences are exhibited by changes in physical properties such as solubility, affinity for oxygen and other characteristics.

Human hemoglobin contains about 0.34 per cent iron, which represents a minimal molecular weight of **16,400**. However, osmotic pressure and ultracentrifugation measurements indicate an actual molecular weight of 63,000 to 67,000 for human hemoglobin, a value four times that of the minimal molecular weight (4 x 16,400 = 65,600). This means that four iron atoms and four heme groups are present in the hemoglobin molecule.

The hemoglobin molecule is made up of four globin peptide chains, each combined with a heme group and all held together in definite arrangement or conformation by hydrogen bonds primarily, through salt linkages and Van der Waals forces are also involved.

Hemoglobins are composed of a colourless protein, globin, which remain combined noncovalently with heme.

Hemoglobin uncombined with oxygen and containing heme with ferrous iron, (Fe^{2+}) is called deoxyhemoglobin, ferrohemoglobin, or reduced hemoglobin and is abbreviated as Hb. The iron atoms in each of the four heme groups in a molecule of Hb can bind reversibly with a molecule of O_2. Fully oxygenated Hb, called oxyhemoglobin (HbO_2), contains four molecules of oxygen (O_2) per molecule of CO to give carboxyhemoglobin (HbCO). Many agents, e.g. peroxides, ferricyanide and quinones can oxidize the Fe^{2+} in Hb to Fe^{3+} to give methemoglobin (met Hb).

Four kinds of globin peptide chain, α, β, γ and δ have been found in various normal and abnormal hemoglobins. Amino acid sequences of the human α, β, and γ chains have been determined and the sequence of the δ chain partially determined. The sequences of α, β, and γ chains are shown in Figure 4.8. α chain contains 141 amino acid residues whereas the β, γ and δ chains contain 146. Numerous segments of the β and α chains have the same sequences.

Four kinds of structure are involved in the organization of the hemoglobin molecule (and of many other proteins). The primary structure is represented by the amino acid sequences of the various chains. Certain portions of the chains are formed into helices and other portions are not helical. This represents secondary structure and is determined by the amino acid sequence for each chain. The folding of each chain and the relations of the various portions of the chain to other portions represents the tertiary structure. The quaternary structure is represented by the organization and conformation of all four chains in complete hemoglobin molecule.

Normal and Abnormal Human Hemoglobins

The blood of a normal human adult contains two well established hemoglobins and apparently traces of others. The major hemoglobin may be designated as $\alpha_2\beta_2$, indicating two α and two β chains of the human, A, type (Fig 7.6). This hemoglobin is referred to as hemoglobin A and makes up 90-95 per cent of the total hemoglobin. Another hemoglobin making up 2-3 percent of the total hemoglobin is hemoglobin α_2, which is made up of two α and two δ chains, and which may be represented by $\alpha_2\delta_2$.

The umbilical cord blood of a newborn infant contains so-called foetal hemogloblin, hemoglobin F, which is made up of two α and two γ chains and which is designated as $\alpha_2\gamma_2$. The infant's blood at birth also contains about 15 percent of hemoglobin A.

An abnormal hemoglobin, hemoglobin Barts, is occasionally found in infant blood, the amount generally being not more than 10 per cent of the total hemoglobin. It rapidly decreases in the blood and often disappears by the time the infants is three months old. Barts hemoglobin is made up

of four γ-chains and is represented by γ_4.

In 1949, Pauling and associates discovered an electrophoretically abnormal hemoglobin in the erythrocytes of persons with sickle-cell anemia, which marked the beginning of systematic searches for abnormal types of hemoglobin. **Hemoglobin found in sickle cell anaemic cases was, named as Hemoglobin S (HbS). The erythrocytes of persons with sickle-cell anaemia contains a mixture of normal hemoglobin (A) and sickle-cell hemoglobin (S) and the sickling process is** *due to deoxygenation of sickle-cell hemoglobin,* **which causes a reversible change in red cell shape from a biconcave disc to a sickle-shaped form.** The rapidity and degree of sickling is proportional to the amount of hemoglobin S in the cells. Ordinarily sickling does not occur unless hemoglobin S represents at least 50 percent of the total cell hemoglobin.

Types of Abnormal Hemoglobin (Hemoglobinopathies)

1. Hemoglobin Barts
2. Hb C
3. Hb D Punjab
4. Hb E
5. Hb G Honolulu
6. Hb G Philadelphia
7. Hb G San Jose
8. Hemoglobin H
9. Hb I
10. Hb M Boston
11. Hb M Milwaukee
12. Hb M Saskatoon
13. Hb Norfolk
14. Hb O Arabia
15. Hb O Indonesia
16. Sickle-cell hemoglobin S
17. Hb Zurich

Today, more than 200 types of abnormal hemoglobins are known.

```
                                                              *10                              20
α , val – leu – ser – pro – ala – asp – lys – thr – asg* – val – lys – ala – ala – try – gly – lys – val – gly – ala – his – ala – gly – glu – tyr –
β , val – his – leu – thr – pro – glu – glu – lys – ser – ala – val – thr – ala – leu – try – gly – lys – val – asg – val – asp – glu – val – gly –
γ , gly – his – phe – thr – glu – glu – asp – lys – ala – thr – ile *thr – ser – leu – try – gly – lys – val – asg – val – glu – asp – ala – gly –

                              30                              40
α , gly – ala – glu – ala – leu – glu – arg – met – phe – leu – ser – phe – pro – thr – thr – lys – thr – tyr – phe – pro – his – phe – asp – leu –
β , gly – glu – ala – leu – gly – arg – leu – leu – val – val – tyr – pro – try – thr – glm* – arg – phe – phe – glu – ser – phe – gly – asp – leu –
γ , gly – glu – thr – leu – gly – arg – leu – leu – val – val – tyr – pro – try – thr – glm – arg – phe – phe – asp – ser – phe – gly – asg – leu –

          50                              60                              70
α , ser – his – gly – ser – ala – glm – val – lys – gly – his – gly – lys – lys – val – ala – asp – ala – leu – thr – asg – ala – val – ala – his –
β , ser – thr – pro – asp – ala – val – met – gly – asg – pro – lys – val – lys – ala – his – gly – lys – lys – val – leu – gly – ala – phe – ser –
γ , ser – ser – ala – ser – ala – ile – met – gly – asg – pro – lys – val – lys – ala – his – gly – lys – lys – val – leu – thr – ser – leu – gly –

                              80                              90
α , val – asp – asp – met – pro – asg – ala – leu – ser – ala – leu – ser – asp – leu – his – ala – his – lys – leu – arg – val – asp – pro – val –
β , asp – gly – leu – ala – his – leu – asp – asg – leu – lys – gly – thr – phe – ala – thr – leu – ser – glu – leu – his – cys – asp – lys – leu –
γ , asp – ala – ile – lys – his – leu – asp – asp – leu – lys – gly – thr – phe – ala – glm – leu – ser – glu – leu – his – cys – asp – lys – leu –

                              110                             120
α , asg – phe – lys – leu – leu – ser – his – cys – leu – leu – val – thr – leu – ala – ala – his – leu – pro – ala – glu – phe – thr – pro – ala –
β , his – val – asp – pro – glu – asg – phe – arg – leu – leu – gly – asg – val – leu – val – cys – val – leu – ala – his – his – phe – gly – lys –
γ , his – val – asp – pro – glu – asg – phe – lys – leu – leu – gly – asg – val – leu – val – thr – val – leu – ala – ile – his – phe – gly – lys –

                              130                             140 141                            46
α , val – his – ala – ser – leu – asp – lys – phe – leu – ala – ser – val – ser – thr – val – leu – thr – ser – lys – tyr – arg.
β , glu – phe – thr – pro – pro – val – glm – ala – ala – tyr – glm – lys – val – val – ala – gly – val – ala – asg – ala – leu – ala – his – lys – tyr – his.
γ , glu – phe – thr – pro – glu – val – glm – ala – ser – try – glm – lys – met – val – thr – gly – val – ala – ser – ala – leu – ser – ser – arg – tyr – his.
```

*asg = asparagine, glm = glutamine and ile = isoleucine

Fig. 7.6 : Amino acid sequences of the α, β, and γ chains of human hemoglobin.

HbS differs from HbA by the change of glutamic acid at position 6 in the β-chain of HbA for valine in HbS.

	HbA	HbS
	Glu	Val
Possible }	GAA	GUA
Codons }	GAG	GUG

In each case A has been changed to U, i.e. only one base has been changed. In fact the base change is GAA to GUA.

The gene of hemoglobin S is derived from that of normal adult hemoglobin A by a simple point mutation.

Rigas and associates discovered an abnormal human hemoglobin whic has been designated hemoglobin H and Jones and associates have shown that hemoglobin H is composed of four β chains, represented as β_4^H.

Many additional abnormal hemoglobins have been discovered, which often have been named according to the place where discovered. These are given in the 'box'.

Ingram has developed a method of detecting hemoglobins called **"fingerprinting"**.

The synthesis of normal and abnormal hemoglobins is controlled by the genes as in the case of other proteins. **The abnormal hemoglobins are formed because of gene mutation.**

Myoglobins

Myoglobin with a molecular weight of about 17,000 consists of a single globin peptide chain combined with heme.

Myoglobins are intracellular tissue pigments (red) which occur in the red muscle fibres of the vertebrates. They combine with oxygen to form oxymyoglobins; which serve as oxygen reservoirs within the cells. Myoglobins bind O_2 more firmly than do the hemoglobins and thus provide oxygen to the tissues at reduced tension.

It is present in large quantities in the skeletal muscle of those mammals that dive deeply in the sea. Human myoglobin is a small globular protein with a molecular weight of 16,700 that contains 152 amino acid residues. It is a single polypeptide chain with L-valine at the NH_2-terminus. Coordinated to the protein is a heme residue as in Fig. 7.7. Heme is an iron-containing *porphyrin* composed of Fe(II); four pyrrole rings linked by methene bridges, and eight side chains attached to the pyrrole rings (Fig. 7.7). The iron is inserted in the centre coordinately linked to the four nitrogen atoms of the pyrrole rings. In myoglobin the Fe(II) is also complexed with an imidazole nitrogen atom of a histidine residue in the protein chain, as shown in Fig. 7.8.

Myoglobin can react with O_2 to form oxymyoglobin (MbO_2), which is in equilibrium with the deoxymyoglobin (Mb).

The equilibrium position of the myoglobin molecule is dependent upon the concentration of O_2 in the system. Therefore, myoglobin may be considered as a storage reserve for O_2, as it is largely in the oxymyoglobin form when the O_2 concentration in the cellular fluid is high but

$$Mb + O_2 \rightleftharpoons Mb\,O_2$$

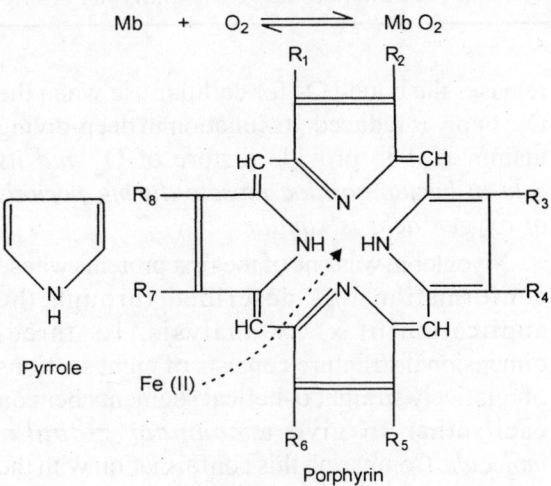

Fig. 7.7 : Porphyrins

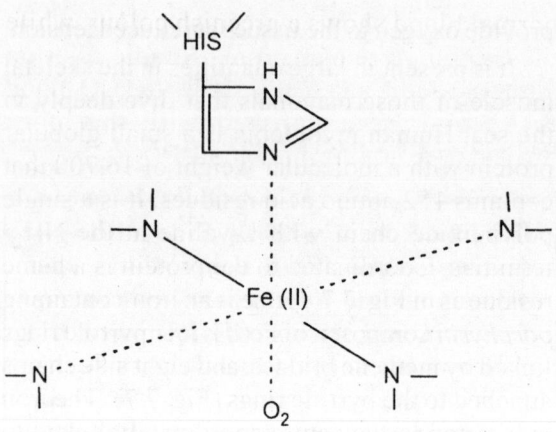

Fig. 7.8 : Representation of oxymyoglobin structure around heme residue

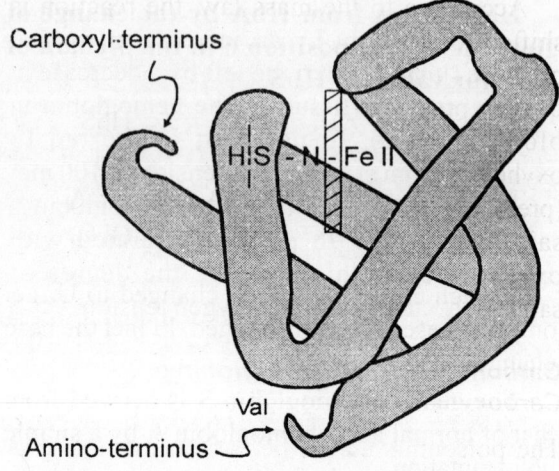

Carboxyl-terminus

HIS - N - Fe II

Val

Amino-terminus

Fig. 7.9 : Myoglobin molecule

Kendrew (U.K.), a Chemist and Perutz (Austria/U.K.), a Chemist were awarded Nobel Prize in 1962 for their studies of the structure of globular proteins.

Kendrew's work produced a three dimensional model of myoglobin at 6 A resolution in 1957 and an almost complete structure in 1960.

Perutz's work determined the structure of haemoglobin by X-ray diffraction technique and three dimensional X-ray analysis.

releases the bound O_2 for cellular use when the O_2 supply is reduced. Its function in deep-diving mammals is to provide a store of O_2 *and its role in human cardiac muscle during periods of oxygen debt is similar.*

Myoglobin was one of the first proteins whose conformation was described through the application of x-ray analysis. Its three-dimensional structure consists of eight sections of relatively straight α-helical segments bent on each other to give a *compact globular molecule*. Comparing this conformation with the amino acid sequence of the primary structure, it is found that the hydrophobic interactions are maximum, as very few hydrophobic side chain residues are exposed to the aqueous solvent medium, The peptide chain is further stabilized by the significant formation of α-helical segments. Breaks in the α-helices are found when L-prolyl or other destabilizing amino acid residues occur in the chain, There is no stability introduced in myoglobin by —S—S— bonds, cysteine being absent from the molecule. The molecule is very compact; there is space for the heme residue in the crevice (Fig. 7.9), but otherwise space exists for only four water molecules in the interior portion of the molecule.

Oxyhemoglobin

The primary function of hemoglobin in blood is to transport O_2 from the lungs, where the oxygen pressure is high, to the tissues, for utilization where the oxygen pressure is low. This is accomplished through the formation of a dissociable hemoglobin-oxygen complex, oxyhemoglobin (ferrooxyhemoglobin):

Hemoglobin + O_2 $\rightleftharpoons$ Oxyhemoglobin

According to the mass law, the reaction is shifted to the right by an increase in oxygen pressure (lungs) and to the left by a decrease in oxygen pressure (tissues). The hemoglobin in blood is 95 to 96 per cent converted to oxyhemoglobin at an oxygen tension of 100 mm (pressure in lung alveoli), and the hemoglobin is said to be 95 to 96 percent saturated with oxygen. Below this pressure the degree of saturation varies with the oxygen tension.

Carbon monoxide hemoglobin or Carboxyhemoglobin

The poisonous action of carbon monoxide is chiefly due to combination with hemoglobin and myoglobin to form carboxyhemoglobin and carboxymyoglobin and thereby to interfere with oxygenation of these substances. Carbon monoxide also combines with ferrous cytochrome oxidase, one of the respiratory enzymes of tissues, and prevents its action, particularly at higher concentrations of the gas.

Carbon monoxide adds on to 'the heme iron atoms exactly as does oxygen, but with much more affinity. The overall reaction of O_2 and CO with hemoglobin (Hb), take place when hemoglobin is

$$O_2 + Hb \rightleftharpoons HbO_2$$

$$CO + Hb \rightleftharpoons HbCO$$

exposed to either gas. When hemoglobin is exposed to a mixture of the gases, there is competition for the hemoglobin according to the equation:

$$HbO_2 + CO \rightleftharpoons HbCO + O_2$$

Various chemical tests for carboxyhemoglobin in blood have been devised. A simple test is to treat the suspected blood with a little NaOH, dilute it greatly, and then compare it with normal blood similarly treated. The normal blood shows a greenish colour, while the CO blood remains pink. Simple dilution without adding alkali also shows the CO blood to be pink, as compared with the more brownish red of normal blood.

> **Carboxy hemoglobin is strikingly distinguished from hemoglobin and oxyhemoglobin by its cherry red colour.** The skin and tissues of victims of CO poisoning are tinged with this colour.
>
> **Haldane has pointed out that the anoxic symptoms caused by CO poisoning are more severe than those of anemia.**

Biosynthesis (Formation) of bile pigments

* When RBCs complete their life span of 120 days, then they get phagocytized in reticuloendothelial system (R.E.S.).
* Haemoglobin is also phagocytized to give haem and globin protein (Fig. 7.10).
* Haem ring gets opened to give a straight chain of 4 pyrrole rings which form substrate for the formation of biliverdin.
* This biliverdin gets reduced to bilirubin.
* Bilirubin combines with albumin in plasma and gets absorbed by hepatic cells, where it combines with yet another protein and after that gets conjugated:
  (a) 80% conjugates with glucuronic acid
  (b) 10% conjugates with some sulphates
  (c) 10% conjugates with other substances

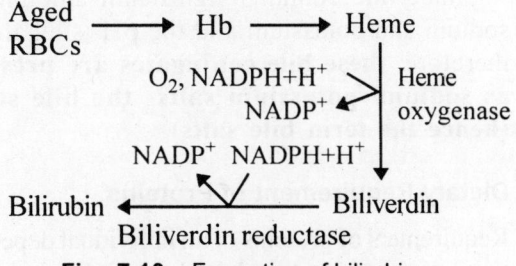

Fig. 7.10 : Formation of bilirubin

Biosynthesis of bile acids (salts) :

These are the biological detergents synthesized from cholesterol in liver. These are secreted with bile into the duodenum. Bile salts possess steroid nucleus, the side chain of which is attached to either glycine (glycocholic acid) or taurine (taurocholic acid). **These are the most effective biological emulsifying agents.** They interact with lipid particles and the aqueous duodenal contents and convert them into smaller particles (emulsified droplets). These also stabilize the smaller particles by preventing them from reuniting. Precursor for the biosynthesis of bile acids is cholesterol. Their synthesis takes place as shown in Fig. 7.11.

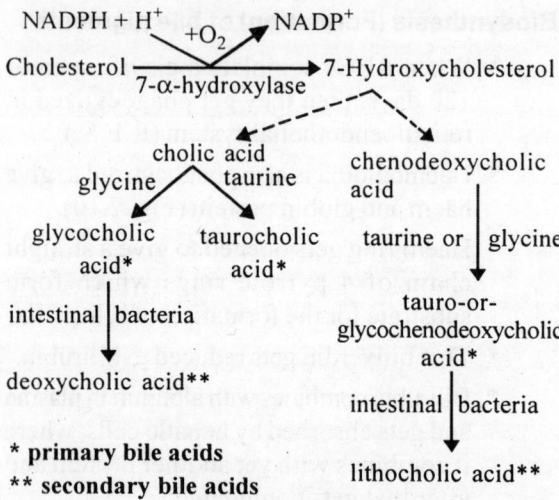

* primary bile acids
** secondary bile acids

Fig. 7.11 : Biosynthesis of bile acids

In human bile, the bile acids are conjugated with glycine and taurine in variable ratios.

Since bile contains significant amount of sodium and potassium and the pH is alkaline, therefore, **these bile conjugates are present as sodium/ potassium salts- the bile salts (hence the term bile salts).**

Dietary Requirement of Proteins

Requirement of proteins of an individual depends upon the age, sex and body weight. It is as mentioned in Table 7.3.

Table 7.3 : Recommended daily dietary protein intake

Category	Description	Daily protein allowance (g)	Nature of diet
Man	Body weight 55 kg	55	Mainly cereals and pulses NPU = 65*
Woman	Body weight 45 kg	45	
Woman	2nd half of pregnancy	55	
Woman	Lactation upto 1 year	65	
Infants	0-3 months	2.3 /kg	Entirely milk NPU=75-100*
Infants	3-6 months	1.8/kg	
Infants	6-9 months	1.8/kg	Milk, cereals and pulses, NPU = 65*
Infants	9-12 months	1.5/kg	
Children	1 year	17	Mostly cereals and pulses NPU = 50*
Children	2 years	18	
Children	3 years	20	
Children	4-6 years	22	
Children	7-9 years	33	
Children	10-12 years	41	
Adolescents: Boys 13-15 years		55	
Adolescents: Boys 16-18 years		60	
Adolescents: Girls 13-18 years		50	

The essential amino acids requirement of adults is less exacting than those of infants and children, therefore, the same dietary has a higher NPU for adults than for children.

Marasmus is predominantly due to the **deficiency of calories.** This is usually observed in children given watery gruels (of cereals) to supplement the mother's breast milk.

Now the chemists have reached the fact that the quantity of protein alone does not solve the entire purpose but the **quality** of a protein has got more significance hence one must give more emphasis on the quality of a protein. **By the quality of a protein, we mean that it must comprise of essential amino acids in it.**

Deficiency Diseases

Protein deficiency is generally encountered during infancy and childhood and is known as protein- energy malnutrition **(PEM)**. There are two severe forms of the disease known as **kwashiorkor** and **marasmus.**

Kwashiorkor is mainly a disease of rural areas, occurring in the second year of life. It occurs most commonly in the infants after weaning (breast feeding) when the diet which replaces mother's milk is markedly deficient in proteins but high in carbohydrate. This disease has its highest incidence **between the age group of 1 to 4 years** when the need for essential amino acids for tissue synthesis is more.

This syndrome is characterized by growth failure, retarded development, loss of appetite, mental apathy, hypoalbuminemia leading to edema, diarrhoea, pellagrous skin lesions, low plasma amino acids, lipids, glucose and potassium levels, gastrointestinal disturbances, dermatosis, fatty liver infiltration and mental disturbances are also frequent.

Marasmus

Marasmus literally means "to waste". It results from a continued severe deficiency of both dietary proteins and the calories i.e. energy.

It generally occurs in the children below one year of age. The symptoms include growth retardation, muscle wasting, anaemia, weakness, and repeated infections. Attitude is irritable. Skin is shrunken, dry and atrophic.

A marasmic child does not show edema or decreased concentration of plasma albumin (usual level in them is 2 to 3 g/dl whereas in kwashiorkor cases it is always less than 2 g/dl) and the level of cortisol in **serum gets increased in marasmic child whereas decreased in kwashiorkor ones.**

Immunoglobulins

Immunoglobulins or *antibodies* **are synthesized in B lymphocytes or their derivatives, plasma cells** and with remarkable specificity bind to *antigenic sites* on their moelcules.

All immunoglobulins are composed of four polypeptide chains, two identical light (L) chains(MW 23,000) and 2 identical heavy (H) chains (MW 53,000-75,000) which are held together as a tetramer (L_2H_2) by disulfide bonds (Fig. 7.12). Each chain can be divided into specific regions that have structural and functional significance. The half of the *light* (L) *chain* towards the carboxyl terminus is referred to as the *constant region* (C_L), whereas the amino-terminal half is the *variable region* of the light chain (V_L). Nearly, one-quarter of the *heavy (H) chain* at the amino terminus is referred to as its variable region (V_H) and the

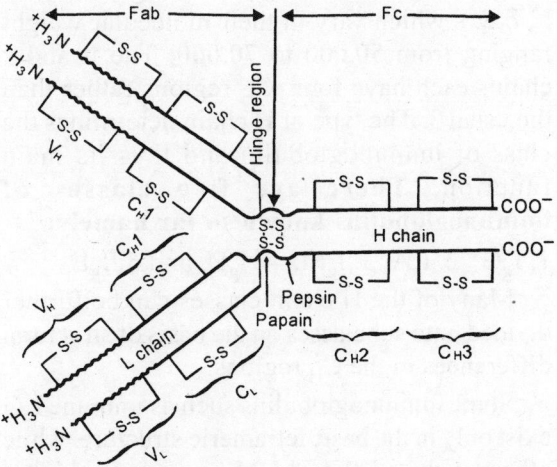

Fig 7.12 : A simplified model for an IgG human antibody molecule showing the 4-chain basic structure and different regions. V, indicates variable region; C, the constant region, and the vertical arrow, the hinge region. Thick lines represent H and L chains; thin lines represent disulfide bonds.

remaining three quarters of the heavy chain are referred to as the constant regions (C_H1, C_H2, C_H3) of that H chain. The function of the immunoglobulin molecule that binds the specific antigen is formed by the amino-terminal portions (variable regions) of both the H and L chains i.e., the V_H and V_L regions.

As made clear in Fig. 7.12, digestion of an immunoglobulin by the enzyme papain produces 2 antigen binding fragments (Fab) and one crystallizable fragment (F_c). The area in which papain cleaves the immunoglobulin molecule i.e., the region between the C_H1 and C_H2 regions is referred to as the **hinge region.**

There are two general types of light chains i.e. *kappa* (k) and *lambda* (λ). A given immunoglobulin molecule always contains two *k* or two λ light chains, never a mixture of *k* and λ. In human the *k* chains are more common than λ chains in immunoglobulin molecules.

In human, 5 classes of H chains have been found which can be easily distinguished from each other by differences in their C_H regions. The 5 classes of H chains are designated γ, α, μ, δ & ε which vary in their molecular weight ranging from 50,000 to 70,000. The μ and ε chains each have four C_H regions rather than the usual 3. The type of H chain determines the class of immunoglobulin and thus its main function. **There are five classes of immunoglobulins known so far namely:**

1. I_gG, 2. I_gA, 3. I_gM, 4. I_gD, and 5. I_gE

Many of the H chain classes can be further divided, into subclasses on the basis of structural differences in the C_H regions.

Some immunoglobulins such as immune I_gG exist only in the basic tetrameric structure, while others such as I_gA and I_gM can exist as higher order polymers of 2, 3 (I_gA) or 5 (I_gM) tetrameric units (Fig. 7.13).

The L and H chains are synthesized as separate molecules and are subsequently assembled within the B cell or plasma cell into

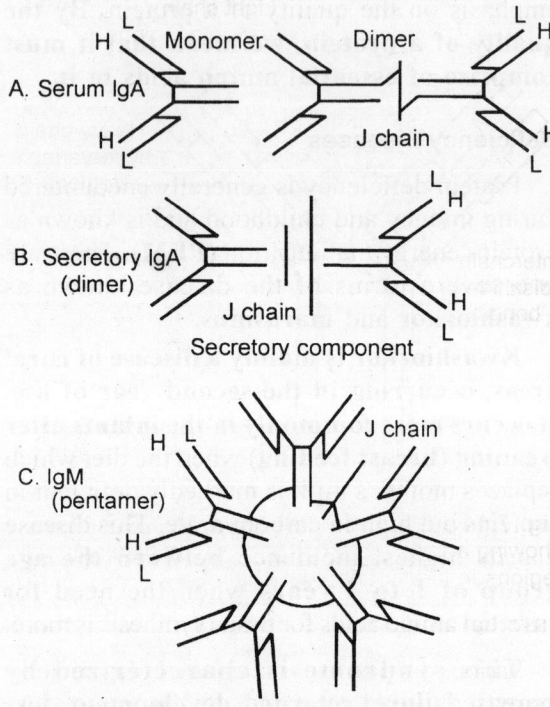

Fig. 7.13 : Highly schematic illustration of polymeric human immunoglobulins. Polypeptide chains are represented by thick lines; disulfide bonds linking different polypeptide chains are represented by thin lines.

mature immunoglobulin molecules, **all of which are glycoproteins in nature.**

Schematic model of I_gG molecule is as shown below in Fig. 7.14.

Each immunoglobulin light chain is the product of at least 3 separate structural genes i.e., a variable region (V_L) gene, a joining region (J) gene (bearing no relation to the J chain of I_gA or I_gM) and a constant region (C_L) gene. Each heavy chain is the product of at least 4 different genes i.e., a variable region (V_H) gene, a diversity region (D) gene, a joining region (J) gene and a constant region (C_H) gene. **In this way, the 'one gene, one protein' concept is no more valid.**

Each person is capable of generating antibodies directed against perhaps one million

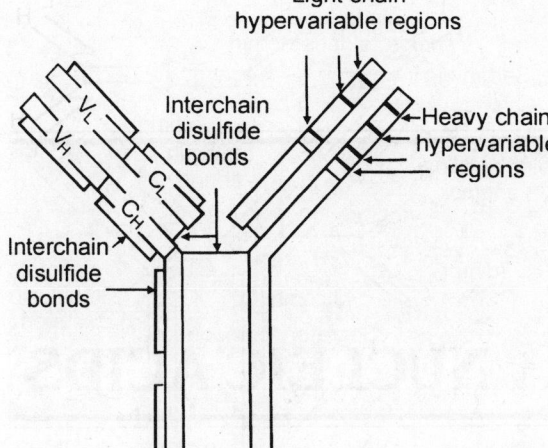

Fig. 7.14 : Schematic model of an I_gG molecule showing approximate positions of the hypervariable regions in heavy and light chains.

different antigens.

Various disorders of immunoglobulins include increased production of specific classes of immunoglobulins or even specific immunoglobulin molecules. **Hypogammaglobulinemia** may be restricted to a single class of immunoglobulin molecules (eg, I_gA or I_gG) or may involve underproduction of all classes of immunoglobulins (I_gA, I_gD, I_gE, I_gG and I_gM).

Plasma Proteins

Normal value of plasma total protein ranges from 6 to 8 gm per 100 ml of blood.

Plasma proteins include albumin, globulin and fibrinogen which can be separated from each other by:

(1) Precipitation method using varying concentrations of salts like sodium sulphate, ammonium sulphate, etc.

(2) Electrophoresis

In normal human plasma six fractions have been separated by electrophoresis as follows:

(a) Albumin, (b) α_1 - globulin, (c) α_2 - globulin, (d) β_1, - globulin, (e) β_2 - globulin, and (f) fibrinogen

Functions of Plasma Proteins

1. **Osmotic Pressure:** Plasma proteins are important in regulating water between blood and tissues, thus they help in maintaining intravascular colloid osmotic pressure.

2. **As carrier of certain metabolites:** They act as a carrier molecule for bilirubin, fatty acids, trace elements and many drugs.

3. **As buffers:** Proteins are amphoteric in nature and thus help in maintaining the pH of blood.

4. The lipoproteins act as **carrier molecule** for different types of lipids and lipid-soluble molecules that are not soluble in the plasma water.

5. Some **metal-binding proteins** for e.g. trnasferrin have the properties of globulins and act as carriers for trace elements.

6. **As immunoglobulins:** The property of antibodies formation resides in the γ -globulin fraction of the proteins.

Proteins	Biological role
Collagen, keratins	Structural proteins
Pepsin, amylase, etc.	Enzymes
Insulin, prolactin	Hormones
Haemoglobin, ceruloplasmin	Transport proteins
Ferritin	Storage proteins
γ - globulins	Immune functions
Hormone receptors	Protein receptors

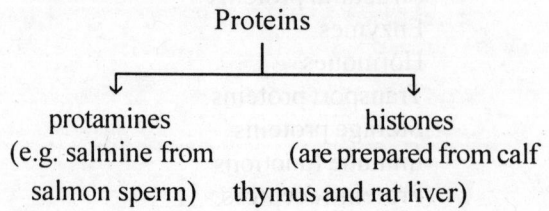

CHAPTER 8

NUCLEIC ACIDS

> We are The carriers of genetic information from one offspring to another. We are very complex molecules. Scientists are pursuing us and shall continue to pursue us till the 'universe' is present as we are very complicated molecules. Many many thanks to the science- stalwarts like James Watson, Francis Crick, Morris Wilkins (forgotten man of DNA), Chargaff, etc., who dedicated their lives for us. Genome technology is only due to us.

If any group of compounds can be said to be 'controller' in biochemistry, it is the nucleic acids which are found in every living cell and these may be defined as the nitrogen containing compounds of high molecular weight, vis-a-vis polymers of nucleotides. These are in fact macromolecules which remain present in most of the living cells, either in the free state or combined with proteins. The nucleic acid protein complexes are known as nucleoproteins, and these can be separated into the component proteins and nucleic acids by treatment with acid or high salt concentration. For the first time, they were reported by the scientist Miescher in 1871. Proteins associated with nucleic acids fall into two major classes as mentioned below:

```
                    Proteins
                       |
         ┌─────────────┴─────────────┐
         ↓                           ↓
    protamines                   histones
 (e.g. salmine from          (are prepared from calf
  salmon sperm)              thymus and rat liver)
```

These proteins are basic in character, for example salmine which consists of 40 arginine

Nucleic acids may be defined as the macromolecules in which the nucleotides remain linked to each other by phosphodiester bonds between the 3' and 5' positions of the sugars.

A portion of a molecule of RNA, therefore, has the structure as given in Fig. 8.1 **where base can either be a purine or pyrimidine.**

Most nucleic acids are very large molecules, therefore, to show the complete formulae is rather very cumbersome. A useful form of shorthand for the structure is therefore employed which exhibits the bases present by using their first letter. The sequence of bases is extremely important so that a nucleic acid may be shown by the first letters of the bases only (Fig. 8.2).

residues out of a total of 120.

As the name suggests, nucleic acids are acidic in character at physiological pH and carry a high density of negative charge. Nucleic acids are mainly of the following two types:

Nucleic acids

Ribonucleic acid   Deoxyribonucleic acid
(RNA)   (DNA)

Hydroiysis of DNA and RNA under controlled conditions yields *nucleotides,* which can be regarded as the basic unit of nucleic acids just as amino acids are the basic unit of the proteins and monosaccharides of the polysaccharides. **Further hydrolysis of *nucleotides* yields *nucleosides*** and eventually phosphate, a sugar and number of purine and pyrimidine bases. Nomenclature and components of nucleic acids have been described in Table 8.1.

Our understanding regarding the nucleic acids has grown tremendously in the recent years. Several top scientists of the world's top laboratories are working day and night on 'nucleic acids', amongst whom good contributories are:

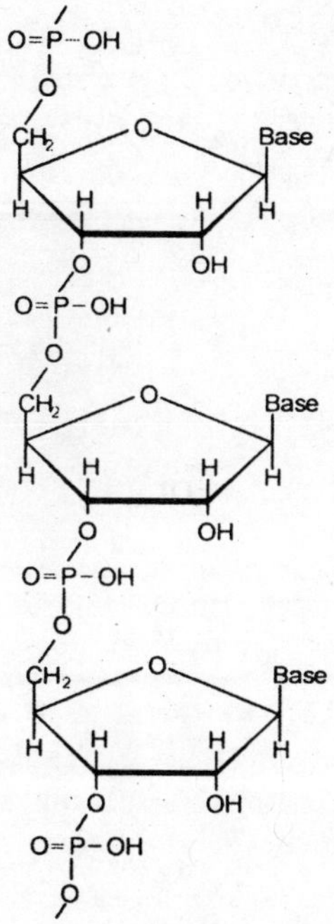

Fig. 8.1 : Part of the molecule of RNA

(i) Miescher,

(ii) A.R Todd,

(iii) **Har Gobind Khorana (Nobel Prize in 1968)***

(iv) Wilkins, (Nobel Prize in 1962)

(v) Watson, (Nobel Prize in 1962)

(vi) Crick, (Nobel Prize in 1962)

Table 8.1 : Nomenclature and Components of nucleic acids

RNA (cytoplasmic nucleic acid)	DNA (nuclear nucleic acid)
Polymer: (base-rib-phosphate)$_n$	(base-deoxyrib-phosphate)$_n$
Nucleotide : base-ribose—O—P—OH with O above (double bond) and OH below	base-deoxyrib — O — P — OH with O above (double bond) and OH below
Nucleoside: base-ribose-OH	base-deoxyrib-OH
Purine : adenine, guanine	adenine, guanine
Pyrimidines : cytosine, uracil and others	cytosine, thymine

* *He succeeded in synthesizing the first wholly artificial gene which contained in it 77 nucleotides. He was of Indian origin, later settled in U.S.*

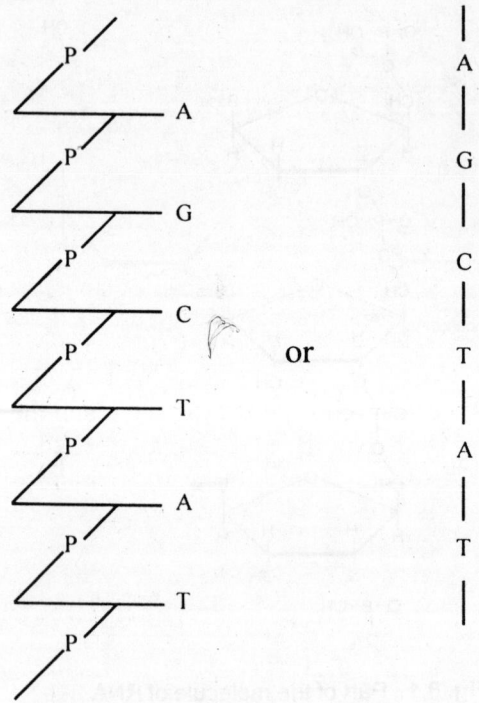

A
|
G
|
C
|
or T
|
A
|
T
|

Fig. 8.2 : Shorthand notation to exhibit the base sequence of a nucleic acid

(vii) Davidson,

(viii) Chargaff, etc.

Functions of the Nucleic Acids

(i) Nucleic acids are responsible for the direction of metabolism throughout the life of a cell.

(ii) They direct the synthesis of proteins.

(iii) They control the synthesis of enzymes.

(iv) They are responsible for the transfer of genetic information from one offspring to another.

(v) Nucleic acids, in fact, contribute the essential substance of the genes and the apparatus by which the genes act.

(vi) For the clinician, they are of major interest as they are undoubtedly involved in the causation of cancers **(malignancies).**

Chemical Composition

Nucleic acids fall into two principal classes according to the nature of the sugar they contain:

(i) the deoxyribonucleic acid, i.e., DNA which contains the sugar known as deoxyribose sugar, and

(ii) the ribonucleic acids i.e., RNAs which contain the sugar known as ribose.

RNA and DNA are polymers of nitrogenous bases, sugars, and phosphoric acid; thus

$$(base\text{-}sugar\text{-}phosphate)_n$$

nucleic acid

where n is a large number.

The link between the polymer units is the phosphate diester bond as shown below:

$$
\begin{array}{c}
O \\
\parallel \\
-\,sugar - O - P - O - sugar - \\
| \\
OH
\end{array}
$$

phosphate diester bond

Nucleotides

When the phosphate diester bond gets hydrolyzed, the monomeric units of nucleic acids are separated which consist of a nitrogenous base, a sugar and a phosphate; such a unit is called as a nucleotide as shown below:

$$
\begin{array}{c}
O \\
\parallel \\
base - sugar - O - P - OH \\
| \\
OH
\end{array}
$$

nucleotide

Nucleotides and nucleosides are named after the bases contained in their structure, as below:

Base	Nucleoside	Nucleotide
Adenine	Adenosine	Adenylic acid
Guanine	Guanosine	Guanylic acid
Uracil	Uridine	Uridylic acid
Cytosine	Cytidine	Cytidylic acid
Thymine	Thymidine	Thymidylic acid

If the base is linked to deoxyribose, then the names are modified so that a nucleoside consisting of adenine and deoxyribose would be called deoxyadenosine. As well as the nucleotides indicated, a number of biologically important nucleotides such as adenosine di- and triphosphate (ADP and ATP), guanosine di- and triphosphate (GDP and GTP) and nicotinamide adenine dinucleotide (NAD) are known to occur in the free state.

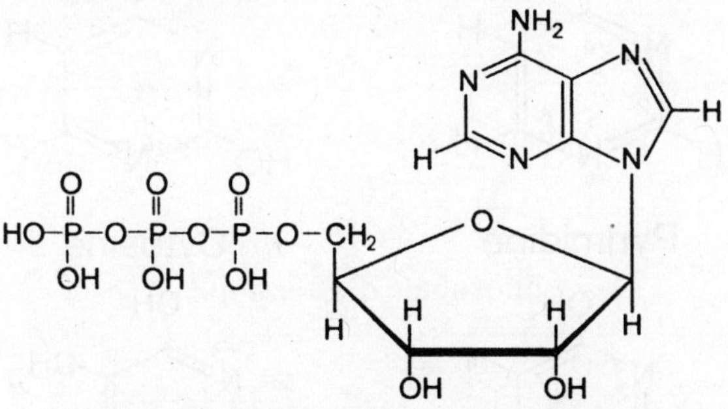

Adenosine 5′- triphosphate (ATP)

Nucleosides

When the ester bond between the sugar and the phosphate group in a nucleotide is hydrolyzed, a fragment consisting of a nitrogenous base and a sugar moiety is obtained which is called as a *nucleoside*,

base — sugar — OH

nucleoside

The important examples of nucleosides include adenosine and uridine whose structures are as given below; others are guanosine, thymidine, cytidine, etc.

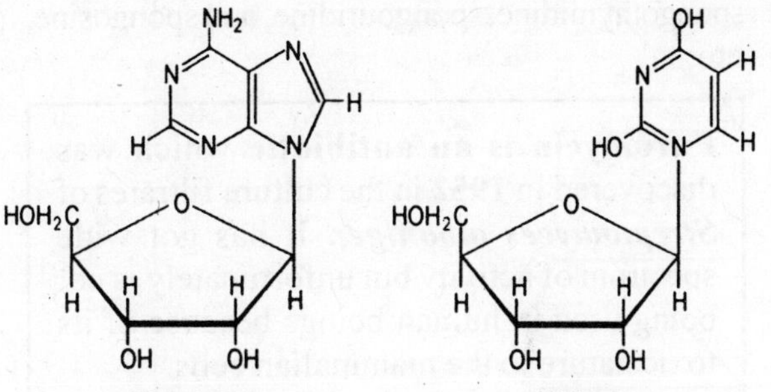

Adenosine

Uridine

Most of the bonds linking the sugar and the base are as shown above, **but transfer RNA does contain an unusual nucleotide pseudouridine in which ribose is linked to the uracil via the 5 position.**

Other examples of nucleosides of natural origin (not derived from nucleic acids) include the important antibiotics like puromycin, tubercidin, nebularine, cordycepin, etc., which are derived from moulds, fungi and also from a group of compounds isolated from sponges, among which the important examples are those of

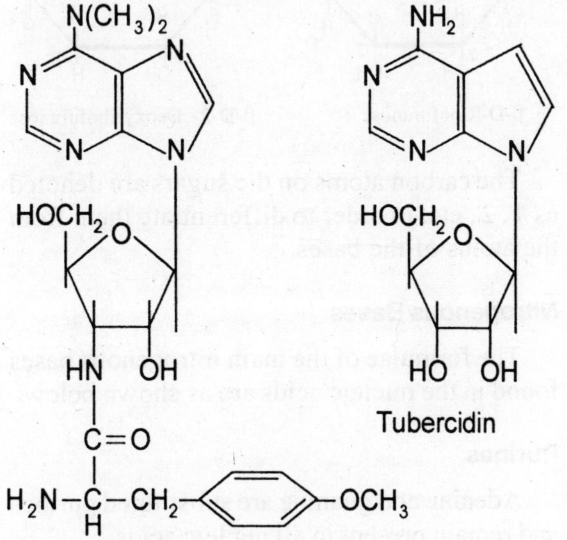

Tubercidin

Puromycin

spongothymidine, spongouridine, and spongosine, etc.

> **Puromycin is an antibiotic** which was discovered in **1952** in the culture filtrates of ***Streptomyces alboniger***. It has got wide spectrum of activity but unfortunately is not being used in human beings because of its toxic nature to the mammalian cells.

The Pentose Sugars

Sugars found in the nucleic acids are either D-ribose as in RNA or D-2-deoxyribose as in DNA, structure of which are as given below. The 'type' of the presence of pentose sugars in nucleic acids is the basis of its classification, **if they contain 'ribose' sugar in its structure, then they are known as ribonucleic acids and if deoxyribose then deoxyribonucleic acid.**

The structures of these sugars are as given below:

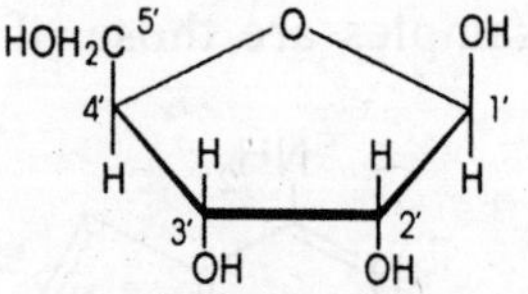

β-D-Ribofuranose 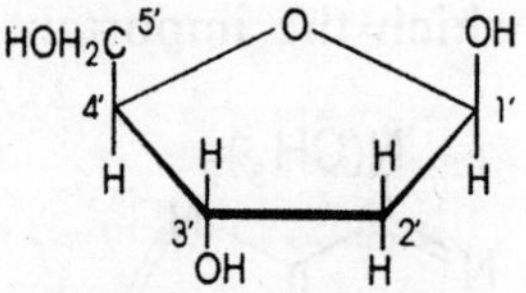   β-D-2- Deoxyribofuranose

The carbon atoms on the sugars are denoted as 1', 2', etc. in order to differentiate them from the atoms of the bases.

Nitrogenous Bases

The formulae of the main nitrogenous bases found in the nucleic acids are as shown below:

Purines

Adenine and guanine are substituted purines and remain present in all nucleic acids.

Small quantities of other bases have been detected in nucleic acids from some sources. It

Purines

Purine

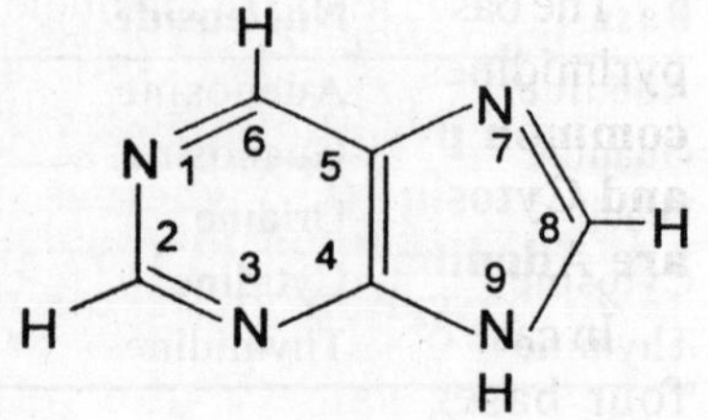

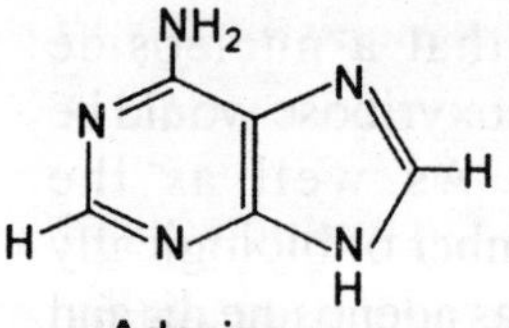

Adenine   Guanine

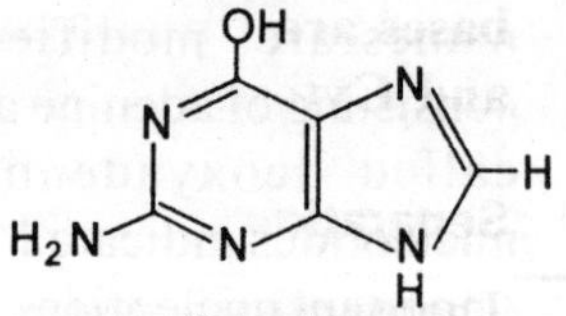

Pyrimidines

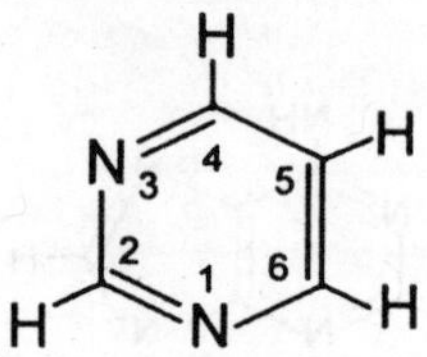

Pyrimidine   Cytosine

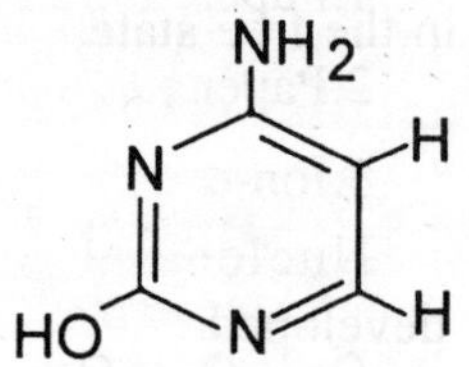

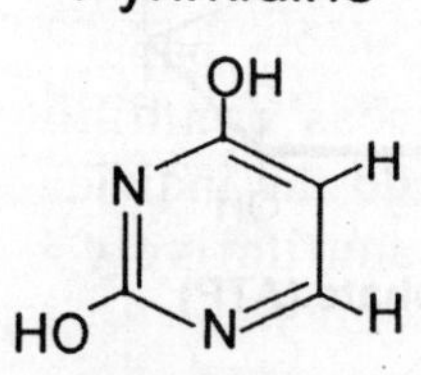

Uracil   Thymine

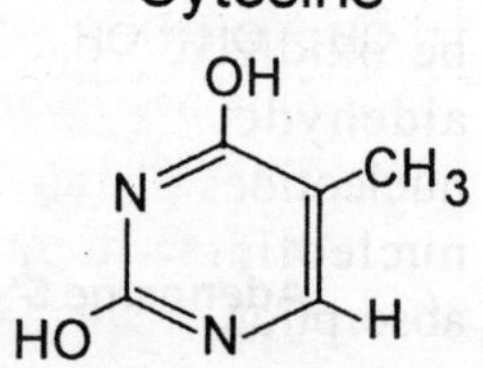

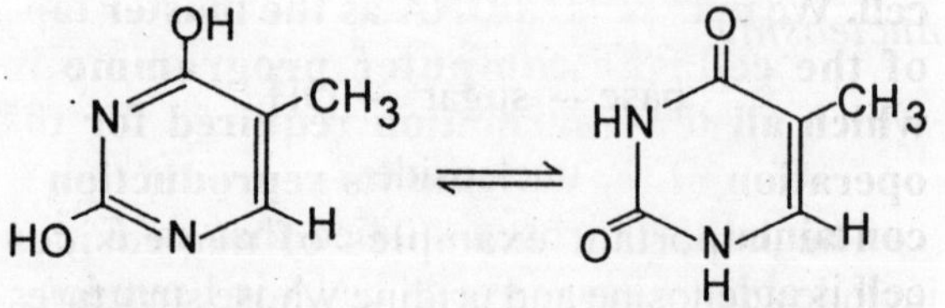

should be noted that both purine and pyrimidine bases can exist in the keto or enol form (Fig. 8.3).

Enol form   Keto form

Fig. 8.3 : The keto and enol forms of thymine

The bases found in the nucleic acids are either pyrimidines or purines. In case of DNA, **the common pyrimidine bases are Thymine (T) and Cytosine (C); whereas the purine bases are Adenine (A) and Guanine (G).**

In case of RNAs, they generally contain only four bases namely, **the purine bases are Adenine and Guanine and the pyrimidine bases are Uracil (not Thymine as in DNA), and Cytosine.**

Separation and Determination of Nucleotides

There are various methods by which nucleotides can be separated and determined, out of which the following three methods are generally used:

1. Paper chromatography,

2. Paper electrophoresis, and

3. Ion-exchange chromatography

Nucleotides can be identified on the developed chromatogram either by ultraviolet (UV) light absorption (dark spots) or fluorescence (light spots). Ribose derivatives can be oxidized by sodium iodate on paper by aldehyde reagents. The areas containing nucleotides can be cut out and the individual nucleotides determined quantitatively by absorption spectroscopy.

DEOXYRIBONUCLEIC ACID (DNA)

The genetic information of a cell is confined in its complement of deoxyribonucleic acid (DNA). This genetic information scientifically is known as the genome of the cell. We may regard DNA as the master tape of the cell, the computer programme in which all the information required for the operation of the cell and its reproduction is contained. It has been studied that an *E. coli* cell is about 1 μm long; its DNA is 1 mm long. **This DNA encodes for atleast 4,000 proteins and contains many regions that regulate the expression of these proteins.**

DNA is intimately associated with the genetic material of the cell. In some micro-organisms, a single strand of DNA seems to be the store for the genetic information; but, in higher organisms, the DNA is present as nucleoprotein in the chromosomes. The amount of DNA in the cell of a particular species is constant, whereas the germ cells with half the number of chromosomes contain half the DNA present in other cells. **The DNA occurs almost exclusively in the nucleus and in minute quantity in the mitochondria.** It plays following *biological roles:*

Biological Roles of DNA

(i) The function of DNA is to act as a *store house of genetic information and to control the synthesis of proteins in the cell.*

(ii) *Cell replication:* Hereditary characteristics are passed on to daughter cells through replication of DNA; during cell division, the two strands of DNA get separated and free nucleotides are attached to each strand according to the *'base pairing'* rule. The nucleotides are then probably 'zipped' together by the action of a DNA polymerase to give two identical molecules of the original DNA (Fig. 8.4).

(iii) *Control of protein synthesis:* It is now clear from a number of experiments that the sequence of bases in the nuclear DNA determines the proteins synthesized in the cytoplasm of the cell. The *'genetic code'* is such that 3 non-overlapping bases known as a *'codon "* code for each amino acid. The code is 'degenerate' in that more than one triplet may code for a particular amino acid. The DNA therefore acts in the first instance as a *'template'* on which the messenger RNA (m-RNA) gets synthesized. The m-

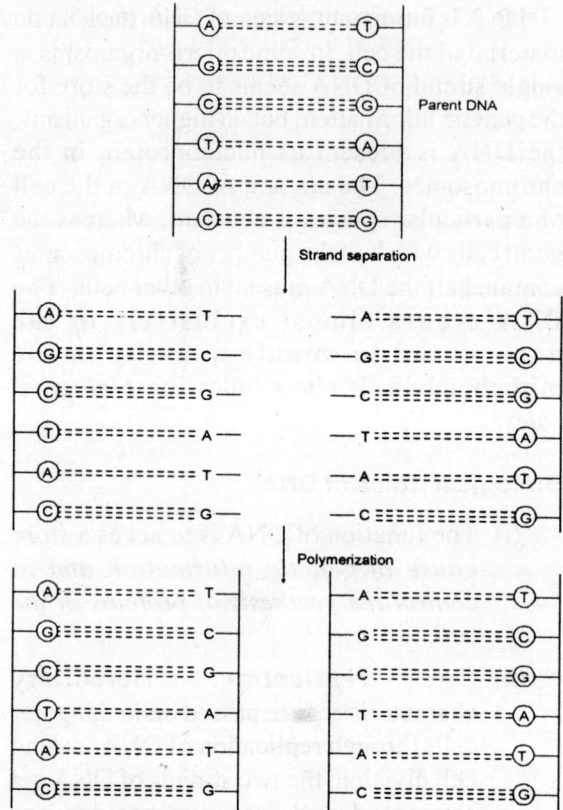

Fig. 8.4 : The replication of DNA (A, G, T and C represent the nucleotides on the newly synthesized strand of DNA)

RNA, with a complementary base sequence to the nuclear DNA, then carries the genetic message from the nucleus to the *protein synthesizing system on the ribosomes.*

Structure of DNA

For convenience, we may study the structure of DNA into three stages namely:

(a) Primary structure,

(b) Secondary structure, and

(c) Tertiary structure

(a) Primary Structure

DNA is a linear polymer (double stranded in its native state) of 21-deoxynucleotide residues which remain linked to each other by phosphodiester bonds between 3' and 5' positions of the 2'-deoxyribosyl moieties (Fig. 8.5).

The most common bases in DNA are:

(a) Adenine

(b) Thymine

(c) Guanine, and

(d) Cytosine

The *primary structure* of DNA is referred to as the linear sequence of nucleotide residues comprising the polydeoxyribonucleotide chain.

The primary structure of DNA molecules from various sources range from a few thousand residues in some viruses to 10^6 residues in bacteria to 10^9 residues in a human chromosomal DNA. A single molecule of bacterial DNA is nearly 1 mm long; whereas the length of a DNA molecule of a human chromosome is estimated to be 8.2 cm. **Molecular weights and lengths of DNA from various sources vary widely.**

Base Composition of DNA

Base composition of DNA remained unidentified after its discovery for nearly a century because of the difficulty of separating the products of DNA hydrolysis from one another. Invention of paper chromatography provided a mean to overcome this difficulty and E. Chargaff was the first scientist to determine the base composition of many species in 1950. The base composition differs widely from one species to another. Each species has a characteristic base composition but every organ of higher organisms has the same base composition. Strikingly, for every organism the ratio of pyrimidines to purines, (A + G)/(C + T), is nearly unity as shown in Table 8.2.

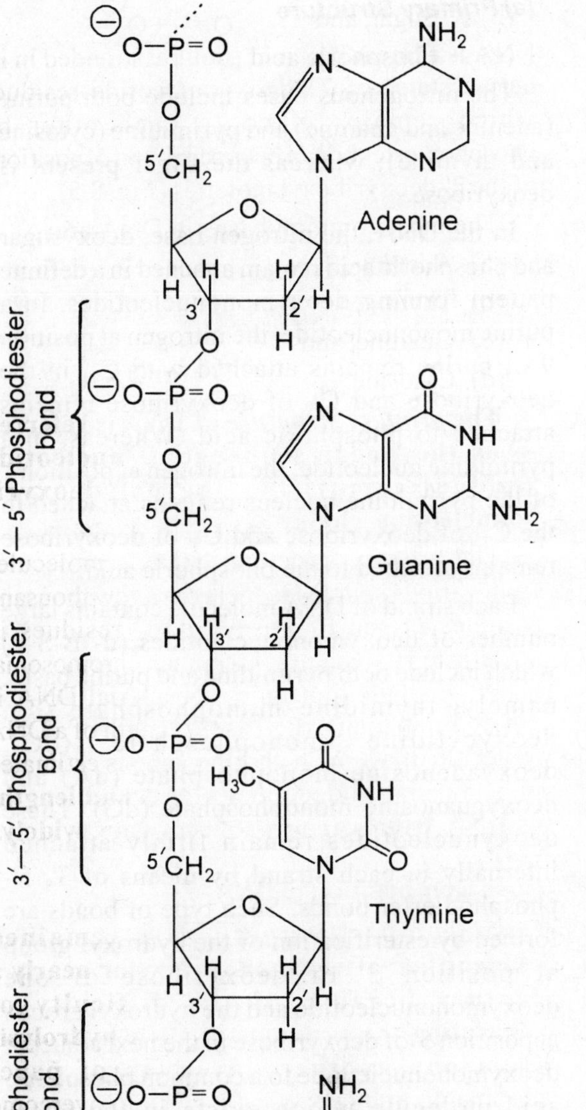

Fig. 8.5 : Covalent backbone of DNA

Table 8.2: Base composition of DNA (mol %) and ratios of various components

Source	A	G	C	T	$\dfrac{A+T}{G+C}$	A/T	G/C	$\dfrac{A+G}{C+T}$
Man	30.4	19.9	19.9	30.1	1.52	1.009	1.000	1.006
Ox	29.0	21.2	21.2	28.7	1.36	1.010	1.000	1.006

The mole percent ratio of guanine to cytosine (G/C) and adenine to thymine (A/T) are also nearly unity in each case as shown above. The (A + T)/(G + C) ratios, however vary widely.

DNA is a very complicated molecule which consists of two chains of polynucleotides which are interwoven in the form of a **spiral structure** which is stabilized by hydrogen bonding between particular base pairs. The stereochemistry of the bases is such that **adenine pairs with thymine and guanine with cytosine** so that the ratio of A/T and G/C is unity (Fig.8.6). This peculiar aspect of the structure of DNA was first of all proposed by the **two very renowned scientists of the field of nucleic acids, i.e., Watson and Crick in 1953** on the basis of the X-ray data of Wilkins and is sometimes known as the **Watson-Crick hypothesis.** This idea has since been confirmed and provides the basis for explaining some of the biological properties of DNA.

Most DNA molecules are of the double helical type although some viruses contain only single stranded DNA and to a great surprise the DNA in the bacteriophage φx 174 is even more unusual as it is **circular in shape.**

It is difficult to arrive at an accurate value for the molecular weight of DNA as the methods used for its isolation may result in breakage in the molecule, but it ranges in millions.

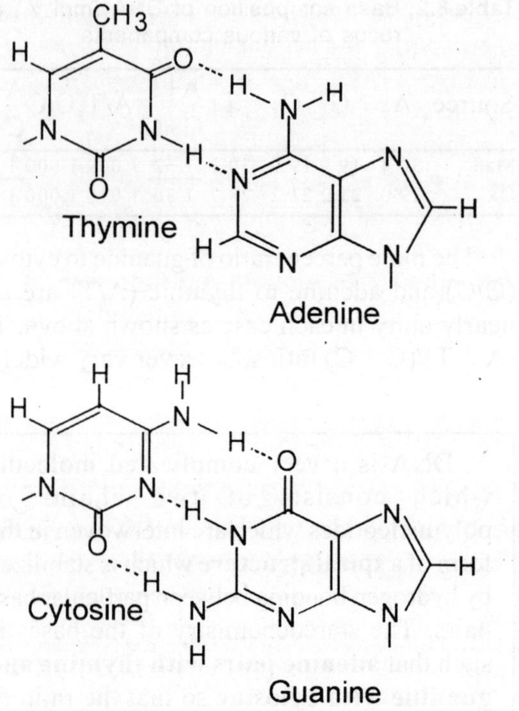

Fig. 8.6 : The pairing of bases by hydrogen bonding (- . - - - - -) as in DNA

(b) Secondary structure

Scientists Watson and Crick were responsible for deducing the structure of DNA in 1953; they were awarded Nobel prize in 1962 for this brilliant discovery. One key to the structure of DNA was Chargaff's observation that purines and pyrimidines are present in DNA in equimolar quantities.

Deoxyribonucleic acids are very complex molecules which possess a molecular weight ranging from 6-100 millions. They are elongated in shape and consist mostly of two strands which remain coiled in a parallel helical manner.

Complete hydrolysis of DNA leads to the formation of the following:

(a)   Various nitrogenous bases,

(b)   Sugar, and

(c)   Phosphoric acid

The nitrogenous bases include both purine (adenine and guanine) and pyrimidine (cytosine and thymine); whereas the sugar present is deoxyribose.

In the DNA, the nitrogen base, deoxysugar and phosphoric acid remain attached in a definite pattern forming deoxymononucleotides. In a purine mononucleotide, the nitrogen at position 9 of purine remains attached with C_1, in the deoxyribose and $C_{5'}$ of deoxyribose remains attached to phosphoric acid. Whereas, in a pyrimidine nucleotide, the nitrogen at position 1 of the pyrimidine nucleus remains attached to the C_1, of deoxyribose and $C_{5'}$ of deoxyribose remains attached to the phosphoric acid.

Each strand of DNA molecule contains large number of deoxymononucleotides (d- B-S-P) which include both pyrimidine and purine bases, namely, thymidine monophosphate (T), deoxycytidine monophosphate (dC), deoxyadenosine monophosphate (dA) and deoxyguanosine monophosphate (dG). These deoxynucleotides remain firmly attached internally in each strand by means of 3', 5'-phosphodiester bonds. Such type of bonds are formed by esterification of the hydroxyl group at position 3' of deoxyribose of one deoxymononucleotide and the hydroxyl groups at position 5' of deoxyribose in the next adjacent deoxymononucleotide to a common phosphoric acid molecule which exists in the latter deoxymononucleotide. The formation of such bonds has been illustrated in Figure 8.7.

The phosphoric acid of the former deoxymononucleotide remains esterified with another deoxymononucleotide existing previous to it. In this manner, a polynucleotide chain gets formed by interlinking of large number of mononucleotides by 3', 5'-phosphodiester bonds. These polynucleotides form the DNA strand.

In different DNAs, the sequence of

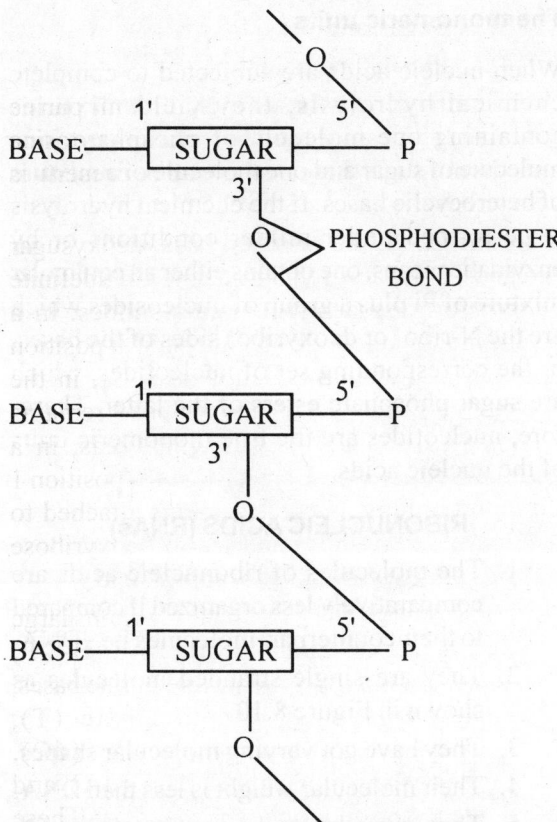

Fig. 8.7 : Formation of 3', 5'-phosphodiester linkages between mononucleotides

deoxymononucleotides is found to vary. The specific properties exhibited by the DNA - molecules are governed by this sequence. The two strands of DNA molecule are complementary to each other. Their base sequence is interdependent which follows the base pairing rule.

In a double-helix, formed by parallel coiling of the two strands along a longitudinal axis, the placing of the bases is such that **adenine is placed in the plane of thymine and guanine is placed in the plane of cytosine or vice versa, the so called base-pairing rule.**

(c) Tertiary structure

The two strands are kept in position and the

structure is stabilized by means of hydrogen bonds, each amino group being joined to a keto group, i.e., adenine to thymine, guanine to cytosine, etc. Formation of two hydrogen bonds between adenine and thymine; and three hydrogen bonds between guanine and cytosine is maximally possible. The formation of the H-bonds between such bases has been shown in Figure 8.8.

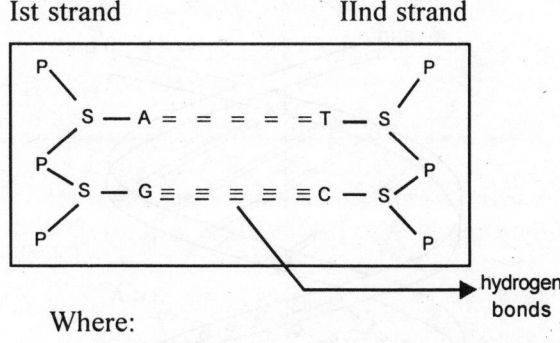

Where:
A = Adenine, G = Guanine, T = Thymine, C = Cytosine, S = 2-deoxyribose, and P = Phosphoric acid

Fig. 8.8 : To show formation of H-bonds between purine and pyrimidine bases

The molar content of adenine equals the molar content of thymine; and the molar content of guanine equals that of cytosine in DNA The ratio of adenine plus thymine to guanine plus cytosine however is not equal and varies from DNA to DNA obtained from different sources.

DNA (Fig. 8.9) helix consists of several million turns. The two strands of a DNA helix run parallel but in opposite directions. **The double helical structure is although quite stable but may be denatured by heat treatment or extremes of pH.** Denaturation of DNA results in uncoiling of the two strands as a result of which two separate chains are formed; the molecular weight also gets halved and absorbance at 260mμ (characteristic of nucleic acids) also gets increased.

DNAs are mainly present in the nucleus of the cells and are the carriers of hereditary characters. DNA can reproduce itself by the phenomenon of replication. Genes are composed of the DNA proteins which are believed to be associated with the mechanism of retention of memory in the brain. Viruses which infect the bacterial cells are also purely DNA-proteins. Double helical structure of DNA is as shown in Figure 8.9.

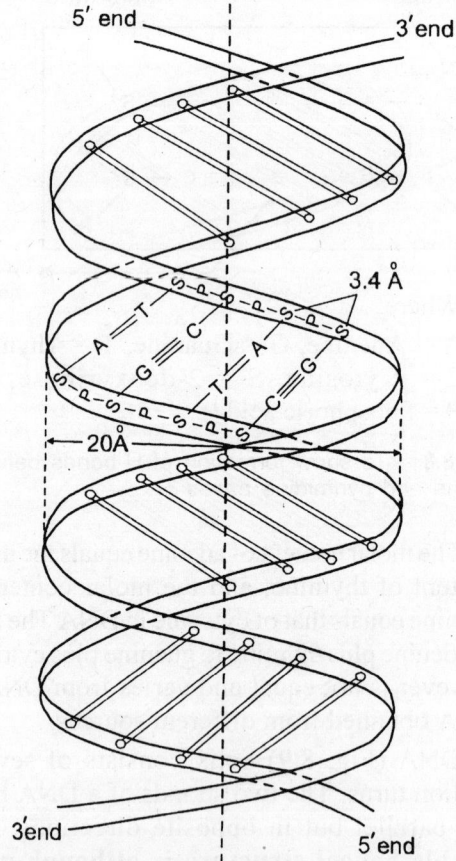

5' end   3'end

3.4 Å

20Å

3'end   5'end

Where: (i)   P means phosphate diester
      (ii)   S means deoxyribose sugar
     (iii)   À = T is the adenine thymine pairing
    (iv)   G = C is the guanine cytosine pairing

Fig. 8.9 : Double helical structure of DNA

The monomeric units

When nucleic acids are subjected to complete chemical hydrolysis; they yield mixtures containing one molecule of phosphate, one molecule of sugar and one molecule of a mixture of heterocyclic bases. If the chemical hydrolysis is performed under milder conditions or by enzymatic means, one obtains either an equimolar mixture of Pi plus a group of nucleosides which are the N-ribo (or deoxyribo) sides of the bases, or the corresponding set of nucleotides, which are sugar phosphate esters of the latter. Therefore, nucleotides are the true monomeric units of the nucleic acids.

RIBONUCLEIC ACIDS (RNAs)

1. The molecules of ribonucleic acids are comparatively less organized if compared to their counterpart molecules i.e., DNA.
2. They are single stranded molecules as shown in Figure 8.10.
3. They have got varying molecular shapes.
4. Their molecular weight is less than DNA.
5. They have been shown to possess 60-6,000 mononucleotides in their molecules.
6. Complete hydrolysis of ribonucleic acids yields a mixture of purines, pyrimidines, sugar and phosphoric acid. The purines found in the hydrolysates are generally adenine and guanine whereas the pyrimidines are cytosine and uracil.
7. Certain purines and pyrimidines are also sometimes found in some RNAs which include:

    (i)   5-methylcytosine,
   (ii)   5-hydroxymethylcytosine
  (iii)   1-methylguanine,
  (iv)   2-methylamino-6-hydroxypurine,
   (v)   6-methylaminopurine, and
  (vi)   6-dimethylaminopurine.

RNA molecule consists of a single strand of nucleic acid in the form of a random coil with only limited regions of base pairing, therefore, the simple relationship of A/U = G/C = 1 does not hold true for most forms of RNA. The molecular weight of transfer RNA is nearly 25,000, whereas other forms of RNA have a high molecular weight of a million or near about.

RNA is distributed throughout the cell, most of which remains present in cytoplasm as soluble and ribosomal RNA, but about 10% is found in the nucleus with minute quantities being also present in the mitochondria. There are three types of RNA present in the cells of higher organisms, viz :

(i) messenger RNA (m-RNA),

(ii) ribosomal RNA (r-RNA),

(iii) transfer RNA or soluble RNA (t-RNA or s-RNA).

All the above RNAs remain actively involved in the synthesis of protein.

8. The sugar in all types of RNAs has been identified to be a pentose sugar named as D- ribose.

9. Different mononucleotides existing ordinarily in the RNAs are:

(i) adenylic acid (A),

(ii) uridylic acid (U),

(iii) guanylic acid (G), and

(iv) cytidylic acid (C)

The sequence of these mononucleotides varies from RNA to RNA. **Different mononucleotides in a RNA strand are interlinked by the 3',5'phosphodiester bonds which are formed in a similar manner as in DNA molecules.**

Types of RNAs

At present, following four types of RNAs are known to exist:

(a) m-RNA (messenger RNA),

(b) t-RNA (transfer RNA) or S-RNA (soluble RNA),

(c) r-RNA (ribosomal RNA), and

(d) viral RNA

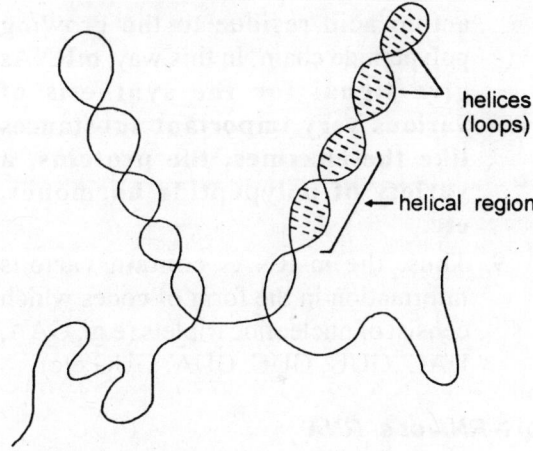

helices (loops)

← helical region

Fig 8.10 : Single stranded helical structure of a RNA molecule. The helical regions are stabilized and maintained in their shapes by A to U & G to C interactions; such interactions (bindings) are maintained by H-bonds.

(a) m-RNA

1. These nucleic acids exhibit highest molecular weight amongst all RNA.

2. Their M.W. ranges from 2-5 lacs.

3. They are highly elongated molecules.

4. They possess varying molecular shapes.

5. They are very short lived.

6. They are synthesized as a result of transcription of the DNA molecules within the nucleus and their base sequence strongly resembles to one of the corresponding DNA strand; the difference occurs only in a pyrimidine base. **In place of thymine, m-RNA**

contains uracil.

7. These have been shown to contain 60-6,000 mononucleotides in their molecules.

8. **They are known as "informational molecules" which carry message from nuclear DNA to the site of protein synthesis i.e. ribosomes,** informing various aminoacyl-t RNAs as to when they should add their particular amino acid residue to the growing polypeptide chain. In this way, **mRNAs give signal for the synthesis of various very important substances like the enzymes, the proteins, a variety of polypeptide hormones, etc.**

9. Thus, the m-RNAs contain various information in the form of codes which consist of nucleotide triplets (e.g., GAA, UAG, GUU, GUC, GUA, GUG etc).

(b) t- RNA or s- RNA

This is also known as soluble RNA (s-RNA); it constitutes nearly 10-20 per cent of total RNAs of the cell. Its M.W. ranges from 20,000 to 40,000 and it bears 70 to 80 mononucleotides in its molecule.

They are found in the soluble fraction of tissue homogenates after centrifugation at high speed i.e. 100,000 x g. There is evidence of the existence of atleast 21 transfer RNAs, each being specific for each naturally existing amino acid. It has been further studied that many amino-acids have more than one different t-RNA. Their main function is just to get attached with the activated amino acid and to carry it to the site of protein synthesis i.e. ribosomes so that it be added to the growing polypeptide chain.

Besides the presence of regular bases i.e. adenine, guanine, uracil and cytosine, t-RNAs have been found to contain some very unusual bases like ribothymidine, dihydrouracil, inosine, dihydrouridine, pseudouridine etc., which possess an unusual linkage between the sugar ribose and the base.

Messenger RNA

The first step in the synthesis of protein is the transfer of genetic message of the DNA to messenger RNA, the process is known as '**transcription**'.

The messenger RNA migrates into the cytoplasm and it is here, in association with ribosome and transfer RNA, **that the 4 letter code is converted to the 20 letter code of proteins. This stage is known as 'translation'.** Part of the DNA strand is only transcribed, so that m-RNA is smaller than the nuclear DNA. The actual molecular weight of a particular m-RNA is determined by the number of amino acid residues in the protein being synthesized, but is often of the order of a million or so. The mRNA, unlike the other forms, is metabolically unstable.

Transfer RNA

Each amino acid has a specific t-RNA which transfers the activated amino acid to the site of protein synthesis. Unlike the other forms of RNA, transfer ribonucleic acids have low molecular weights and are made up of relatively few nucleotides. The complete sequence of nucleotides has been determined for some t-RNAs and speculations made about the '**recognition sites**' on the molecule. There are two of these sites on each t-RNA molecule, one that identifies a particular amino acid and the other which recognizes and binds to the triplet base on the codon. This triplet of bases on the t-RNA is known as an **anti-codon.** All t-RNAs have the same terminal group of bases CCA and it is the adenine that reacts with the activated amino acid.

The molecule of alanine-t-RNA has been fully studied which is a single stranded molecule. Its structure resembles to that of clover-leaf (clover is a kind of grass) and is as shown below. This has been confirmed by x-ray diffraction techniques.

All transfer RNAs have been found to possess a terminal adenosine which bears a free hydroxyl group at 2' or 3' position of ribose and cytidylic acid at second and third positions. (Fig. 8.11).

Studies have also revealed that t-RNA molecules have a complex structure with extensive internal base-pairing (Figure 8.11). The following points are common to all known t-RNA structures:

1. Guanosine at the 5'-terminal, and the sequence of CCA at the 3'-terminal. The amino acid becomes attached through its carboxyl group, by an ester link to a ribose hydroxyl group of the 3'-terminal adenosine.

2. A 'DHU' loop of 8-12 unpaired bases, which always contains an unusual base called as dihydrouracil.

3. A loop of 7 unpaired bases, containing the sequence Ψ CG, where Ψ is pseudouridine.

4. A loop of seven unpaired bases containing the anticodon which always has uridine base at its 5'-side, and a purine, often methylated on its 3'-side.

5. A smaller loop of variable size is found between the T ψ CG loop and the anticodon loop as shown in the Fig. 8.11).

(c) r-RNA

These RNAs constitute nearly 50 to 60 per cent of the total ribonucleic acid of the cells and are single stranded molecules which are highly elongated. The r-RNA strands are found to be helical at certain portions. The helical portion exhibits hydrogen bonding as per base-pairing rule.

Most of the r-RNA is found to be combined with proteins in macro molecular aggregates called as ribosomes which are found in the cytoplasm and on the cytoplasmic surface of granular endoplasmic reticulum. They are also often called *cytoribosomes*. On the granular endoplasmic reticulum, 5-8 ribosomes are linked by a m-RNA strand to form a linear cluster called **polyribosome** or **polysome** (Fig. 8.12).

Ribosomes may be characterized by their sedimentation constant. Ribosomes possess a sedimentation constant of 80 S and mass of 4.4×10^6 daltons. The 80 S ribosome is made up of two subunits namely a large subunit of 60 S and a small subunit of 40 S.

Primary structure of r-RNA referred to

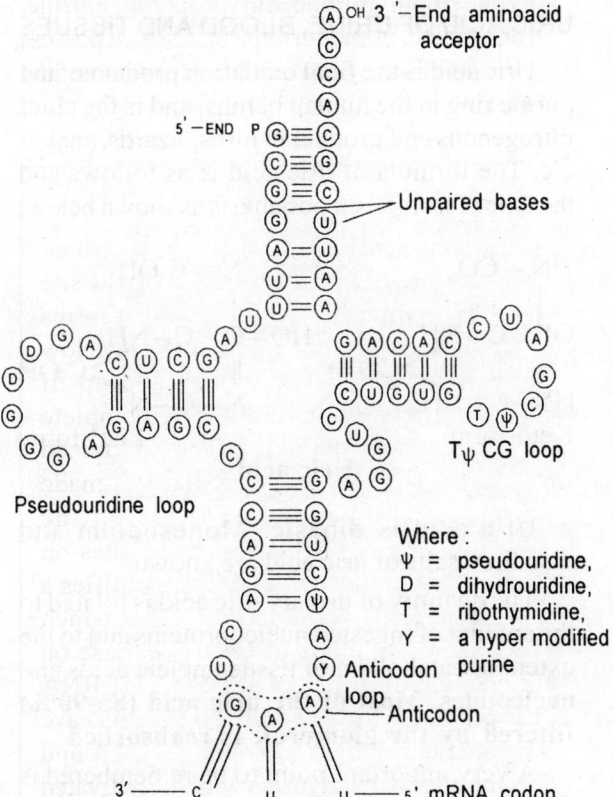

Fig. 8.11 : A possible structure of alanine-t-RNA

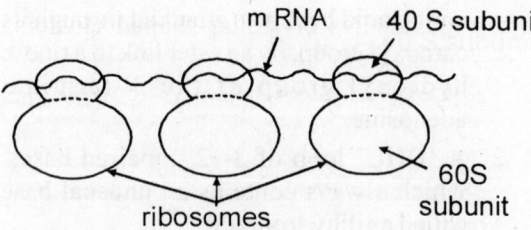

Fig. 8.12 : Polyribosome

the number and sequence of nucleotide (i.e., their bases). For instance, mammalian 5 S, 5.8 S, 18 S and 28 S rRNAs consist of about 120, 160, 1900 and 4,700 bases respectively

---

Ribosomal RNA

Ribosomes are microscopic particles in the cell which are visible only under the electron microscope with a fairly uniform composition of about 60% protein and 40% RNA. These are made up of two parts which can be separated in vitro. In animal cells, the 80 S ribosomes consist of 60 S and 40 S subunits of different chemical composition. Several ribosomes may be attached to a particular strand of m-RNA to form a **'polysome'**, rather like beads on a string.

---

which include mainly adenine, guanine, cytosine and uracil and a few pseudouridines. Besides the major bases, some minor nitrogenous bases may also be found.

Secondary structure of r-RNA consists of many short double-helical stems interconnected by single stranded loops. Each double-helical stem is formed by hydrogen bonds.

(d) Viral-RNA

Viruses which infect the animal and plant cells are mostly ribonucleoproteins. The percentage of RNA in such viruses ranges from 1 to 44. So far, the most studied viral-RNA is that of tobacco mosaic virus (TMV). **TMV is rod like in shape,** approximately 3,000 Å in length and 170

Å in diameter.

Viral-RNAs are single stranded helical molecules which generally possess molecular weight of nearly 2.2×10^6. However, the M.W. of different types of viral-RNAs may range from 1.2×10^6 to 32×10^6. They have been found to have 6,400 mononucleotides in their molecules. Each helix has a radius of 40 Å and has been found to contain some 49 nucleotides per turn. Adenylic acid remains present at the terminal nucleotide at each end. The fact that the RNA molecule remains covered by the protein molecule has been established. Careful separation of the protein part of viral nucleoproteins by the sophisticated latest techniques has revealed that it is the nucleic acid portion which is infective and not the protein portion.

URIC ACID OF URINE, BLOOD AND TISSUES

Uric acid is the final oxidation product of the purine ring in the human beings, and is the chief nitrogenous end product in birds, lizards, snakes etc. The formula of uric acid is as follows and the type of isomerism possible is as shown below:

$$
\begin{array}{cc}
\begin{array}{l}
HN-CO \\
\quad | \qquad | \\
OC \quad C-NH \\
\quad | \qquad \| \qquad \rangle CO \\
HN-C-NH
\end{array}
\rightleftharpoons
&
\begin{array}{l}
N=C.OH \\
\quad \| \qquad | \\
HO-C \quad C-NH \\
\quad \| \qquad \| \qquad \rangle C.OH \\
N-C-N
\end{array}
\end{array}
$$

Keto-form   Enol-form

Uric acid

Uric acid is dibasic. Monosodium and disodium salts of uric acid are known.

The quantity of urinary uric acid is related to the amount of ingested nucleoproteins and to the extent of catabolism of tissue nucleic acids and nucleotides. **Most of the uric acid (85-90%) filtered by the glomeruli is reabsorbed.**

A very important point to be remembered is that in leukemia where the destruction of leukocytes takes place rapidly, output of uric acid gets tremendously increased. This is also true in the diseases of the liver and organs rich in nucleoproteins. There is always found disturbed metabolism of uric acid in the disease **'gout'**, the biochemistry of which is not yet very clear. It is seen that prior to an attack of gout, the urinary output of uric acid gets somewhat decreased and after the attack, it gets increased and remains increased for several days. Uric acid forms salts with sodium, calcium, magnesium, ammonium and potassium to give corresponding urates. Uric acid crystals may be easily distinguished in a sediment of urine sample under microscope (Figs. 8.13 and 8.14).

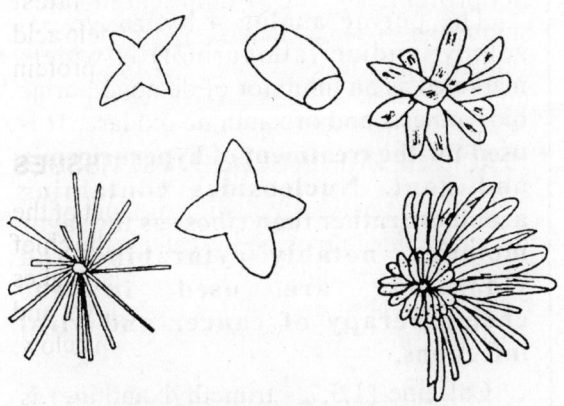

Fig. 8.13 : Uric acid crystals

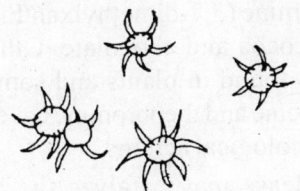

Fig. 8.14 : Ammonium urate crystals

Uric acid crystals when aggregate to form clusters, give rise to troublesome stones either in the kidneys or the bladder. The largest contribution in the formation of stones in the kidneys is that of calcium oxalate crystals; then phosphate crystals and then the least contribution is of uric acid crystals. The acid sodium urate may form

clusters of needles or stellar-shaped clusters. Ammonium urate crystals are often spherical and generally covered with spikes. They are also referred to as **"thorn apple" crystals.** (Fig. 8.14). These are usually pigmented. In addition, they may exhibit many **'bizarre'** shapes. **The range of uric acid in normal human plasma is from 2 to 6 mg per cent, averaging 4 mg%. Values for females is a little on lower side averaging to about 3.5 mg% than their counterparts i.e. males who have an average value of about 4.5 mg%.** Red blood cells appear to contain about half as much uric acid as in plasma. Uric acid appears to be very irregularly distributed in tissues.

Following are the four types of "Gout'

1. *Primary metabolic gout:* This is caused due to an overproduction of uric acid, **due to genetic defects which promote the *de novo* purine synthesis. It is characterized by high levels of blood and urinary urates, rise in the miscible uric acid pool, accumulation of uric acid and urates in cartilages and joints, urate calculi in kidneys and renal damage.** These urate deposits are referred to as *tophi.* Such deposits in the joints provoke a painful inflammatory condition; for some reason it has been observed that the joints at the base of the big toe get especially susceptible; such a condition is known as **acute gouty arthritis.** The chronic inflammatory changes induced by the depositions of sodium urate tophi can generate **chronic gouty arthritis,** eventually resulting in the destruction of joints. The exact mechanism for the deposition of such urates is not yet clear.

2. *Secondary metabolic gout:* **It results from a secondary increase**

in the catabolism of purines in various states like prolonged fasting, leukaemia and polycythaemia etc. In this type, more breakdown of tissues takes place as a result of which system gets loaded with unusually high amount of nucleotides.

3. **Primary renal gout: This is caused due to the failure of urate excretion by the renal tubules which is due to the genetic deficiency of the urate transport system in renal tubules.** This type of gout does not involve any over production of uric acid.

4. **Secondary renal gout: This results from a failure of urate elimination in the glomerular filtrate** which is due to a generalized renal failure in the kidney disorder called **glomerulonephritis.**

Effect of Diet (Also consult Chapter 15)

Excretion of uric acid continues at a rather constant rate during starvation and purine-free diet due to the so-called endogenous (tissue) purine metabolism. **The ingestion of foods high in nucleoproteins, such as glandular organs, produce a marked increase; whereas a diet of milk, eggs, and cheese (very low in purine content), causes practically no elevation in uric acid excretion.**

Treatment of Gout (Also consult Chapter 15)

The classic treatment for gout is the administration of **colchicine, a drug which has got the tendency to interrupt the mitosis of leucocytes** and thus prevents development of inflammation. It is believed that the inflammation is a consequence of phagocytosis of urate crystals by the leucocytes that invade the

Cancers are made up of cells that continue to divide indefinitely. Since cell division requires a net synthesis of nucleic acids, there has been considerable effect made to find compounds that will selectively inhibit the formation of nucleic acids and check the uncontrolled growth of cancer.

Synthetic analogs of nucleobases, nucleosides and nucleotides are widely used in medical sciences and clinical medicine. One of the most important components of the oncologist's pharmacopeia is the group of synthetic analogs of purine and pyrimidine nucleobases and nucleosides.

The purine analog 4-hydroxypyrazolopyrimidine (allopurinol) is widely marketed as an inhibitor of de novo purine biosynthesis and of xanthine oxidase. **It is used for the treatment of hyperuricemia and gout. Nucleosides containing arabinose rather than ribose as the sugar moieties, notably cytarabine and vidarabine are used in the chemotherapy of cancer and viral infections.**

Caffeine (1,3,7 - trimethylxanthine) is found in coffee, tea and other plants; theobromine (3,7-dimethylxanthine) occurs in tea, cocoa and chocolate. Other purines are also found in plants and some of these like caffeine and theobromine have important pharmacological actions.

Nuclease may catalyze the hydrolysis specifically of DNA and RNA or they may attack both kinds of polynucleotide. These enzymes are generally of two types:

(i) **Exonucleases:** Which require a terminus at which to initiate hydrolysis, and

(ii) **Endonucleases:** Which do not require a terminus and which may attack at one or many sites within a polynucleotide.

affected area. Various compounds which promote the excretion of urate by the kidneys have been introduced as a means of controlling gout.

More recently, **a competitive inhibitor of xanthine oxidase has been developed to control gout by preventing the formation of urate** so that excess purines are excreted as hypoxanthine and xanthine; **this compound is known as allopurinol** and differs from hypoxanthine in the distribution of ring nitrogens. The rationale for its use is that hypoxanthine and xanthine will not precipitate in the joints. Hypoxanthine is more soluble than urate, although xanthine is not. Allopurinol also is not a completely safe drug.

Allopurinol

LESCH-NYHAN SYNDROME

Rare patients afflicted with a condition named as **Lesch-Nyhan Syndrome** may be met with once in a while; **this disease is caused by a hereditary deficiency of GMP pyrophosphorylase. This x-linked recessive disease is peculiarly horrifying because children suffering from it mutilate (damage their own organs/body parts) themselves.** Characteristically, they will bite off the tips of their own fingers or bite their lips if their hands are protected i.e. tied upon with some string/ rope etc. The aggressive attacks may be of serious nature like biting of others or as age advances, may use obscene abusive language. The pathos of the affliction is accentuated by the tendency of the children to be very likable and open, quick to laugh and capable of warm affection. The climax is that such children get sometime terrified of their own aggression; they may even scream under the cover of fear and may bite their fingers seriously. Patients suffering from this disease have a tendency to excrete large quantities of uric acid - more per unit of body mass than is seen in any other condition. Their synthesis of purines is extraordinarily rapid (of course, they also become gouty as an additional distress).

The missing enzyme i.e. GMP pyrophosphorylase is responsible for the salvage (protection from loss) of free guanine and hypoxanthine by converting them to the corresponding nucleoside monophosphates. This enzyme is found to be more active in brain, which has over 10-fold more enzyme than does the liver.

Genetic Tracing of Fatherhood

DNA finger printing technology now available in our country in various upgraded well equipped laboratories is a very good mean in establishing **paternity.**

This technology is responsible in establishing fatherhood while dealing with cases where a husband has abandoned his wife. Previously there did not exist any specific law to take action against culprits who abandoned their wives and children taking advantage of absence of any legally admissible evidence of their marriage to these women. **This technology is a 'full proof' method in establishing paternity scientifically.**

ENZYMES AND ISOENZYMES

ENZYMES

Enzymes are biological catalysts (biocatalysts) which bring about chemical reactions in living cells. They accelerate the rate of the reaction and are usually present in very small amount in various cells. They can also exhibit their activity when they have been extracted from the source. They are organic compounds and a number of them have been obtained in crystalline form. **Today, more than 840 enzymes are known.**

General properties of the enzymes:

1. They are proteinous in nature.
2. They accelerate the rate of the reaction by:
   (a) not altering the reaction equilibrium.
   (b) being required in minute quantity.
   (c) being not consumed in the overall reaction.
3. They act as catalysts, deficiency of which may diminish the rate of a particular reaction; whereas complete absence of it may completely block a particular reaction.
4. They are very specific for their substrates.

5. They possess active sites at which interaction with substrate occurs.
6. They are responsible for lowering the activation energy.
7. **Some enzymes are regulatory in function.**

Enzyme Cofactors, Coenzymes, Prosthetic Groups

In addition to the protein component, many enzymes require nonprotein constituents for their proper functioning. In some cases these components, broadly described as cofactors, may be metal ions and, in other cases, organic molecules of relatively low molecular weight. When the small organic molecules are tightly bound either by covalent or coordinate bonds, they are called as **prosthetic groups. The heme group of the cytochromes is an example of a prosthetic group.**

Pyridoxal phosphate, a slightly modified form of vitamin B_6 (pyridoxine), is an essential cofactor or coenzyme, for an important group of enzymes known collectively as *transaminases*. As the name implies, these enzymes transfer α-amino group from an amino acid to a α-keto acid.

Coenzymes

Coenzymes are organic molecules, often derived from the B vitamins, that participate directly in enzymatic reactions. Some coenzymes are attached to their companion enzymes as tightly bound prosthetic groups, whereas others can be easily removed by dialysis. The complete functional complex of enzyme and cofactors is called a *holoenzyme;* the protein part, free of the cofactors, is called an *apoenzyme.*

Characteristics of coenzymes:

1. They are stable towards heat.
2. Generally derived from vitamins.
3. Function as co-substrates.
4. They participate in:
   - (a) Electron transfer reactions, e.g. NAD^+, NADH, FMN, FAD, etc.
   - (b) Group transfer reactions e.g., CoA, TPP, pyridoxal phosphate, tetrahydrofolic acid, etc.

Coenzymes	Functions performed
1. NAD^+	Hydrogen transfer
2. $NADP^+$	Hydrogen transfer
3. FAD	Hydrogen transfer
4. FMN	Hydrogen transfer
5. TPP (Thiamine pyrophosphate)	Acetyl group transfer
6. PP (Pyridoxal phosphate)	Amino group transfer
7. Biotin	Carboxyl group transfer
8. Coenzyme A	Acyl group transfer

Nicotinamide nucleotides

NAD^+, $NADP^+$ and their reduced forms are involved in a great variety of dehydrogenase reactions in the mitochondria, cytosol and endoplasmic reticulum of the cell. They are water soluble, and are usually free to diffuse away from the enzyme after conversion to the oxidized or

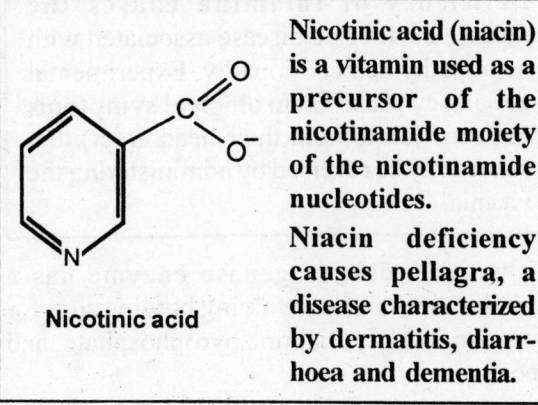

*NADP⁺ has PO₄ here

Nicotinamide adenine dinucleotide (NAD); NADP is nicotinamide adenine dinucleotide phosphate.
* $NADP^+$ has got PO_4 in place of OH

reduced form, to take part in another dehydrogenase reaction catalysed by another enzyme.

Nicotinic acid (niacin) is a vitamin used as a precursor of the nicotinamide moiety of the nicotinamide nucleotides.

Niacin deficiency causes pellagra, a disease characterized by dermatitis, diarrhoea and dementia.

Nicotinic acid

Flavin nucleotide coenzymes:

FAD is the coenzyme of a class of dehydrogenases known as flavoproteins. The flavin moiety of the molecule is derived from riboflavin (vitamin B_2).

Flavin mononucleotide (FMN) is an important coenzyme in some flavoproteins, including NADH coenzyme Q reductase, etc.

FMN consists of riboflavin phosphate (i.e., FAD without the adenosine monophosphate moiety).

Flavin coenzymes remain tightly bound to the enzyme protein throughout the reaction, in contrast to the nicotinamide coenzymes that bind reversibly to the enzyme.

A number of mitochondrial dehydrogenases are flavoproteins; for example, NADH dehydrogenase, succinate dehydrogenase and fatty acyl CoA dehydrogenase.

Thiamine pyrophosphate

Thiamine (Vitamin B_1) is the precursor of thiamine pyrophosphate, the coenzyme for some important oxidative decarboxylation reactions (pyruvate dehydrogenase, oxoglutarate dehydrogenase).

In oxidative decarboxylation, loss of CO_2 is accompanied by oxidation of an aldehyde to an acid.

Deficiency of thiamine causes the disease beriberi, a disease associated with neuropathy and cardiopathy. Experimental deficiency causes **neurological symptoms** (pigeons fail to hold their head erect) that can readily be reversed by administering the vitamin.

Pyruvate dehydrogenase enzyme has a complex mechanism involving binding sites for pyruvate, NAD^+, thiamine pyrophosphate and lipoic acid.

Pyridoxal phosphate

Pyridoxal phosphate (derivative of vitamin B_6) acts as a coenzyme in transamination and decarboxylation reactions. In a transamination reaction the aldehyde group of pyridoxal phosphate first forms a Schiff's base with the amino group of the amino acid, which is then converted to keto acid. Pyridoxal phosphate is thereby converted to pyridoxamine phosphate which transfers the amino group to another keto acid to form an amino acid.

Pyridoxal phosphate also acts as a coenzyme in decarboxylation reactions of amino acids such as :

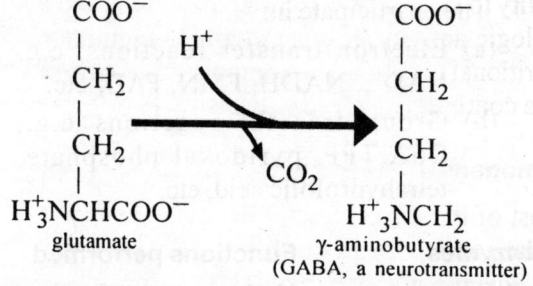

$$
\begin{array}{c}
COO^- \\
| \\
CH_2 \\
| \\
CH_2 \\
| \\
H_3^+NCHCOO^- \\
\text{glutamate}
\end{array}
\xrightarrow[\ \ \ CO_2\ \ \ ]{H^+}
\begin{array}{c}
COO^- \\
| \\
CH_2 \\
| \\
CH_2 \\
| \\
H_3^+NCH_2 \\
\gamma\text{-aminobutyrate} \\
\text{(GABA, a neurotransmitter)}
\end{array}
$$

Vitamin B_6 deficiency is rare in man, because the vitamin is widely distributed in common foodstuffs and in addition is synthesized in appreciable quantities by intestinal flora. The main abnormality seen in B_6 deficiency is dermatitis which is readily cured by the administration of the vitamin.

Biotin

It is an essential food factor and is a coenzyme for carboxylation reactions (e.g. pyruvate carboxylase). These reactions involve ATP, which is necessary in the first step of the reaction; this is the conversion of biotin to carboxybiotin by the addition of CO_2 to C-1 of biotin.

Pantothenic acid is an essential food factor which forms part of coenzyme A.

Coenzyme A

It is a complex molecule which contains a free sulfhydryl (-SH) group. This group can react with a carboxyl group to form a thioester. Such thiolesters are involved in many reactions involving acyl groups, including acetyl and fatty acyl groups.

Enzyme and cofactor turnover

Like all biologic materials, enzymes have a finite half-life; that is, they are subject to turnover and replacement. Therefore, a diet must include sufficient essential amino acids, metals and vitamins to provide enzyme replacement, among other needs. Human beings have only a limited ability to store most essential metal ions and the biologic activity of most vitamins requires the nutritional needs for the components of enzymes on a continuing everyday basis.

Zymogens or proenzymes

Most of the intracellular enzymes are secreted in their active forms known as **Zymase** form of the enzyme but side by side few enzymes are secreted in their inactive forms known as **proenzymes** or **zymogens**.These enzymes (proenzymes/zymogens) have a tendency to undergo prior change in structure after coming into contact with certain activating agents.Activating agent may be H^+, another enzyme on the active form of the zymogen itself. For instance gastric juice contains pepsin which is secreted by pepsinogen (a zymogen). **Pepsinogen (Fig 9.1) is changed into its active form pepsin by H^+ of the gastric juice.**

Once formed pepsin itself acts on pepsinogen and catalyses its own conversion into pepsin;such a process is called as **autocatalysis** (Fig 9.1)

Thus, **zymogens** are inactive precursors of enzymes that are primarily concerned with proteolytic activity. The important examples of this category are the enzymes found in the gastrointestinal tract that act on dietary proteins. This unique process is probably involved with the protection of tissues from digestion by their own proteolytic enzymes.

Important examples of the enzymes that occur as zymogens are as follows:

Zymogem	activator	active enzyme
Pepsinogen	H^+, pepsin	pepsin
Trypsinogen	trypsin, enterokinase	trypsin
Chymotrypsinogen	trypsin	chymotrypsin
Procarboxy-peptidase	trypsin	carboxy-peptidase
Proelastase	trypsin	elastase
Prorennin	H^+, rennin	rennin

> **Pepsin is the major proteolytic enzyme found in the stomach. Pepsinogen has a M.W. of 42,500 and is converted by acid or pepsin itself to active pepsin with a M.W. of 34,500.** The conversion is accompanied by the removal of one-fifth of the peptide chain(in the form of six peptides).

Allosteric Enzymes

Some of the enzymes possess additional sites known as allosteric sites (Greek:allo-other) besides the active site. Such enzymes are known as allosteric or regulatory enzymes. The allosteric sites are the unique places on the enzyme molecule.

These enzymes are regulated by certain substances called allosteric modulators (effectors) which reversibly bind to the enzyme at the allosteric site. An interaction with the

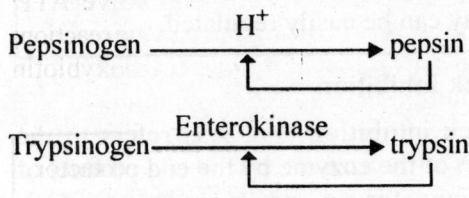

Fig. 9.1 : Activation of a zymogen

effector molecule brings about conformational changes in the catalytic site of the enzyme. The binding of the effector molecule may inhibit the enzymatic reaction (called as allosteric inhibition); such an effector molecule is called as a negative effector (allosteric inhibitor). Contrarily, an effector may also activate the enzymatic reaction (called as allosteric activation) and is called a positive effector (allosteric activator).

Examples of this category are (i) HMG CoA reductase is a regulatory enzyme of cholesterol biosynthesis, where as aspartate transcarbamoylase is the regulatory enzyme for pyrimidine synthesis.

If the effector substance is the substrate itself then it is called as **homotropic effect;** contrarily, if the effector molecule is a substance other than the substrate then it is called as the **hetrotropic effect.** Removal of inhibition can be brought about by increasing the amount of the inhibitor. Mechanism of action of allosteric enzymes can be very well understood by the following Figure 9.2.

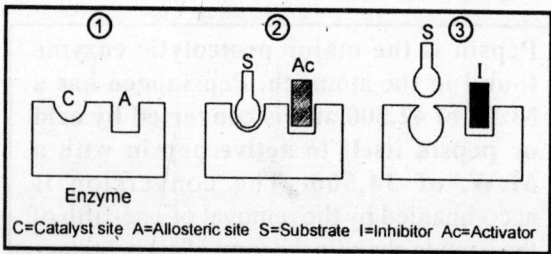

Enzyme

C=Catalyst site A=Allosteric site S=Substrate I=Inhibitor Ac=Activator

Fig. 9.2 : Action of allosteric enzymes: (1) The enzyme has separate catalytic (C) and allosteric (A) sites (2) When activator (Ac) is fixed, the catalytic site assumes correct three dimensional structure, so that substrate(S) can combine, (3) When inhibitor (I) is attached, catalytic site is altered, so that substrate is not engaged.

A few examples of allosteric enzymes are as follows:

(a) succinylCoA+glycine $\xrightarrow{\text{ALA synthase}}$ δ-amino-levulinic acid (ALA)

This is the first step in the synthesis of heme. Here the end product i.e.,

heme will allosterically inhibit the enzyme ALA synthase which is the key enzyme of heme synthesis.

(b) Carbamoyl phosphate + asparate

$\downarrow$ Asparate transcarbamoylase

carbamoyl asparate

This is the first step in the biosynthesis of cytidine triphosphate(CTP).Here ,the end product i.e.,CTP will allosterically inhibit the enzyme asparate transcarbamoylase.

(c) Inhibition of enzyme HMG CoA reductase by cholesterol (the end product of cholesterol biosynthesis) is another example of allosteric inhibition.

(d) **Phosphofructokinase (PFK) which catalyzes the phosphorylation of fructose-6-phosphate to fructose- 1, 6 -diphosphate is the rate limiting enzyme of glycolysis. This enzyme is allosterically inhibited by ATP and citrate but allosterically activated by AMP and fructose-6-phosphate.**

Allosteric enzymes are utilized by the body for regulating various metabolic pathways. Such a regulatory enzyme in a particular pathway is called as a **key enzyme or rate limiting enzyme.** The flow of the whole pathway is constrained as if there is a bottle-neck at the level of the key enzyme. The allosteric inhibitor is most effective when substrate concentration is low. This is metabolically very significant. When more substrate molecules are available, automatically there is less necessity for stringent regulation. In this way, the whole pathway can be easily regulated.

Feedback inhibition

Feed back inhibition (Fig 9.3) refers to the inhibition of the enzyme by the end product of the reactions, for e.g., when a substrate (A) is converted to a product (P) through various intermediates (B, C,D, E, etc), the end product of the reaction inhibits the first enzyme of the pathway (Fig 9.3). In this type of inhibition, the accumulation of the end product slows down the whole reaction sequence and since the end product continues to be consumed, its synthesis continues. Since it is partially competitive, both V_{max} and K_m are altered.

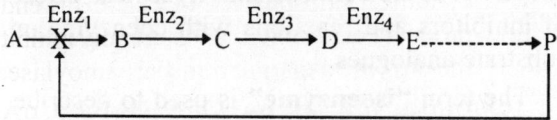

Fig. 9.3 : Feedback Inhibition

As it is a mixed type of inhibition, the inhibitor binds to the enzyme at a site other than the active site called as **allosteric site** which is encountered in **allosteric enzymes.**

Feedback inhibition is a type of regulatory mechanism which has been identified in many instances and is especially interesting since it is a self- regulatory device allowing a cell to adjust the rate of synthesis of a metabolic intermediate to its everchanging needs. One important classical example of it involves the synthesis of CTP in **Escherichia coli.** Early in this reaction sequence, carbamoyl phosphate is converted to carbamoyl aspartate by the enzyme **aspartate transcarbamoylase.** This reaction is crucial, since its inhibition affects the subsequent reactions leading to CTP. This enzyme is sensitive to inhibition by CTP. As the reaction sequence produces CTP, and when the CTP is not used rapidly enough in subsequent reactions (e.g., incorporation into nucleic acids), a critical concentration of CTP is reached, which inhibits aspartate transcarbamoylase. The result is a decrease in the synthesis of CTP until its concentration is lowered below the level at which the enzyme is inhibited.

Classification of Enzymes

As per international classification, **the enzymes** have been classified into six major classes, each with several subclasses; within each subclass, formal names have been assigned to the known enzymes to describe the reactions they catalyze. Trivial names for many enzymes, for example, pepsin, trypsin, urease, etc. are still very common and easy to remember as well. Many enzymes are still easier to recognize them by their trivial names. The newer nomenclature has been less widely adopted due to its own complications.

No.	Major classes	Examples
1.	Oxidoreductases	Alcohol dehydrogenase, xanthine oxidase.
2.	Transferases	Hexokinase, etc.
3.	Hydrolases	Glucose-6-phosphatase, pepsin, carboxypeptidase
4.	Lyases	Aldolase, pyruvate decarboxylase
5.	Isomerases	Phosphotriose isomerase, phosphoglucomutase
6.	Ligases	Glutamine synthetase, glutathione synthetase

Six major classes are:

1. *Oxidoreductases:* They catalyze a wide variety of oxidation-reduction reactions and frequently employ coenzymes such as NAD^+, $NADP^+$, FAD, or lipoate as the hydrogen acceptor. Other acceptors include coenzyme Q or molecular oxygen. **Common trivial names include dehydrogenase, oxidase, peroxides, and reductase.**

2. *Transferases:* They catalyze various kinds of group transfers. Many important steps in metabolism require transfer from one molecule to another of amino, carboxyl, carbonyl, methyl, acyl, glycosyl, or phosphoryl groups. **Common trivial names include amino transferase (transaminase), acyl carnitine transferase and transcarboxylase.**

3. *Hydrolases:* They catalyze cleavage of

bonds between a carbon and some other atom by addition of water. **Some common trivial names include esterase, peptidase, amylase, urease, phosphatase, pepsin, trypsin and chymotrypsin.**

4. *Lyases:* They catalyze breakage of carbon-carbon, carbon-sulphur and certain carbon-nitrogen (excluding peptide bonds. **Common trivial names include decarboxylase, aldolase, citrate lyase and dehydratase.**

5. *Isomerases:* They catalyze racemization of optical or geometric isomers and certain intramolecular oxidation-reduction reactions. **Trivial names include epimerase, racemase, and mutase.**

6. *Ligases:* These catalyze the formation of bonds between carbon and oxygen, sulphur, nitrogen and other atoms. The energy required for bond formation is frequently derived from the hydrolysis of ATP. **Some trivial names include synthetase and carboxylase.**

Isomeric enzymes or isoenzymes or isozymes (Multiple molecular forms of enzymes)

A particular enzyme obtained from different times often has certain physicochemical properties which are characteristic of the tissue

---

of origin, although the same chemical reaction is catalyzed in each case. Electrophoresis and chromatography in particular are the two techniques which are most frequently used to separate and 'finger print' these multiple molecular forms. Different physicochemical properties of the enzymes frequently affect their catalytic activity, so that they often differ in such properties as their Km, sensitivity to heat, effect of inhibitors and reactions with coenzyme or substrate analogues.

The term **"isoenzyme"** is used to describe the multiple form of an enzyme which are distinct proteins, such as those of lactate dehydrogenase, creatine phosphokinase, alkaline phosphatase etc. A single tissue may contain more than one form of an enzyme, for instance, kidney contains isoenzymes of alkaline phosphatase which may be separated from each other with the help of column chromatography on diethylaminoethyl-cellulose (DEAE-Cellulose).

Lactate dehydrogenase which has thoroughly been studied is composed of four subunits. There are two different subunits that can be combined into tetramers in five ways. The possible combinations can be separated by electrophoresis as shown in Figures 9.4 and 9.5. If one subunit type is identified as "M" (the major form found in muscle or liver) and the second as "H" (the major form found in heart), then the tetramers could have the compositions M_4, M_3H, M_2H_2, MH_3, or H_4. These can be separated from each other by electrophoresis.

Examples of Isoenzymes are:
1. Lactate dehydrogenase **(LDH)**
2. Creatine phosphokinase **(CPK or CK)**
3. Alkaline phosphatase **(ALP)**
4. Malate dehydrogenase
5. Carbonic anhydrase
6. Hexokinase
7. Phosphorylase
8. Glucose-6-phosphate dehydrogenase, etc.

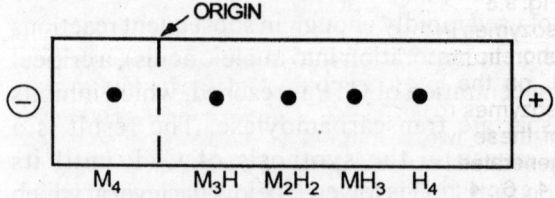

Fig. 9.4: Electrophoresis of lactate dehydrogenase isoenzymes at pH 8.6

In man, the content of several isoenzymes differs in heart and liver. Although the reason for this is not known, use is made of the fact in diagnostic differentiation of diseases of the liver and myocardium. In both types of disease states, lactate dehydrogenase leaks out of the damaged cells and increases the concentration of the enzyme in blood serum. Differentiation can be based in part on the pattern that appears on electrophoresis and in part on the fact that some of the isoenzymes from the myocardium are

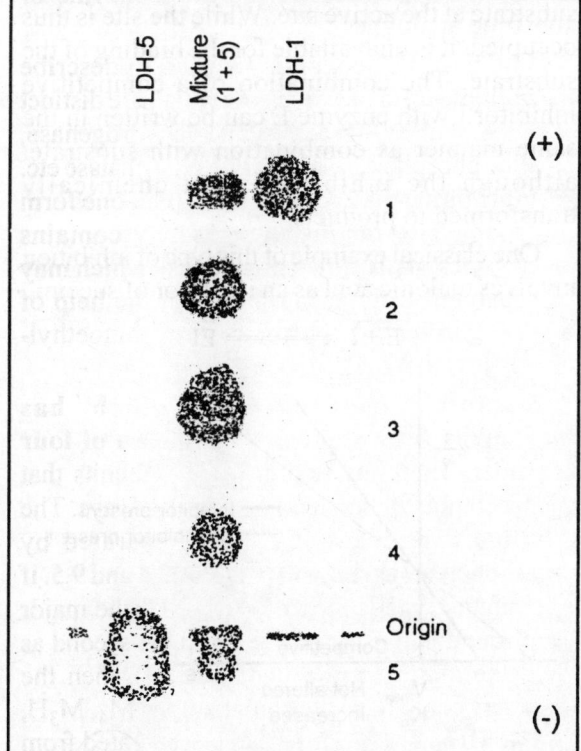

Fig. 9.5: This photograph shows the LDH isozymes in each of three preparations after electrophoretic resolution in starch gel. On the right is LDH-1, on the left LDH-5, and in the middle are the isozymes resulting from a mixture of equal quantities of these two preparations. All five isozymes were generated in the mixture in the approximate ratio of 1 : 4 : 6 : 4 : 1, the expected distribution after random reassociation of subunits. The total enzyme activity in the mixture was the sum of the activities of the single isozyme preparations. All three preparations were placed in 1 M NaCl and frozen overnight before electrohoretic resolution.

more resistant to heat denaturation than the corresponding hepatic isozymes. In the simpler differential test situation, a serum sample may be analyzed twice, once before and once after heat denaturation under carefully controlled conditions.

Clinically Important Enzyme Inhibitors

Enzymes may also be inactivated or denatured by a variety of chemical means, several of which have clinical importance. Many enzymes depend on essential sulfhydryl groups, which form tight covalent bonds with various heavy metals. For this reason mercury, lead, silver, etc are extremely toxic. **Even iron and copper, although they are classed as essential minerals, can produce intoxication when ingested in excess.**

Another class of inhibitors affects enzymes by introducing foreign alkyl groups into the structure. Most of these substances were initially developed as chemical warfare agents and are highly toxic in nature. Two best known are:

(a) diisopropylfluorophosphate (DFP), and

(b) the so called nitrogen mustards, for example, methachloramine and 2, 2'-dichloro-N-methyldiethylamine.

These, so called, nitrogen mustards are now employed clinically as enzyme inhibitors in the treatment of certain types of neoplastic diseases.

Enzyme inhibitors are:
1. Mercury
2. Lead
3. Silver
4. DFP
5. Various insecticides used in agriculture
6. Nitrogen mustards

The organic phosphates, of which DFP is only one example, are particularly good inhibitors of acetylcholinesterase, which breaks down the neurotransmitter substance known as acetylcholine. **Inactivation of acetylcholinesterase produces violent spasms of the pulmonary system and interferes with normal neuromuscular and cardiac functions.** Similar agents employed as insecticides in agriculture may be severely or fatally toxic.

Enzyme Inhibition

The rate of an enzyme-catalyzed reaction can be decreased by specific inhibitors, i.e., compounds that combine with the enzyme and prevent normal enzyme substrate interactions in the active site, thus diminishing the rate of the reaction. Certain enzymic inhibitors are poisonous for living organisms, including cyanide, hydrogen sulfide and carbon monoxide. Many drugs are also inhibitors of metabolic reactions and molecular pharmacology is largely dependent on the knowledge of inhibition of enzymes.

Application of enzyme inhibition

1. Studies on enzyme inhibition have led to the development of hundreds of new drugs for use in medicine and veterinary science.
2. Enzyme inhibition studies have been directed specifically toward increasing our understanding of specific reactions or metabolic pathways in animals and plants.
3. Enzyme inhibition studies have also led to the development of nerve gases, insecticides and herbicides (weed killers).

Types of Inhibition

Many substances inhibit enzymes and reduce the initial velocity (increase 1/v). The Lineweaver-Burk plots reveal the mechanism of the inhibition. **Following four types of inhibitions are known:**

1. **Competitive inhibition,**
2. **Non-competitive inhibition,**
3. **Partially competitive inhibition, and**
4. **Uncompetitive inhibition.**

1. Competitive Inhibition

In this type of inhibition (Fig. 9.6), competitive inhibitors can combine reversibly with the active site of the enzyme and compete with the substrate at the active site. While the site is thus occupied, it is unavailable for the binding of the substrate. The combination of a competitive inhibitor I with enzyme E can be written in the same manner as combination with substrate, although the inhibitor is not chemically transformed to products.

One classical example of this type of inhibition involves malonic acid as an inhibitor of succinic

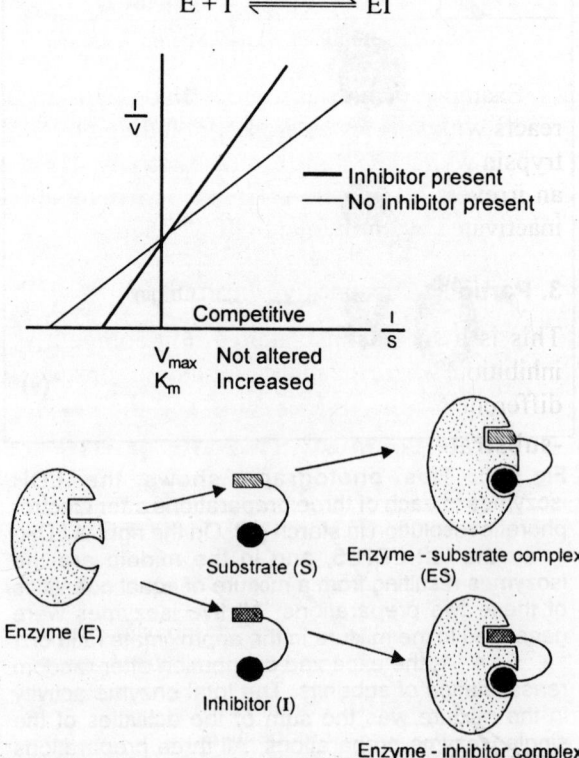

$$E + I \rightleftharpoons EI$$

Inhibitor present
No inhibitor present

Competitive

V_{max} Not altered
K_m Increased

Enzyme (E)
Substrate (S)
Inhibitor (I)
Enzyme - substrate complex (ES)
Enzyme - inhibitor complex **(EI)**

Fig. 9.6 : Showing Competitive Inhibition of an enzyme

dehydrogenase. This enzyme forms complexes and with the proper concentrations of reactants, succinate is not dehydrogenated (oxidized) to fumaric acid. On the other hand, with sufficient succinate present, the inhibition by malonate can be completely overcome.

2. Noncompetitive Inhibition

In this type, inhibition occurs when the inhibitor binds to a site on the enzyme other than the active site or binds irreversibly to the active site.

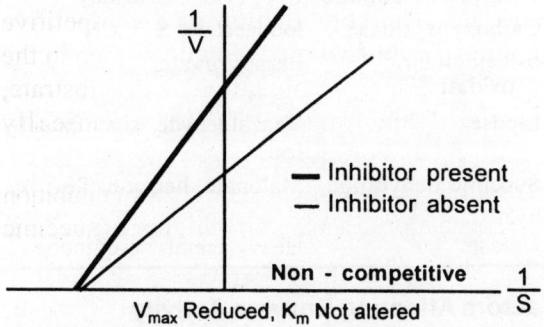

— Inhibitor present
— Inhibitor absent

Non - competitive

V_{max} Reduced, K_m Not altered

Examples include diisopropylfluorophosphate reacts with various esterases including chymotrypsin which has some esterase activity. This is an irreversible reaction. Urease is irreversibly inactivated by ultraviolet light.

3. Partially Competitive Inhibition

This is a special instance of non-competitive inhibition, where the inhibitor binding constant is different for the free enzyme and the enzyme -substrate complex. Two alternatives are

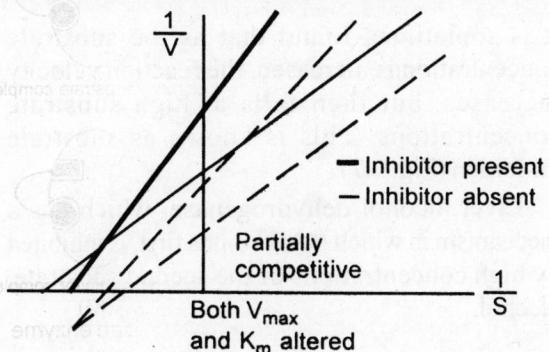

— Inhibitor present
— Inhibitor absent

Partially competitive

Both V_{max} and K_m altered

indicated by the solid and broken lines.

4. Uncompetitive Inhibition

It occurs when the inhibitor binds after the substrate has bound to the enzyme, and then stops the reaction from occurring; eventually no product is formed. This type of inhibition is not reversed by increasing substrate concentration. This type of inhibition is most frequently found in enzymic reactions with two or more substrates.

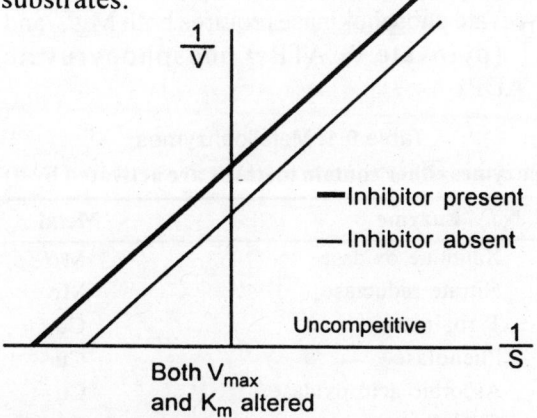

— Inhibitor present
— Inhibitor absent

Uncompetitive

Both V_{max} and K_m altered

Enzyme Activators

Many ions and molecules have the capacity to activate some enzymes. Metal ions are activators of a number of enzymes. Following Table 25.1 shows this relationship. **Pepsin (as proenzyme pepsinogen) is activated by H^+ to form the active enzyme.** Many reducing agents (cysteine, glutathione) act as enzyme activators of-SH enzymes. Enzymes themselves activate other enzymes or proenzymes; i.e., enterokinase activates trypsinogen to form active trypsin.

Enzyme activators are :	
1. Mg^{++}	2. Mn^{++}
3. Cobalt	4 Molybdenum
5. Calcium	6. Copper
7. Iron	8. Zn^{++}
9. Cysteine	10. Glutathione

Many enzymes require a metal ion (Table 9.1) for activity. In some cases, the requirement is specific for a particular metal. Carbonic anhydrase shows no activity upon removal of zinc, and no other metal is known to replace zinc in this enzyme. In other cases, more than one metal is able to bring about activation; for example, Mg^{++}, Mn^{++}, or Zn^{++} activate enolase (2-phosphoglycerate$\rightarrow$phosphoenolpyruvate + H_2O). In a few cases it appears that two metal ions may be required by the enzyme; for example, pyruvate phosphokinase requires both Mg^{++} and K^+ (pyruvate + ATP$\rightarrow$ phosphopyruvate + ADP).

Table 9.1: Metalloenzymes
(Enzymes either contain metal or are activated by it)

Sl. No.	Enzyme	Metal
1.	Xanthine oxidase	Mo
2.	Nitrate reductase	Mo
3.	Tyrosinase	Cu
4.	Phenolase	Cu
5.	Ascorbic acid oxidase	Cu
6.	Cytochrome enzymes	Fe
7.	Catalase	Fe
8.	Peroxidases	Fe
9.	Tryptophan oxidase	Fe
10.	Homogentisicase	Fe
11.	Lecithinases A and C	Ca
12.	Lipases	Ca
13.	Carbonic anhydrase	Zn
14.	Lactic dehydrogenase	Zn
15.	Carboxypeptidase	Zn
16.	Peptidases	Mg
17.	Phosphatases	Mg
18.	ATP-enzymes, such as hexokinases	Mg
19.	Arginase	Mn
20.	Phosphoglucomutase	Mn
21.	Dipeptidases	Mn
22.	Peptidases	Co

Enzyme inhibitors are those which have a tendency to inhibit/ retard or stop the activity of an enzyme.

Some important examples of enzyme inhibitors are as given in Table 9.2:

Table 9.2 : Enzymes and their inhibitors

Enzyme	Inhibitors
Arginase	Ornithine, lysine, L- amino acids
Alkaline phosphatase	Chelating compounds, arsenate, F^-
Carboxylase	$HCHO$, CH_3CHO, C_6H_5CHO
Cholinesterase	Physostigmine, neostigmine
Carbonic anhydrase	CO, sulfanilamide
Cytochrome oxidase	CN^-, H_2S, CO, azide
Carboxypeptidase	Iodoacetate, S^{--}, CN^-
α-Ketoglutaric oxidase	Parapyruvate
Lipase	Benzaldehyde, some metal ions
Succinic dehydroge-nase	Malonate, hematin, Se
Urease	Heavy metals, o-quinone

Factors Affecting Enzyme Activity

Major factors responsible to affect the enzymic activity are the following:

1. Concentration of substrate
2. Concentration of enzyme
3. Concentration of reaction products
4. Effect of pH
5. Effect of temperature and
6. Effect of time

Substrate concentration

It is sometimes found that as the substrate concentration is increased, the reaction velocity increases, but then falls at high substrate concentrations. This is known as substrate inhibition (Fig. 9.7).

Liver alcohol dehydrogenase, which has a mechanism in which NAD^+ binds first, is inhibited by high concentrations of the second substrate, alcohol.

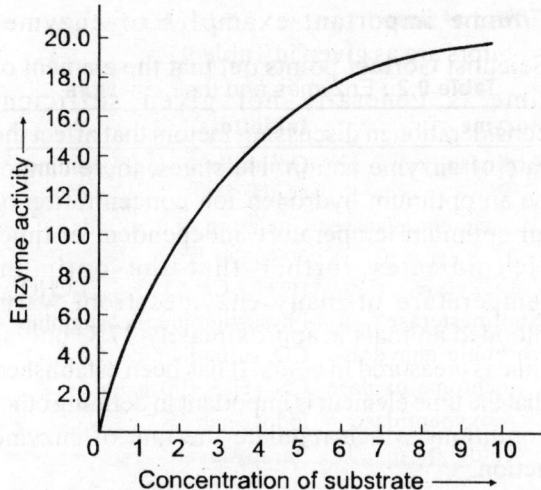

Fig. 9.7 : Effect of substrate concentration on enzyme activity

Concentration of enzyme

Within fairly wide limits the speed of an enzymatic reaction is proportional to the enzyme concentration. This can be shown to hold for many enzyme systems, provided interfering conditions do not develop and the substrate concentration is maintained constant (Fig. 9.8).

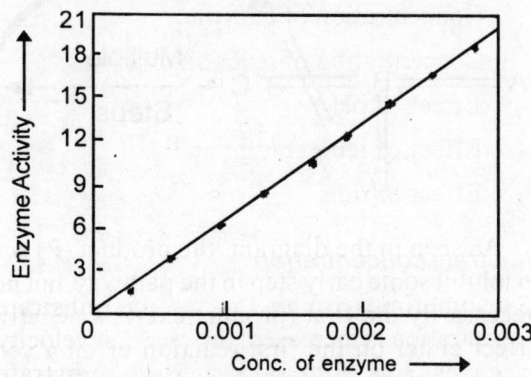

Fig 9.8 : Effect of enzyme concentration on enzyme activity

Concentration of reaction products

An enzyme-product complex is part of the reaction sequence of enzyme-catalysed reactions. In the presence of large concentrations of product, this complex is dominant and product inhibition is observed. This is one of the reasons why the velocity of the reaction falls as the equilibrium is approached and it is of physiological importance in controlling pathways by negative feedback. In single-product enzymes as shown below in equation, addition of the product causes reversal of the reaction, but if there are two or more products, both are needed for reversal to occur, so inhibition of the forward reaction by each can be studied separately.

$$E + S \underset{k_2}{\overset{k_1}{\rightleftharpoons}} ES \xrightarrow{k_3} E + P$$

Usually each product is competitive with the substrate from which it is derived, e.g. see 'box'.

Effect of pH

Each enzyme has a pH optimum- i.e., a H^+ concentration at which the enzyme reacts at maximum speed. Very slight changes toward either side of the pH optimum may result in profound alterations of reaction rates, (Fig. 9.9).

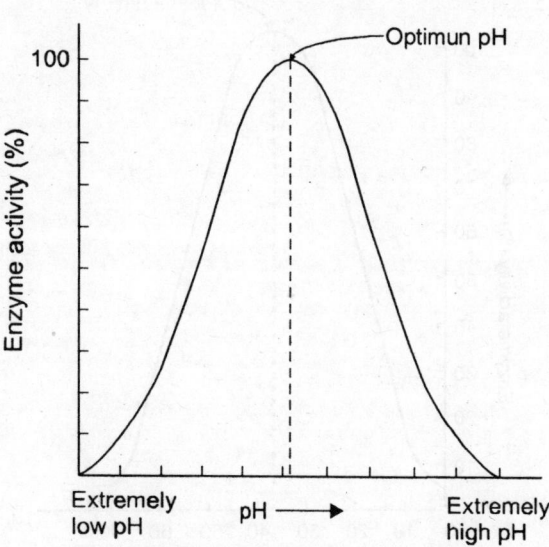

Fig. 9.9 : Effect of pH on enzyme activity

Hexokinase reaction is an example of product inhibition. In this reaction, ADP is competitive with ATP, and glucose -6-phosphate is competitive with glucose.

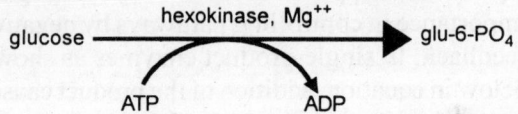

G-6-P may also act as a product inhibitor if it is not removed rapidly.

Effect of temperature

Chemical reactions, both catalyzed and noncatalyzed proceed at a faster rate as the reaction temperature is increased. This is true of enzymatically catalysed reactions in general only up to about 50°C. Above this temperature, heat inactivation of enzymes becomes a more important factor than the increased reaction rate and in all but a few exceptional cases, the speed of reaction slows and ceases around 70^0 to 80°C.

The optimum temperature of an enzyme is that temperature at which the greatest amount of substrate is changed in unit time. (Fig. 9.10).

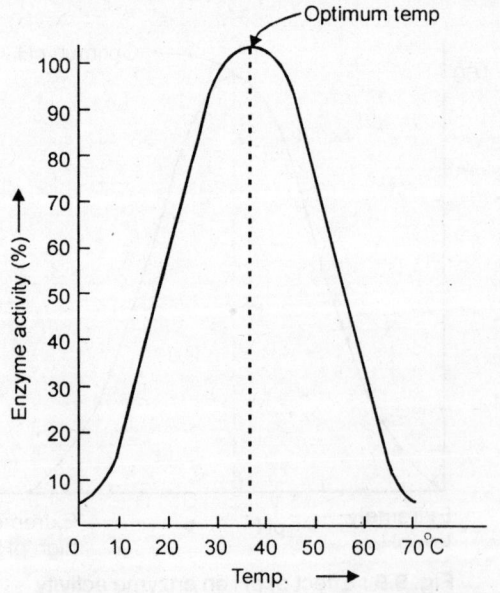

Fig 9.10: Effect of temp. on enzyme activity

Effect of time

Scientist Gortner points out that the element of time is generally not given sufficient consideration in discussing factors that affect the rate of enzyme action. He states, there cannot be an optimum hydrogen ion concentration or an optimum temperature independent of time. He indicates further that the optimum temperature of many enzymes from warm blooded animals is approximately 37°C only if time is measured in hours. It has been established that the time element is important in defining other conditions which regulate the rate of enzyme action.

Feedback Inhibition or Feedback Control

A significant control mechanism operating in living cells is known as feedback inhibition or control of enzymes. Specifically, this refers to the inhibition of the activity of an enzyme in a biosynthetic pathway by an end product of that pathway. A general representation of this kind of control is shown below:

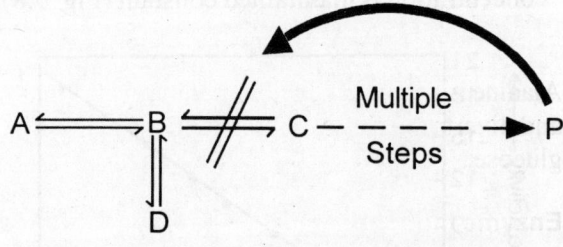

As seen in the diagram, the product (P) acts to inhibit some early step in the pathway, but not necessarily the first (product exerts a negative effect either on the first reaction or on a very early reaction). Frequently, substance B can be converted to more than one product; in this case the intermediate products are C and D. By feedback control it is possible not only to inhibit the production of P, but also to divert the flow of B from one pathway to another.

Several examples of this type have been studied in some detail. One of these systems involves the synthesis of pyrimidines. In this case, cytidine triphosphate (CTP) is an end product in a series of reactions and CTP markedly inhibits the enzyme concerned with the first specific step in this biosynthesis, namely, aspartate transcarbamoylase, which catalyzes the reaction between aspartate and carbamoyl phosphate to form ureidosuccinate. A series of further reactions leads to the synthesis of cytidine triphosphate.

Cholesterol synthesis is also regulated by feedback inhibition.

Yet another example of this phenomenon is the scheme involving pyruvate kinase, which converts phosphoenolpyruvate (PEP) to pyruvate. Major isoenzymes of this enzyme are found in muscle (M) and liver (L). The L-isozyme is subject to negative feedback, as shown below:

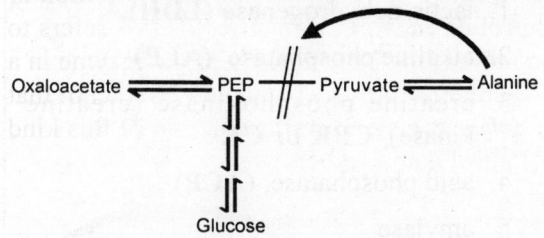

Alanine is a feedback inhibitor of pyruvate kinase and diverts the flow of pyruvate from alanine to glucose.

Enzyme Induction

Cellular enzymes can be divided into two primary classes:

   (a) Constitutive Enzymes,

   (b) Inducible Enzymes.

Constitutive enzymes

Enzymes of this class are present at virtually a constant concentration during the life of the cell. Presumably this is caused by a more or less constant relationship between the processes of enzyme synthesis and those of enzyme degradation.

Inducible enzymes:

Enzymes of this class are variable in the cell and as the need for the particular enzyme increases, the rate of synthesis gets increased or induced with respect to the rate of enzyme degradation. Thus, some of the enzymes responsible for glucose metabolism may be induced by increasing the load of glucose that an animal is required to metabolize. **Similarly, some of the enzymes involved in amino acid metabolism are inducible either by loading doses of the amino acid itself or by certain hormones.** During the wasting process, it is possible to measure increased serum concentrations of creatine phosphokinase, aldolase and other enzymes not regarded as inductive in the normal sense of the term.

The Michaelis-Menten Equation

The Michaelis constant (K_m) corresponds to the substrate concentration that produces half-maximal velocity. K_m is independent of enzyme concentration (Fig. 9.11).

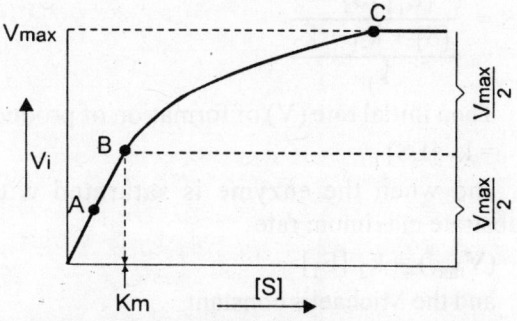

Fig. 9.11 : Determination of Km and V max

Derivation of the Michaelis-Menten equation

A mathematical analysis of the kinetics of an enzyme-catalysed reaction was proposed by Michaelis and Menten, whose names are always associated with the equation derived below. The derivation is based on a model of enzyme action in which the enzyme (E) binds to a single substrate (S) to form an enzyme-substrate complex (ES), which breaks down to form products (P) and to liberate free enzyme (E):

$$E + S \underset{k_{-1}}{\overset{k_1}{\rightleftharpoons}} ES \xrightarrow{k_2} E + P$$

k_1, k_{-1} and k_2 are rate constants for the various reactions as indicated above.

It is assumed that the reaction is in the steady state, with the concentration of ES constant, and the analysis applies only to the start of the reaction, at which point negligible amounts of products have been formed, so that the reverse reaction E+P→ES is also negligible. Then

$$\frac{d[ES]}{dt} = k_1([E_1] - [ES]) [S] - k_{-1}[ES] - k_2[ES]$$

$$k_1[E_1] [S] - k_1 [ES] [S] - k_{-1} [ES] - k_2 [ES] = 0$$
$$k_1 [E_1] [S] = [ES] (k_1[S] + k_{-1} + k_2)$$
$$\frac{k_1[E_1] [S]}{k_1[S] + k_{-1} + k_2} = [ES]$$

Divided by k_1

$$ES = \frac{[E_1] [S]}{\dfrac{[S] + k_{-1} + k_2}{k_1}}$$

Then initial rate (V) of formation of product
= k_2 [ES]

and when the enzyme is saturated with substrate maximum rate

$$(V_{max}) = k_2 [E_1]$$

and the Michaelis constant

$$K_m = \frac{k_{-1} + k_2}{k_1}$$

Therefore,

$$\upsilon = k_2 [ES] = \frac{k_2 [E_1] [S]}{[S] + K_m}$$

$$\upsilon = \frac{V_{max} [S]}{[S] + K_m}$$

Strictly, this derivation is restricted to a single substrate reaction.

ISOENZYMES OR ISOZYMES

The term isoenzymes or isozymes may be defined as the enzymes existing in multiple forms having different mobilities on electrophoresis, different relative activities towards different substrates, and being differently depressed by inhibitors.

It has been shown that the relative amounts of the isoenzymes of a particular enzyme differ in different organs so that in diseases different enzyme patterns are found according to the organ from which they have come. Examples of isoenzymes are cited in 'box'.

Examples of isoenzymes are:
1. lactic dehydrogenase **(LDH)**,
2. alkaline phosphatase **(ALP)**
3. creatine phosphokinase (creatine kinase), **CPK or CK**
4. acid phosphatase, **(ACP)**
5. amylase
6. malate dehydrogenase,
7. cholinesterase,
8. hexokinase,
9. phosphoglucomutase,
10. pyruvate kinase, etc.

In clinical biochemistry till date most of the work has been done on the following isoenzymes:

(a) lactic dehydrogenase (LDH),

(b) alkaline phosphatase (ALP) and

(c) creatine kinase i.e. creatine phosphokinase (CK or CPK)

Today, nearly 100 enzymes have been detected to exist as 'isoenzymes'. Starch gel gives a clear electrophoretic separation than any other media. The vertical form is recommended. Other media include cellulose acetate, agar gel, etc.

Clinical significance of enzymes

The relative abundance of certain enzymes or their isoenzymes in serum has found application in the diagnosis of several diseases as mentioned below:

Alkaline Phosphatase

Measurement of the activity of alkaline phosphatase in serum in the investigation of bone diseases constituted one of the earliest applications of enzyme tests in diagnosis and has remained one of the most useful. The value of serum alkaline phosphatase assays in various disorders of bone has been confirmed by more than 50 years' experience, while isoenzyme studies have demonstrated that bone is indeed the source of the raised serum enzyme activity in these conditions. In contrast, no other enzyme test has emerged of comparable value in bone diseases, inspite of the systematic attention which has been devoted to the development of diagnostic enzymology in recent years.

Raised serum alkaline phosphatase was shown to accompany rickets of various aetiologies, **Paget's disease,** and **hyperparathyroidism with skeletal involvement.**

γ-glutamyl transferase is probably the most sensitive enzymic test of liver function yet described.

The normal range of serum alkaline phosphatase activity in adults is usually taken as **3-13 King-Armstrong units/100 ml.**

The serum alkaline phosphatase activity of the new-born infant is rather above the normal adult level, and it rises rapidly to as much as two and a half to three times the adult upper limit of normal during the first year of life. The activity falls somewhat by the end of the second year to values which are of the order of one and a half to two and a half times of 20-30 King-Armstrong units/100ml. These elevated values are maintained approximately constant throughout childhood and early adolescence with perhaps some upturn at the onset of puberty, typically declining to adult levels during the later teenage years.

When hepatobiliary disease is suspected, it is advisable to resort to an alternative enzyme test. The activities of several enzymes in serum reflect impaired biliary function in ways similar to (but not completely identical with) the behaviour of alkaline phosphatase in this situation. These enzymes typically show normal activities in osteoblastic bone disease. **Two such enzymes, i.e., 5'-nucleotidase and γ-glutamyltransferase,** have been shown to exhibit serum activities within the adult normal range in children and their use has therefore been recommended as a liver function test in young patients.

The highest serum alkaline phosphatase levels are generally encountered in Paget's disease of bone (Osteitis deformans) and the raised enzyme activity is often the only abnormality in the composition of the serum seen in this condition. The activity in serum may reach levels of 100-200 King-Armstrong units/100 ml or more, **the higher values being associated with cases in which a greater proportion of the skeleton is involved.**

While, determination of serum alkaline phosphatase activity is of great value in the detection of osteomalacia and rickets, the same is not true of hyperparathyroidism, in which an increased serum alkaline phosphatase is only seen in those cases in which bone changes are present.

Successful treatment of hyperparathyroidism (e.g. by the removal of a parathyroid adenoma) is followed by a fall in serum alkaline phosphatase activity which may, however be preceded by an initial rise due to healing of the bony lesions: this contrasts with the immediate fall in serum calcium.

Infiltration of the bones by malignant disease is accompanied by a rise in serum alkaline phosphatase activity whenever the process stimulates osteoblastic activity.

ISOENZYMES OF ALKALINE PHOSPHATASE (ALP)

On careful electrophoresis of plasma, four isoenzyme bands of ALP can be distinguished (liver, placenta, intestine, bone), but unfortunately there is a major difficulty in distinguishing the bone enzyme from the liver enzyme, as they migrate very close together in the support systems used. With these difficulties ALP isoenzyme detection has so far had to remain as a semi research procedure.

Acid Phosphatase

Acid phosphatase is an important enzyme and is found to be in abundance in adult prostate and seminal fluid, while significant amounts are found in several other tissues such as red cells, liver, kidney, bone, spleen and pancreas.

Normal Range

1 to 3.5 K.AU./100 ml or

1.8 to 6.5 I.U./litre

Most of the activity in normal serum is nonprostatic in origin and is found in both sexes at all stages. Less than 0.8 K.A. units is tartarate labile and so represents prostatic fraction.

Elevation

Clinical significance of acid phosphatase is chiefly in metastatic cancer of prostate, both in detection and following the progress of disease. **Raised values mostly between 5 to 50 K.A.U. are seen in over 75% cases of metastasizing prostatic carcinoma. Some times, values over 100 and very rarely even over 1,000 may be found.** Most of the increased enzyme activity is tartarate labile. Very high levels may be found in some cases of malignant prostate with secondaries (most often in bones).

A small increase has also been found in acute retention and following prostate massage, but values soon return to normal. Similar increases are noticed in Paget's disease and carcinoma of breast but in such cases the determination is not of much clinical significance.

If the increase in tartarate labile fraction is not significant and the total level is found raised, the increase may be due to red cells or other sources of acid phosphatase.

Isoenzymes of Acid Phosphatase

By polyacrylamide gel electrophoresis, various isoenzymes designated arbitrarily as 0, 1, 2, 3, 3b, 4 and 5 have been identified from different sources in normal and disease conditions. Zero represents the slowest moving and 5 the fastest moving fraction. Most of these isoenzymes are labile even at the room temperature and become inactivated. Therefore, in the serum only stable isoenzyme is found. The isoenzyme pattern in the leukocytes found is as follows:

Isoenzymes	Sources
1,2,4	in neutrophils
1,4	in monocytes
3	in lymphocytes and platelets
3b	in primitive blasts
5	in reticulum cells of leukaemic reticuloendothelosis

ISOENZYMES OF ACID PHOSPHATASE (ACP)

At the most, there do exist 14 isoenzymes on electrophoresis. One finds clear cut 14 bands on electrophoretogram. **The only isoenzyme of clinical importance is prostatic acid phosphatase.**

Normal plasma contains a tartarate resistant isoenzyme 5.

In variety of diseases, other isoenzymes may appear in plasma.

In metastatic prostatic cancer —changes in plasma enzyme activity are due to the presence of isoenzyme 2, which is tartarate labile.

Many acid phosphatase isoenzymes are cell specific i.e. derived from a specific type of cell.

Aminotransferases (Transaminases)

The enzymes which are involved in the transfer of an amino group (CH_2-NH_2) from an alpha amino acid to a alpha keto acid are called as transaminases and the process is called as transamination. Transamination reaction is an important step in the metabolism of amino acids.

Two enzymes occur in human tissues which catalyze reaction of this type:

(a) Aspartate aminotransferase, popularly known as **GOT (glutamic-oxaloacetic transaminase)** and

(b) Alanine aminotransferase, **popularly known as GPT (glutamic-pyruvic transaminase).**

Both transaminases are widely distributed in human tissues, GOT activity almost always being greater than GPT activity.

Serum GOT and GPT catalyse the following reactions of transaminations respectively:

α KG + Aspartic acid

$\Updownarrow$ GOT

Glutamic acid + Oxaloacetic acid

α KG + Alanine

$\Updownarrow$ GPT

Glutamic acid + Pyruvic acid

Interpretation

The normal range for serum GOT is 4-17 IU/l or 8-40 units/ml and for GPT 3-15 IU/l or 5-35 units/ml.

According to Wroblewski, in the newborn, values upto 120 units for GOT and 90 units for GPT must be considered normal.

Determination of GOT is particularly useful in myocardial infarction (M.I.) when ECG findings are not very clear. GOT rises rapidly after myocardial infarction; peak values which may be 2-20 times of normal, are reached within 24-48 hours and return to normal levels typically within 3-5 days.

Elevated level of GOT has been observed in almost 97% clinically proved cases of M.I.

Normal values have been reported in heart conditions without infarction, such as angina and pericarditis, in patients with pulmonary embolism and also in patients with acute abdominal attacks.

Foulk and Fleisher found an increase in over 50% patients with acute pancreatitis.

SGPT is not usually elevated in M.I. unless the lesion is a large one or there is associated liver damage.

Both the enzymes exhibit raised levels in hepatocellular damage e.g. due to hepatotoxic drugs, infective hepatitis and primary or secondary liver cancer. Raised levels are also seen in **Lannec's cirrhosis,** biliary cirrhosis and obstructive jaundice. In infective hepatitis, the increase is particularly marked and highest values are obtained. In early stage GOT is more increased than GPT, but SGPT exceeds SGOT in advanced stage. In infective hepatitis, estimation of serum transaminases is the most sensitive diagnostic index.

Very high values are obtained in toxic hepatitis due to carbontetrachloride poisoning.

Serum transaminases particularly SGOT gets elevated in certain muscular disorders, e.g. progressive muscular dystrophy, dermatomyositis and also following extensive muscle trauma, but is usually normal in progressive muscular atrophy, myasthenia gravis and rheumatoid arthritis.

Recommendations on the Use of Serum Enzyme Assays in the Diagnosis of Acute Myocardial Infarction

1. A single set of cardiac enzyme values in the emergency room is not sufficiently sensitive to exclude myocardial infarction. **Although a single, markedly positive CK-MB value will greatly increase the probability of acute infarction,** data are insufficient to support or reject a policy whereby low-risk patients, who otherwise would be sent home, would be observed until one or more CK-MB values are obtained.

2. If a myocardial infarction is inspected, then samples of total CK and CK-MB levels should be measured on admission and about 12 and 24 hours later, although condensed versions of this strategy may ultimately prove to be equally efficacious and more cost effective. If MI may have occurred more than 24 hours before admission, and if CK and CK-MB levels are not diagnostic, a total LDH level should be ordered. If the total LDH level is elevated, an assay of LDH isoenzymes should be obtained. If the first LDH1/LDH2 ratio is only slightly less than 1.0, a second assay is probably indicated.

3. If chest pain occurs after admission, CK and CK-MB assays should be done at 0, 12 and 24 hours.

4. **Routine use of enzyme assays other than those for CK, CK-MB, and LDH isoenzymes is not recommended.**

5. If more than 2 hours may pass before CK isoenzymes will be assayed, the serum sample should be preserved on ice.

Other Laboratory Measurements

Blood sugar

Hyperglycemia occurs frequently following AMI (acute myocardial infarction), not only in diabetic patients, in whom ketoacidosis may be precipitated, but also (with a lower frequency) in nondiabetics, in whom several weeks may elapse before carbohydrate tolerance returns to normal.

Serum lipids

These are often determined in patients with AMI. However, the results may be misleading, since numerous factors that can alter the values are operating at the time of the patient's admission to the hospital; for example, **stress increases serum cholesterol, whereas recumbency (the state of taking rest by lying down) decreases it.** Serum triglycerides are affected by calorie intake, intravenous and recumbency.

During the first 24-48 hours after admission, total cholesterol and HDL cholesterol remain at or near baseline values but generally fall precipitously after that. The fall in HDL cholesterol after AMI is greater than the fall in total cholesterol, thus the ratio of total cholesterol to HDL cholesterol is no longer useful for risk assessment early after MI. Therefore, unless values are obtained very early in patients admitted for AMI, it is the best to defer determinations of serum lipid levels until at least 8 weeks after the infarction has occurred.

Serum Amylase

Amylase is a starch splitting enzyme which hydrolyses starch and other high molecular dextrins to maltose at an optimum pH of 7.1. It is present in the pancreas and parotid gland. The major activity of this enzyme, called amylopsin, is in pancreatic juice, some is also found in saliva.

Interpretation

Normal range of serum amylase is given as 80-180 Somogyi units/100 ml. **The clinical significance of this enzyme chiefly lies in the diagnosis of acute pancreatitis in which values frequently exceed 2000 units.** Usually activities over 550 units strongly suggest a diagnosis of acute pancreatitis. The rise is rapid and transient, reaching a peak within the first 12-24 hours after the onset and returning to normal usually in 2 to 3 days.

In chronic disease of the pancreas, whether due to neoplasm or due to chronic pancreatitis, such high values are not seen (rarely exceeds 200 units/100 ml). In these conditions either duct obstruction is more gradual or progressive destruction of secreting tissues largely counteracts its effect.

High activities may also occasionally occur in variety of conditions in which pancreatic damage is secondary to other abdominal disturbance such as perforated gastric ulcers, peritonitis, intestinal obstruction. In these conditions values over 500 units may be found. These usually develop 5 to 10 days after the onset of symptoms and appear to be due to increased pressure on pancreatic duct.

ISOENZYMES OF AMYLASE

Although techniques are becoming available for the separate estimation of amylase isoenzymes (pancreatic, salivary), the measurement of isoenzymes is unlikely to resolve the major diagnostic problem of differentiating acute pancreatitis from non-pancreatic abdominal emergencies (perforated peptic ulcer, gut obstruction, etc.). This is because in the later situation, the pancreatic amylase that is normally present in the gut lumen leaks through the intestinal wall into the peritoneal cavity and from there it is absorbed into the blood stream.

Drugs such as morphine which cause contraction of sphincter of oddi increase serum amylase.

Creatine Kinase (CK or CPK)

CPK is a dimer consisting of one subunit which is found in the brain (designated as B) and another in muscle (designated as M). It exists in the following three isozymic forms namely:

1. **MM (found in skeletal and heart muscle)**
2. **MB (found in cardiac muscle, also found in striated muscle)**
3. **BB (found in brain and a variety of other tissues)**

About 15% of the heart CK is in the form of MB isoenzyme, the remaining 85% being MM. It should be noted that skeletal muscle also contains some MB isoenzyme (<0.4%). The amount of MB isoenzyme increases in the plasma after a myocardial infarct, and therefore

---

MB isoenzyme of CK increases in plasma after a myocardial infarction.

---

in theory provides a fairly specific test.

The most useful application of estimating plasma MB activity is in the investigation of those patients suspected of having an infarct.

Heart and skeletal muscles are the richest sources of serum creatine phosphokinase, an enzyme which reversibly catalyzes the phosphorylation of creatine with ATP to form adenosine diphosphate and creatine phosphate.

$$\text{Creatine Phosphate} + \text{ADP} \xrightleftharpoons{\text{CPK}} \text{Creatine} + \text{ATP}$$

This enzyme is also found in cerebral tissue. Consequently, damage or disease (e.g. myocardial infarction, acute cerebrovascular disease, muscular dystrophy or injury) of these tissues will result in elevated serum CK levels.

High levels of CPK are also found after

> In the wake of myocardial infarction, CK activity begins to rise within 4 to 6 hours; reaches to peak between 18 to 30 hours and returns to normal by the third day. Marginally increased levels may be found due to severe exercise and by large multiple intramuscular injections. Besides the diagnostic importance in M.I, it's also of diagnostic importance in progressive muscular dystrophy of Duchenne type, polymyositis and in other muscular dystrophies.

severe exercise, in hypothyroidism, acute cerebrovascular accidents and strokes and motor neuron disorders.

Normal levels in men and women differ with the methods employed. Normal values in men and women according to the method of Hughes (modified) are as given below:

Men : 20 - 50 IU/litre

Women : 10 - 37 IU/litre

The magnitude of elevation of CK in M.I. is found to be greater than those of SGOT and LDH elevations. CPK may be a more sensitive indicator of myocardial ischaemia than the other enzymes and may be potentially more useful in subendocardial infarctions. No increase in activity is noted in heart failure cases.

CPK activity is not elevated in liver disease, blood dyscrasia, chronic pulmonary diseases and chronic renal diseases. Minimal elevation has been infrequently noted in isolated cases of pulmonary infarction. Rarely, positive reactions have been reported associated with gangrene of the gallbladder, carcinoma of the pancreas, and diabetic acidosis. CPK activity levels may be altered by the presence of thyroid disease. Extremely high enzyme values are found more frequently in severe myxoedema than in the milder forms. When the disease is controlled with thyroid hormone, the enzymic activity returns to the normal range.

In contrast to SGOT and LDH, CPK is not elevated in patients with primary hepatic disease or with hepatic congestion from heart failure. In rare instances of pulmonary embolism or pulmonary infarction, one may find abnormal serum CPK activity, but the elevation in CPK is slight and may be due to local irritation of skeletal muscle by phlebitis.

Lactic Dehydrogenase (LDH or LD)

Lactic dehydrogenase is an enzyme which catalyzes the reversible conversion of lactic acid to pyruvic acid (Fig. 9.12).

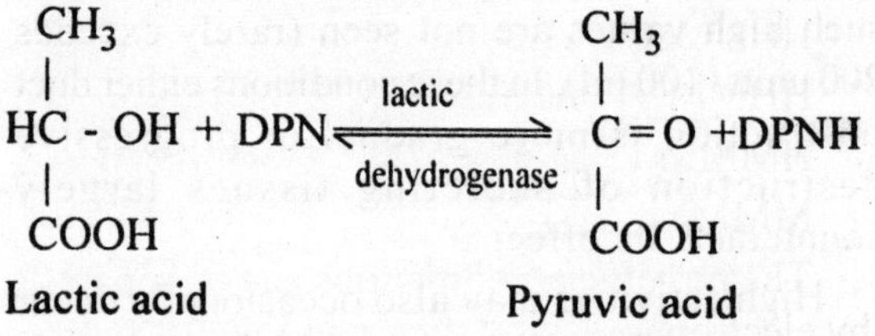

$$
\begin{array}{ccc}
CH_3 & & CH_3 \\
| & \text{lactic} & | \\
HC - OH + DPN \rightleftharpoons & & C = O + DPNH \\
| & \text{dehydrogenase} & | \\
COOH & & COOH \\
\text{Lactic acid} & & \text{Pyruvic acid}
\end{array}
$$

Fig. 9.12 : Biochemistry of lactic dehydrogenase

This enzyme is found in varying concentration in all the tissues of the body, namely in decreasing order-liver, skeletal muscle, kidney, heart muscle, lung, serum etc.

LDH rise is usually noted within the first 12 to 24 hours after myocardial infarction, peak is reached in two to four days and gradual return to normal is seen from the eighth to the fourteenth day. The peak elevations in LDH are roughly proportional to the extent of injury to the myocardial tissue. In myocardial infarction, LDH elevations above 3,000 units suggest a grave prognosis.

> LDH levels get increased in megaloblastic anaemia, carcinomatosis, acute leukaemia, granulocytic leukaemia, heart failure, pulmonary infarction, renal necrosis, muscle disease and sickle cell anaemia. Less pronounced LDH increases are seen in inflammatory hepatic disease.

The disadvantage of LDH determinations is that this enzyme is also relatively non-specific for myocardial tissue. It is so widespread in body cells that coexistent disease processes in other organ systems can cause elevations.

Isoenzymes of Lactic Dehydrogenase (LD)

Mammalian lactic (lactate) dehydrogenases are tetramers composed of two types of subunits, designated as M (the major form found in muscle or liver) and H (the major form found in heart). Five combinations of subunits are possible i.e.,

HHHH (H_4)

HHHM (H_3M)

HHMM (H_2M_2)

HMMM (HM_3)

MMMM (M_4)

The possible combinations can be separated by electrophoresis as shown in Fig. 9.13.

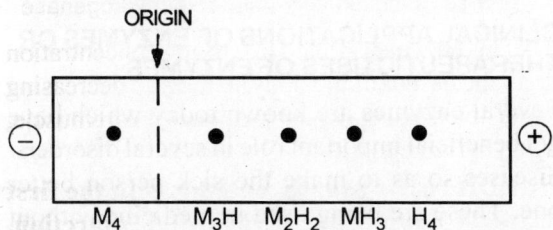

Fig. 9.13: Electrophoresis of lactate dehydrogenase isoenzymes at pH 8.6

It is clear from the Fig 9.13 that the net charge on the isozyme differs, those with an increasing content of the H subunit have an increasingly larger negative charge, while M_4 isozyme has a slightly positive net charge. These five forms of lactate dehydrogenase are isozymes that catalyze the same reactions, but they are found to different extents in different tissues. In man, the context of the several isozymes differs in heart and liver. Although the reason for this is not yet known, use is made of the fact in diagnostic differentiation of various diseases of liver and myocardium (heart). In both types of disease states, LD leaks out of the damaged cell

and increases the concentration of the enzyme in blood serum.

In liver and heart muscle the predominant isozyme has subunit composition H_4 whereas in skeletal muscle, the predominant isozyme is M_4. The H_4 and M_4 isozymes have different K_m values for pyruvate. **Raised levels of LD_1 and LD_2 are characteristic of myocardial infarction; whereas LD_4 and LD_5 get elevated in liver disorders.**

Five isoenzymes of LD are known to exist:

LD_1, LD_2, LD_3, LD_4 and LD_5 (based on electrophoretic mobility)

1. Heart-LD_1 and LD_2
2. Liver-LD_5
3. Skeletal muscle-variable

Plasma LD may be elevated in:

(a) **Myocardial disease**

(b) **Liver disease**

(c) **Skeletal muscle disease**

(d) **Miscellaneous**

LDH of serum and various tissues consists of five different components which are separable by electrophoresis. These fractions are known as isoenzymes because they catalyze the same chemical reaction, i.e; the reduction of pyruvate to lactate.

Cellular damage to tissues such as myocardium and liver results in characteristic abnormalities in the relative proportions of various isoenzymes, demonstrable by electrophoresis. The plasma of normal adults contains five plasma isoenzymes, i.e. LDH_1, LDH_2, LDH_3, LDH_4 and LDH_5. These isoenzymes may be differentiated by physical (thermal stability), chemical (mobility on starch gel) and immunological characteristics.

LDH_1 and LDH_2 fractions of lactic

dehydrogenase become predominated in cases of myocardial infarction during electrophoresis. These isoenzyme changes occur earlier in the course of infarction and persist longer than the total plasma LDH enzyme activity.

Haemolyzed specimens cannot be used and the amount of serum subjected to electrophoresis must contain an adequate amount of enzyme activity.

Normal range

It differs with the method employed. For the spectrophotometric method, Wroblewski has given the normal range as 200-650 units (85-300 I.U. per litre), Elliot and Wilkinson as 150-500 units (72 to 240 I.U. per litre) whereas King, using his own method as 70-240 I.U. per litre.

> There is a marked increase in the proportion of LD_1 in serum in myocardial infarction and LD_5 in liver disease.
>
> An increase in the level of lactate dehydrogenase activity in cerebrospinal fluid has been reported in cases of tumours of the Central Nervous System. The normal range has been given as 10-25 I.U./l by King and as 3-20 by Wroblewski.

Antienzymes

Antienzymes may be referred to as the enzymes possessing antagonistic property to the proteolytic enzymes of the human system. Such enzymes are synthesized within our body. **Because of the availability of such enzymes,**

> Some well known antienzymes are:
> 1. Anti-trypsin
> 2. Anti-pepsin
> 3. Anti-rennin
> 4. Anti-urease etc.

the wall of the alimentary canal is not digested itself by its own proteolytic enzymes. Likewise, intestinal parasites (which are very common especially amongst children for example round-worms, hook-worms, pinworms, etc.) are also not digested by the proteolytic enzymes present in the alimentary canal. **Reports are also available regarding production of antienzymes in the serum when certain enzyme preparations are given parenterally.** The mucous membrane is also believed to contain anti-proteolytic enzymes. **Ascaris has been shown to contain anti-trypsin and anti-pepsin activity.**

> **Radioimmunoassay can also be used to measure serum trypsin activity in suspected cases of cystic fibrosis.**

CLINICAL APPLICATIONS OF ENZYMES OR THERAPEUTIC USES OF ENZYMES

Several enzymes are known today which have got beneficial important role in several disorders/diseases so as to make the sick person better one. These are being used in medicine without any hesitation. Their use in medicine is on increase day by day. More and more researches are going on in this direction. Since, the enzymes are inactivated in gastrointestinal tract, hence these are administered parenterally. Some of the important examples of such enzymes are as follows:

Trypsin

This has proved to be of value in the treatment of several clinical conditions. The purified enzyme has been administered parenterally, orally and intramuscularly. **In the treatment of acute thrombophlebitis (a blood clot and inflammation in a vein), small recurrent injections have been beneficial in many patients.**

Some types of ulcers have responded well to trypsin therapy, as have some specific traumatic injuries, such as boxers' black-eye and a number of other injuries to athletes and others.

Streptokinase

It is a bacterial enzyme obtained principally from β-hemolytic streptococci. **It causes fibrinolysis and dissolution of clot. It is used in the treatment of haemothorax and haematoma.**

Hyaluronidase

It is prepared from mammalian testes. It acts by depolymerizing hyaluronic acid and increasing tissue permeability. **It is used in the treatment of traumatic or postoperative edema.**

Pepsin

It is obtained from hog stomach. It is used in the treatment of gastric achylia (congenitally undeveloped gastric glands).

Thromboplastin

This is prepared by lysis of blood platelets and is used for blood coagulation.

Urokinase

It is prepared from human urine and is used in the treatment of pulmonary embolism and in myocardial infarction to dissolve the clot.

Fibrinolysin

It is prepared by activating fibrinolysinogen by streptokinase and is used in the treatment of venous thrombosis, pulmonary and arterial embolism.

Rennin

It is obtained from the glandular layer of calf stomach and is used in the therapy of gastric achylia.

DIAGNOSTIC IMPORTANCE OF ENZYMES (AT A GLANCE)

The assay of serum enzymes is used as an important aid to diagnosis. The level of enzymic activity of a number of enzymes gets raised in different pathological conditions. With the advancement of 'Biochemistry', it is now preferable to take into account the level of serum enzymes in certain diseases before starting the treatment. Timely enzymic investigations are of great value and significance to the physicians/ surgeons.

Some enzymes of diagnostic importance with principal conditions involved are as follows: (in alphabetical order, Table 9.3).

The great significance of enzymes is that the thousands of chemical transformations going on continually in living matter would not be possible without enzymes, which are the most important tools of the living cell. For the hydrolysis or the oxidation of such substances like fats and proteins, in the laboratory we commonly employ strong acids or alkalies or oxidizing agents and high temperatures.

Enzymes are organic catalysts produced by living organisms. They are generally soluble and colloidal substances, characterized by great activity, specificity and susceptibility to the influence of pH, temperature, and other environmental changes.

All the enzymes which have been isolated in pure condition to date are proteins. (The converse of this statement, i.e., that all proteins are necessarily enzymatically active is, however, not true).

All enzymes are proteins in nature does not hold true 100% as now there do exist few enzymes that are made up of RNA; **such enzymes are called as ribozymes. Thomas Cech** and **Sidney Altman** discovered ribozymes for which they were awarded Nobel Prize in Physiology and Medicine in the year **1989.**

Table 9.3 : Enzymes of diagnostic importance with principal conditions involved

Enzymes	Principal conditions in which level of activity in serum gets elevated
Amylase	Acute pancreatitis
Acid phosphatase (optimum pH 5)	Prostatic carcinoma *
Alkaline phosphatase (optimum pH 10)	Diagnosis of liver diseases, especially biliary obstruction and detection of osteoblastic bone disease, e.g. rickets.
Aspartate transaminase (AST-previously GOT)	Myocardial infarction. Liver diseases, especially with liver cell damage.
Alanine transaminase (ALT-previously GPT)	Liver diseases especially with liver cell damage.
Lactate dehydrogenase (LDH or LD)	Myocardial infarction, but also increased in many other diseases (liver disease, some blood diseases).
Creatine phosphokinase (CPK) or Creatine kinase (CK)	Myocardial infarction and skeletal muscle diseases (muscular dystrophy, dermatomyositis).
γ-glutamyl transferase (γ-GT) * *	Diagnosis of liver diseases, particularly biliary obstruction and alcoholism.
Urinary Elevation N -acetyl glucosaminidase in Urine can be used to indicate renal transplant rejection.	

* *Determination by radioimmunoassay technique which gives good results, is the choice of estimation these days, therefore, it should be carried at least in cases of suspected prostatic carcinoma.*

* * *γ - GT is elevated in the plasma of alcoholics, and also of epileptics taking barbiturates. This is because consumption of alcohol or barbiturates causes considerable proliferation of the endoplasmic reticulum inducing high levels of the enzyme.*

Table 9.3: enzymes of aliphatic ionorhance with principal conditions involved
methecnolonic acid cycle-wise.

CHAPTER 10

HUMAN NUTRITION/BALANCED DIET

(Longer the belt, shorter the life; few people die by taking less calories but many times more from excess; check the obesity from the very begining of life, do not depend upon fast foods, do atleast moderate exercise/yoga daily and enjoy the life till the last respiration)

Nutrition deals with the needs of the organism for sustenance. Food is the basic requirement for all the living beings whether microorganisms or plants or animals, without which the existence of life is not possible. The modern science of nutrition deals mainly with the requirement of the body, both in kind and amount, and the choice of food to meet these needs. **Main three functions of food are to:**

(a) supply energy

(b) form (or maintain) body tissues and

(c) preserve a suitable internal environment so that enzymes bringing about hundreds of metabolic reactions and the hormones regulating various processes might function properly.

Following is the nutritional requirement of human beings:

(a) **carbohydrates**   (b) **lipids**

(c) **proteins**   (d) **minerals**

(e) **vitamins, and**   (f) **sufficient amount of water**

Excess intake of such foods should be taken care of which contain various food toxins (Table 10.1).

* a south american plant with thick roots that is grown for food; its roots are used as food; synonym: tapioca

Table 10.1 : Various food toxins found in routine edibles.

Sl. No.	Food toxin	Source(s)
1.	5-dehydroxytryptamine	Banana and some other fruits
2.	Tyramine	Some cheeses
3.	Cyanide	Almonds, cassava* and other plants
4.	Cycasin	Cycad nuts
5.	Nitrosamines	Some fishes, meat or cheese
6.	Sanguinarine	Mustard oil
7.	Hemagglutinins	Legumes
8.	Oxalate	Rhubarb
9.	Solanine	Green potatoes
10.	Various mycotoxins	Fungi
11.	Aflatoxin B_1	Produced by the species of
12.	Aflatoxin G_1	fusarium

ENERGY REQUIREMENT

The energy requirement of the animal body may be divided into two functional classifications, viz., **that for basal metabolism and that for active work. (Table 10.2). Basal metabolism includes the energy expended in respiration, blood circulation, intestinal contractions, activities of various organs, maintenance of muscular tonus, thermal**

Table 10.2 : Energy requirement for basal metabolism and active work.

Energy Requirement	
Basal metabolism	**Active work**
(It covers involuntary actions like respiration, blood circulation, intestinal contractions, activities of various organs, maintenance of muscular tonus, thermal equilibrium, etc.)	(It covers voluntary actions like playing, running, swimming, walking, pulling rikshaw, ploughing fields manually, wood-cutting manually, etc.)

equilibrium, etc. **The basal metabolic rate is influenced by the amount of active protoplasmic mass (hence by height, weight, surface area, age, sex, composition of the tissues, etc.) and is governed by endocrine organs, particularly the thyroid and pituitary glands.**

The energy consumed in work, play and indeed all forms of voluntary activity, imposes an additional requirement for fuel over the basal which depends upon the nature and extent of the muscular work. Whereas an average man expends about 100 Cal per hour while sitting at rest, his/her metabolism may increase to as high as six times this value with extreme physical effort.

Mary, Swartz and Rose summarised the hourly expenditure of calories of an average 70 kg man under various conditions as follows :

1.	Sleeping	: 65
2.	Awake lying still	: 77
3.	Sitting at Rest	: 100
4.	Standing relaxed	: 105
5.	Dish washing	: 144
6.	Light exercise	: 170
7.	Walking slowly to moderately fast	: 200-300
8.	Carpentry or painting	: 240
9.	Active exercise	: 290
10.	Walking down stairs	: 364
11.	Sawing wood	: 480
12.	Swimming	: 500
13.	Running 5.3 miles per hour	: 570
14.	Very severe exercise	: 600
15.	Walking up stairs	: 1100

From the above estimates one may predict the calorie requirement of the individuals. **The total energy requirement for different types of workers ranges from:**

(a) a minimum of **2000 to 2500** Cal per day (White - collar workers)

Break-up of calories per day by a normal adult individual may be considered as:

(i)   Carbohydrates
(400 g) x 4 = 1600 Calories

(ii) Lipids
(80 g) x 9 = 720 Calories

(iii) Proteins
(45 g) x 4 = 180 Calories
_____
2500 Calories

(b) **to a maximum of 4000 to 6000 (lumbermen, excavators, etc),** of which about 1400 to 1900 Cal are consumed in basal metabolism and the balance in various forms of activity.

Calorie intake must be adjusted to specific needs. The proper allowance is that which will maintain body weight and rate of growth at the desired levels over extended periods. **When disease is present, calorie supply must provide energy for tissue repair, for the immunological mechanisms and for the wasting effects of fever.**

The Food and Nutrition Board, National Research Council, recommended daily calorie intake as given in Tables 10.3 (a & b) The calorie allowances apply to the individual normally engaged in model rate physical activity, under usual environmental stresses.

For a long time, emphasis in the study of nutrition was laid on calorie requirements. **Animal calorimeter was developed by Atwater, Rosa and Benedict. Human calorimeter developed by Du Bois revealed that a normal 70 kg man expends, on an average, energy equivalent to about 3,000 calories per day.** There is yet another calorimeter which is known as Bomb calorimeter; this can be used to determine the caloric value of various foods. Composition and energy content of various common food stuffs are as given in Table 10.3.

On the basis of the definition of a large calorie (Cal or kcal), the quantity of heat necessary to raise the temperature of 1kg of water through 1°C, the following values are obtained:

1 gm of carbohydrate   =   4.1 kcal
1 gm of fat (lipid)   =   9.4 kcal
1 gm of protein   =   5.6 kcal

However, in the body, protein is not completely utilized, although carbohydrates and lipids are. On this basis, the following round figures are commonly used in Medicine/Science.

1 gm of carbohydrate   =   4 kcal
1 gm of fat   =   9 kcal
1 gm of protein   =   4 kcal

Daily Requirement

The average normal man needs 2,500 to 3,000 calories (see above break-up of calories) per day and the normal woman some what less, usually, 1,700 to 2,100 calories per day. Recommended daily-dietary allowance for various categories of human beings is given in Table 10.4 (a and b).

Following is the nutritional requirement of human beings:

(a)   carbohydrates
(b)   lipids
(c)   proteins
(d)   minerals
(e)   vitamins, and
(f)   sufficient amount of water

High fat consumption has been found to be associated with **cancer of breast and colon.**

The main sources of saturated fat in the human diet are the meat of ruminants, dairy products and hard margarine. Cholesterol is found only in foods of animal origin, particularly in egg yolk.

Carbohydrates

Principal carbohydrates in the human diet are the starches and the sugars. Grains and vegetables constitute the primary sources of the starches, while fruits of sugars. Carbohydrates make up some 40-80 per cent of total calories furnished by the diet. Less than 1 percent of the carbohydrate intake is found in the tissues, emphasizing its ready utilization as a source of energy or its conversion to fat stores in adipose tissues as a potential energy source.

When ingested in amount in excess of that required to produce energy, carbohydrate is converted to fat, e.g., glycogen, a principal carbohydrate of the human body, gets firstly converted to pyruvic acid **via 'glycolysis' and then to acetyl CoA which is the precursor for the biosynthesis of fatty acids vis-a-vis fats in the human body.**

No definite amount of the intake of carbohydrates is known today but it has been established so far that at least **100 grams of carbohydrates are required per day by a normal healthy adult in order to avoid ketosis, excessive protein catabolism and other undesirable responses.** These carbohydrates remain confined to almost all kinds of foodstuffs which we consume daily in a normal course i.e., all types of vegetables (potatoes, carrots, chillies, arums, beans, pumpkin etc.), spices, condiments, corns (wheat, maize, oat, millet, gram, etc.), pulses, meat, egg, milk, fish etc.

The paper with which we come across daily

Table 10.3 : Composition and energy content of various common foodstuffs

Sl. No.	Foodstuff	Food energy (calories/ 100 gm)	Composition of foods, 100 gm. edible portion					
			Water %	Protein 'gm'	Fat 'gm'	Carbohy-drate 'gm'	Calcium 'mg'	Phosphorus 'mg'
1.	Bread, white	275	34.7	8.5	3.2	51.8	79	92
2.	Bread, toasted	313	25.5	9.7	3.7	59.0	90	105
3.	Whole wheat	240	36.6	9.3	2.6	49.0	96	263
4.	Barley	349	11.1	8.2	1.0	78.8	16	189
5.	Millet	350	9-13	7-13	2.2±	73.0	-	-
6.	Rice (brown, raw)	360	12.0	7.5	1.7	77.0	39	303
7.	Rice (milled, cooked)	119	70.5	2.5	0.1	26.2	8.0	45
8.	Wheat flour (whole)	333	12.0	13.3	2.0	71.0	41	372
9.	Wheat germ	361	11.0	25.2	10.0	49.5	84	1096
10.	Butter	720	15.5	0.6	81.0	0.4	20	16
11.	Cheese	398	37.0	25.0	32.2	2.1	725	495
12.	Milk (cow's whole)	69	87.0	3.5	3.9	4.9	118	93
13.	Milk (cow's skimmed)	36	90.5	3.5	0.1	5.1	123	97
14.	Eggs, fresh, whole	165	74.0	12.8	11.5	0.7	54	210
15.	Eggs, fresh, white	50	87.8	10.8	0	0.8	6.0	17
16.	Eggs, fresh, yolk	361	49.4	16.3	31.9	0.7	147	586
17.	Apple	66	84.1	0.3	0.4	14.9	6.0	10
18.	Banana	88-132	74.8	1.2	0.2	23.0	8.0	28
19.	Orange	45	87.2	0.9	0.2	11.2	33	23
20.	Peach	46	86.9	0.5	0.1	12.0	8.0	22
21.	Carrots, raw	42	88.2	1.2	0.3	9.3	39	37
22.	Poatoes, peeled, boiled	83	77.8	2.0	0.1	19.1	11	56
23.	Tomatoes, raw	20	94.1	1.0	0.3	4.0	11	27
24.	Almonds	600	4.7	18.6	54.1	19.6	254	475
25.	Groundnuts (roasted)	560	2.6	26.9	44.2	23.6	74	393
26.	Walnuts	650	3.3	15.0	64.4	15.6	83	380

is a form of cellulose, which, chemically has got as much glucose in it as starch has, but this paper can not be digested by the human beings because of the lacking of the corresponding enzyme i.e. **'cellulase'** in the digestive tract. On the other hand, this enzyme remains present in ruminants, therefore, they are able to digest cellulose which is found in abundance in their diet. Be it known that the main food of the ruminants is different types of grasses.

Potato consists of starch granules surrounded by an envelope of cellulose. If a raw potato is eaten, even if it is chewed thoroughly, it will pass as such through the digestive tract without yielding any calories and appear undigested in the faeces. **A raw potato, therefore, has got no food value. On the other hand, if the potato is heated, then the cellulose**

Table 10.4 (a) : Recommended daily calories intake and other dietary allowances for different categories

	Age years	Weight kg (lbs)	Height cm (In)	Calories	Protein 'g'	Calcium 'g'	Iron 'mg'	Vitamin 'A' 'I.U.'	Thiamine 'mg'	Riboflavin 'mg'	Equiv. Niacin 'mg'	Vitamin 'C'mg'	Vitamin 'D''I.U.'
Men	18-35	70(154)	175 (69)	2906	70	0.8	10	5000	1.2	1.7	19	70	
	35-55	70(154)	175 (69)	2600	70	0.8	10	5000	1.0	1.6	17	70	
	55-75	70(154)	175 (69)	2200	70	0.8	10	5000	0.9	1.3	15	70	
Women	18-35	58(128)	163 (64)	2100	58	0.8	15	5000	0.8	1.3	14	70	
	35-55	58(128)	163 (64)	1900	58	0.8	15	5000	0.8	1.2	13	70	
	55-75	58(128)	163 (64)	1600	58	0.8	10	5000	0.8	1.2	13	70	
Infants	0-1	8 (18)		kg x 11.5 ± 15	kg x 2.5 ± 0.5	0.7	kg x 1.0	1500	0.4	0.6	6	30	400
Children	1-3	13 (29)	87 (34)	1300	32	0.8	8	2000	0.5	0.8	9	40	400
	3-6	18 (40)	107 (42)	1600	40	0.8	10	2500	0.6	1.0	.11	50	400
	69	24 (53)	124 (49)	2100	52	0.8	12	3500	0.8	1.3	14	60	400
Boys	9-12	33 (72)	140 (55)	2400	60	1.1	15	4500	1.0	1.4	16	70	400
	12-15	45(98)	156(61)	3000	75	1.4	15	5000	1.2	1.8	20	80	400
	15-18	61 (134)	172(68)	3400	85	1.4	15	5000	1.4	2.0	22	80	400
Girls	9-12	33 (72)	140 (55)	2200	55	1.1	15	4500	0.9	1.3	15	80	400
	12-15	47 (103)	158 (62)	2500	62	1.3.	15	5000	1.0	1.5	17	80	400
	15-18	53 (117)	163 (64)	2300	58	1.3	15	5000	0.9	1.3	15	70	400

Table 10.4 (b) : Important daily allowances of nutrients for expectant and nursing mothers

Nutrient	Normal Women			Pregnant	Lactating
	Sedentary	Moderately active	Very active		
Calories (Cal)	1900	2200	3000	+ 300	+ 500 to 700
Proteins (g)	45	45	45	55	65
Calcium (g)	0.4-0.5	0.4-0.5	0.4-0.5	1.0	1.0
Iron (mg)	30	30	30	40	30
Vitamin 'A' as					
(i) retinol (µg)	750	750	750	750	1150
(ii) carotene (µg)	3,000	3,000	3,000	3,000	4,600
Thiamine (mg)	1.0	1.1	1.5	+ 0.2	+ 0.4
Riboflavin (mg)	1.0	1.2	1.7	+ 0.2	+ 0.4
Folic acid (µg)	100	100	100	150-300	150

envelope will burst, and the content is then available for digestion. This is an example of a food which has got no food value in the raw state, but has a very high food value in the cooked state. Calorie values of some of the important routine items (foods) are as mentioned in Table 10.5.

Table 10.5 : Calorie values of some important common foods

1. Cow's milk	: 69 Cal/100 ml
2. Buffalo's milk	: 109 Cal/100 ml
3. Human milk	: 67 Cal/100 ml
4. Butter	: 720 Cal/100 g
5. Desi ghee	: 830-890 Cal/100g
6. Fishes	: 50-150 Cal/100g
7. Meats	: 100-450 Cal/100g
8. Egg	: 165 Cal/100g
9. Curd (cow's)	: 69 Cal/100 ml
10.Curd (buffalo's)	: 109 Cal/100 ml
11.Apple, one medium size	: 66 Cal
12.Banana, one	: 88-132 Cal
13.Potato, boiled, 1 medium size	: 83 Cal
14.Tomato, raw, 1 medium size	: 20 Cal
15.Peas, green, cooked, 1/2 cup	: 56 Cal

Lipids

Lipids are the principal energy yielding substances and the per unit heat production from lipids (fats) is more than double in comparison to carbohydrates and proteins which are other two major food stuffs for the human beings. Fat is rather slowly digested and the large amounts of it in a meal tend to slow down the digestion process of other foods as well.

There is no rule for the proportion of fat and carbohydrate in a diet. For a normal person, 80gm fat is recommended. Of course, the essential fatty acids(Table 10.6) must be supplied, the requirement of which is small and these fatty acids are found in many food oils. The deficiency of the so called essential fatty acids in the diet of rats causes retarded growth, scaly skin, kidney lesions, and bloody urine formation (haematuria).

These fatty acids are also believed to control the rate of cholesterol biosynthesis in animals.

Linoleic, linolenic and arachidonic acids are considered to be essential fatty acids (EFA) in the mammals as they are not synthesized in them, hence, must be supplied in the diet. They all are polyunsaturated fatty acids.

Although, the synthesis of fatty acids from intermediates in the catabolism of carbohydrates and amino acids has been demonstrated in many species of animals and plants, most mammals are unable to synthesize in adequate amounts fatty acids containing more than one double bond in the carbon chain. When rats are fed a diet not containing polyunsaturated fatty acids for two to three months, they develop deficiency symptoms, characterized by scaliness of the skin, desquamation and sloughing of the tail, lesions in the kidneys, and ultimately death. All these symptoms can be prevented or cured by the addition of 10 drops of lard oil or a small amount of linoleic acid to the diet. Other polyunsaturated fatty acids are also curative, **but linoleic acid is considered to be the essential fatty acid, since it cannot be synthesized but is the precursor for the biosynthesis of other polyunsaturated fatty acids.**

Table 10.6: Essential fatty acids

Sl No.	Name	Sources
1.	Linoleic acid	linseed oil, cottonseed oil, peanut oil, corn oil, soyabean oil, egg-yolk, etc.
2.	Linolenic acid	linseed oil, rapeseed oil, soybean oil, fish viscera, etc.
3.	Arachidonic acid	lecithin*, cephalin*
* these are phospholipids which are found both in plants and animal tissues, viz; plant seeds (soyabean etc.), egg yolk etc.		

Although the deficiency of linoleic acid in the diet of humans is very rare, there have been reported some cases of dermatitis in infants and animals that responded to the addition of a few drops of lard oil to the diet (Fig. 10.1).

Polyunsaturated fatty acids also decrease the biosynthesis of cholesterol from either saturated fatty acids or nonfat sources. As little as 2 to 3

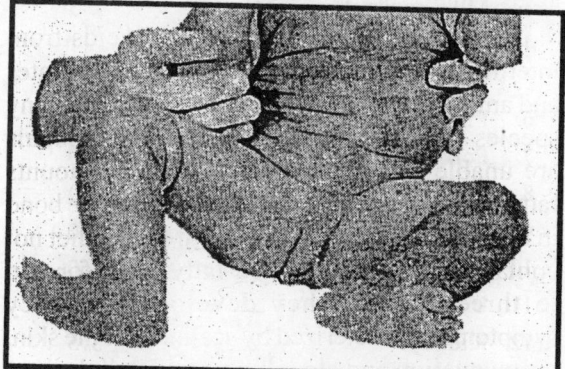

Fig 10.1 : Essential fatty acid deficiency

grams of fats per day like cottonseed, corn, and safflower (Kusumbh) oils will inhibit the cholesterol-promoting effect of 1 gram of fat consisting of saturated fatty acids, such as beef tallow (animal fat melted down) or butter.

The hydrogenation of fats, which is carried out extensively in order to convert liquid oils into a more solid state, **results into considerable reduction in the amount of essential unsaturated fatty acids.**

An outstanding problem of lipid nutrition these days is the relationship of dietary fat to hyper-cholesterolaemia and that of hypercholesterol-aemia to atherosclerosis which remains unclear even to day.

Atherosclerosis is a disease primarily concerned with the integral layer of the artery and is characterized by the thickening and loss of elasticity of the arterial wall by the excessive deposits of cholesterol and other lipids. When narrowing of a vessel occurs (Figures 10.2, 10.3,

10.4 and 10.5), serious impairment of the blood supply to important structures may result. **Atherosclerosis, for instance, in the coronary arteries, is responsible for angina pectoris (pain in the heart i.e., heart attack), and in the cerebral arteries for many mental changes in the old age.** In the vessels of the legs it may be responsible for intermittent claudication (limping, lameness). Complete obstruction of blood flow, usually due to thrombosis results in cardiac infarction, hemiplegia or senile gangrene.

Streptokinase and urokinase are the enzymes being used to disintegrate thrombus (clots) in the cardiac arteries and elsewhere.

Normal amount of the cholesterol in serum is in the range 0f 150-250 mg. It's still on safer side if the level of cholesterol is maintained between **150 to 200 mg%** in blood as per the latest recommendations of the Nutrition Board

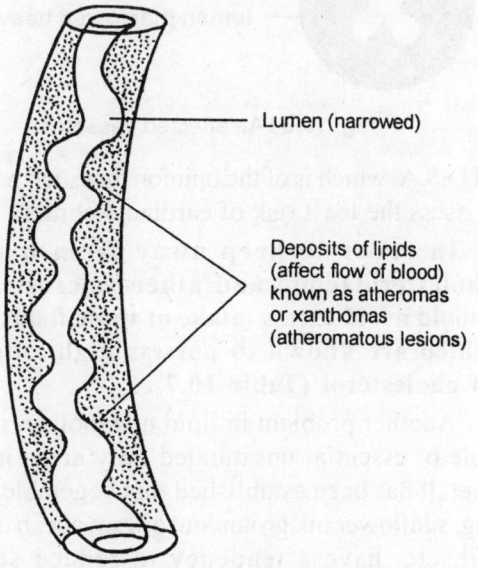

Lumen (narrowed)

Deposits of lipids (affect flow of blood) known as atheromas or xanthomas (atheromatous lesions)

Fig 10.2 : A vessel in which lumen has become narrow due to haphazard deposit of lipids (cholesterol, TG etc.). Sick artery / vessel.

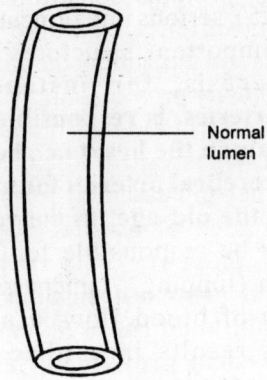

Fig 10.3 : A vessel in which blood flow is normal

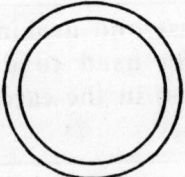

Fig. 10.4 : A normal vessel in which blood flow is normal

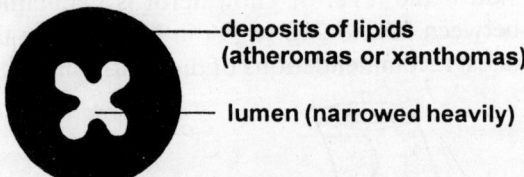

Fig. 10.5 : An affected vessel

of U.S.A. which is of the opinion that such people possess the least risk of cardiac disorders.

In order to keep away from hyper-cholesterolaemia and atherosclerosis one should avoid excess intake of those foodstuffs which are known to possess high amount of cholesterol (Table 10.7).

Another problem in lipid metabolism is the role of essential unsaturated fatty acids in the diet. It has been established that vegetable oils, e.g. sunflower oil, groundnut oil, soyabean oil, til oil, etc. have a tendency to reduce serum cholesterol level in human beings in contrast to the effect of dietary animal fat i.e. desi ghee

Table 10.7 : Cholesterol content of some important human foods

Sl. No.	Food	Cholesterol (mg per 100 gm edible portion)
1.	Vegetable oils	nil
2.	Margarine (imitation butter)	nil
3.	Milk, cow's skimmed	3
4.	Milk, cow's whole	11
5.	Chicken	60
6.	Fish	70
7.	Pork	70
8.	Beef	70
9.	Cheese	100
10.	Butter	250
11.	Liver	300
12.	Kidney	375
13.	Egg, whole	550
14.	Egg, yolk	1,500
15.	Brain	2,000

etc.

Habitual consumption of too much mustard oil is also not good for the heart, according to the researches conducted by the Indian Council of Medical Research (ICMR) as it causes myocardial fibrosis(growth of fibrous tissue). The mechanism by which mustard oil leads to **'myocardial fibrosis'** is not clear but the agent suspected is erucic acid, which is a major component of mustard oil. The ICMR bulletin says, it may be necessary to cultivate mustard varieties with low levels of erucic acid or no erucic acid. Consumption of too much coconut oil and mustard oil can lead to an increase in the level of blood cholesterol; contrarily gingily oil (til oil) can actually reduce cholesterol content.

Percentage of linoleic acid, the so called essential fatty acid in fats and oils of plant and animal origin is as follows :

1. Safflower oil (Kusumbh)   80%
2. Sunflower oil   70%
3. Corn oil   55%
4. Soyabean oil   50%
5. Cottonseed oil   45%
6. Sesame oil (Til oil)   45%
7. Peanut oil   30%
8. Coconut oil   5%

Those having a tendency of obesity/family history of obesity or hypercholesterolaemia should avoid the food items summarised in 'box'.

FAT CONTROLLED DIET: FOODS TO BE AVOIDED

Whole milk, ice cream sour cream, cheese, commercial biscuits, beef, pork, chicken, lamb, kidney, brain, liver, butter, lard, coconut oil, olive oil, chocolate, custards, puddings, etc.

Lipids play an important role in the diet by helping in the absorption of fat soluble vitamins i.e. A, D, E and K. Lecithins prevent development of fatty livers. **Nutritional cirrhosis of liver is caused due to the deficiency of dietary choline which remains present in lecithin.**

Lipids serve as the more important source of energy in the diet of the hard workers such as wrestlers, athletes, labourers, wood-cutters, etc. Ordinarily, excess fat intake should be avoided because this causes an increase in adiposity, hypercholesterolaemia, ketosis, etc. which all are undesirable.

Proteins

Nature of Proteins and their role in nutrition

Proteins are complex nitrogenous substances present in all living tissues. They are built up of simpler molecules called **'amino acids'**. There are **22** different amino acids which occur in an infinite variety of combinations in proteins.

Together with carbohydrates, fats, minerals and vitamins, proteins constitute one of the essential ingredients of our diet. While, carbohydrates and fats supply the calorific needs of the body, dietary proteins supply the building blocks for the formation of blood and tissue proteins, enzymes, antibodies, and certain hormones. They are essential for body growth and maintenance of normal physiological processes. **Recent researches have indicated that protein deficiency in infancy and early childhood (upto 5 years) impairs not only physical growth but also mental development, the damage being permanent and irreversible.**

Protein is required by every cell and is the basis of protoplasm. Moreover, it is the most expensive of the foodstuffs.

Protein's Quality

Now, the chemists have reached the fact that the quantity of protein alone does not solve the entire purpose but the quality of a protein has got more significance, hence, one must give emphasis on the quality of a protein. By the quality of a protein, we mean that it must comprise of essential amino acids in it. This came about with the realization by chemists that proteins from various sources differ widely in their amino acid make up and that their value in nutrition depends largely upon the presence of specific amino acids.

It should be known that the requirement of animals and man is not for proteins, but for specific amount of specific amino acids, the so called essential, or indispensable amino acids.

Casein of milk has been respected as a complete biological protein. It supplies sufficient quantity of all the amino acids required for growth and other needs of the body (Table 10.8). Proteins have been classified into two categories i.e. adequate and inadequate (Table 10.9).

The adult human body can maintain nitrogenous equilibrium on a mixture of eight pure amino acids as its sole source of nitrogen. These eight are as given in Table 10.7. **For growth in infants, histidine is also needed.**

Are all dietary proteins equally good?

No, it is a common fallacy to consider all dietary proteins to be equally good. Actually, proteins differ widely in their nutritional value. The variations are due to differences in digestibility and more particularly the amino acids' composition (Figures 10.6 and 10.7). The nutritive value of a protein is largely determined by the relative concentrations of the **'essential amino acids'** it contains.

Studies of various investigators have shown that an intake of about 0.9 gm of protein per kg body weight is adequate for all ordinary needs in the normal adult. In childhood, this allowance must be increased considerably to permit growth of new tissues. The same applies in pregnancy and lactation. The recommended daily dietary allowance for protein for an average man weighing about 70 kg is 70 g and for an average woman 58 grams.

What are 'essential' amino acids?

The human organism has the ability to synthesize all except **eight** amino acids, utilizing the available sources of nitrogen. The **eight** amino acids should be supplied ready-made by the diet and are, therefore, called **'essential amino acids'. They are the following: Tryptophan, Lysine, Methionine, Threonine, Phenylalanine, Leucine, Isoleucine and Valine (Table 10.8).**

Table 10.8 : Nutritive classification of the amino acids

Essential (Indispensable)	Semi-essential (semi-indispensable)	Non-essential (dispensable)
1. Lysine	1. Arginine	1. Glutamic acid
2. Leucine	2. Tyrosine	2. Aspartic acid
3. Isoleucine	3. Cystine	3. Alanine
4. Methionine	4. Glycine	4. Proline
5. Valine	5. Serine	5. Hydroxyproline,
6. Phenylalanine	6. Histidine*	etc.
7. Tryptophan		
8. Threonine		

* It's treated to be an essential amino acid for the infants

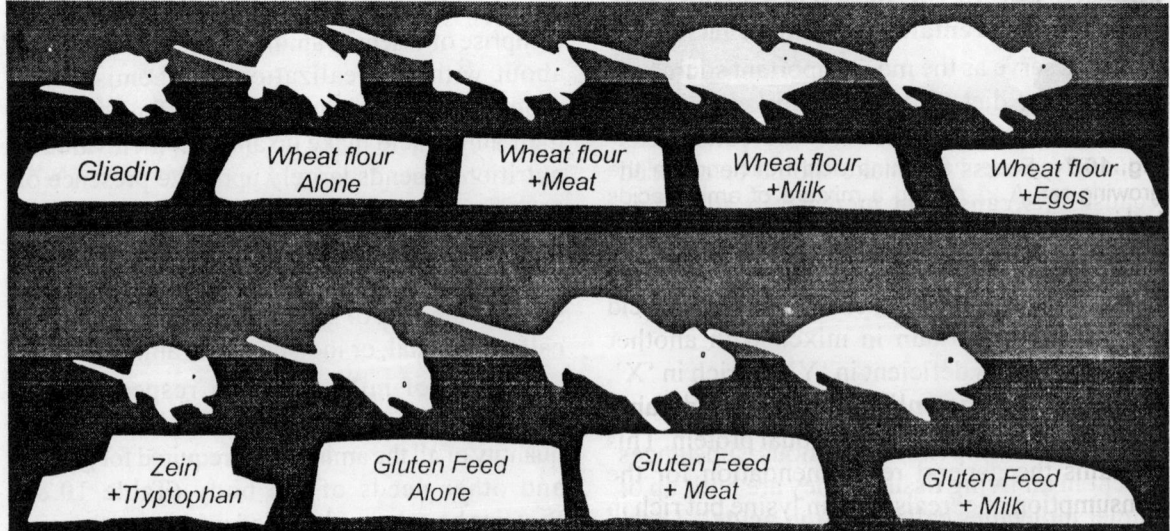

Gliadin   Wheat flour Alone   Wheat flour +Meat   Wheat flour +Milk   Wheat flour +Eggs

Zein +Tryptophan   Gluten Feed Alone   Gluten Feed + Meat   Gluten Feed + Milk

Fig. 10.6 : These rats were all of the same age and had been fed for the same length of time on diets containing the same proportion of protein. The variation in size is due to differences in the chemical constitution of the proteins eaten.

Table 10.9 : Proteins for the growth of rats

Sl. No.	Adequate (Sufficient)	Sl. No.	Inadequate (insufficient)
Animal Proteins			
1.	Casein of milk	1.	Gliadin of wheat
2.	Lactalbumin of milk	2.	Legumin of pea
3.	Ovalbumin of egg	3.	Zein of corn
Vegetable Proteins		4.	Hordein of barley
4.	Globulin of cottonseed	5.	Gelatin of horn
5.	Glutenin of wheat	6.	Legumelin of soyabean
6.	Edestin of hempseed		
7.	Excelsin of Brazil nut		

Can the deficiency of one protein be made good by another?

Yes, this is known as mutual complementation between proteins. Although one protein is deficient in one essential amino acid 'X', it may

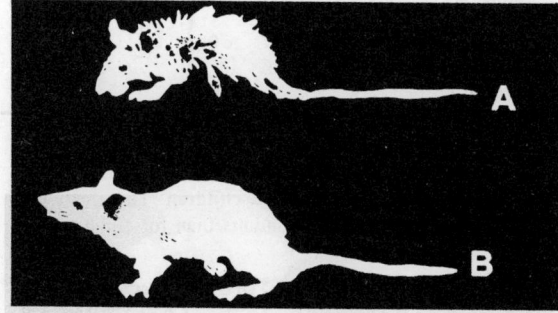

Fig. 10.7 : Essential amino acid deficiency in the growing rat. A. A rat fed a mixture of amino acids lacking valine. B. The same rat after receiving valine added to the amino acid mixture.

contain an excess of another essential amino acid 'Y'. If such a protein in mixed with another protein which is deficient in 'Y' but rich in 'X', the NPU of the combination is considerably higher than that of either individual protein. This explains the general recommendation for the consumption of cereals (low in lysine but rich in methionine) together with pulses (rich in lysine but low in methionine).

Relation between calorie intake and protein utilization

Carbohydrates and fats are the main sources of energy (i.e. calories). Proteins are primarily of value in the formation and regeneration of tissues but they too can serve as a source of energy. When the calorie needs of the body are not adequately met from the intake of carbohydrates and fats, part of the dietary protein is diverted towards energy production. To prevent such wastage of proteins, therefore, care should be taken to raise the intake of carbohydrates and fats to the required levels when offering protein supplements to cover a dietary protein gap.

1. Protein content of the product should be sufficiently high to facilitate the administration of atleast 10-20 grams of protein daily.

2. Nutritive value of the protein should be high. Adequate (first class proteins) are given in table 9.9.

3. Product should be palatable enough to enable the easy administration of the required quantity of protein.

4. Product should not have been baked or toasted at high temperature which damages the nutritive value of the protein.

5. Its protein should preferably be in intact condition and not predigested, i.e. not in the form of protein hydrolysate or mixture of amino acids.

6. It has been established that amino acids mixture cannnot be utilized as efficiently as equivalent amount of proteins.

7. Abnormally high concentration of amino acids in the intestines may also provoke diarrhoea while the elevated blood amino acids levels may cause nausea and vomiting.

Protein foods in slimming regimens

The sheet anchor of any weight reduction course consists in reducing the carbohydrates' content of the diet and limiting the calorie intake by restricting the quantity of the diet. As protein has a high satiety value, protein-rich foods with low carbohydrate content find an important place in slimming regimens.

Daily Protein Requirements

The protein requirements of an individual depend upon the age, sex and body-weight. Primarily, it is expressed in terms of the **"ideal reference protein"**. Infants, whether breast-fed or bottle-fed, receive only the reference protein (NPU = 75-100) until they are weaned. But the mixed proteins of the diets of children and adults are of lower quality and, therefore, due allowance should be made for this factor in calculating the protein requirements. For instance, if the requirement of an adult, in terms of the ideal reference protein, is 0.5 g. per kg bodyweight, it will be 1 g per kg in terms of a dietary protein with an NPU of 50. This is the basis of the official recommendations made recently regarding the dietary allowances for Indian subjects.

Recommended Dietary Protein Allowances for Indians

The following are the daily protein allowances for Indians recommended by the Expert Group of th Indian Council of Medical Research.

Nature of the "Protein Gap" in India

The considered opinion of nutrition authorities is that the protein content of the average Indian diet is adequate but the actual quantity of food consumed by the majority is insufficient. An increased consumption of the normal diets would serve to make up the calorie deficit and also ensure a satisfactory level of protein intake. However, this does not apply to some cases, e.g. weaned infants, pre-school children and pregnant

Category	Description	Daily protein allowance (g)	Nature of diet
Man	Body weight 55 kg	55	
Woman	Body weight 45 kg	45	Mainly cereals and pulses NPU = 65*
Woman	2nd half of pregnancy	55	
Woman	Lactation upto 1 year	65	
Infants	0-3 months	2.3/kg	Entirely milk
Infants	3-6 months	1.8/kg	NPU = 75-100
Infants	6-9 months	1.8/kg	Milk, cereals and
Infants	9-12 months	1.5/kg	pulses;NPU= 65
Children	1 year	17	
Children	2 years	18	
Children	3 years	20	
Children	4-6 years	22	Mostly cereals and pulses
Children	7-9 years	33	NPU = 50*
Children	10-12 years	41	
Adolescents:	Boys 13-15 years	55	
Adolescents:	Boys 16-18 years	60	
Adolescents:	Girls 13-18 years	50	

* The essential amino acid requirements of adults are less exacting than those of infants and children. Therefore, the same diet has a higher NPU for adults than for children

or lactating mothers, whose protein needs in both quality and quantity are considerably higher than those of the general adult population. For such vulnerable groups, the average diets consisting mostly of cereals and pulses cannot satisfy the needs, as the persons find it inconvenient or physically difficult to eat enough of such diets. Therefore, they need more concentrated sources of proteins as dietary supplements.

Effect of Heat on Protein Quality

Under normal condition of cooking, the digestibility of food proteins is generally improved and no damage occurs to the availability of the amino acids. **In the raw state, some vegetable foodstuffs, e.g. peas and beans, contain trypsin- inhibitors which lower the**

digestibility of their proteins. Mild heating destroys these inhibitors and improves the protein digestibility and thereby the nutritive value.

However, proteins suffer serious damage in nutritive value when they are subjected to drastic conditions of heating, especially in presence of sugars and other carbohydrates in the dry state, as in the baking of biscuits. **The damage is due to the formation of an indigestible linkage between the essential amino acid lysine and a reducing sugar.** The deterioration can be detected only by biological tests but not by chemical analysis. As lysine is the most limiting essential amino acid in cereal proteins, even a slight reduction in its availability results in a conspicuous fall in the nutritive value af cereal-based products. It is, therefore, imperative to avoid any drastic process of heating such as baking or toasting in the manufacture of protein foods.

How Useful are Protein Hydrolysates and Amino Acid Preparations for Oral Administration?

The practical value of 'oral" amino acid preparations (predigested proteins) has been seriously overemphasized. Their use was originally based on a misconception, concerning the digestive capacities of the human gastro-intestinal tract. **Actual feeding trials have proved that, even in extreme starvation or diseases like peptic ulcer, ulcerative colitis or regional enteritis,** protein digestion and amino acid absorption are normal and the use of hydrolysed protein seems unnecessary. **It was observed that being unpalatable, protein digests were often rejected and vomited by the patients.** It is also established that amino acid mixtures cannot be utilized as efficiently as equivalent amounts of proteins. The main reason for such poor utilization seems to be the extremely rapid absorption of free amino acids and the consequent flooding of the tissues with excessive

amounts af amino acids which cannot be utilized equally rapidly and are therefore partially wasted. The abnormally high concentration of amino acids in the intestines may also provoke diarrhoea while the elevated blood amino acid levels may cause nausea and vomiting. On the other hand, in the course of normal protein digestion, the amino acids are released in a slow and regulated manner, keeping pace with absorption and utilization, there being neither accumulation of amino acids in the intestines nor unduly high level in the blood.

The recent craze for the addition of lysine to multivitamin and mineral preparations intended as supplement to children has no rational basis. Being in the free form, it is rapidly absorbed but is largely wasted as the other essential amino acids are not supplied simultaneously. Further, although lysine content of cereals is low, **the most limiting essential amino acid in the average mixed diets consumed in our country may be either methionine, threonine or tryptophan but not lysine.**

Increased Protein Needs of Diabetics and the Elderly

Additional protein upto 0.5 g per kg body weight per day is recommended to diabetics because it has a more sustained effect in maintaining blood sugar than carbohydrate. A protein rich snack at bed time serves as a precaution against morning hypoglycaemia.

In old age, the calorie requirements are considerably reduced but not those of proteins and other nutrients. **Owing to the increased proneness to illness with the resulting tissue break-down and negative nitrogen balance, speedy recovery demands a higher protein intake than that provided by the normal diet. Therefore, the elderly should receive, protein-rich foods fortified with minerals and vitamins:**

Conclusion

In view of the scientific data presented in the earlier pages, the following consideration should be borne in mind while selecting a protein food as a dietary supplement.

1. The protein content of the product should be sufficiently high to facilitate the administration of at least 10-20 grams of protein daily.

2. The nutritive value of the protein should be high equivalent to a Net Protein Utilization of at least 60.

3. The product should be palatable enough to enable the easy administration of the required quantity of protein.

4. The product should not have been baked or toasted at high temperatures which damage the nutritive value of the protein.

5. Its protein should preferably be in the intact condition and not predigested, i.e. not in the form of protein hydrolysate of mixture of amino acids.

Kwashiorkor

It is mainly a disease of rural areas, occurring in the second year of life. It occurs most commonly in the infants after weaning (breast feeding) when the diet which replaces the mother's milk is markedly deficient in protein (Figures 10.8 & 10.9) but high in carbohydrate. Kwashiorkor disease has its highest incidence between the age group of **1 to 4 years** when the need for essential amino acids for tissue synthesis is great. No age is immune, but in elders, clinical manifestations not so obvious and usually less severe, because both protein and energy requirements are relatively reduced as age advances.

The disease is characterized by growth failure, retarded development, loss of appetite, mental apathy, hypoalbuminemia leading to edema, diarrhoea, pellagrous skin lesions, low plasma amino acids, lipids, glucose and potassium.

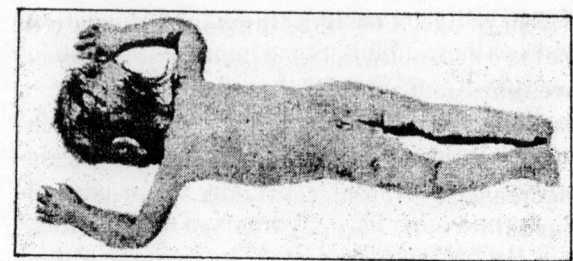

Fig. 10.8 : Symptoms of protein deficiency : Boy, 2 years 1 month old on admission. Note widespread distribution of skin lesions and edema.

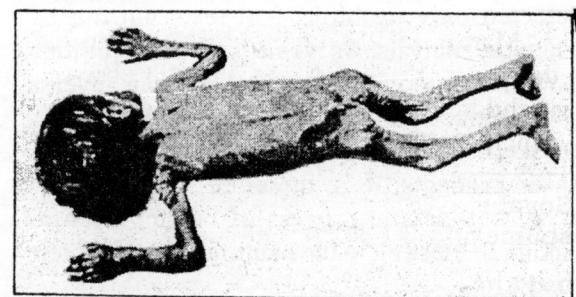

Fig. 10.9 : Same child two weeks after starting the treatment, showing disappearance of the edema and improvement in the skin lesions. Note the degree of muscular wasting, which had been concealed by the edema.

Gastrointestinal disturbances, dermatosis, fatty liver infiltration and mental disturbances are also frequent. The condition is usually complicated by dietary deficiencies other than protein and calories. It has been observed in children that protein malnutrition causes a reduction of the circumference of the head which may lead to impaired growth of the brain and its development and mental retardation. Malnutrition may likewise reduce resistance to infection. Treatment consists in instituting more adequate diet, with special reference to protein and correction of electrolyte and water balance.

Marasmus

Marasmus literally means **"to waste"**. It results from a continued severe deficiency of both **dietary proteins** and the **calories** i.e. **energy.** It generally occurs in the children below

1 year of age. **The symptoms include growth retardation, muscle wasting, anaemia, weakness, and repeated infections. Attitude is irritable.** Skin is shrunken, dry and atrophic.

A marasmic child does not show edema on decreased concentration of plasma albumin **(usual level in them is 2 to 3g/dl whereas in kwashiorkor cases it is always less than 2g/dl)** and the level of cortisol in serum gets increased in marasmic child whereas decreased in kwashiorkor.

> Marasmus is predominantly due to the **deficiency of calories.** This is usually observed in children given watery gruels (of cereals) to supplement the mother's breast milk.

Soyabean (Glycine hispida - a very good source of proteins for vegetarians).

Soyabean is being eaten in China for several thousands of years. The whole dry grain contains about **40-43 percent of protein** (twice as much as in most other pulses) and also upto **20% fat.** Soyabean forms the basis of the great variety of the sauces and pastes with which Chinese cooks garnish their food. Contrarily, in India and Europe the people have not yet been attracted by it because of its peculiar bitter flavour.

It has been observed that the nutritive value of the wheat flour is increased by several folds if the soyabean flour is mixed with it in the ratio of 50:50. Such a flour has been proved to be very useful for the growing children. Effect of a single protein on the growth of rats has been shown in Figure 10.10, whereas supplementation effect (supplemented with amino acids and protein) has been shown in Figures 10.11 and 10.12 respectively.

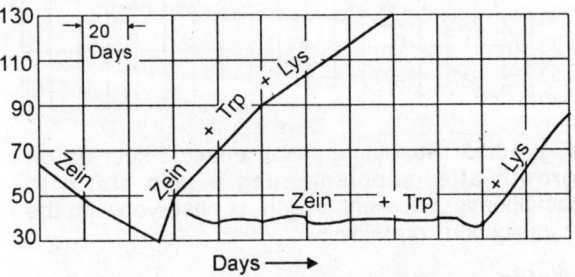

Fig. 10.11: Graph showing supplementation effect. When zein supplemented with tryptophan and lysine, excellent growth is obtained. With tryptophan as the only supplement, body weight alone is maintained, there is no remarkable gain in body weight; growth takes place only after further addition of lysine.

Minerals

These have equally important role in the human body for proper growth and maintenance. Living organisms contain at least 29 elements. among these, **13 are non metals** i.e. C, H, O, N, S, P, Cl, F, Br, I, B, Si and As. The metals are Ca, Mg, Na, K, Fe, Cu, Zn, Ni, Co, Mn, Al, Pb, Sn, Mo, V and Ti.

Among the elements needed in quantities **greater than 100 mg daily are** Ca, Mg, Na, K, P, and Cl; these are called the **macroelements.** The others are needed in very minute quantities (less than 100 mg daily) and are termed as **microelements or oligoelements or trace elements.**

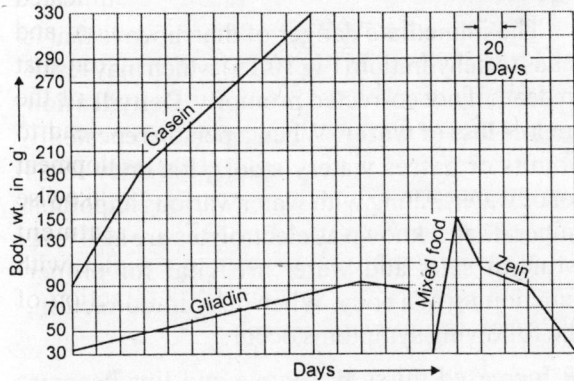

Fig. 10.10: Growth curve of rats maintained on diets containing a single protein. Poor growth is observed with gliadin as the protein (lysine deficient), and with zein (lysine and tryptophan deficient). Excellent growth is obtained with a casein diet.

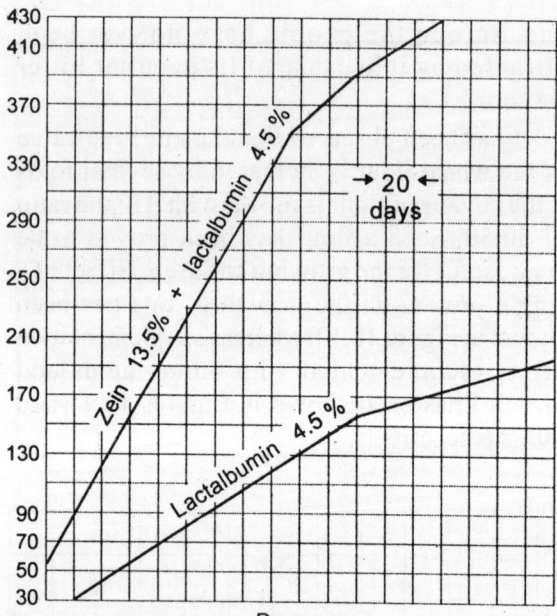

Fig. 10.12: Supplementation effect. Effect on rat growth after supplementing a zein diet with lactalbumin. Excellent growth is observed with the combination proteins.

Water

It constitutes nearly 70% of the total body weight and may be roughly compared to the ratio of water and land on the earth (Figures 10.13 and 10.14) where again water covers nearly 75% of the total area of the earth, thus emphasizing the

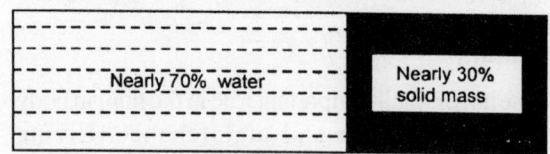

Fig. 10.13: Exhibiting ratio of water and solid mass in human body

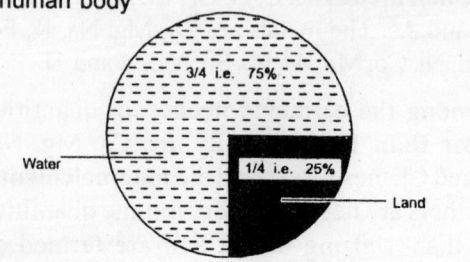

Fig. 10.14: Exhibiting the ratio of water and land on the earth

contribution of water in the human body and on the earth.

Loss of about 10% of body water causes illness and loss of about 20% may cause death. All the enzymatic reactions proceed in the human body in an aqueous phase of which water is the important component. Nearly 75% of the total diseases of the infants are caused due to giving them deficient and uncleaned water.

Diarrhoea and oral rehydration

Young children in our country suffer from various health problems. **Malnutrition and diarrhoeal diseases cause a large proportion of illness and death in young children**. Repeated attacks of diarrhoea often produce and worsen malnutrition.

What is diarrhoeal disease?

When a person passes liquid watery stools more than three times in 24 hours, he or she is said to have diarrhoea. It is very often accompanied by vomiting, fever and loss of appetite. This disease is caused by a variety of bacterial and viral agents which usually come from unclean surroundings. **Food, water, dirty hands and clothing carry these bacterial and viral agents.**

The immediate danger of diarrhoea is that it leads to dehydration (Fig 10.15) which may result in death if not corrected promptly. **Dehydration means loss of water.** When a person repeatedly vomits or passes watery stools, his body loses lot of water. Along with water, various important mineral salts, known as electrolytes are also lost. Mineral salts and water are vital for proper functioning of a body. When dehydration sets in, the following symptoms occur:

■ Increased thirst ■ Tongue and lips become dry ■ Weakness ■ Skin loses its elasticity ■ Eyes become sunken ■ In children below 18 months, the depression on their head - bone becomes more sunken ■ Urine output decreased

In diarrhoea in children, oral rehydration therapy (a mixture of pinch of sugar and salt in a cup of boiled and cooled water) should be started immediately (Fig 10.16) without any delay.

When liquid from the body is lost in large quantities and rapidly, particularly in very young children, dehydration can be very severe. This can lead to sudden death.

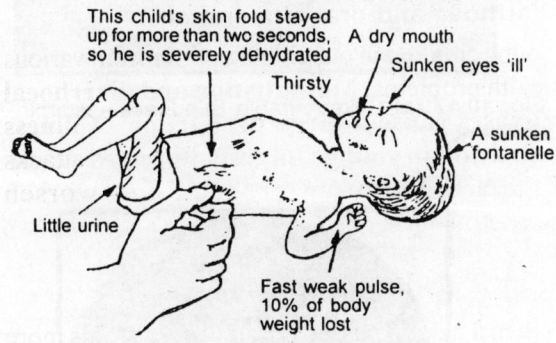

Fig. 10.15: Effect of dehydration

Vitamins

In addition to carbohydrates, lipids, proteins, inorganic salts and water, normal growth and good health in the mammals require the presence of additional compounds in the diet. These are organic in nature and are called vitamins. Not all living organisms require vitamins (some bacteria do not), nor do they necessarily need the same number or kind, since some vitamins can be synthesized by the organism. **For example, the guinea pig, man and other primates cannot synthesize vitamin C (ascorbic acid) due to the absence of enzyme L-gulono-oxidase and are therefore susceptible to scurvy,** whereas the rat can synthesize vitamin C and therefore does not require it in the diet. We do not know the biochemical functions of all the known vitamins, although many, especially those of the vitamin B group, are known to be precursors of coenzymes.

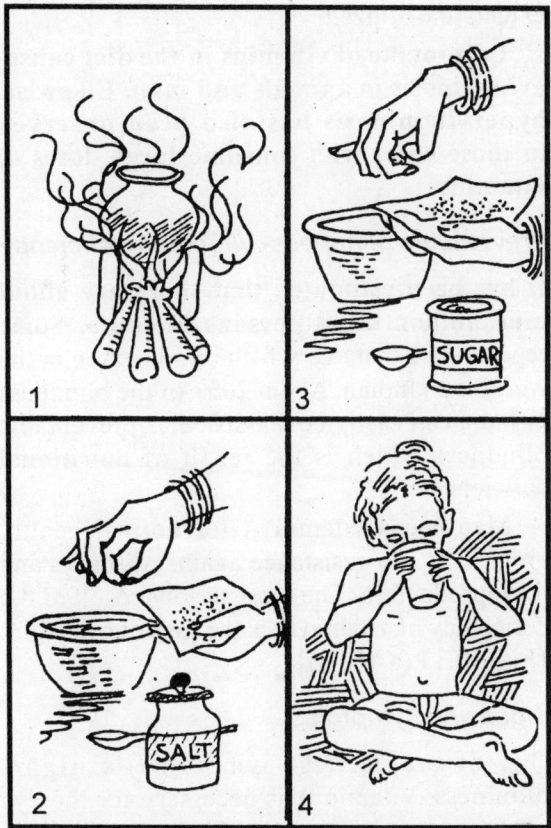

Fig. 10.16 : To show oral rehydration therapy

Vitamins are usually divided into two categories: those that are fat soluble and those that are water soluble. **Fat soluble vitamins are A, D, E and K; the water soluble vitamins are members of the B and C groups.** Nearly, all these vitamins are found in the consumable articles for instance vegetables, milk, meat, fish, pulses, corns(wheat, millet, gram, etc), fruits, cereals, etc.

Intestinal organisms play a role in the vitamin quota available to the animal or man. They may synthesize vitamins in significant amount. Vitamin K is an important example of a vitamin synthesized by intestinal organisms. Folic acid, nicotinic acid, pyridoxine, biotin, thiamine and riboflavin are other examples. These may be absorbed to varying extents and utilized.

Less intake of vitamins in the diet causes avitaminosis in animals and man. Likewise, hypervitaminosis has also been observed in those cases who consume large doses of vitamins.

Preventable Blindness- Vitamin A deficiency

It has been estimated that there are about nine million blind persons in India. Some reports state that every fifth blind person in the world is an Indian. About 20% of the blindness in India can easily be classified as preventable blindness which is the result of nutritional deficiencies.

Man needs vitamin A for normal health, growth, for the resistance against diseases and for reproduction. The most serious result of the deficiency of vitamin A is the loss of eye sight. {Fig. 10.17 (a and b)}.

Signs and Symptoms

One of the earliest symptoms is **night-blindness.** Vitamin A is necessary for the eye to respond or become sensitive to changes in light. If vitamin A is lacking, the person is unable to see clearly in dimlight or at night. Such children may be able to see perfectly well during day time. The condition is commonly known as night blindness. In addition, there are some visual changes in the eye. The white portion of the eye becomes dry and flaky. As a result, the thin membrane loses its lustre and appears rough and dry. This condition is known as **xerophthalmia** which means 'dry-eye'. Wrinkled pearly grey spots, triangular or round in shape may appear on the white portion in chronic cases. These are known as 'Bitot spots'.

These lesions by themselves do not affect vision. If the condition is not treated promptly, the black portion of the eye, that is the cornea also gets involved, resulting in keratomalacia and permanent blindness. This is a condition wherein the black portion of

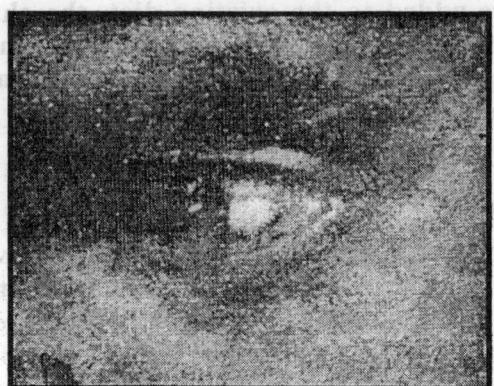

Fig. 10.17 (a) : Preventable Blindness - vitamin A deficiency

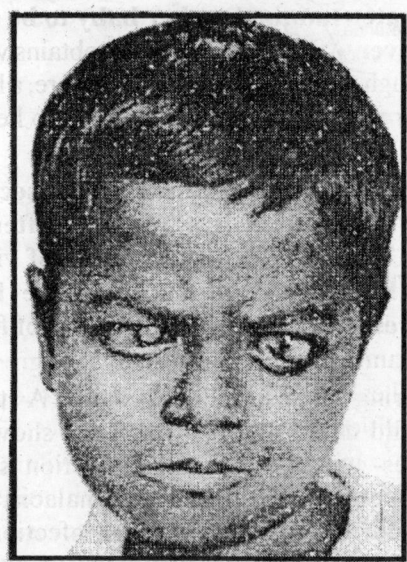

Fig. 10.17 (b) : To show the effect of vitamin A deficiency

the eye becomes softened into a cloudy, opaque mass.

In India, we have abundant sources of vitamin A that are easily and cheaply available. These include foods such as carrot, green leafy vegetables, namely drumstick leaves, amaranth, spinach and fruits like mango and papaya. Studies conducted by National Institute of Nutrition have shown that **if 40 g of green leafy vegetables** are added to the existing diet, the child would get the required amount of vitamin A. This is because leafy vegetables are good sources of carotene which can be converted into vitamin A in the body.

Causes

However, intake of vitamin A by children as well as women is' very low. In some areas, it is believed that children should not be given green leafy vegetables as it may cause diarrhoea. Others believe that pregnant women should not eat papaya; Thus, some of the rich sources of this vitamin are denied to those who need it most.

A well - nourished mother provides adequate vitamin A to her baby to be stored in its liver. After birth, the infant obtains vitamin A through the mother's milk. Therefore, a healthy mother provides enough vitamin A to her baby before birth as well as after birth.

Colostrum is the thick milky secretion of the breast in the first few days after child birth. This is a very rich source of vitamin A. Infants fed colostrum have better reserves of vitamin A. The practice of feeding colostrum should be encouraged.

During acute infections, vitamin A status of the child deteriorates. It has been shown that measles- common childhood infection is one of the important causes of keratomalacia. Acute respiratory and gastrointestinal infections also aggravate vitamin A deficiency. Intestinal parasites, especially round worms are common among children belonging to poor communities. Incidence of vitamin A deficiency is higher among the children having round worms in their gastrointestinal tracts.

Prevention and treatment

Even the most severe cases of vitamin A deficiency can be successfully treated. The usual practice is to administer intramuscular injections of 30,000 µg of vitamin A for two or three consecutive days. This is followed by oral doses for a few more days till the body reserves are built up. Conjunctival lesions and night blindness respond well to relatively small doses of vitamin A. Oral administration of 1,000 µg daily for about a week usually reverses the changes.

Corneal lesions should be treated as a medical emergency. 30,000 µg of water miscible vitamin A can be injected intramuscularly followed by 1000 µg of vitamin A orally for a period of 15 days. This helps in rapid clinical and biochemical improvement. Oil soluble vitamin A should not be injected as the absorption of this compound from the site of injection is poor.

Diet improvement

The most logical method of prevention would be to improve the diet of the vulnerable groups.

Consumption of adequate amount of vitamin A is essential to keep the eyes bright. Drumstick leaves, spinach, amaranth, carrots and pumpkin contain large quantities of carotene. The substance is converted into vitamin A in our body. Even children suffering from mild forms of malnutrition are able to absorb carotene from amaranth. The presence of even small amount of fat helps in the absorption. Carotene is also present in large quantities in fruits like mango and papaya. Consumption of such food [Fig. 10.18 (a & b)] should be encouraged. Particularly pregnant and lactating women should eat sufficient quantities of foods rich in vitamin A. They can meet requirements easily if they eat atleast one medium sized bowl full of cooked greens every day.

As a short- term measure, periodical oral administration of vitamin A has been suggested for the prevention of vitamin A deficiency in children.

Based on the recommendations of the National Institute of Nutrition (NIN), Hyderabad, the Government of India has launched a massive prophylaxis programme against vitamin A deficiency from 1970 in several states. In this programme children between 1-5 years are being given an oral dose of 2,00000 I.U. of vitamin A once in six months. The programme is implemented through the existing public health set up. Evaluation carried out in some states has shown a significant reduction in the incidence of xerophthalmia wherever the programme was well implemented.

A few paise spent on inexpensive foods rich in vitamin A can make all the difference between **good vision and no vision** (Fig. 10.19).

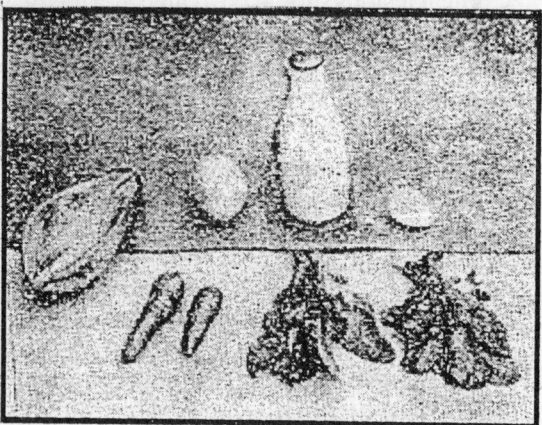

(a)

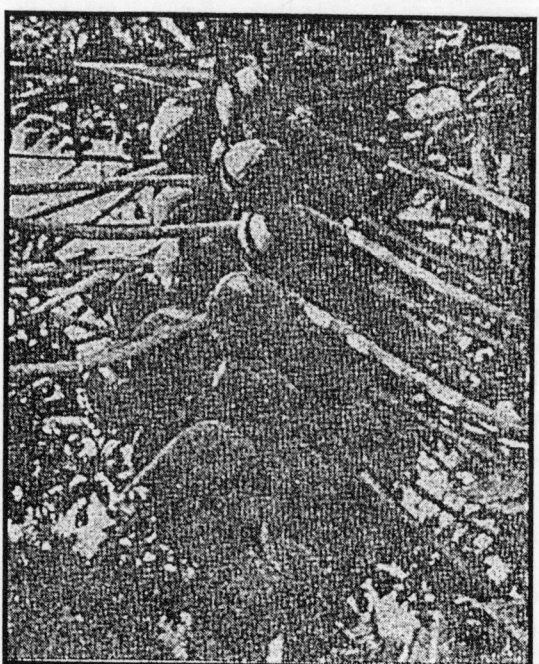

Fig. 10.18 (a & b) : Treatment part of vitamin `A' deficiency

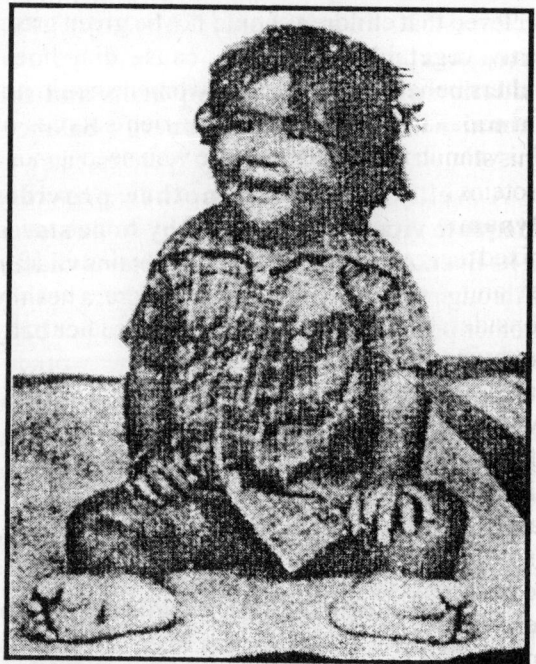

Fig. 10.19 : Normal child with good vision

TIPS FOR HEALTHY EATING

- **Eat whole grain cereals, millets and pulses.**
- Eat plenty of seasonal vegetables and one seasonal fruit daily.
- **Consume green leafy vegetables.**
- **Milk and milk products, fruits and vegetables are essential for healthy ageing.**
- Foods of animal origin, oil, fat and sugar are good for growing children, adolescents, pregnant and lactating women.

Specific Dynamic Action (S.D.A.) of Foods or calorigenic action of foods:

Scientist Rubner observed that carbohydrates, fats and proteins fed to a fasting dog, stimulated the energy metabolism over the basal level to varying extents. For example, he found that in a fasting dog requiring 400 KCal, feeding of 100g. of carbohydrates produces 425 KCal, 44.4 g. of fat produces 416 KCal and 100 g. of protein produces 520 KCal of heat (Table 10.10). **The extra heat produced is obtained by the oxidation of the tissue constituents and the animal will be in negative energy balance.** This stimulating effect of carbohydrates, fats and proteins on energy metabolism is called **'Specific Dynamic Action' (S.D.A.).** The S.D.A. of a mixed diet containing 62.5 g. carbohydrates, 10g. fat and 10g. protein is about 8 per cent. A considerable amount of work has been carried out by Scientist Lusk and several other workers on the causes of the high S.D.A. of proteins. When different amino acids were fed, alanine, glycine, and phenylalanine were found to produce high S.D.A. According to Krebs, two main factors responsible for the high S.D.A. of proteins are: (1) The energy required for deamination of amino acids which again is derived by the oxidation of other metabolites; and (2) The energy required for the synthesis of urea which is obtained by the oxidation of other metabolites present in the tissues.

POLYSACCHARIDES (FIBRES) NOT UTILISED IN THE HUMAN BODY

The polysaccharides not utilised in the human body are cellulose, hemicelluloses, fructosans, galactans, mannans, pentosans, dextrans, levans and pectins; **such polysaccharides are called as fibres:**

Cellulose

Cellulose is a polysaccharide made up of β-glucose molecules. The β-glucose molecules are linked by 1:4 linkage. In starch, α-glucose units are linked by 1:4 linkage. Due to this difference in chemical structure, cellulose is not acted upon by amylases present in the digestive juices. **Pure forms of cellulose are cotton and paper pulp.**

Hemicelluloses

Hemicelluloses are polysaccharides containing pentoses, hexoses and uronic acids. **They are present in small amounts in all vegetables and in large amounts in husks of cereals and pulses, corn cobs and straws.** They are not acted upon by enzymes present in human digestive juices.

Table 10.10: Energy output in a fasting dog fed carbohydrates, fats, proteins and their blends (SDA of food)

Sl. No.	Nature of food	Energy value of food (KCal)	Energy output (KCal)	Extra energy produced due to SDA of food	
				(KCal)	(percent)
1.	Fasting	-	400	-	-
2.	100 g. of carbohydrates	400	425	25	6.2
3.	44.4 g. of fat	400	416	16	4.0
4.	100 g. of protein (casein)	400	520	120	30.0
5.	62.5 g. carbohydrate + 10 g. fat + 10 g. protein	400	432	32	8.0

Fructosans

Fructosans are polysaccharides formed by the combination of large number of fructose molecules. The well- known example is inulin present in Jerusalem artichoke. **Inulin is used for testing kidney function**. When inulin is injected into the blood, it is readily excreted in urine. The inulin molecule is small enough to be filtered by renal glomerular membrane and is not reabsorbed in the tubules. **Some foods, e.g., onions contain large amounts of fructosans.**

Galactans

Galactans are polysaccharides composed of galactose molecules. In addition, they contain small amounts of D-mannonic acid and sulphuric acid in combination. **The well- known polygalactan is agar-agar.** Agar- agar is insoluble in cold water but is soluble in hot water. Solutions containing 1 to 4 percent of agar-agar set to a jelly on cooling. Agar- agar is used in media for culturing bacteria. Sea weeds contain polygalactans.

Mannans

Mannans are polysaccharides composed of mannose. They occur in yeast, bacteria and some plants. The most abundant source of mannans is ivory nuts, i.e., seeds of Tagua palm.

Pentosans

Pentosans are polysaccharides formed by the combination of large number of pentoses. The common examples are xylan (composed of xylose) and Araban (composed of arabinose). They occur in grasses, straw, wood, gums and mucilages. They are not hydrolysed by enzymes present in digestive juices of human beings.

Dextrans and Levans

Dextrans and levans are polysaccharides obtained by the action of bacteria on glucose and fructose, respectively. Dextrans consist of chains of 1:6 glycoside linkage with cross linking between chains by 1:4 linkage. They have high molecular weights and form rather viscous colloidal solutions in water. They have attracted considerable clinical interest because of their possible use as plasma substitutes since they form non- toxic solutions, with high colloidal osmotic pressure suitable for intravenous administration as a temporary replacement of plasma proteins lost by haemorrhage. Dextrans so administered are slowly metabolised and disappear from the circulation. Levans are composed of fructose units with 2:6 linkages, thus differing from inulin which has 1:2 linkages.

Pectins

pectins are compounds formed by the combination of a large number of galacturonic acid units. A part of the carboxyl groups exists as methyl esters. In the presence of sucrose and citric acid, pectin forms a jel. **This is the basis of the preparation of jams and jellies.**

CARBOHYDRATES NOT UTILISED BY THE BODY (Role of fibres in the diet)

It is known for a long time that foods from plants contain indigestible polysaccharides called as **'Fibre'** or **'Crude fibre'**. The role of this fibre in human nutrition was not well understood except its function as bulk agent in preventing constipation. **Recent researches have shown that many other cell wall polysaccharides e.g., hemicelluloses, mucilages, pectin, gums, etc., are not digested by human beings.** Crude fibre gives only an approximate estimate of cellulose and lignin and does not estimate other unavailable carbohydrates such as hemicelluloses, pectin, mucilages, etc. It is evident that the actual non-available carbohydrate contents of plant foods are greather than the **'Crude fibre'** contents. During the past few years, there has been a renewed interest in the role of dietary fibre in nutrition.

Low fibre diets have been reported to be associated with ischemic heart disease, diabetes, diverticular disease, cancer of the colon, etc. A number of observations on the beneficial as well as adverse effects of dietary fibre are on the record. **Some of the important findings are as follows:**

Effect on Carbohydrate metabolism: The results of recent studies indicate that incorporation of fibre in the diet improves the glucose tolerance in diabetic humans. Certain types of dietary fibre, such as pectin and guar gum decreased the blood glucose concentration in diabetic patients by decreasing digestion and rate of absorption in the intestines. It has been found that the carbohydrates present in ragi (Eleucine coracana) are digested and absorbed more slowly than the carbohydrates of rice as the former contains about 11 percent available carbohydrates while rice contains only 1 percent.

Protein Utilization: Digestion and absorption of proteins are adversely affected when fibre contents of the diet is increased. The endogenous excretion of nitrogen has been found to be high on diets rich in fibre. Digestibility of protein decreases and there is a greater loss of nitrogen in faeces when fibre in the diet is increased. For example, the true digestibility of ragi proteins was very much less (65 percent) than that of rich proteins (85 percent) in humans due to the high unavailable carbohydrates (11 percent) in the former.

Fat Metabolism: Studies by several workers have shown that incorporation of fibre in the diet, in general, brings about a reduction in the serum cholesterol by preventing the absorption of cholesterol. Many types of fibre have been shown to lower the serum cholesterol and lipid levels. **Pectin is the only material which has shown a definite hypocholesterolemic effect.** The hypocholesterolemic effect of fibre is greater in cases of diets rich in cholesterol.

Mineral Absorption: A number of reports reveal that absorption of calcium, magnesium and phosphorus is decreased by the presence of fibre in the diet.

Prevention of Constipation: **The inclusion of fibre in the diet increases the faecal bulk and prevents constipation.** Faecal bile acid excretion increases with increase in the level of fibre in the diet.

Comparison of human milk versus cow's				
	Human		**Cow's**	
	Range (percent)	Average	Range (percent)	Average
Water	82-90	87	82-90	87
Protein	1.0-2..0	1.3	2.5-4.5	3.4
Caseinogen	-	0.8	-	2.85
Albumin (along with little globulin)	-	0.5	-	0.55
Fats	2.0-4.5	3.3	2.5-5.5	3.7
Lactose	5.6-7.8	0.8	3.5-5.6	4.8
Ash	0.1-0.4	0.25	0.6-0.9	0.73
Calcium	0.018-0.042	0.03	0.09-0.17	0.125
Phosphorus	0.010-0.020	0.016	0.07-0.12	0.095

Food irradiation is a cold process for killing microorganisms.

In irradiated food no significant change in appearance, smell or taste is observed.

Irradiated food is very safe to eat, wholesome and nutritious.

So far 33 countries have cleared irradiated foods for human consumption and about 20 apply this technology on a commercial scale.

CHAPTER 11

WATER AND ELECTROLYTES BALANCE

WATER

The chief constituent of living matter is water. Its importance in both the structure and functioning of the tissues is enormous.

The body of a healthy adult male consists of some 65 to 70 percent of water and about 15 percent of fat; the remainder is accounted for by the solid parts of cells and supporting structures. The considerable variations in total body water (TBW) between one person and another are due to differences in fat content since the amount of **water in the fat-free parts of the body is remarkably constant. This reveals the fact that the water content of the body of the female ranges from 50 to 55 percent which is rather less than that of the male. In very fat people, the body water may not be more than 40 percent of the total body weight.**

In its capacity as a solvent, water plays a very important role in the cellular reactions. A very large number of substances are soluble in water and many others such as fats and fat - soluble compounds can be carried in fine emulsions or be rendered water - soluble by combination with hydrophilic substances.

Owing to the high heat capacity of water, large changes in heat production can take place in the body with very little alteration in the body temperature. Since the latent heat of evaporation of water is high, the loss of a small amount of water in evaporated sweat means a relatively large loss of heat. **Moreover, the high latent heat of solidification is a protection against the freezing of the tissues.**

Water is received by the body from the two main sources. Most of it is taken by mouth in the form of food and drinks but a small amount of water is normally formed in the tissues as a result of oxidation of the hydrogen of foodstuffs. **The amount of water ingested by an individual varies according to the habit, climate and occupation.**

The amount of **metabolic water** formed in the tissues as a result of oxidation processes is nearly **300-350 ml in man,** that is nearly 14 percent of his total daily fluid intake. This water is formed in the cells and is of great significance to the organism. **It is of utmost importance to the hibernating animals who live for longer periods on metabolic water and to organisms such as the moths of the clothes who do not normally have ready access to water.**

Following Table 11.1 gives an idea of turnover of fluid which occurs in the body during

24 hours. **In 24 hours, a man secretes 1 to 1.5 litre(s) of saliva, 1 to 2 litre(s) of gastric juice, 0.5 to 1 litre of bile, 0.6 to 0.8 litre of pancreatic juice and 3 litres of intestinal juice.** All this fluid except about 100 ml which is escaped through faeces is reabsorbed.

Table 11.1 Water balance of an adult man in a temperate climate

Daily intake		Daily output	
Drinks	1300 ml	**Urine**	1500 ml
Food	850 ml	**Expired air**	400 ml
Formed in the body by		**Skin**	500 ml
Oxidation	350 ml	**Faeces**	100 ml
Total	2500 ml	**Total**	2500 ml

Water Metabolism

Since most biochemical reactions of the body take place in an aqueous medium, control of water balance is an important requirement for **homeostasis.**

Although water is freely permeable across the cell membrane but contrarily other solutes are less mobile because of several barriers imposed by membrane systems. These barriers give rise to fluid pools or compartments i.e., **intracellular fluid and extracellular fluid.**

Intracellular fluid makes up 30-40% of the body weight, or about two-thirds of total body water. **Potassium and magnesium are the predominant cations. The anions are mainly proteins and organic phosphates with chloride and bicarbonate at low concentrations.**

Extracellular fluid contains sodium as the predominant cation and accounts for 20-25% of body weight or one-third of total body water. It contributes to vascular, interstitial, transcellular and dense connective tissue fluid pools. Vascular fluid is the circulating portion, is rich in proteins and does not readily cross endothelial membranes, whereas interstitial fluid surrounds the cells and accounts for 18-20% of total body water. It exchanges with vascular fluid via the lymph system. Transcellular fluid remains present in digestive juice, intraocular fluid, cerebrospinal fluid (CSF), and synovial (joint) fluid. These fluids are secretions of specialized cells. Their composition differs considerably from that of the rest of the extracellular fluid, with which they rapidly exchange contents under normal conditions. Dense connective tissue (bone, cartilage, etc) fluid exchanges slowly with the rest of the extracellular fluid and accounts for nearly 15% of total body water.

Movement of water is mainly due to **osmosis** and **filtration.** In osmosis, water moves to the area of higher solute concentration. Thus, active movement of salts into an area creates a concentration gradient down as a result of which water flows passively. In filtration, hydrostatic pressure in atrial blood moves water and nonprotein solutes and through specialized membranes to produce an almost protein - free filtrate; **this process occurs during the formation of renal glomerular filtrate.** Besides, filtration also accounts for the movement of water from the vascular space into the interstitial compartment which is opposed by the osmotic (oncotic) pressure of plasma proteins.

Cells move ions (especially Na^+ and K^+) against a concentration gradient by a **'sodium pump'** that actively transports sodium across the plasma membranes.

Kidneys are the major organs to regulate the extracellular fluid composition and volume. **The three main processes which occur in the nephrons are:**

a) **Formation of a virtually protein - free ultrafiltrate in the glomerulus.**

b) **Active reabsorption (principally in the proximal tubule) of solutes from the glomerular filtrate; and**

c) **Active excretion of substances such as hydrogen ions into the tubular lumen, usually in the distal portion of the tubule (Fig 17.1).**

The normal glomerular filtration rate (GFR) is 100 - 120 ml/min which means nearly 150 litre of fluid passes through the renal tubules each day. Since the **average daily urinary output is 1-1.5 litres, 99% of** the glomerular filtrate is reabsorbed. Approximately 80% of the water is reabsorbed in the proximal tubule, a consequence of active absorption of solutes. Reabsorption in the rest of the tubule varies according to the individual's water balance in contrast to the **obligatory reabsorption** which occurs in the proximal tubule.

The facultative absorption of water depends upon the establishment of an osmotic gradient in the **loop of Henle** by the secretion of Na^+ from the ascending loop and their uptake by the descending loop. As a result, the proximal end of the loop is hyperosmotic (1200 mosm/kg) and the distal end hypoosmotic with respect to blood. The collecting ducts run through the hyperosmotic region. **In the absence of antidiuretic hormone (ADH), the cells of the ducts are relatively impermeable to water.** They become permeable to water in the presence of ADH, however, and the urine becomes hyperosmotic with respect to blood.

Water as a Solvent

For a solid to dissolve, three following points must happen:

a) The molecules (or ions) of the solid must separate from one another.

b) The molecules of the solvent must also undergo a separation to admit the molecules (or ions) of the solute. This causes the breaking of some of the linkages holding the solvent molecules together.

c) Some sort of linkages must be formed between the solvent molecules and the solute molecules to balance the attraction which the solute molecules exert on one another.

Homeostatic Controls

The composition and volume of extracellular fluid are regulated by the following two complex mechanisms i.e;

a) **Hormonal mechanism**

b) **Nervous mechanism**

which interact to control its osmolality, volume and pH.

The osmolality of extracellular fluid is mainly due to Na^+ and accompanying anions; this is kept within narrow limits (285-295 mosm/kg) by the regulation of water intake **(via a thirst centre)** and water excretion by the kidney through the action of ADH. The volume is kept relatively constant, provided the individual's body weight remains constant to within $\pm$ 1 kg. **Volume receptors** sense the effective circulating blood volume which when decreased, stimulates the renin-angiotensin- aldosterone system and results in retention of Na^+. The increased Na^+ level leads to a rise in osmolality and secretion of ADH with a resultant increase in water retention. Side by side, **antagonistic systems** also exist that cause an increased Na^+ excretion. **Atrial natriuretic peptide (ANP), also called atrial natriuretic factor (ANF) or hormone,** is released by the cardiocytes of the cardiac atria in response to mechanical stretch caused by the plasma volume expansion.

ANF has got the following two functions:

a) **Induces diuresis, and**

b) **Induces natriuresis**

These effects result from renal hemodynamic changes associated with increases in GFR and inhibition of Na^+ reabsorption from inner medullary collecting ducts.

ANP is a 28 amino- acid peptide and possesses only one disulfide linkage in its

structure. The precursor and the storage form of ANP in cardiocytes is a 126 - amino acid polypeptide. Following are the stimuli of ANP:

   (i)   Blood volume,

   (ii) High blood pressure,

   (iii) Elevated serum osmolality,

   (iv) Increased heart rate and

   (v) Elevated levels of plasma catecholamines

Activation of the ANP gene in cardiocytes by glucocorticoids leads to increased synthesis of ANP which also regulates Na$^+$ and water homeostasis by different mechanisms that include inhibition of steps in the renin- angiotensin- aldosterone pathway and inhibition of ADH secretion from posterior pituitary cells.

Electrolytes Balance

   Major electrolytes are the following:

   (a) Na$^+$,

   (b) K$^+$,

   (c) Cl$^-$, and

   (d) HCO$_3^-$

Sodium:

The average sodium content of the human body is 60 mEq/kg, of which 50% is in extracellular fluid, 40% is in bone and 10% is intracellular. The chief dietary source of Na$^+$ is salt added during cooking and in the preparation of pickles. Excess sodium is largely excreted via urine, whereas some is lost via perspiration. Gastrointestinal losses are little except in diarrhoea.

   Sodium balance is integrated with the regulation of extracellular fluid volume. Depletion hyponatremia (i.e., sodium loss greater than water loss) may result from less intake of sodium, excessive loss of fluid from vomiting or diarrhoea, diuretic abuse and adrenal insuffi-ciency. Hyponatremia can cause decreased extracellular fluid volume, as occurs in congestive heart failure, uncontrolled diabetes mellitus, nephrosis, cirrhosis and inappropriate ADH secretion, etc.

Hypernatremia is caused by the loss of hypoosmotic fluid which occurs in burns, fevers, high environmental temperature, **diabetes insipidus,** kidney diseases, exercise, etc or **by the increased Na$^+$ intake** as takes place during adminstration of hypertonic NaCl solution, ingestion of NaHCO$_3$, etc.

Potassium:

The average K$^+$ content of the human body is 40 mEq/kg which is found mainly in intracellular space. **It is required for the metabolism of carbohydrates and increased cellular uptake of K$^+$ also occurs during catabolism of glucose.** Potassium is widely distributed in plant sources and animal foods, **the human requirement is nearly 4 g/ day.** Insulin and catecholamines accelerate a shift of K$^+$ into the cells. **Excess K$^+$ is excreted via urine, a process regulated by aldosterone.**

Plasma potassium plays a role in the irritability of excitable tissues. A high concentration of plasma K$^+$ causes electrocardiographic (ECG) abnormalities and possibly to cardial arrhythmia, which may be due to lowering of the membrane potential.

Low concentration of plasma K$^+$ (hypokalemia) increases the membrane potential, decreases irritability, and produces other ECG abnormalities and **muscle paralysis too.**

Hyperkalemia may take place in renal diseases and adrenal insufficiency. Metabolic acidosis, particulauly in diabetic acidosis and catabolism of celluar protein in starvation or fever cause K$^+$ release from cells. **Treatment consists in correction of acidosis and promotion of cellular uptake of K$^+$ by administration of insulin which increases intake of glucose. In severe cases, ion exchange resins given orally bind K$^+$ in intestinal secretions.**

Hypokalemia may occur from loss of

gastrointestinal secretions (which contain large amounts of K^+) and from excessive loss via urine because of increased aldosterone secretion or diuretic therapy. **Hypokalemia is usually associated with alkalosis.**

Chloride:

It is the major extracellular anion. **Nearly, 70%** is found in extracellular fluid. The average Cl^- content of the human body is 35 meq/kg. Chloride obtained from food is almost completely absorbed. **Plasma levels of Na^+ and Cl^- in general undergo parallel alterations; however, in metabolic alkalosis, chloride concentration gets increased.**

Dehydration

When a person passes liquid watery stools more than three times in 24 hours, he or she is said to have diarrhoea. It is very often accompanied by vomiting, fever and loss of appetite. This disease is caused by a variety of bacterial and viral agents which usually come from unclean surroundings. **Food, water, dirty hands and clothing carry these bacterial and viral agents.**

The immediate danger of diarrhoea is that it leads to dehydration which may result in death if not corrected promptly. **Dehydration means loss of water.** When a person repeatedly vomits or passes watery stools, his body loses lot of water. Along with water, various important mineral salts, known as electrolytes are also lost. Mineral salts and water are vital for proper functioning of a body. When dehydration sets in, the following symptoms occur:

■ Increased thirst ■ Tongue and lips become dry ■ Weakness ■ Skin loses its elasticity ■ Eyes become sunken ■ In children below 18 months, the depression on their head - bone becomes more sunken ■ Urine output decreased

In diarrhoea in children, oral rehydration therapy (a mixture of pinch of sugar and salt in a cup of boiled and cooled water) should be started immediately without any delay.

When liquid from the body is lost in large quantities and rapidly, particularly in very young children, dehydration can be very severe. This can lead to sudden death.

Properties of water

Acid and base concentrations in living system are fully regulated to maintain conditions compatible with normal life. Biochemical reactions involving acids and bases occur in the body water, whereas buffer systems protect the body from significant variations in the concertrations of acids and bases.

Life can not be sustained without water. Water constitutes 45-73% of total human body weight. It is distributed in intracellular (55%) and extracellular (45%) compartments and provides a continous solvent phase between body compartments. As the biological solvent, water plays a major role in all aspects of metabolism: **absorption, transport, digestion,** and **excretion of inorganic and organic substances as well as maintenance of body temperature.** The unique properties of water are due to its structure.

Physical properties of water

Density (at 4^oC)	1.0 g/mL
Molecular weight	18
Liquid range	0° - 100^oC
Melting point	0^oC
Boiling Point	100^oC
Heat of fusion	80 cal/g
Heat of vapourization	540 cal/g
Dipole moment	1.86 Debye unit
Dielectric constant (E)	78.4
Solid / liquid density ratio	0.92

CHAPTER 12

METABOLISM OF CARBOHYDRATES

We have a beautiful scene in intermediary metabolism. We include very important anabolic and catabolic pathways. Our anabolic pathways include glycogenesis (synthesis of glycogen) and gluconeogenesis (synthesis of glucose or glycogen); whereas catabolic ones include glycogenolysis, glycolysis, TCA cycle and pentose phosphate pathway. Ours catabolic routes have a tendency to liberate energy which is used for various purposes in the human body whereas ours anabolic routes have a tendency to synthesize glycogen/glucose and then store it so that the same may be utilized in odd situations.

We include in ourselves the only hypoglycaemic hormone i.e., insulin, the deficiency of which leads to a very fierceful disease of carbohydrate metabolism called as Diabetes Mellitus.

The major function of carbohydrate metabolism is to provide energy for various metabolic processes of the body. In this role, carbohydrates are utilised by the cells mainly in the form of glucose. Carbohydrates have the advantage of being cheap, easily digestible and rapidly metabolizable.

Carbohydrates' metabolism is basically the metabolism of glucose and substances related to it.

The sugar of the blood is glucose. The digestion of carbohydrates such as starch, sucrose and lactose produces glucose, fructose and galactose respectively which pass into the blood circulation. Conversion of fructose and galactose into glucose occurs in the liver.

under aerobic conditions, i.e.

$$\text{glucose} \xrightarrow{\text{glycolysis}} \text{pyruvic acid}$$

in the presence of O_2: acetyl CoA $\xrightarrow{\text{TCA Cycle}} CO_2 + H_2O$

under anaerobic conditions i.e. in the absence of O_2: lactic acid

Carbohydrates supply nearly 2/3 energy requirement of the body.

Glycolysis

The oxidation of glucose to pyruvate is termed as glycolysis (Fig 12.1).

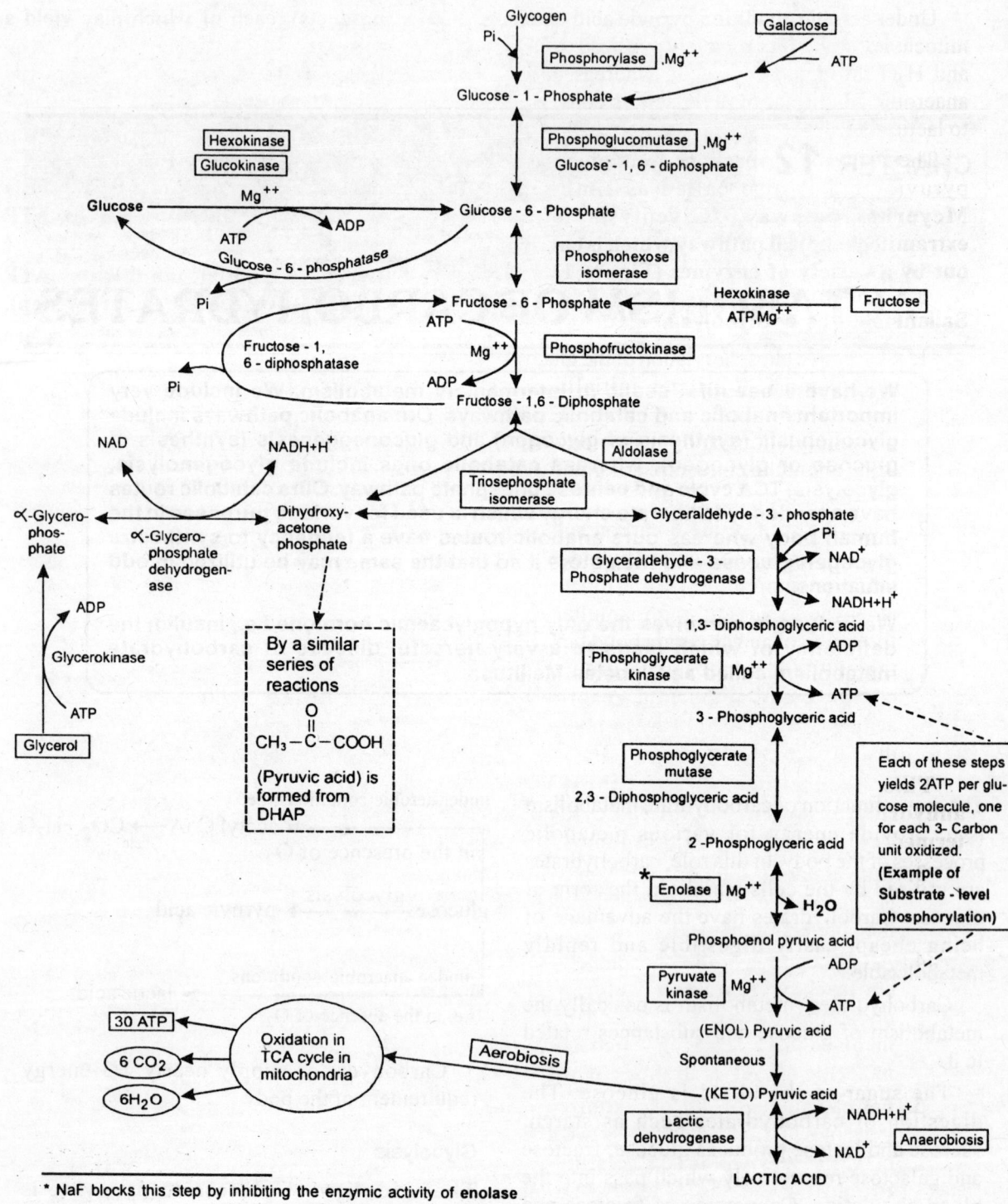

* NaF blocks this step by inhibiting the enzymic activity of **enolase**

Figure 12.1 : Glycolytic Pathway (Glycolysis)

Under aerobic condition pyruvic acid enters mitochondria and is completely oxidized to CO_2 and H_2O through TCA cycle, whereas under anaerobic condition, pyruvic acid is converted to lactic acid.

The sequence of reactions from glucose to pyruvic acid is also called as **Embden-Meyerhof** pathway. **'Glycolysis is an extramitochondrial pathway which is carried out by a variety of enzymes (Figure 12.1).**

Salient features of Glycolysis

1. Successive phosphorylation of the glucose at C-1 and C-6 utilizes initially two molecules of ATP. These phosphorylations and an isomerization bring about the conversion of glucose to fructose 1,6-diphosphate.

2. After the split of the 6-carbon sugar to two 3- carbon molucules (by aldolase), there is immediate oxidation of the aldehyde to an acid with simultaneous formation of an anhydride bond between the acid and a phosphate group, this complex and important reaction is achieved by glyceraldehyde phosphate dehydrogenase, utilizing NAD^+.

This formation of the phosphate anhydride by an enzyme of the cytosol is termed as substrate level phosphorylation.

3. Conversion of the phosphate anhydride to a carboxylic acid is then combined with the conversion of ADP to ATP.

4. After the move of the phosphate to C-2, enolase, by removing water, yields phosphoenolpyruvate, which is then involved in a reaction in which a further molecule of ATP is formed from ADP.

5. For each mole of glucose oxidized, the yield of ATP from glycolysis is two moles of ATP (4 ATP produced, 2 ATP utilized). In addition, 2 moles of NADH are produced (one for each of the 3- carbon products), each of which may yield a further two moles of ATP, if oxidized by the electron transport chain via the glycerol phosphate shuttle.

6. **The first rate limiting step (regulatory step) in glycolysis is catalysed by enzyme PFK. This enzyme is inhibited by citrate, ATP and NADH.**

7. **Pyruvate kinase is inhibited by ATP and NADH (second regulatory step).**

8. All the reactions of glycolysis are reversible except which are catalysed by
   (i) Hexokinase,
   (ii) PFK, and
   (iii) PK

9. Enzyme enolase is inhibited by fluoride. Since RBCs do not possess mitochondrial enzymes to oxidise glucose aerobically, they depend upon glycolysis only for their energy requirement, that is why, NaF is used in the collection of blood sugar samples because it prevents glycolysis by inhibiting the enzyme enolase, **otherwise a low value (low blood sugar) will be obtained due to glycolysis.**

10. It is a major pathway by which glucose is metabolized in RBCs.

11. Glycolysis gives rise to certain important compounds which are very important for other biochemical processes; those produced include:
    (i) Glyceraldehydade 3-PO_4: Required for the biosynthesis of triglycerides and phospholipids.
    (ii) Acetyl Co-A: Required for the biosynthesis of cholesterol.
    (iii) Pyruvate: Required for the biosynthesis of alanine by transamination.

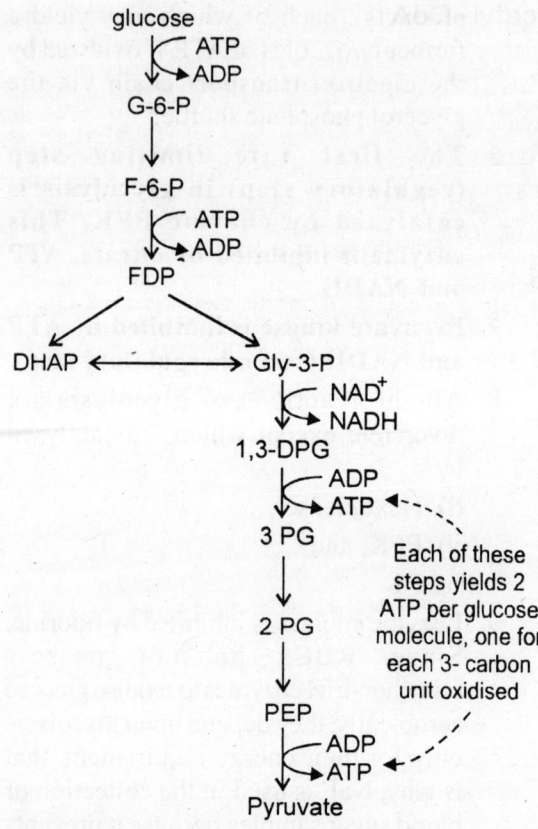

Figure 12.2 : Simplified schematic presentation of 'glycolysis'.

Simplified schematic presentation of glycolysis is given in (Figure 12.2).

Further metabolism of Pyruvate

Pyruvate produced by glycolytic pathway and the other metabolic pathways can be converted either to oxaloacetate or acetyl CoA as shown in Figure 12.3.

Citric acid cycle

This cycle is also known as TCA cycle or Krebs cycle (Figure 12.4). As the first product of this cycle i.e., citric acid contains three carboxyl groups, hence the name **'Tricarboxylic Acid Cycle'** has been given to this cyclic process.

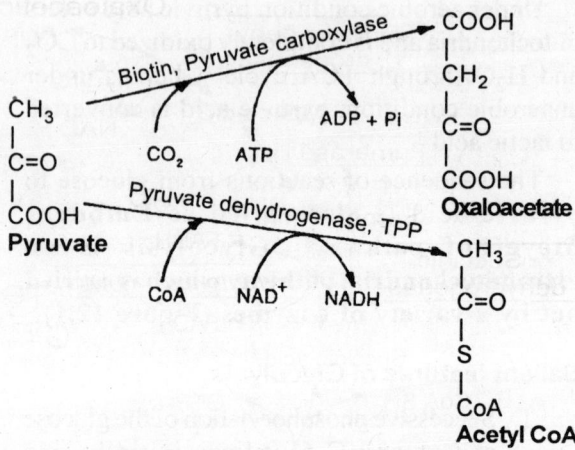

Figure 12.3 : Pyruvate metabolism

No hereditary disorders of TCA cycle enzymes are known. This cycle continuously operates in all the cells. Enzymes of this cycle remain mainly confined in the mitochondrial fraction of the cell.

Salient features of TCA cycle

1. This cycle operates only under aerobic conditions i.e. in the adequate supply of oxygen because it requires supply of NAD^+ and FAD which are regenerated when NADH and $FADH_2$ transfer their electrons to O_2 through the electron transport chain.

2. Before pyruvate gets entry into TCA cycle, it is oxidatively decarboxylated to acetyl CoA.

3. This cycle may be referred to as a mechanism whereby acetyl coenzyme A may be completely oxidized to CO_2 and H_2O.

4. The very first reaction of the cycle, which occurs in the presence of an enzyme called the **"condensing enzyme" (citrate synthetase)** is a condensation between acetyl CoA and oxaloacetic acid to form citric acid and coenzyme A. This

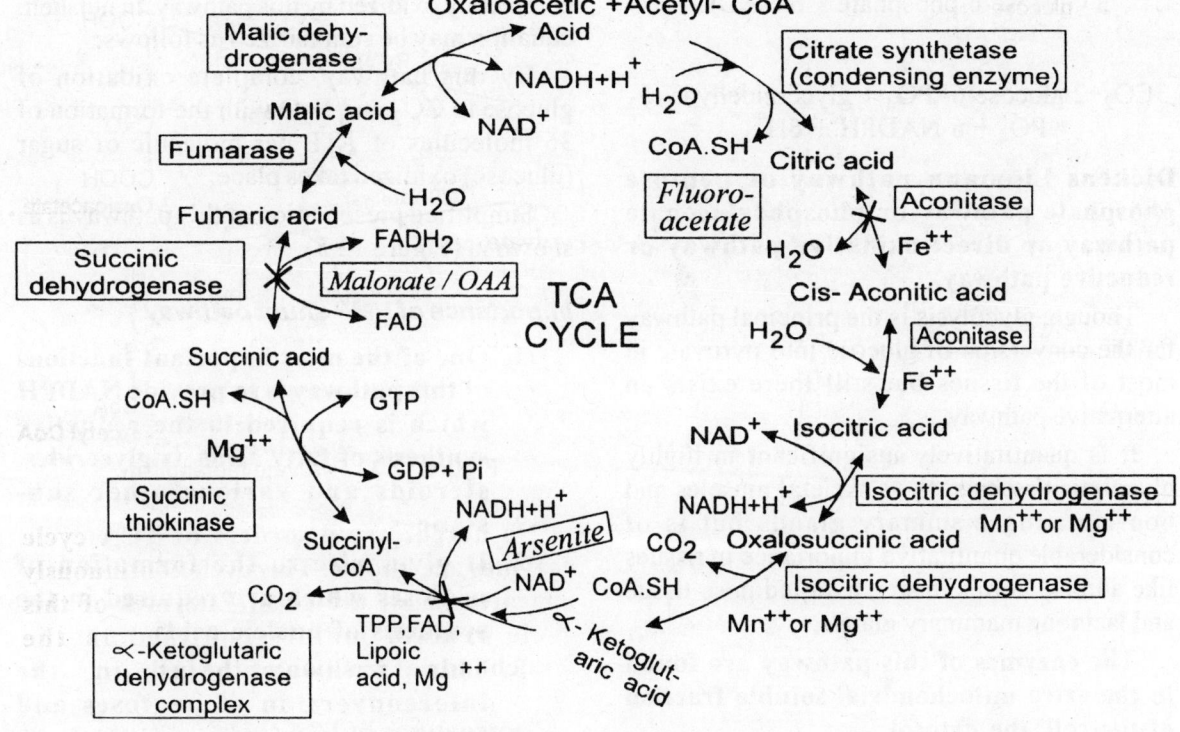

Figure 12.4 : TCA cycle (Krebs cycle)

reaction may be considered to be irreversible.

5. Aconitase and isocitric dehydrogenase play role as shown in the cycle.

6. α-ketoglutaric acid (α-keto acid) gets oxidatively decarboxylated forming succinyl CoA in the presence of TPP, NAD^+, FAD, CoA, lipoic acid and Mg^{++}.

7. The importance of this pathway lies in the fact that it is one of the pathways that generates the major part of the ATP and NADH in the cell.

8. NADP can be formed from $NADP^+$ and NADH by a mitochondrial trans-hydrogenase.

9. **ATP thus produced is utilized by the cell for its functions which are numerous and the NADPH for the biosynthesis of fatty acids, steroids** and other important substances of the human body.

Energetics of TCA cycle

(i) Pyruvic acid to acetyl CoA $2 \times 3 = 6$

(ii) Isocitric acid to oxalosuccinic acid $2 \times 3 = 6$

(iii) α-KGA to succinyl CoA $2 \times 3 = 6$

(iv) Succinyl CoA to succinic acid $2 \times 1 = 2$
 (substrate level phosphorylation)

(v) Succinic acid to fumaric acid $2 \times 2 = 4$

(vi) Malic acid to oxaloacetic acid $2 \times 3 = 6$

Total 30 ATP

Thus, total number of ATP molecules generated in TCA cycle under aerobic conditions is 30.

Hexose Monophosphate Shunt Pathway

This pathway is also known as **Warburg-**

$$3 \text{ Glucose-6-phosphate} + 6 \text{ NADP}^+$$

$$\downarrow$$

$$3CO_2 + 2 \text{ glucose-6-} PO_4 + \text{glyceraldehyde-3-}PO_4 + 6 \text{ NADPH} + 6H^+$$

Dickens Lipmann pathway or pentose phosphate pathway or phosphogluconate pathway or direct oxidative pathway or reductive pathway.

Though, glycolysis is the principal pathway for the conversion of glucose into pyruvate in most of the tissues but still there exists an alternative pathway.

It is quantitatively insignificant in highly glycolytic tissues such as skeletal muscles and non-lactating mammary glands but is of considerable quantitative importance in tissues like adrenal cortex, testis, liver, adipose tissue and lactating mammary glands.

The enzymes of this pathway are found in the extra mitochondrial soluble fraction of the cell, the cytosol.

Besides the above tissues, it also operates in leucocytes and erythrocytes.

It is a multicyclic process in which 3 molecules of glucose-6-phosphate give rise to 3 molecules of CO_2 and three-5- carbon residues (namely: ribulose-5-PO_4). The latter are arranged to regenerate 2 molecules of glucose-6-phosphate and one molecule of the glycolytic intermediate i.e. glyceraldehyde-3-PO_4. Since 2 moles of glyceraldehyde-3-PO_4, can regenerate glucose-6-PO_4, glucose may be

---

Genetic Error: Genetic deficiency of glucose-6-P dehydrogenase enzyme, supposed to be a key enzyme of PPP may enhance fragility of RBCs as a result of which several disorders like hemolysis of RBCs, anemia and jaundice, particularly after the administration of vitamin K, sulpha drugs, favabeans and quinine may take place.

---

completely oxidized by this pathway. In nutshell, equation may be summarized as follows:

By this pathway, complete oxidation of glucose to CO_2 and H_2O with the formation of 36 molecules of ATP per molecule of sugar (glucose) oxidized takes place.

Simplified presentation of this pathway is as shown in (Figure 12.5).

Importance of HMP shunt pathway

1. **One of the most important functions of this pathway is to provide NADPH which is required in the reductive synthesis of fatty acids, triglycerides, steroids and various other substances.**

2. **It gives rise to the formation of pentoses which are required in the synthesis of nucleic acids.**

3. **This pathway helps in the interconversion of pentoses and hexoses.**

Energetics: By this pathway, complete oxidation of glucose to CO_2 and H_2O yields 36 **molecules of ATP** whereas complete oxidation of each molecule of glucose through the combined two pathways namely glycolysis and TCA cycle yields 38 moles of ATP which means that the ATP yield via PPP is almost equal to what is obtained by the combined effect of glycolysis and TCA cycle. Moreover, PPP is a shorter route for the yield of ATP than the combined routes of glycolysis + TCA.

GLYCOGENESIS

This process may be referred to as the synthesis of glycogen from glucose or other sugars.

In the very first reaction glucose gets phosphorylated to form glucose-6-PO_4 in the presence of ATP; this reaction is catalysed by glucokinase. In the next step, mutation of the phosphate group of glucose-6-PO_4 from position 6 to the position 1 takes place in the presence of

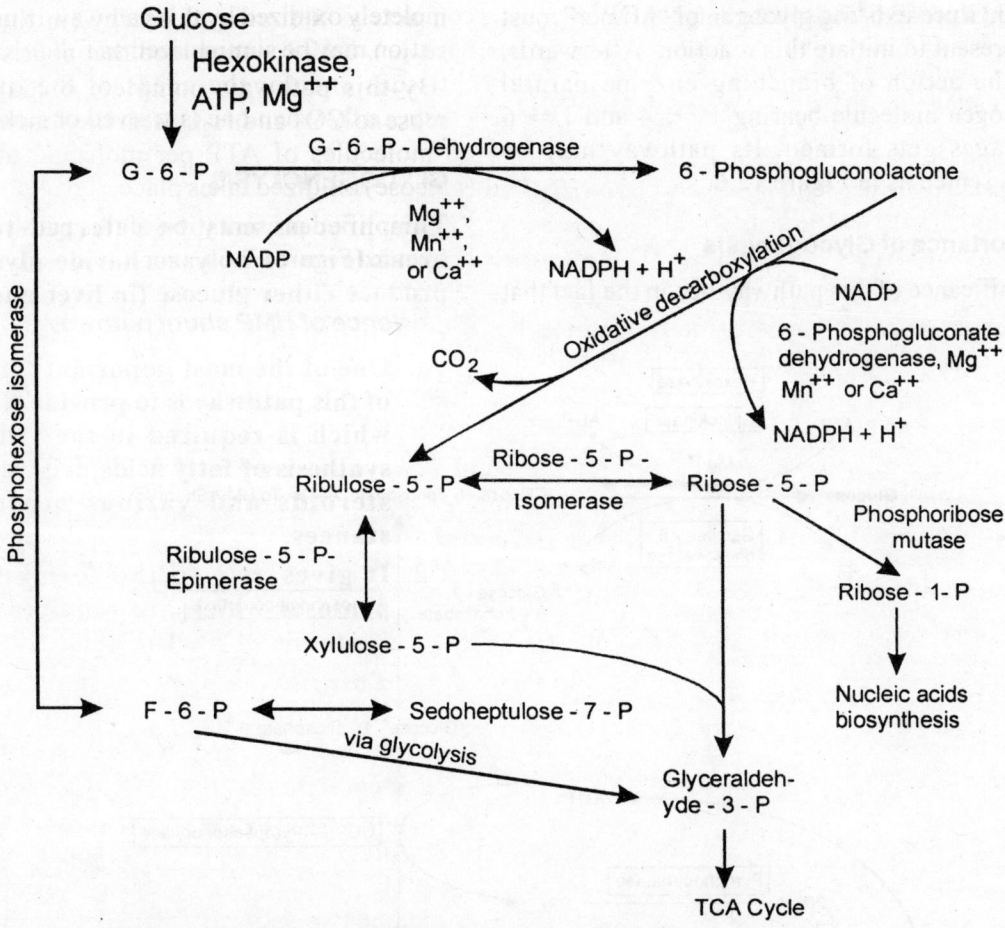

Figure 12.5 : Pentose phosphate pathway (simplified presentation)

a cofactor glucose 1,6 diphosphate; this reaction is catalysed by the enzyme phosphoglucomutase. In the next reaction, glucose-1-PO_4 reacts with UTP to form active nucleotide i.e., uridine diphosphate glucose in the presence of enzyme UDPG pyrophosphorylase; in this process, two terminal phosphates are removed from UTP as inorganic pyrophosphate, while the remaining UMP portion gets joined by a pyrophosphate bridge to glucose-1-phosphate to form UDP-glucose.

The next reaction is catalysed by the enzyme glycogen synthetase, in this reaction, the C_1 of the activated glucose of UDPG forms a glycosidic bond with the C_4 of a terminal glucose residue of glycogen, liberating UDP with the formation of unnatural glycogen i.e., straight

> *Glycogen* in fact, is a reservoir of energy. After a heavy intake of carbohydrates, as much as 1/10th of the liver mass may consist of this storage form of glucose, whereas in starvation or during illness when there is loss of appetite, the **glycogen reserve** may be almost depleted in order to meet out the energy requirements of the body.

chain; a pre-existing glycogen or "primer" must be present to initiate this reaction. Afterwards, by the action of branching enzyme natural glycogen molecule bearing $1 \rightarrow 4$ and $1 \rightarrow 6$ linkages gets formed. Its pathway may be represented as in Figure 12.6.

Importance of Glycogenesis

Significance of this pathway lies in the fact that it acts as a source of energy (in the form of sugar), both for the blood that nourishes other tissues and for the needs of the liver itself especially when one is starved or sick.

GLYCOGENOLYSIS

This process may be referred to as the breakdown of polysaccharide glycogen to produce either glucose (in liver and kidney

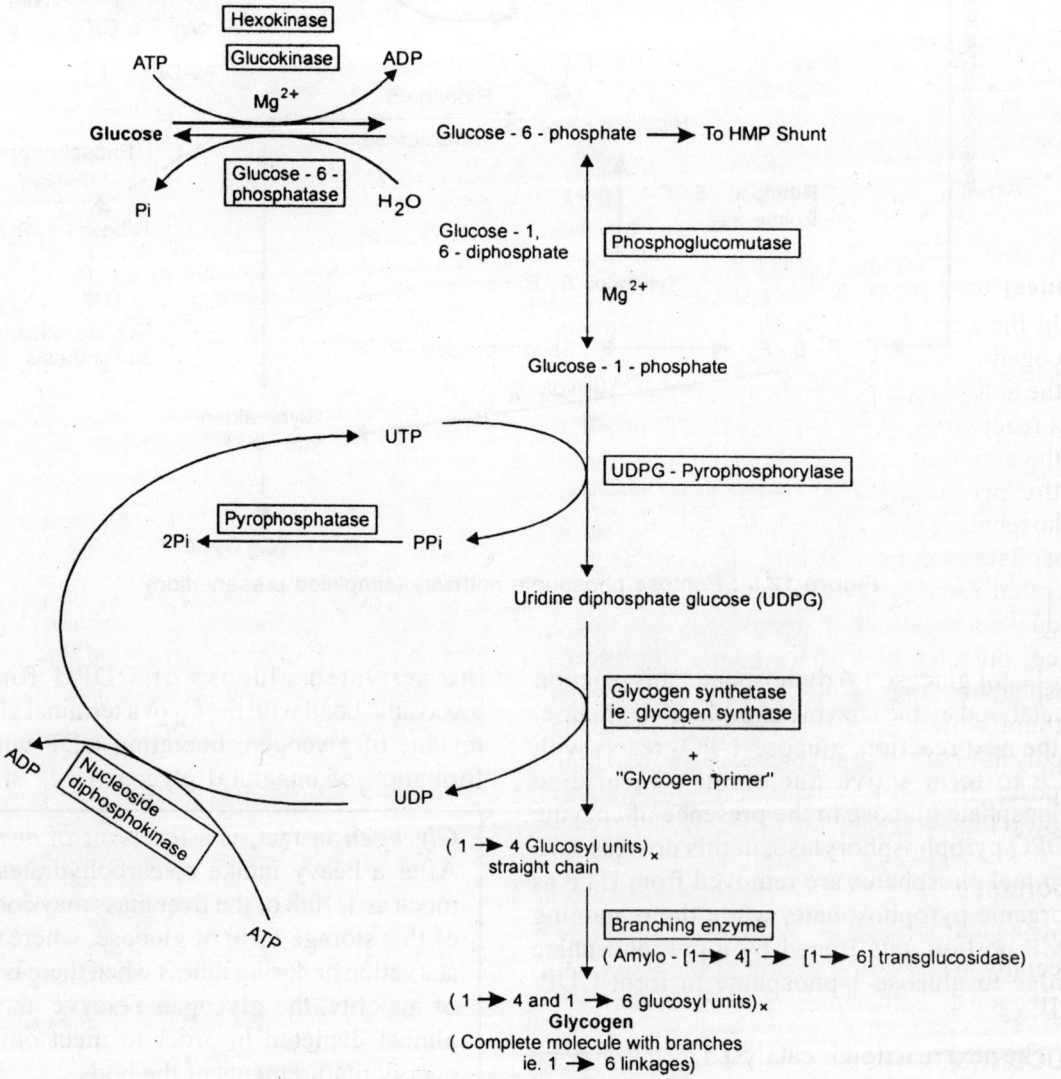

Figure 12.6 : Pathway of Glycogenesis

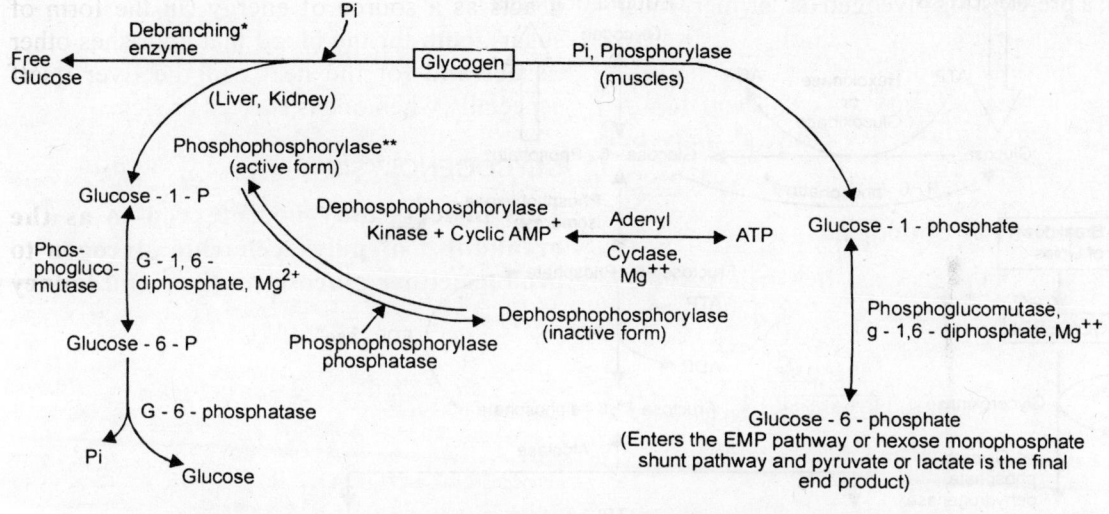

Figure 12.7 : Pathway of Glycogenolysis

tissues) or glucose-6-PO$_4$ (in muscles).

In the very first reaction of this pathway, glycogen is broken down to form glucose-1-P by the action of enzyme phosphorylase. In the next reaction g-1-PO$_4$ is converted to g-6-PO$_4$ by the action of enzyme phosphoglucomutase in the presence of cofactor glucose-1-6-diphosphate. Then, by the action of glucose-6-phosphatase upon g-6-PO$_4$, phosphate gets liberated forming glucose which is the end product of hepatic and renal glycogenolysis. Since, muscles lack the enzyme glucose-6-phosphatase, hence g-6-PO$_4$ is the end product in them which enters finally either in the glycolysis or HMP shunt pathway for oxidation purposes. Its pathway may be represented as follows (Figure 12.7):

Importance

It gives energy to various tissues of the body, especially in starvation, sickness, carbohydrate deprivation and other similar conditions.

GLUCONEOGENESIS

This process may be referred to as the synthesis of glucose or glycogen from non-carbohydrate sources like α-amino acids, α-keto acids, lactate, etc. The mechanism involved in this pathway is essentially the reversal of TCA cycle and the glycolytic pathway. Since, some of the reactions are not reversible, such reactions do take place by alternative routes.

Main sites of this pathway are liver and kidneys but liver is the main site.

Such substances which are responsible for this phenomenon are termed as **gluconeogenic substances which include several amino acids like alanine, serine, aspartic acid, valine, isoleucine, threonine, glutamic acid, histidine, arginine, proline, etc., and lactate and glycerol (formed from the metabolism of fats).**

Very little gluconeogenesis takes place in brain, skeletal muscle and the heart muscle.

Its pathway may be represented as given in Figure 12.8.

Regulation of Gluconeogenesis

It's regulated by the following intracellular and

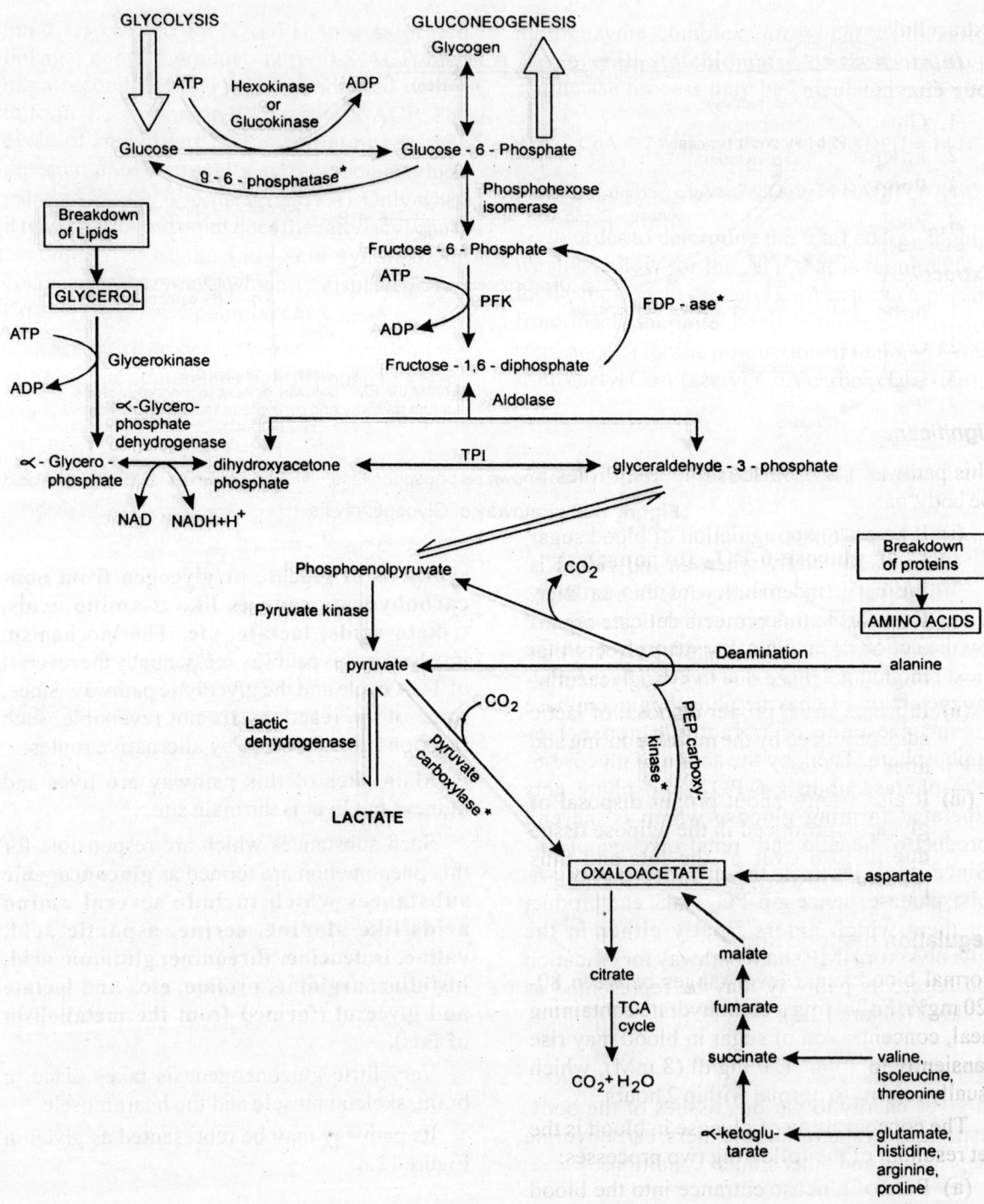

Fig. 12.8 : Pathway of gluconeogenesis showing the synthesis of glucose from (a) lactate (b) gluconeogenic amino acids and (c) glycerol

extracellular regulators :

Intracellular Regulators: **These include four enzymes viz:**

1. Glucose-6-phosphatase
2. Fructose 1,6-diphosphatase
3. Pyruvate Carboxylase
4. Phosphoenolpyruvate carboxykinase

Extracellular Regulators

1. Insulin
2. Glucocorticoids
3. Glucagon, etc.

Significance

This pathway plays various important roles in the body, namely:

(i) It helps in the regulation of blood sugar level especially when an individual is taking less carbohydrates via diet. Eventually, this protects delicate organs e.g. brain against harmful effects that might take place due to hypoglycaemia.

(ii) It brings about proper disposal of lactic acid, produced by the muscles during and after exercise.

(iii) It also brings about proper disposal of glycerol, produced in the adipose tissue due to turn over of the fats and thus prevents its wastage.

Regulation of blood sugar

Normal blood sugar level ranges between 80-120 mg%. Following a carbohydrate containing meal, concentration of sugar in blood may rise transiently to about 150 mg/dl (8 mM), which usually returns to normal within 2 hours.

The concentration of glucose in blood is the net resultant of the following two processes:

(a) Rate of glucose entrance into the blood stream.

(b) Rate of glucose removal from the blood stream.

Means by which sugar is added to the blood

1. By absorption from the intestines
2. By glycogenolysis (by breakdown of liver glycogen)
3. By gluconeogenesis

Means by which sugar is removed from the blood

1. Glycogenesis (conversion to liver glycogen and muscle glycogen)
2. In the synthesis of fats (i.e., triglycerides)
3. In the synthesis of glycoproteins, nucleic acids, lactose (during lactation), etc.
4. Loss in urine

A balance of above these two processes will keep the blood sugar within normal range.

Balance between the 'in' and 'out' of sugar may be summarised as follows:

These two processes are influenced by a number of factors under physiological conditions.

The blood glucose level is most efficiently regulated by a mechanism in which liver, extrahepatic tissues and a battery of hormones play an important role.

1. *Role of Liver:* Liver, being the centre of all metabolic activities is mainly responsible for the regulation of blood glucose level. In liver, exist:

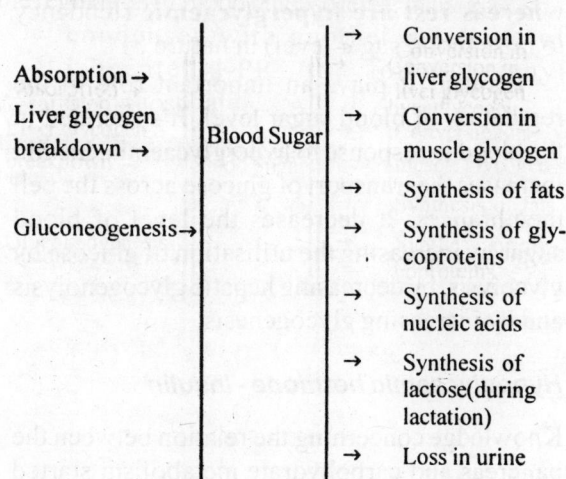

Absorption →			→	Conversion in liver glycogen
Liver glycogen breakdown →	Blood Sugar		→	Conversion in muscle glycogen
			→	Synthesis of fats
Gluconeogenesis→			→	Synthesis of glycoproteins
			→	Synthesis of nucleic acids
			→	Synthesis of lactose (during lactation)
			→	Loss in urine

(i) the developed mechanism for uptake of glucose from the blood.

(ii) mechanism for the conversion of glucose to glycogen (glycogenesis).

(iii) mechanism for the release of glucose from glycogen (glycogenolysis), and

(iv) mechanism for the denovo synthesis of glucose from non-carbohydrate precursors (gluconeogenesis).

2. Role of extrahepatic tissues

(a) *Role of muscles:* Muscle glycogen does not contribute directly to the blood sugar due to the absence of the enzyme i.e. glucose-6-phosphatase. **Glycogenolysis in the muscles provides glucose to blood only through the formation of lactic acid which by Cori's cycle is converted to glucose in the liver.**

(b) *Role of kidneys:* These also exert a regulatory effect by reabsorbing glucose through the reabsorptive system of the renal tubules. When the blood glucose level rises above the renal threshold, **then the excess glucose is expelled through urine (glucosuria).**

3. *Role of hormones:* Several hormones play an important role in the homeostatic mechanism of blood sugar level. **Out of these, insulin is the only hypoglycaemic hormone whereas rest are hyperglycaemic** (tendency to raise blood sugar level) in nature.

Insulin: It plays an important role in the regulation of blood sugar level. It's secreted in the blood in response to hyperglycaemia. Insulin increases the transport of glucose across the cell membrances. It decreases the level of blood sugar by increasing the utilisation of glucose by glycolysis, by decreasing hepatic glycogenolysis and by increasing glycogenesis.

Hypoglycaemic hormone - Insulin

Knowledge concerning the relation between the pancreas and carbohydrate metabolism started with the classical research of two Scientists namely *Von Mering* and *Minkowski* who in 1889 could demonstrate that the removal of the pancreas in the dog was the sole cause of diabetes mellitus. Later on, in 1921, three scientists i.e. *Banting, Best* and *Macleod discovered* the active principle of the pancreas which they named as insulin. Administration of insulin to a normal animal leads to a profound hypoglycaemia which may result in convulsions or unconciousness (insulin shock). Whereas, in the diabetic, a maintained administration of *insulin* completely brings down the blood sugar level within normal range.

Pancreas contains about 2 million (20 lacs) interalveolar cell islets (islets of Langerhans or islands of Langerhans, Fig. 12.9) which together weigh about 1 g. Each of these small, highly vascular bodies contains three types of cells viz:

(a) Many β-cells which are responsible for the secretion of insulin.

(b) A smaller number of α-cells which are responsible for the secretion of glucagon.

(c) A few D cells which are responsible for the secretion of gastrin and somatostatin.

A normal human pancreas contains about 8 mg insulin and the per day secretion of it is nearly 2 mg or 50 units. Insulin is a small protein (molecular weight being 5,734) which consists of two chains as shown below: .

(i) **A chain : It consists of 21 amino acid residues (Fig. 12.10).**

(ii) **B chain: It consists of 30 amino acid residues.**

A and B chains remain linked to each other with the help of disulphide bonds (Fig. 12.10). Human insulin is a derivative of a much larger single polypeptide chain which consists of 86 amino acids and is known as pro-insulin. A trypsin like enzyme has got the capability to split pro-insulin into active hormone

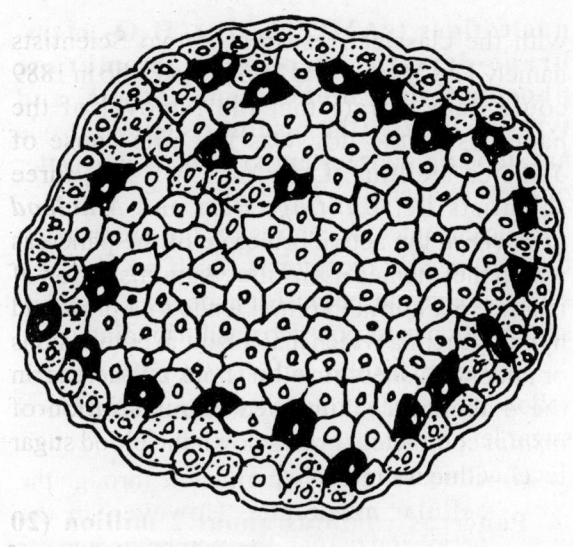

α - cells (•••) Glucagon

D - cells (•) Gastrin and somatostatin

β - cells (●) Insulin

Fig. 12.9 : Schematic representation of an **islet of Langerhans** showing distribution of glucagon, somatostatin, and insulin containing cells.

i.e. insulin. Pro-insulin has a low biological activity (nearly 5%) if compared to insulin.

Insulin has been isolated from different species like beef, bovine, pig, sheep, ox, etc. and it differs slightly in its amino acid make up from one another. Insulins obtained from pig and ox are very similar to the human hormone, that is why, the patients treated with these insulins develop measurable amounts of antibodies, they exhibit little or no adverse antigenic reactions. Insulin has been synthesized in the laboratory but it is not yet being synthesized commercially on a large scale, that is why, we are still dependent upon insulins from animal species. **Isolated natural insulins may contain zinc, which is often deliberately added because of the fact that it increases the insolubility of the hormone, probably by causing aggregation of the molecules.**

Insulin is rapidly metabolized in the liver and has a half-life of about 5 minutes. The disulfide (-s-s-) bonds present between the two chains are cleaved by an enzyme called as GIT **(glutathione-insulin transhydrogenase)** which remains present in liver and probably also in renal tubules.

Insulin gets easily destroyed by the enzymes of the alimentary tract, therefore, to give it orally is meaningless. In severe diabetic patients, it must, therefore, be

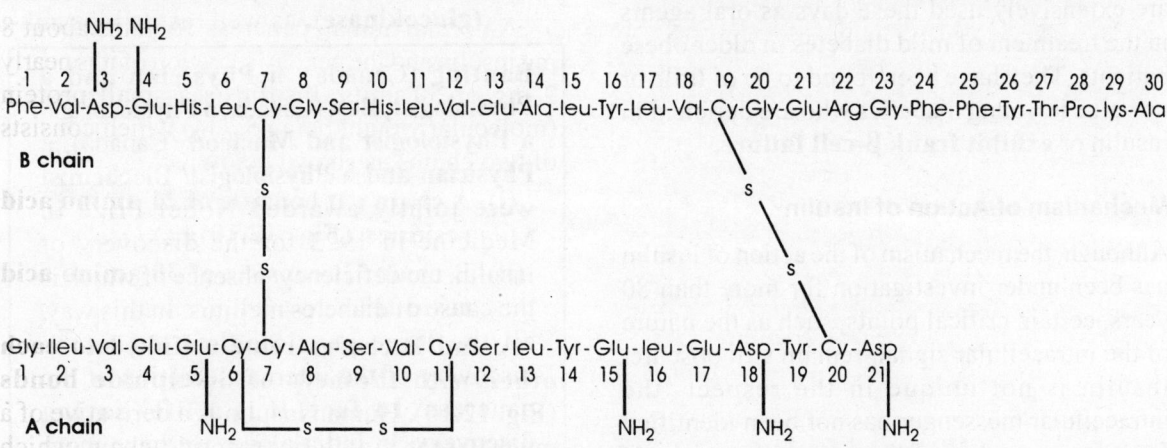

Fig.12.10 : Structure of bovine insulin

administered by injection, usually subcutaneously. It diffuses freely from the site of injection and its duration of action is only 6 to 12 hours. Since, its duration is less, therefore, two or three injections are required per day. In order to increase its duration, or say, **to make it long acting, it has been combined with either zinc or basic fish sperm protein protamine or some other suitable agent.** Be it known, insulin is an acidic protein. Such insulins are long acting and may be able to keep the blood sugar within satisfactory normal range throughout the entire day.

Hyperinsulinaemia is a state which is recognized by the excessive secretion of insulin.

Estimation of insulin is carried out by a sophisticated technique called as **'Radio immunoassay'**. Its normal range in fasting individuals is nearly 20 micro units per ml (25 units=1 mg). Shortly after taking carbohydrate meal, these values may be increased by several folds. After oral administration of 50 g glucose, values of 85, 74, 37, and 19 micro units have been found after 30, 60, 90 and 120 minutes respectively.

Insulin secretion may be stimulated by **sulphonylureas such as tolbutamide** which are extensively used these days as oral agents in the treatment of mild diabetes in older obese patients. They have been found to be of little or no value in young diabetics who are deficient in insulin or **exhibit frank β-cell failure.**

Mechanism of Action of Insulin

Although, the mechanism of the action of insulin has been under investigation for more than 80 years, certain critical points, such as the nature of the intracellular signal, remain still obscure. Insulin is not unique in the respect- the intracellular messenger has not been identified for a large number of hormones. A variety of different molecules have been proposed **as the intracellular second messenger or mediator which include insulin itself, calcium, cyclic nucleotides (cAMP, cGMP), H_2O_2 membrane-derived peptides, membrane phospholipids, monovalent cations, and tyrosine kinase (the insulin receptor).** None has stood rigorous testing so far but it is a matter of great concern.

Current interest centres on the observation that the insulin receptor is, itself an insulin - sensitive enzyme, because it undergoes autophosphorylation in response to insulin binding.

However, insulin is believed to act in the following ways in order to lower down the blood sugar level.

(i) Glucose is freely permeable through the cellular membrane. However, in the peripheral tissues, the membrane imparts a sort of resistance in glucose transport across it. Insulin, in such peripheral tissues, is responsible for increasing the permeability of the cell membrane for glucose and thus increases the transport of sugar from extracellular fluids to intracellular compartments, as a result of which more glucose becomes available for oxidation.

(ii) Insulin has been noticed to promote the enzymic activity of **hexokinase (glucokinase),** as well as its biosynth-

Banting (Canada), **a Physician and a Physiologist; Best** (Canada) **a Physician and a Physiologist and Macleod** (Canada), **a Physician and a Physiologist/ Biochemist** were jointly awarded Nobel Prize in Medicine in 1923 for the discovery of insulin, the deficiency/ absence of which is the cause of diabetes mellitus. In this way, all the three physiologists led to the discovery of the internal secretion of the pancreas. **In fact, it is a life- saving discovery.** In India alone, we have more than five crores diabetics, out of which severe diabetics require insulin therapy and are dependent upon it- no other treatment.

Discovery of Insulin (Journey of Insulin)

■ Knowledge concerning the relation between the pancreas and carbohydrate metabolism started by **Von mering & Minkowski- 1889.**

■ **Isolation of Insulin** by Banting, Best and Macleod - **1921**

■ **Nobel Prize** to **Banting, Best and Macleod - 1923**

■ **Crystallization** of Insulin by **Abel - 1926**

■ **Structure** discovered by **Sanger- 1952**

■ **Sanger** won the Nobel Prize - **1958**

■ **Proinsulin** was discovered by **Steiner-** 1967

✳ Banting and Best, first of all detected initial hyperglycemic activity in their original pancreatic extracts, and in 1923 Murlin called the substance responsible for this hyperglycemic activity as glucagon i.e., **mobiliser of glucose.**

✳ **Glucagon** is a straight chain polypeptide having **29** amino acids.

✳ **Molecular weight of glucagon** is **3,485.**

✳ It contains no cysteine residues and thus has no disulfide bonds.

✳ Glucagon is synthesized from its precursor **proglucagon (M.W. 9000).**

✳ Its plasma **half-life** is very short (five minutes).

✳ It circulates in plasma in free form.

esis. In this way, more enzyme becomes available for the metabolism of glucose (remember the first step of glycolysis).

(iii) It increases the amount of glucose-6-

✳ Insulin is the hormone secreted by the β cells of the islets of Langerhans **and derives its name from the Latin word 'insula' which means an island.**

✳ The gene for the synthesis of insulin hormone remains located on chromosome No.11

✳ **β-cells contain insulin and zinc.**

✳ Human insulin is a polypeptide having **51 amino acids (molecular weight 5,734)** arranged in two chains, namely:

(a) an acidic (A) chain containing 21 amino acids, and

(b) a basic (B) chain containing 30 amino acids

✳ **Two chains remain joined together by two disulphide bonds** which are essential for the biological activity.

✳ **Daily requirement of insulin is 1-2 mg (25- 50 units).**

✳ **Half-life of insulin is about five minutes.**

✳ Excessive secretion of insulin occurs in cases of **insulinoma,** tumour of the pancreas.

phosphate entering into HMP shunt.

(iv) It promotes the process of lipogenesis by forming more fatty acids, fats and glycerol from glucose as a result of which glucose is diverted to the formation of these substances; eventually blood sugar level gets reduced.

(v) It counteracts the inhibition, caused by the hormones of anterior pituitary gland on the activity of enzyme hexokinase, thereby nullifies their hyperglycaemic effect.

(vi) Insulin has also been reported to augment

Hypoglycaemia **may be considered to be present when the blood sugar is below 40 mg per 100 ml** (true glucose). It occurs most frequently as a result of over-dosage with insulin in the treatment of diabetes. Insulin secreting tumours (insulinoma) of the pancreas, which are extremely rare, produce a severe hypolyglycaemia, in which glucose may be almost completely absent from the blood.

Hyperglycaemia is another opposite state of hypoglycaemia in which one finds raised blood sugar level. The highest values of fasting blood sugar are obtained in diabetes mellitus, in which it may vary from normal upto 500 mg per 100 ml and even more depending upon the severity of the condition. **As the blood sugar level gets raised above 500 mg per 100 ml, there are chances of some degree of coma.** Except in diabetes, the fasting blood sugar rarely exceeds 200 mg per 100 ml. Hyperactivity of the thyroid, pituitary, adrenal glands and the states of emotional stress may give small increases not exceeding fasting blood sugar level more than 150 mg per 100 ml. However in diabetes associated with either hyperthyroidism or hyperpituitarism, still much higher figures are obtained.

A rise in blood sugar, which may be quite appreciable, can occur in sepsis and in a number of infectious diseases. A moderate hyperglycaemia may also be encountered in some intracranial diseases such as meningitis, encephalitis, tumours and haemorrhage.

One may say that a fasting blood sugar between 150 and 200 mg per 100 ml is very suggestive of diabetes mellitus whereas over 200 is almost diagnostic.

the biosynthesis of following three enzymes:

(a) **Glycogen synthetase:** responsible for promoting glycogenesis pathway.

(b) **Phosphofructokinase:** responsible for the phosphorylation of F-6-P into F-1, 6-diP (see glycolytic pathway)

(c) **Pyruvate kinase:** responsible for the conversion of phosphoenolpyruvic acid into enolpyruvic acid and finally to pyruvic acid (glycolytic pathway)

The net result of the induction of these enzymes is more conversion of glucose into glycogen and more degradation of glucose by way of glycolytic pathway.

(vii) It suppresses the biosynthesis of *glucose-6-phosphatase* and *fructose-1, 6-disphosphatase* as a result of which phenomenon of reversal of glycolysis to form glucose gets thus suppressed.

(viii) It promotes the **biosynthesis of proteins from amino acids** as a result of which less gluconeogenic amino acids are available for the phenomenon of gluconeogenesis; eventually formation of glucose gets affected.

(ix) It depresses the activity of enzyme adenyl cyclase as a result of which, the formation of cyclic-AMP is reduced which eventually is responsible to promote hepatic and renal glycogenolysis by activating enzyme dephosphophosphorylase kinase. Ultimate result is the less breakdown of glycogen to form glucose in such tissues.

(x) Insulin acts in an antagonistic manner to other hyperglycaemic hormones like cortisol, adrenaline, etc. Hyperglycaemia stimulates insulin secretion whereby hypoglycaemia inhibits it.

♦ The pancreas remains located within the curve of duodenum.

♦ **Insulin, for the first time was isolated in 1921 by Banting, Best and Macleod from pancreas.**

♦ For the discovery of insulin, three scientists namely, Banting, Best & Macleod were awarded **Nobel Prize in 1923.**

♦ Crystallized insulin was prepared by Abel in 1926.

♦ **Action of insulin is to increase the rate of transfer of glucose into cells for oxidation.**

♦ It is secreted by the β-cells of the islets of Langerhans of pancreas (Fig. 12.9).

♦ Pancreas contains about two million inter alveolar cell islets (islets of Langerhans) which together weigh about 1 g. Each of these small, highly vascular bodies contains many β-cells which secrete insulin, a smaller number of α-cells secrete glucagon, whereas a few D-cells secrete gastrin and somatostatin.

♦ A normal human pancreas contains about 8 mg insulin and, secretes about 2 mg or 50 units of insulin per day.

♦ The structure of insulin was discovered by **Sanger in 1952,** for this novel work he was awarded **Nobel Prize in the year 1958**

♦ **Sanger is the only Chemist to win Nobel Prize for the second time in the year 1980 for his work on base sequence of Nucleic Acids.**

♦ Insulin is a small protein (M.W. 5,734) containing A chain of 21 amino acid residues and a B chain of 30 residues. The chains are linked by disulphide bonds.

♦ Insulin is a derivative of a much larger single polypeptide chain of 86 amino acids known as pro-insulin (M.W. 9,000) in humans.

♦ **Proinsulin was discovered by Steiner in 1967.**

Side by side, if carbohydrates are being consumed frequently in excess, then, they result into active lipogenesis. Excess carbohydrates get converted into lipids and stored in adipose tissues. The process of lipogenesis, therefore, is responsible to lower down the blood sugar level.

■ Whenever blood sugar gets raised, insulin is secreted which induces the synthesis of glucokinase and glycogen synthetase in the liver, thus gears up glycolysis and glycogenesis.

■ Simultaneously, insulin supresses the synthesis of key gluconeogenic enzymes, meaning by, it retards the activity of gluconeogenesis pathway.

■ It also inactivates glycogen phosphorylase, the rate-limiting enzyme for glycogenolysis.

■ In carbohydrate deprivation, hypoglycaemia induces the secretions of epinephrine, glucagon, glucocorticoids and other hyperglycaemic hormones which increase **'gluconeogenesis'** by inducing key gluconeogenic enzymes. Induction of glucose-6-phosphatase by glucocorticoids and the activation of liver glycogen phosphorylase by epinephrine are also responsible for increasing the rate of **'glycogenolysis'**

■ Kidneys do also play a vital role in the regulation by absorbing or not-absorbing glucose as per the requirement.

CHAPTER 13

METABOLISM OF LIPIDS

Blood lipids

The normal level of total serum cholesterol is from 150-200 mg/dl; normal level of HDL-cholesterol in serum is from 30-63 mg/dl (men) and 35-75 mg/dl (women); normal level of VLDL is upto 28 mg/dl, normal level of LDL-cholesterol in serum is upto 150 mg/dl; normal level of serum triglycerides is from 30-140 mg/dl; normal level of total lipids in serum is from 400 - 700 mg/dl; even then the intake of lipids via diet is very essential for various reasons. However, periodical checkup of various lipid fractions (lipid profile) in blood is also very essential and demand of the day especially in the society 40 plus in age because of the alarming rising trend in the incidence of cardiovascular disorders/ diseases.

In contrast to the blood glucose level, the normal fasting level of total blood lipids of about 500 mg/100 ml may be subject to much wide fluctuations ($\pm$ 200 mg/100 ml) and will return much more slowly to baseline levels after a meal.

Since probably no absolute tissue demand for blood lipids exists, the consequences of lowered lipid levels are insignificant in comparison to the effects of hypoglycaemia. The pathology of the disorders in blood lipid metabolism tends to be related, rather, to excessive concentrations of lipids i.e., hyperlipidaemia.

Plasma lipoproteins

Virtually, all the phospholipids in liver or other

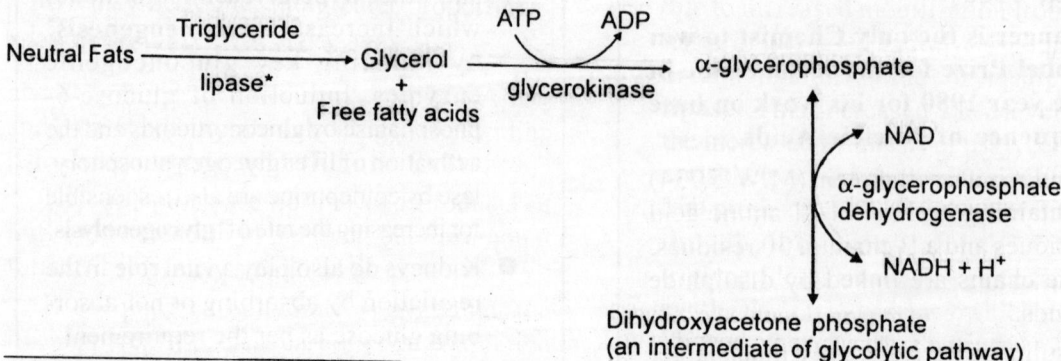

*also known as lipoprotein lipase

tissues exist in the membranes, with very few of them occurring in the form of solutions or micelles.

Lipids are water insoluble and are transported in the body in an aqueous medium in combination with various specific proteins. This results in lipid: protein complex called as lipoproteins, synthesis of which takes place in the liver.

Lipoproteins (phospholipid-carrier protein complex) are the important vehicles for the transfer of phospholipids.

Plasma lipoproteins occur in four major forms which are:

1. High or heavy density lipoproteins (HDL)
2. Low density lipoproteins (LDL)
3. Very low density lipoproteins (VLDL)
4. Chylomicrons.

Plasma lipoproteins always remain in dynamic state which are being continuously synthesized and degraded with rapid exchange of both lipid and protein among themselves. **Two enzymes namely, lecithin cholesterol acyl transferase (LCAT) and lipoprotein lipase (also called triglyceride lipase)** play a significant role in the catabolism of lipid fraction of lipoproteins.

Tangier Disease: An inability to carry normal amount of phospholipids and cholesterol in the blood is encountered in Tangier disease, which results from a congenital defect in the formation of a transport protein by the liver. A deficiency in the liver's capacity for the synthesis of albumin; which causes **analbuminemia**, leads to a decrease in the plasma's capacity to carry the fatty acids released from the fat depots.

Oxidation of fatty acids

The action of hormonally controlled lipase results in the hydrolysis of neutral fats to glycerol and free fatty acids. Glycerol enters the glycolytic pathway as shown below via the formation of glycerophosphate:

Fatty acids tightly bound with albumin are carried to various tissues for oxidation via blood.

Fatty acids oxidation takes place in mitochondria. Fatty acids are also oxidized to CO_2 and H_2O in the human body by the following three mechanisms:

(a) β-oxidation

(b) α-oxidation, and

(c) ω-oxidation

Out of the above, β-oxidation is the principal pathway, by which bulk of fatty acids gets oxidized liberating energy.

(a) β-*Oxidation Theory:* The term oxidation means that the oxidation takes place in the β-carbon of the fatty acid with the removal of two carbon atoms at a time from the carboxyl end of the molecule.

Fatty acids containing both the even number and the odd number of carbon atoms and as well as unsaturated fatty acids are oxidized by this theory. **Knoop** was the first who in 1904 invented this theory. In order to study the fate of fatty acids, he prepared a homologous series of phenyl fatty acid derivatives, which he fed to the animal; then he was able to isolate the phenyl labelled compounds in the urine. The simplest is benzoic acid, which is eliminated in the form of hippuric acid after combination with glycine.

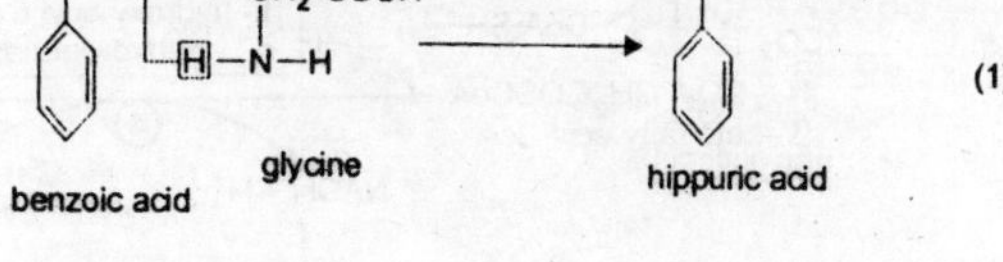

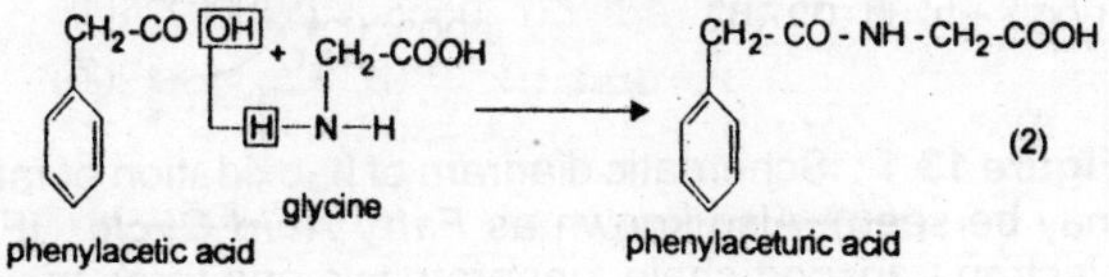

However, the next higher derivative i.e. phenylacetic acid is eliminated as the corresponding glycine derivative i.e., phenylaceturic acid.

With higher fatty acids, the products isolated were either hippuric acid (1) or phenylaceturic acid (2) for example,

$C_6H_5.CH_2 \, CH_2 \, COOH$ yields   (1)

$C_6H_5.CH_2. \, CH_2. \, CH_2. \, COOH$ yields   (2)

$C_6H_5.CH_2. \, CH_2. \, CH_2. \, CH_2.COOH$ yields   (1)

$C_6H_5.CH_2.CH_2.CH_2.CH_2.CH_2.COOH$ yields   (2)

etc.

From the results, he was able to draw the conclusion that oxidation of fatty acids occurred in such a way that at each stage in the degradation process there was a loss of two carbon atoms because of the oxidation at the β carbon atom, for example (Figure 13.1).

Mechanism of β-Oxidation of fatty acids

Five reactions are involved in the β-oxidation process as described below. All

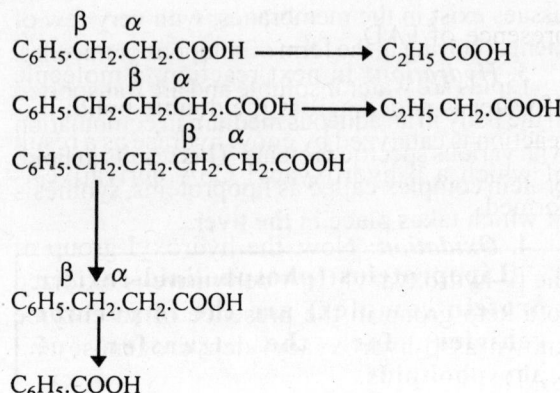

these reactions take place in the mitochondria of the cell.

1. *Activation*: The very first reaction consists in the formation of an acyl coenzyme-A derivative from the free fatty acid; this reaction is catalysed by a **thiokinase** which required the presence of ATP and CoA (Figure 13.1).

2. *Desaturation* : Once the fatty acid has been activated, it can now be dehydrogenated in the α, β position by acyl dehydrogenase in the

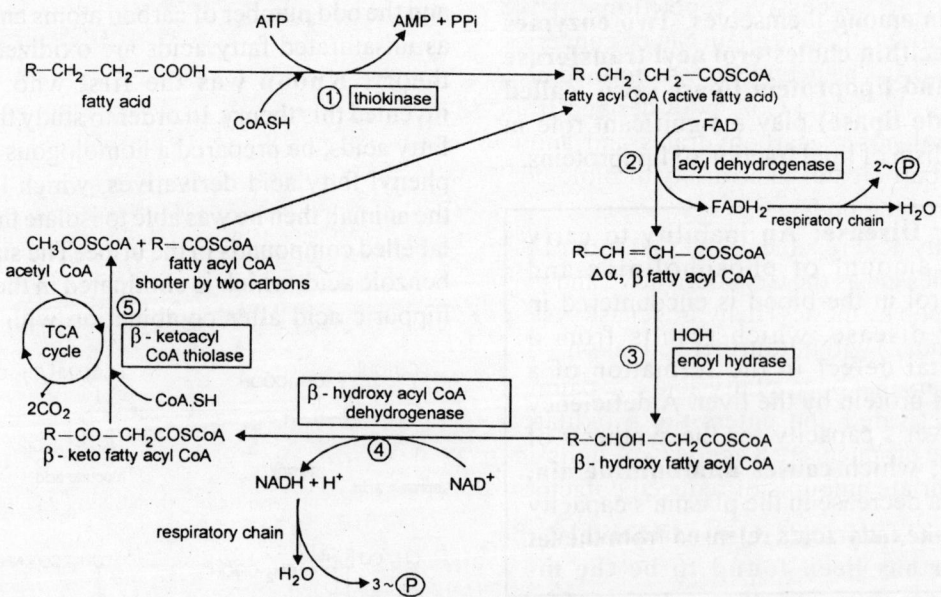

Figure 13.1 : Schematic diagram of β–oxidation of fatty acids (removal of one acetyl CoA unit from a fatty acid may be seen). Also known as ***Fatty Acid Cycle*** . [FADH$_2$ and NADH$_2$, when oxidized by the mitochondrial electron transport chain, generate two and three moles of ATP per mole of FADH$_2$ and NADH$_2$ respectively].

presence of FAD.

3. *Hydration:* In next reaction, a molecule of water is added across the double bond; this reaction is catalyzed by enoyl hydrase as a result of which a β-hydroxyacyl CoA derivative is formed.

4. *Oxidation:* Now, the hydroxyl group of the β–hydroxyacyl CoA derivative is oxidized to a keto group in the presence of an enzyme known as β-hydroxyacyl dehydrogenase and NAD.

5. *Thiolytic cleavage:* The final step in the process of β-oxidation is the cleavage of the β-keto derivative by a molecule of coenzyme in the presence of enzyme β-ketoacyl CoA thiolase.

The products of the reactions are a molecule of acetyl CoA and a molecule of an activated fatty acid which is two carbon shorter than the fatty acid at the start. Now, the activated fatty acid can be further degraded by repetitions of the process, starting at the second reaction; reaction no. 1 i.e. activation step is not necessary at all. By the successive repetitions of the process, entire fatty acid chain can be converted to acetyl CoA. The acetyl CoA so formed now mixes with the acetyl CoA pool derived from the metabolisms of carbohydrates and amino acids and participates in a variety of biological processes of the body.

The fatty acid residue of the first turn of the cycle is released as the CoA derivative and may be acted upon by the acyl dehydrogenase system (reaction no. 2) without further activation.

It appears that once a fatty acid e.g. palmitic acid, is activated and enters the β-oxidative system, the products are 8 acetyl CoA units and the appropriate amounts of reduced cofactors.

(b) α-*Oxidation:* **Quantitatively, β-oxidation has been found to be the most important pathway for the oxidation of fatty acids. However, α-oxidation, i.e. the removal of one carbon at a time from the carboxyl end of the molecule, has been** found to occur in the brain tissue. **It does not require CoA intermediates and does not generate high-energy phosphates.**

(c) *Omega Oxidation (ω-Oxidation)* **: It is normally a very minor pathway and takes place with the help of hydroxylase enzymes. The CH_3 group is converted to a CH_2OH group that subsequently is oxidized to-COOH, thus forming a dicarboxylic acid.** This dicarboxylic acid is then β-oxidized usually to adipic (C_6) and suberic (C_8) acids, which are then excreted through urine.

Generation of ATP by the complete oxidation (β-oxidation +TCA cycle) of Stearic acid (18 carbon fatty acid)

The schematic diagram of fatty acid oxidation sequence in brief is as shown in Figure 13.2.

The net overall reaction involved in degrading a fatty acid by two carbons can be represented as follows:

By repetition of these reactions, the entire fatty acid molecule gets converted into acetyl CoA, which may enter the TCA cycle and be oxidized to CO_2 and H_2O liberating many molecules of ATP for energy purposes.

Steps	Moles of ATP
1. Stearate + ATP + CoASH	
$\downarrow$	
Stearyl~SCoA --------------------------------	- 1
2. Stearyl~SCoA → 9 Acetyl-SCoA	
(a) 8 $FADH_2$ → 8 FAD (8 x 2=16)	
(b) 8 NADH → 8 NAD^+ (8 x 3=24)-----	+ 40
3. 9 Acetyl~SCoA + 18 O_2	
(9 x 12=108)	
$\downarrow$	
18 CO_2 + 9 H_2O + 9 CoASH--------------------	+ 108
	147

Overall reaction

$C_{17}H_{35}$ COOH + $18O_2$ +147 ADP +147 Pi
Stearic acid $\downarrow$
$18CO_2$ + $18H_2O$ + 147 ATP

Depending upon the needs of the organism for energy, **the remaining amounts of acetyl~SCoA may be diverted for the synthesis of important substances like cholesterol, acetylcholine, etc.**

As shown in Figure 13.2 the pathway is used a total of 8 times to convert an **18-carbon fatty acid (e.g., stearic acid) to 9 moles of acetyl S~CoA. Upon oxidation of the acetyl groups, a total of 147 molecules of ATP can be generated in the mitochondria,** which contain all enzymes required for the TCA cycle, oxidative phosphorylation and electron transfer system as well as for β–oxidation. The steps can be

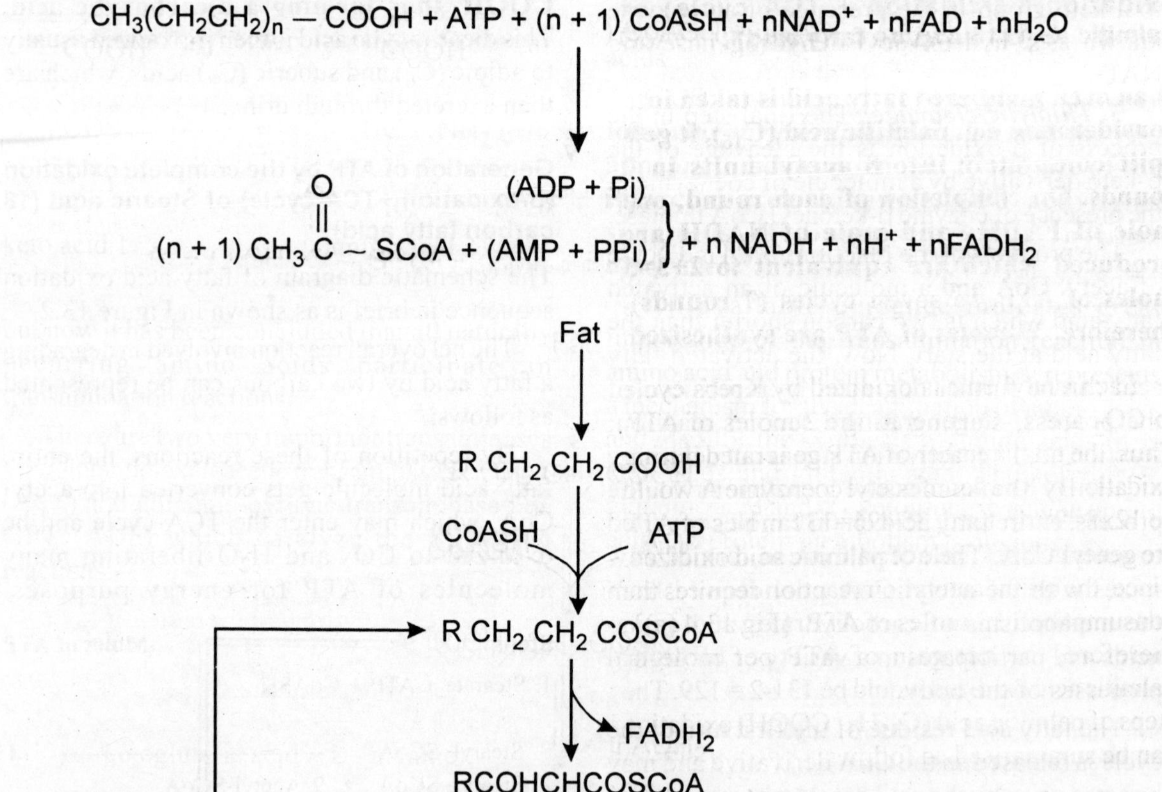

$$CH_3(CH_2CH_2)_n - COOH + ATP + (n + 1) \ CoASH + nNAD^+ + nFAD + nH_2O$$

$$\left.\begin{array}{l} (n + 1) \ CH_3 \overset{\overset{\displaystyle O}{\|}}{C} \sim SCoA + (AMP + PPi) \end{array}\right\} + n \ NADH + nH^+ + nFADH_2$$

(ADP + Pi)

Fat

$$R \ CH_2 \ CH_2 \ COOH$$

CoASH   ATP

$$R \ CH_2 \ CH_2 \ COSCoA$$

FADH_2

$$RCOHCHCOSCoA$$

NADH + H^+

$$R - \overset{\overset{\displaystyle \,}{C}}{\underset{\overset{\displaystyle \|}{O}}{}} - CH_2COSCoA$$

$\left(\dfrac{n}{2}-2\right)x$

$$RCOSCoA + CH_3COSCoA$$

Fig. 13.2 : Fatty acid oxidation sequence. The pathway is used (n/2-1) times for each fatty acid. For instance, an 18 carbon chain would go through the cycle 8 times, i.e., once through and 7 repeats-to yield the nine two - carbon fragments as acetyl CoA.

summarised as follows:

Since the total free energy decrease is nearly 2600 kcal per mole, the "efficiency" of conversion of energy to ATP is :

$$\frac{147 \times 8}{2600} \times 100 = 45\%$$

Generation of ATP by the complete oxidation(β-Oxidation + TCA cycle) of palmitic acid (16-carbon fatty acid) :

If an even numbered fatty acid is taken into consideration e.g. palmitic acid (C_{16}), it gets split completely into 8 acetyl units in 7 rounds. On completion of each round, one mole of $FADH_2$ and mole of NADH are produced which are equivalent to 2+3=5 moles of ATP. In seven cycles (7 rounds), therefore, 35 moles of ATP are synthesized.

Each acetyl unit is oxidized by Krebs cycle to CO_2 and H_2O generating 12 moles of ATP. Thus, the total number of ATP generated during oxidation of 8 moles of acetyl coenzyme A would be 12x8=96. In total, 35+96=131 moles of ATP are generated per mole of palmitic acid oxidized. Since, the initial activation reaction requires the consumption of 2 moles of ATP {Fig 13.4 (a)}, therefore, the net gain of ATP per mole of palmitic acid oxidized would be 131-2 = 129. The steps of palmitic acid ($C_{15}H_{31}$ COOH) oxidation can be summarised as follows:

Energetics of palmitic acid oxidation :

Mechanism (steps)	ATP yield
I. β- oxidation 7 cycles	
7 $FADH_2$ (oxidized by electron transport chain (ETC), each $FADH_2$ yields 2 ATP	: 14
7 NADH (oxidized by ETC, each NADH liberates 3 ATP	: 21

II. From 8 acetyl CoA

Oxidized by citric acid cycle, each acetyl CoA generates 12 ATP	: 96
Total energy from one molecule of palmitoyl CoA	: 131
Energy utilized for activation (formation of palmitoyl CoA)	: –2
Net yield of oxidation of one molecule of palmitate	: 129

The ultimate aim of fatty acid oxidation is to generate energy. The energy obtained from the complete oxidation of palmitic acid (16 carbon) is as mentioned above.

The standard free energy of palmitate = 2,340 Cal. The energy yield by its oxidation is 129 ATP (129x7.3 Cal) = 940 Cal.

The efficiency of energy conservation by fatty acid oxidation

$$= \frac{940}{2,340} \times 100 = 40\%$$

Oxidation of fatty acids with an odd number of carbon atoms

In natural fats, the straight-chain, even-carbon

$$CH_3 CH_2.COOH \xrightarrow[\quad +CoA.SH \quad]{ATP \quad AMP+PPi} CH_3.CH_2.CO.SCoA$$

propionic acid   propionyl CoA

$$CH_3CH_2.CO.SCoA \xrightarrow[\quad + CO_2, biotin \quad]{ATP \quad ADP+Pi} CH_3.CH(COOH).CO.SCoA$$

methyl malonyl CoA

$$CH_3. CH(COOH). CO.SCoA$$

$$\downarrow \; B_{12} \; | \; Coenzyme$$

$$HOOC. CH_2. CH_2.CO.SCoA$$

succinyl CoA

fatty acids are found in abundance but they also contain odd carbon and branched chain fatty acids in minor quantity. The odd-carbon fatty acids e.g. propionic acid is oxidized as follows:

Succinyl CoA, so formed can now be oxidized via succinic acid and the TCA cycle to CO_2 and H_2O.

Heart mitochondria cannot oxidize propionyl CoA. The involvement of biotin in the CO_2 fixation reaction is a clear example of the function of this vitamin as a conenzyme.

FATTY ACID SYNTHESIS

Apart from the essential polyunsaturated fatty acids, the human body is capable of synthesizing all the other fatty acids required either for structural lipids in membranes or for storage purposes. **Thus, the 'lipogenesis' may be referred to as the process by which fatty acids are synthesized. Liver is the main active site for this process i.e. lipogenesis. Although any substance whose metabolism yields acetyl CoA as an end product is a potential precursor for lipogenesis, the most important source is the carbohydrate.**

Carbohydrates when consumed in excess than the body's energy requirement, then, they get converted to fats; during conversion first of all acetyl CoA and CO_2 are formed from glucose which both are important prerequisites for fatty acids formation.

Lipogenesis is not simply a reversal of the oxidation pathway. As in glycogenesis and glycogenolysis, entirely different pathways are followed in case of anabolism and the catabolism of fatty acids. One difference is that the synthetic process occurs outside the mitochondria in the cytosol. Another is that although coenzyme A is important for lipogenesis, the intermediate compounds become attached to the sulfhydryl group of a protein known as the *acyl carrier protein* **(ACP)**. Third, lipogenesis requires a carboxylation reaction involving CO_2, ATP, and the coenzyme biotin, none of which is needed for β-oxidation. Finally, the reversal of the oxidation stages, which in β-oxidation utilize the coenzymes FAD and NAD^+, shows an absolute specificity for NADPH to provide the reducing equivalents for lipogenesis. For convenience, let us consider fatty-acid biosynthesis in its three constituent phases (Fig 13.3): (1) the provision

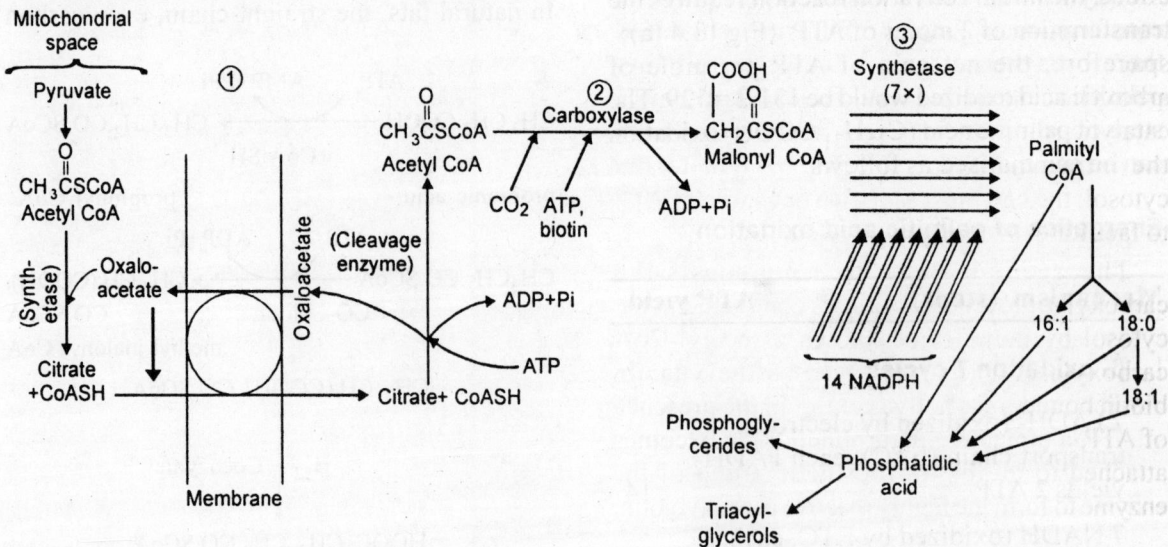

Fig. 13.3 : The three stages of fatty acid biosynthesis

of the starting material, acetyl CoA, which originates inside the mitochondrion and must be transported out to the cytosol; (2) the carboxylation of acetyl CoA to the true substrate of lipogenesis, malonyl CoA; and (3) the condensation of the two-carbon units and their reduction to long-chain, saturated acids, chiefly palmitic acid.

Although the reactions of lipogenesis occur in the cytosol compartment, the starting material, acetyl CoA, is generated within the permeability barrier of the mitochondrion. Since the inner mitochondrial membrane is impermeable to coenzyme A or its derivatives, the acetyl CoA must first be converted to a form that can cross the membrane. This may be accomplished by combining the acetyl CoA with oxaloacetate to form citrate; the mitochondrial membrane possesses a specific transport site or translocase system for tricarboxylic acids such as citrate and isocitrate. Once the citrate reaches the cytosol, it may be reconverted to acetyl CoA plus oxaloacetate, by the citrate-cleavage enzyme, a reaction which is not simply the reverse of that of the condensing enzyme, but which requires energy input in the form of ATP as well as coenzyme A. The oxaloacetate may be transferred back into the intra mitochondrial space by a specific translocase for this dic-arboxylic acid. In this way, oxaloacetate plays a catalytic role that carries the acetyl group from the intramitochondrial compartment to the cytosol; the cell must sacrifice one mole of ATP to facilitate this transport cycle.

The second stage in lipogenesis-the carboxylation of acetyl CoA-is conducted in the cytosol by the enzyme known as acetyl-CoA carboxylase. The latter contains the vitamin biotin bound to its active centre. In the presence of ATP, a molecule of carbon dioxide becomes attached to the biotin prosthetic group of the enzyme to form the highly reactive carboxybiotin:

1. CO_2 + Biotin - Enzyme + ATP
   $$\downarrow$$
   Carboxybiotin - Enzyme + ADP + Pi

In this activated form, the carboxyl group may be readily transferred to acetyl CoA to form the free carboxyl of the product, malonyl CoA:

2. Carboxybiotin - Enzyme + CH_3CO - SCoA
   COOH
   |
   CH_2CO - SCoA + Biotin - Enzyme

This reaction is identical in form to the carboxylation of pyruvate by pyruvate carboxylase. Again, a molecule of ATP is spent by the cell in order to activate acetyl CoA for its condensation role in lipogenesis. The carboxylation step is a primer regulator of fatty-acid synthesis in as much as it controls the entry of two-carbon units into the process.

All the subsequent steps in lipogenesis involve either the malonyl or the acetyl group; though their activated carboxyls are transferred from CoASH to ACP-SH (Fig. 13.4).

All the carbons of the fatty acid produced, other than the two in the terminal CH_3CH_2— position that come from acetyl ACP are derived from the malonyl ACP. Moreover, although the carboxylation process is an important priming step for lipogenesis, the — COOH that is added is stripped off from the malonyl CoA as CO_2 during condensation reactions. Therefore, in reality all the fatty-acid carbons ultimately are derived from acetyl CoA, and none of the CO_2 taken up by carboxylation is incorporated into the fatty acids.

The subsequent steps in the cytoplasmic synthesis of fatty acids are similar to the reversal of the reactions in mitochondrial β-oxidation. The keto group in the β-position is first reduced by NADPH to a hydroxyl group; a double bond is introduced by a dehydration reaction; the double bond is reduced by NADPH to a saturated linkage; and the product, butyryl-S-ACP, then has a second malonyl group condensed with it to form the six-carbon β-keto acyl-S-ACP. The cycle of reductions and dehydrations is thus repeated until eventually a 16-carbon product, palmityl-S-ACP is formed (Fig 13.4). Only when it reaches this end point does the fatty-acyl chain becomes free of the fatty-acid synthesizing complex of enzymes, which is displaced with CoA SH to release palmityl CoA.

This entire process is performed with all the intermediate compounds tightly bound to a large multienzyme complex, *fatty-acid synthetase*. The overall stoichiometry of the fatty-acid synthetase process may be calculated.

Acetyl CoA + 7 Malonyl CoA + 14 NADPH + 14 H$^+$
↓
Palmityl CoA + 7 CoA + 7 CO$_2$ + 14 NADP$^+$ + 7H$_2$O

In order to determine the total energy input, we must allow for the ATP that is required (1) for the movement of acetyl CoA to the cytoplasm from inside the mitochondria (citrate-cleavage step) and (2) for the production of malonyl CoA from acetyl CoA (acetyl-CoA carboxylase step):

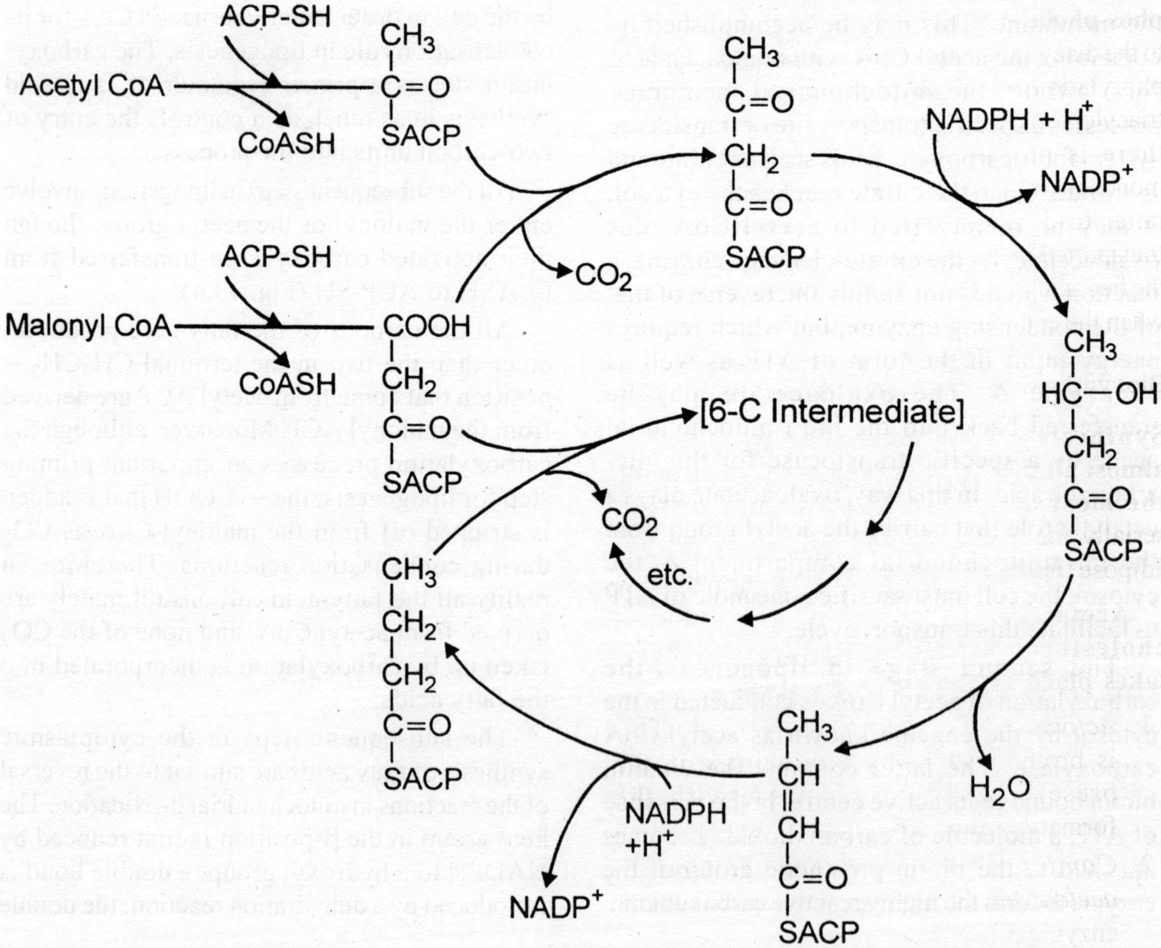

Fig. 13.4 : Role of acyl carrier protein (ACP) and NADPH in the reductive biosynthesis of fatty acids

$$8 \text{ Acetyl CoA} + 15 \text{ ATP} + 14 \text{ NADPH} + 14 \text{ H}^+$$
$$\downarrow$$
$$\text{Palmityl CoA} + 15 \text{ ADP} + 15 \text{ Pi} + 7 \text{ CoA} + 14 \text{NADP}^+$$
$$+ 7 \text{ H}_2\text{O}$$

Many different metabolic fates may befall the palmityl CoA molecule (Fig 13.3). It may be further elongated by two carbons at a time in either the mitochondria or the endoplasmic reticulum. Palmitate or its elongation product stearic acid (18:0) may be desaturated in the endoplasmic reticulum to form the monounsa-turated fatty acids, palmitoleic (16:1) and oleic (18:1) acids, respectively. **It may be esterified to the hydroxyl groups of a glyceropho-sphate to form a phosphatidic acid which is the key intermediate in both fat and phos-pholipid biosynthesis.** It may be esterified to the diacylglycerol that is formed by the dephosphorylation of phosphatidic acid to produce a triacylglycerol(in the liver, as in most body tissues, there is no pathway for the formation of monoacylglycerols nor for the esterification of the latter to diacylglycerols). Finally, it may be transported back into the mitochondria, either as the free acid or as the carnitine ester, for β-oxidation when the energy supplies in the cell are low.

Biosynthesis of cholesterol

Synthesis of cholesterol takes place in almost all the tissues of the body, liver being the most active site. Less important sites serially include skin, adrenal glands, gonads, adipose tissue, muscles, aorta, adult brain etc.

Acetate is the principal precursor of cholesterol biosynthesis. Its synthesis takes place as shown in Figure 13.5 :

1. *Activation of acetate to acetyl CoA* : This is brought about by a thiokinase in the presence of ATP and CoA with the formation of acetyl CoA.
2. *Condensation of two acetyl CoA to acetoacetyl CoA* : This is brought about by enzyme thiolase.
3. *Formation of β-hydroxy-β-methylgl-utaryl CoA* : Acetoacetyl CoA further condenses with another molecule of acetyl CoA in the presence of HMG CoA synthetase forming β-hydroxy-β-methylglutaryl CoA.
4. *Formation of mevalonic acid:* Now, β-hydroxy β-methylglutaryl CoA is reduced to mevalonic acid; the reaction is catalysed by the enzyme HMG-CoA reductase in the presence of reduced NADP.

Side-by-side, b-OH- b-methylglutaryl CoA (HMG—CoA) may also give rise to ketone bodies.

5. *Phosphorylation of mevalonic acid:* Mevalonic acid is phosphorylated to 5-phosphomevalonic acid in the presence of ATP and Mg^{++} ions. Reaction is catalysed by mevalonate kinase.

   5-phosphomevalonic acid is further phosphorylated to form 5-diphosphomevalonic acid in the presence of ATP and Mg^{2+}; the reaction is catalysed by the enzyme phosphomevalonate kinase.
6. Diphosphomevalonate loses CO_2 and H_2O to form isopentenyl pyrophosphate in the presence of an enzyme decarboxylase.
7. Isopentenyl pyrophosphate is now isomerized by a liver enzyme to form 3,3-dimethylallyl pyrophosphate which later on condenses with another molecule of isopentenyl-PP to form geranyl pyrophosphate.
8. Now, a molecule of isopentenyl-PP (C_5) reacts with geranyl-PP (C_{10}) to give rise to farnesyl pyrophosphate (C_{15}).
9. Now, in the presence of squalene synthetase reduced pyridine nucleotide and Mg^{++}, Mn^{++}, or Co^{++}, two moles of farnesyl-PP condense to form squalene.
10. Squalene in the presence of oxydocyclase I and a pyridine nucleotide undergoes cyclization process forming a steroid like structure called lanosterol (Figure 13.5).

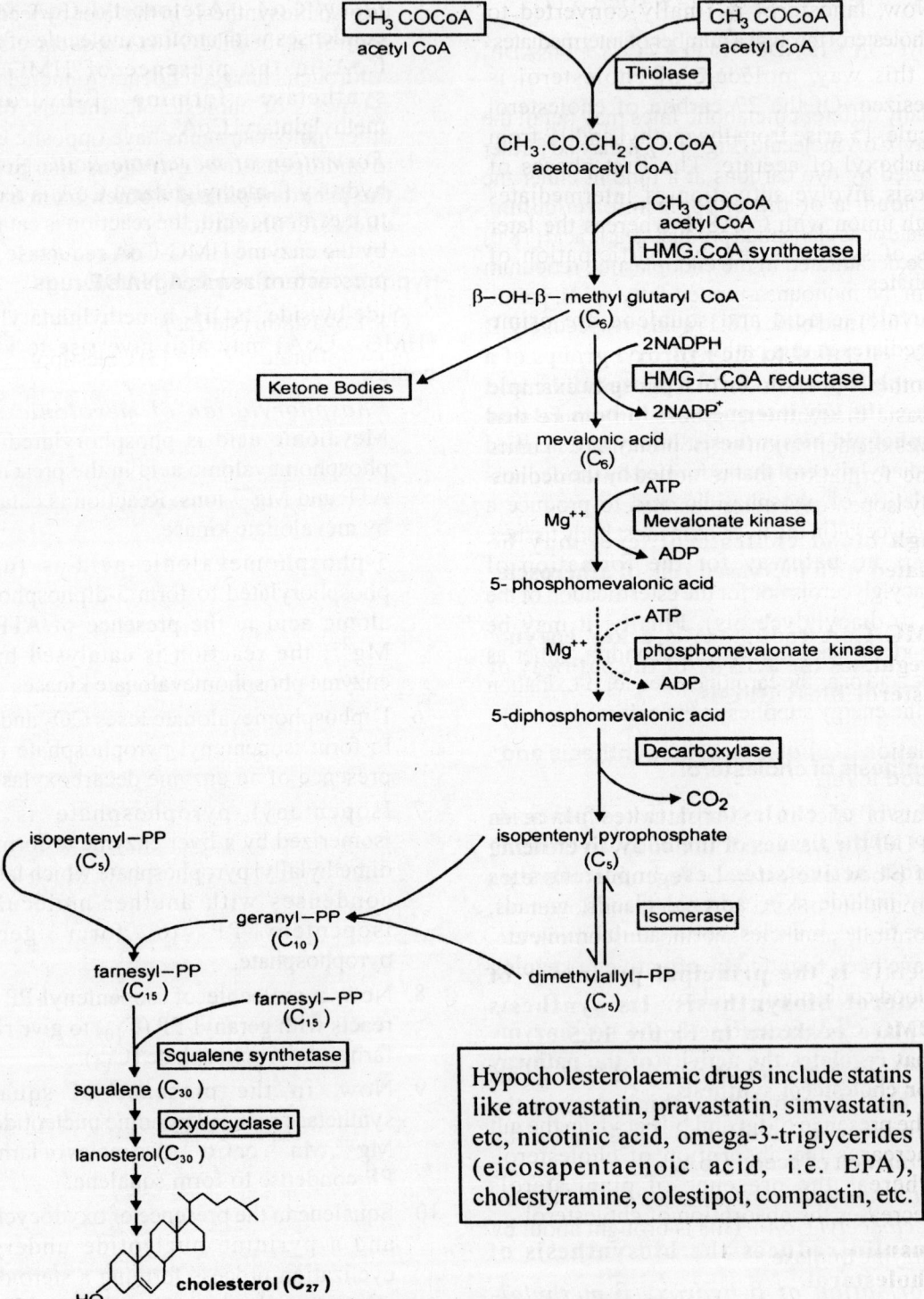

Figure 13.5 : Biosynthesis of Cholesterol

11. Now, lanosterol is finally converted to cholesterol through a number of intermediates.

In this way, molecule of cholesterol is synthesized. Of the 27 carbon of cholesterol molecule, 15 arise from the methyl and 12 from the carboxyl of acetate. The first phases of synthesis involve activation of intermediates through union with CoASH, whereas the later stages of synthesis involve participation of phosphates.

Mevalonic acid and squalene are prime intermediates in this pathway.

Synthesis of cholesterol is the only example of a basic biosynthetic process in nature that involves condensation of isoprenoid (C_5) units and the formation of the active intermediate namely isopentenyl pyrophosphate.

High blood cholesterol level may be associated with increased risk of atherosclerosis.

HMG-CoA reductase is a key enzyme that regulates the activity of the pathway of cholesterol biosynthesis.

Regulation of cholesterol biosynthesis and its blood level

1. Fats/oils rich in polyunsaturated fatty acids (PUFA) have been found to lower the level of blood cholesterol. Vegetable oils e.g., groundnut oil, safflower oil, sunflower oil, corn oil, soyabean oil and linseed oil, etc. have been found to be effective in keeping blood cholesterol level low.

2. **HMG CoA reductase is the key enzyme that regulates the activity of the pathway for cholesterol synthesis.**

3. The presence of fat and bile acids in the gut increases the absorption of cholesterol, whereas the presence of plant sterols decreases the absorption of cholesterol.

4. **Insulin reduces the biosynthesis of cholesterol.**

5. Cholesterol itself has been found to decrease its own biosynthesis in the liver by feedback control at the HMG-CoA reductase stage.

6. Androgens have a tendency to increase the synthesis of cholesterol, whereas, on the other hand, estrogens have opposite effect to androgens, thus **estrogens also protect the premenopausal women from hypercholesterolaemia.**

Hypocholesterolaemic Agents/Drugs

(1) Lovastatin (statins)

(2) Clofibrate   (3) Colestipol

(4) Cholestyramine   (5) Compactin, etc.

Catabolism of cholesterol may be regarded as the "mother" of the following so many valuable compounds of the body.

(i) Bile acids

(ii) Androgenic hormones, e.g. testosterone

(iii) Oestrogenic hormones, e.g. oestradiol and oestrone

(iv) Glucocorticoid hormones, e.g. cortisol

(v) Mineralocorticoid hormones, e.g. aldosterone and others.

Level of cholesterol gets increased in the following conditions:

(i) Diabetes mellitus

(ii) Hypothyroidism

(iii) Obstructive jaundice

(iv) Cirrhosis of liver

(v) Nephrotic syndrome

(vi) Atherosclerosis, etc.

And gets decreased in :

(i) Acute hepatitis

(ii) Malnutrition

(iii) Anaemia

(iv) Occasionally in hyperthyroidism

(v) Gaucher's disease, etc.

Catabolism of cholesterol and its excretion

Cholesterol is formed by many tissues of the body, but is catabolized by only a few tissues. The main catabolic fate of cholesterol is its oxidation to cholanic acids (cholic acids) and side by side, the main route of excretion is into the GI (gastrointestinal) tract via bile or through mucosal cells. Besides, gonads and the adrenals also utilize cholesterol for the biosynthesis of hormones (Figures 13.6 a & b).

The formation of bile acids from cholesterol in the liver represents the most important fate of cholesterol. Nearly, 80-90% of body's cholesterol is ultimately metabolized to bile acids for example cholic acid and chenodeoxycholic acid.

Cholesterol is transported in the blood as lipoproteins. The highest proportion of cholesterol is found in the low density lipoprotein fraction, **i.e. β-lipoprotein fraction (LDL).**

Cholesterol cannot be catabolised to straight chain molecule or to acetyl CoA, therefore, can't be used as a source of energy by the cells.

The combined risk factors of coronary heart disease (CHD) can be determined following the estimations of serum cholesterol and HDL-cholesterol. The ratio of cholesterol to HDL-cholesterol has predictive value in determining

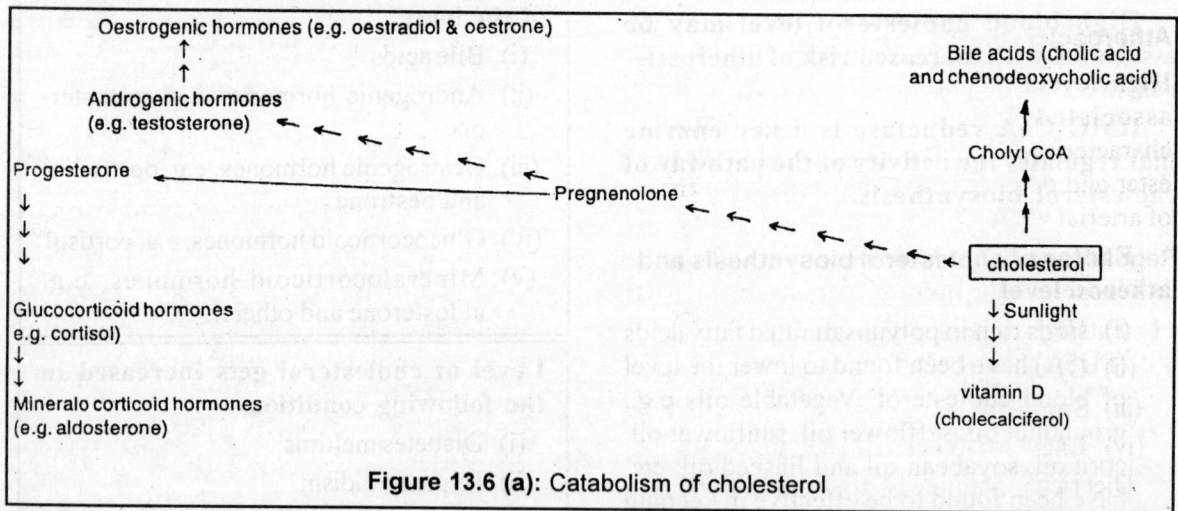

Figure 13.6 (a): Catabolism of cholesterol

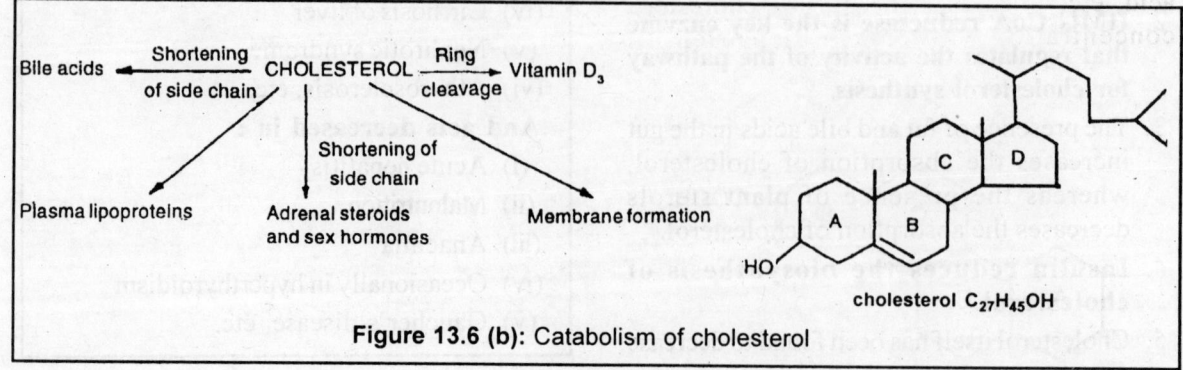

Figure 13.6 (b): Catabolism of cholesterol

the risk of CHD more accurately. For normal males, the ratio of 5 : 1 and for normal females, the ratio of 4.5 : 1 are considered as average risk. Lower ratios significantly reduce the risk, whereas ratios 9.5 : 1 and 7:1 for males and females respectively, are believed to double the risk of CHD. An inverse relationship has been observed between the risk of CHD and the concentration of HDL-cholesterol.

HDL-cholesterol represents approximately 20-25% of the total cholesterol in serum.

HDL-cholesterol may act as a scavenger(sweeper) of cholesterol from the tissues overloaded with extra cholesterol, whereas, low HDL-cholesterol may be predictive of risk of CHD and high HDL-cholesterol is protective one.

Atherosclerosis

High levels of cholesterol are found to be associated with atherosclerosis which is characterized by the deposition of cholesterol ester and other lipids in the connective tissues of arterial walls.

Factors which play a vital role in atherosclerosis include:
  (i) **High blood pressure**
  (ii) **Obesity**
  (iii) **Smoking**
  (iv) **Lack of exercise, etc.**

Diet rich in saturated fatty acids (butyric acid, caproic acid, caprylic acid, palmitic acid, stearic acid, etc.) increases the plasma cholesterol concentration, whereas diet rich in

polyunsaturated fatty acids (PUFA) such as linoleic acid, linolenic acid and arachidonic acid decreases the plasma cholesterol concentration.

Corn oil, linseed oil, soyabean oil, peanut oil, cottonseed oil, sunflower oil etc. have a tendency to lower blood cholesterol level whereas butter fat and coconut oil, etc. raise it.

PUFA exert their effect by :
  (i) stimulating the excretion of cholesterol into the intestines.
  (ii) stimulating the oxidation of cholesterol to bile acids.
  (iii) increasing the metabolic rate of cholesterol esters.

Bile acids

Bile acids are the following three, namely:
  (i) Cholic acid
  (ii) Deoxycholic acid, and
  (iii) Lithocholic acid.

They remain present in the bile in conjugation with glycine and taurine as glycocholic and taurocholic acids. Bile acids are the derivatives of cholanic acid.

Cholic acid is 3,7,12 trihydroxy cholanic acid; deoxycholic acid is 3,12 dihydroxy cholanic acid; and lithocholic acid is 3-hydroxy cholanic acid.

Salts of bile acids have a tendency to lower the surface tension and are good emulsifying agents and hence play an important role in the absorption of fats from the intestines.

Ketone bodies (acetone bodies)

Ketone bodies are the three, namely:
  (i) acetoacetic acid
  (ii) β-hydroxybutyric acid, and
  (iii) acetone

The principal ketone body is acetoacetic acid which gives rise to β-hydroxybutyric acid by reduction and acetone by decarboxylation.

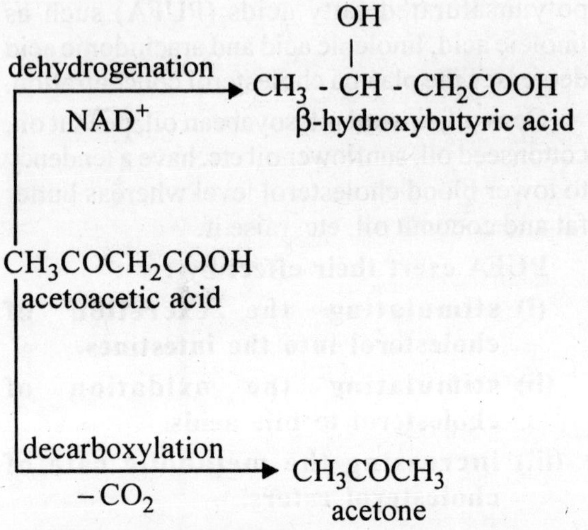

$$\xrightarrow[\text{NAD}^+]{\text{dehydrogenation}} \quad \overset{\displaystyle \text{OH} \atop |}{\text{CH}_3 - \text{CH} - \text{CH}_2\text{COOH}}$$
β-hydroxybutyric acid

CH₃COCH₂COOH
acetoacetic acid

$$\xrightarrow[-\text{CO}_2]{\text{decarboxylation}} \quad \text{CH}_3\text{COCH}_3$$
acetone

Ketone bodies are acidic in nature and when produced in excess over long period, as happens in diabetes mellitus, causes ketoacidosis which is ultimately fatal.

Ketone bodies are the intermediate breakdown products of fatty acid metabolism. Under normal conditions, fatty acids are oxidized to CO_2; these intermediates do not appear to any great extent either in the blood or urine.

Ketosis

Significant accumulation of ketone bodies in the blood (ketonaemia) and their excretion in urine (ketonuria) give rise to a condition known as **ketosis**.

Normal level of ketone bodies in blood is upto 3 mg per 100 ml and upto 50 mg in urine per day.

Under certain metabolic conditions such as starvation, high fat diet, severe diabetes mellitus, more fat is metabolized for energy purposes giving rise to increased formation of ketone bodies.

Increased fatty acid oxidation is a characteristic of starvation and diabetes mellitus, leading to the production of ketone bodies by the liver.

Under normal metabolic conditions, most of the acetyl CoA formed from the oxidation of fatty acids, pyruvate and other sources get condensed with oxaloacetic acid and oxidized through the TCA cycle. However, in circumstances when the metabolism of carbohydrate gets impaired or operating at a low level, such as in the diabetes mellitus, starvation, or prolonged living on a low carbohydrate diet, the fate of acetyl CoA gets altered for two reasons.

1. the oxaloacetate available to condense with acetyl CoA is in limited supply, and
2. a much greater proportion of the body's energy needs is being supplied by the oxidation of fatty acids, leading to the production of acetyl CoA in greater than normal amounts.

Because of this combination circumstances (large amount of acetyl CoA and small amounts of oxaloacetate), the metabolism of acetyl CoA instead of a normal route takes place through a different route in which the condensation of two molecules of acetyl CoA to form acetoacetyl CoA takes place; this reaction is catalysed by β-ketothiolase in which one molecule of coenzyme A gets liberated. Next reaction is catalysed by the enzyme HMG CoA synthetase forming β - hydroxy - β - methyl glutaryl CoA in

> **The three compounds, namely acetone, acetoacetic acid and β-hydroxybutyric acid are called as 'ketone bodies' or 'acetone bodies' and the process of their formation is known as 'ketogenesis'.**

which again one molecule of coenzyme A is liberated. Further reaction is catalysed by the enzyme HMG CoA lyase forming acetoacetic acid (Figure 13.7) in which one molecule of acetyl coenzyme A is liberated. The final reaction takes place forming acetone and β-hydroxybutyric acid; first of all in a spontaneous reaction, acetoacetic acid gets decarboxylated forming **acetone** and side by side acetoacetic acid gets

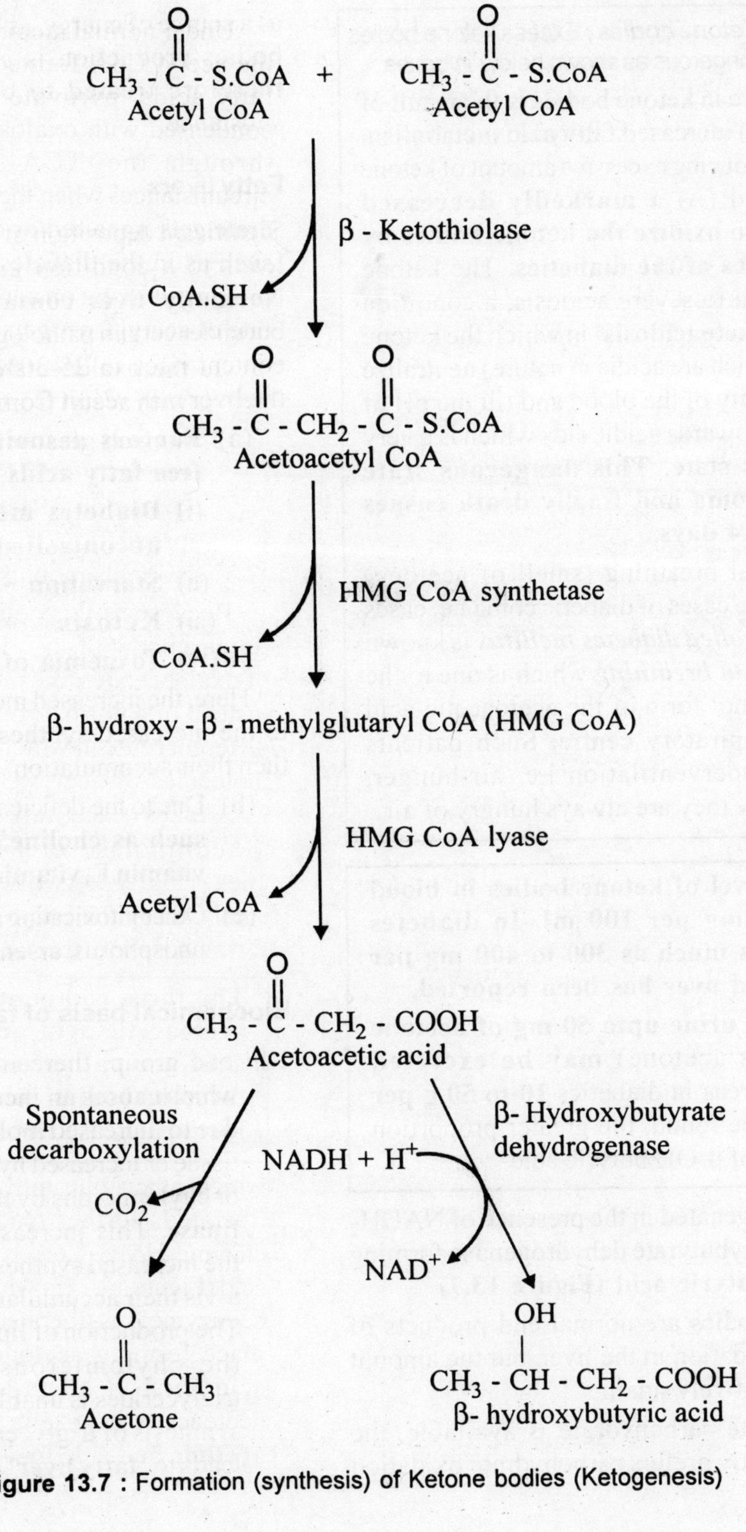

$$CH_3 - \overset{\overset{\displaystyle O}{\|}}{C} - S.CoA \quad + \quad CH_3 - \overset{\overset{\displaystyle O}{\|}}{C} - S.CoA$$

Acetyl CoA   Acetyl CoA

β - Ketothiolase

CoA.SH

$$CH_3 - \overset{\overset{\displaystyle O}{\|}}{C} - CH_2 - \overset{\overset{\displaystyle O}{\|}}{C} - S.CoA$$

Acetoacetyl CoA

HMG CoA synthetase

CoA.SH

β- hydroxy - β - methylglutaryl CoA (HMG CoA)

HMG CoA lyase

Acetyl CoA

$$CH_3 - \overset{\overset{\displaystyle O}{\|}}{C} - CH_2 - COOH$$

Acetoacetic acid

Spontaneous decarboxylation

CO_2

$NADH + H^+$

β- Hydroxybutyrate dehydrogenase

NAD^+

$$CH_3 - \overset{\overset{\displaystyle O}{\|}}{C} - CH_3$$

Acetone

$$CH_3 - \overset{\overset{\displaystyle OH}{|}}{CH} - CH_2 - COOH$$

β- hydroxybutyric acid

Figure 13.7 : Formation (synthesis) of Ketone bodies (Ketogenesis)

Danger of Ketone bodies : Excess ketone bodies are very dangerous as shown below 'in boxes':

An increase in ketone bodies is the result of both i.e. (i) increased fatty acid metabolism in liver producing excessive amount of ketone bodies and (ii) **a markedly decreased capacity to oxidize the ketone bodies by the muscles of the diabetics.** The ketone bodies lead to severe acidosis, a condition called as 'ketoacidosis' in which the ketone bodies (which are acidic in nature) neutralize the alkalinity of the blood and tilt the pH of the blood towards acidic sic' which is a very dangerous state. **This dangerous state leads to coma and finally death ensues within 4-14 days.**

The typical breathing (smell of acetone) found in the cases of diabetic coma i.e. cases of *uncontrolled diabetes mellitus* is known as *Kussmaul breathing* which is due to the effect of enol form of the acetoacetic acid on the respiratory centre. Such patients exhibit hyperventilation i.e. air-hunger, meaning by they are always hungry of air.

Normal level of ketone bodies in blood is upto 3 mg per 100 ml. In diabetes mellitus as much as 300 to 400 mg per 100 ml and over has been reported.

In normal urine upto 50 mg of acetone bodies (as acetone) may be excreted daily, whereas in diabetics **10 to 50 g per litre** may be found, the greater proportion being that of β-OH butyric acid.

---

also dehydrogenated in the presence of $NADH_2$ and β-hydroxybutyrate dehydrogenase forming **β-hydroxybutyric acid (Figure 13.7).**

Ketone bodies are normal end products of fatty acid oxidation in the liver, but the amount formed is relatively small.

If adequate carbohydrate is available, the liver apparently prefers carbohydrate oxidation as a source of energy, as a result of which ketone bodies production is small. Carbohydrate is therefore treated to be an **'antiketogenic'** substance.

Fatty livers

Significant deposition of triglycerides in the liver leads to a condition known as **'fatty liver'. Normally, liver contains 5% of the lipids,** but under certain pathological conditions, the lipid content rises to 25-30%. The increased fat in the liver may result from:

(a) **Factors associated with increased free fatty acids (FFA) level are:**
  (i) **Diabetes mellitus (severe uncontrolled)**
  (ii) **Starvation**
  (iii) **Ketosis**
  (iv) **Toxaemia of pregnancy,** etc.

Here, the increased mobilization of FFA leads to the increased synthesis of triglycerides and then their accumulation.

(b) Due to the deficiency of **lipotropic factors such as choline, lecithin, methionine, vitamin E, vitamin B_6 i.e. pyridoxine, etc.**

(e) Other intoxicating agents like $CHCl_3$, CCl_4, phosphorus, arsenic, lead, alcohol, etc.

Biochemical basis of fatty liver

1. In one group, there is some primary factor which causes an increase in the FFA either due to increased mobilisation from adipose tissue or increased hydrolysis of lipoproteins or chylomicrons by the enzyme **lipoprotein lipase.** This increased FFA level leads to the increased synthesis of triglycerides, vis-a-vis their accumulation later or in the liver. The production of lipoproteins (specifically the chylomicrons and VLDL) from triglycerides is unable to keep pace with the synthesis of triglycerides, which eventually leads to **'fatty liver'.** This is the mechanism

in disorders like uncontrolled diabetes mellitus, toxaemia of pregnancy, ketosis and starvation, etc.

2. In the other group, the defect lies in the production of plasma lipoproteins. Such a defect/blockade may be at one or more of the following sites:

   (i) **Synthesis of apoproteins**

   (ii) **Synthesis of lipoproteins from lipid and apoproteins**

   (iii) **Synthesis of lipids-specifically the phospholipids.**

   (iv) **Secretory mechanism of the lipoproteins.**

Substances which have got the capability to prevent or relieve such abnormal deposition of lipids in the liver are termed as **lipotropic factors** which are as mentioned just above.

Role of liver in the metabolism of lipids

Liver is the main site for the metabolism of lipids because it contains complete enzyme system to carry out the following major activities which are very important:

   (i) **Synthesis of triglycerides**

   (ii) **Synthesis of phospholipids**

   (iii) **Synthesis of plasma lipoproteins such as VLDL, HDL, etc.**

   (iv) **Synthesis of cholesterol and its derivatives such as bile acids, etc.**

   (v) **Synthesis and degradation of fatty acids (β- oxidation)**

   (vi) **Formation of ketone bodies**

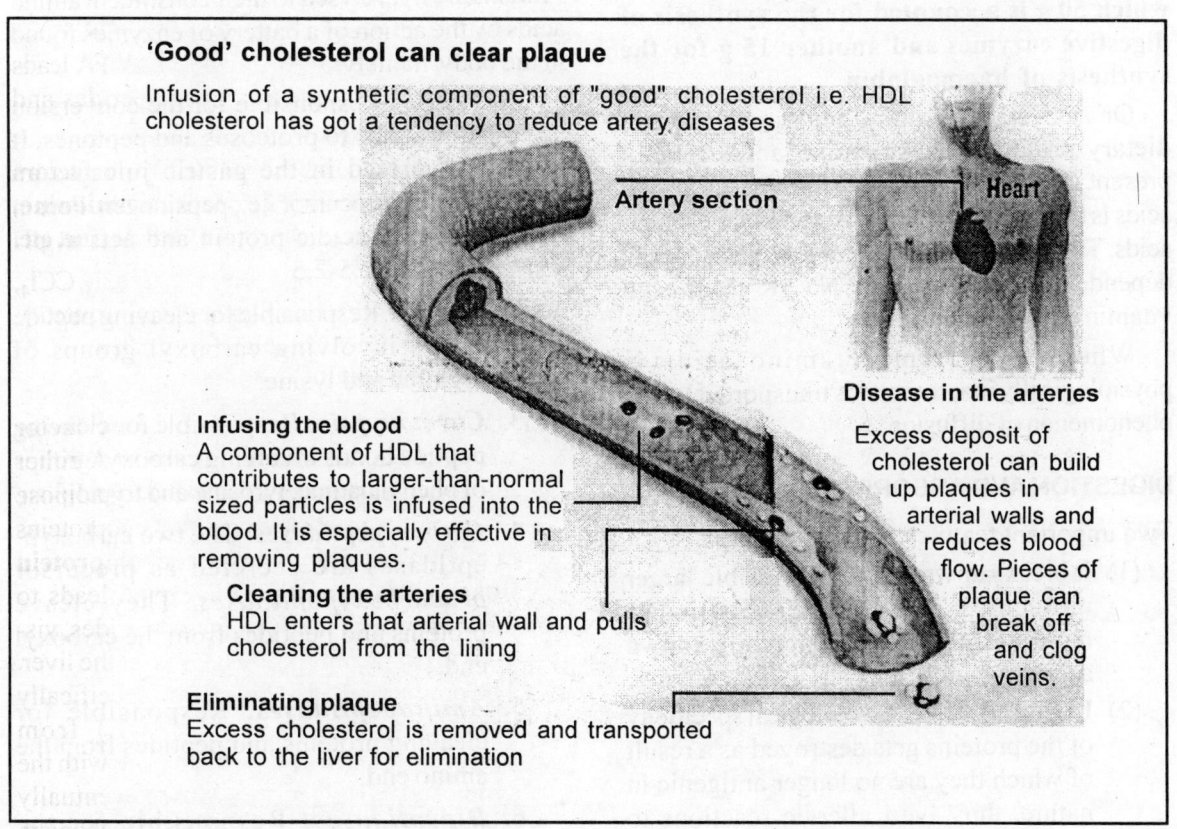

'Good' cholesterol can clear plaque

Infusion of a synthetic component of "good" cholesterol i.e. HDL cholesterol has got a tendency to reduce artery diseases

Artery section

Heart

Disease in the arteries

Excess deposit of cholesterol can build up plaques in arterial walls and reduces blood flow. Pieces of plaque can break off and clog veins.

Infusing the blood
A component of HDL that contributes to larger-than-normal sized particles is infused into the blood. It is especially effective in removing plaques.

Cleaning the arteries
HDL enters that arterial wall and pulls cholesterol from the lining

Eliminating plaque
Excess cholesterol is removed and transported back to the liver for elimination

Sources of amino acids in the body pool

Role of their in the metabolism of lipid

Absorption

CHAPTER 14

METABOLISM OF PROTEINS

The total protein turnover of an adult male is estimated to be around 400 g/day, of which 50 g is accounted for the synthesis of digestive enzymes and another 15 g for the synthesis of haemoglobin.

On an overall, 20 amino acids are present in dietary proteins. These amino acids remain present in L-configuration. L-form of the amino acids is the physiological active form of the amino acids. The transport of such amino acids is energy dependent and requires ATP, Na^+, K^+, Mn^{++} and vitamin B_6.

Whereas D- form of amino acids is physiologically inactive and is transported by the phenomenon of diffusion.

DIGESTION AND ABSORPTION

Two important features of digestion are:

(1) It breaks down the non-diffusible larger molecules into smaller diffusible molecules which are commonly known as amino acids.

(2) During digestion, the biological specificity of the proteins gets destroyed as a result of which they are no longer antigenic in nature, thus avert allergic reactions to food.

Digestion of Proteins by various enzymes

Proteins are hydrolysed to their constituent amino acids by the action of a battery of enzymes found in the body, namely:

1. **Pepsin:** Responsible for the conversion of proteins to proteoses and peptones. It is secreted in the gastric juice as an inactive precursor i.e., pepsinogen. Pepsin is a very acidic protein and acts at pH between 1.5-2.5.

2. **Trypsin:** Responsible for cleaving peptide bonds involving carboxyl groups of arginine and lysine.

3. **Chymotrypsin:** Responsible for cleaving peptide bonds involving carboxyl groups of phenylalanine, tyrosine and tryptophan.

4. **Carboxypeptidases:** The two carboxypeptidases are secreted as precursor procarboxypeptidases. They cleave proteins and peptides from the carboxyl end.

5. **Aminopeptidases:** Responsible for cleaving proteins and peptides from the amino end.

6. **Dipeptidases:** Responsible for the cleavage of dipeptides.

Absorption

It is known that absorption is very rapid in man. The extent of hydrolysis of the food protein is low in the stomach which is nearly 10-15% but quickly reaches upto 50-60% in the duodenum. In the duodenal contents, the enzymes trypsin and chymotrypsin remain present at the concentrations of 200-800 µg per ml of fluid within a short time of stimulation. These high concentrations of enzymes are capable of rapidly hydrolyzing food proteins to small peptides. Absorption of protein fragments takes place in the duodenum and the jejunum, most of it is absorbed as di-and oligopeptides.

L- form of the amino acids is absorbed at much faster rate than the D-form. All amino acids are absorbed by active process which requires ATP, Na^+, K^+, Mn^{++} and pyridoxal phosphate.

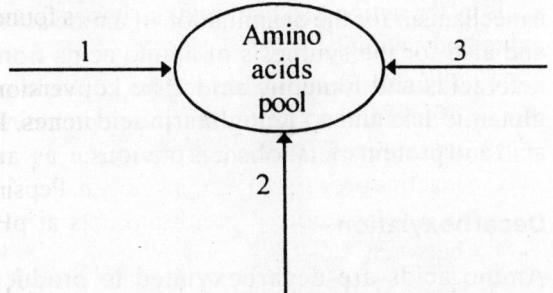

Sources of amino acids in the body pool include:

1. Dietary proteins
2. Intracellular synthesis $\}$ Metabolism
3. Tissue protein breakdown $\}$ (Table 14.1)

Transamination

It is a combined process of deamination and amination according to which the amino group of one amino acid may be reversibly transferred to the keto acid of another amino acid, thus effecting amino acid-keto acid interconversion. This phenomenon was for the first time discovered by two scientists namely **Braunstein and Kritzmann.**

The process represents intermolecular transfer of amino groups without the splitting of ammonia. The reaction is reversible and is catalyzed by *transaminase enzymes,* which remain confined to almost every tissue or the animal but the major sites are heart, brain, kidney, testicle and liver.

The general process of transamination may be represented as follows:

It was earlier found that glutamic acid and its keto acid i.e., α - ketoglutaric acid participate in a large proportion of transamination reactions

---

Table 14.1 : Metabolism of amino acids within the cell

Anabolic phase	*Catabolic phase*
It is a synthetic process	**It is a breakdown process**
1. Biosynthesis of proteins which includes tissue proteins, blood proteins, enzymes and hormones.	1. Transamination
	2. Decarboxylation
	3. Oxidative deamination
2. Biosynthesis of non-protein nitrogen substances takes place for e.g., creatine, purines, pyrimidines, glutathione, choline, etc.	4. Utilization of nitrogen residue i.e., (i) Synthesis of glutamine (ii) Urea cycle

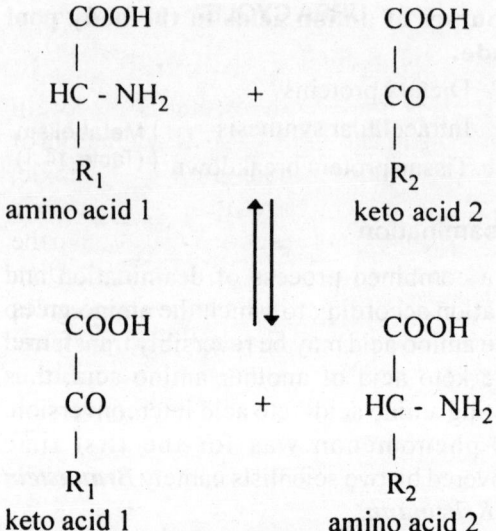

amino acid 1   keto acid 2

keto acid 1   amino acid 2

but now it has been concluded that all naturally occurring amino acids participate in transamination reactions.

There are two very important transaminases viz., glutamic-oxaloacetic transaminase i.e., GOT (AST) and glutamic-pyruvic transaminase i.e., GPT (ALT) which catalyze the following reactions:

L - glutamic acid + pyruvic acid

$\updownarrow$ transaminase

α - ketoglutaric acid + L - alanine

L - glutamic acid + oxaloacetic acid

$\updownarrow$ transaminase

α - ketoglutaric acid + L - aspartic acid

The transaminases require pyridoxal phosphate as cofactor. GOT is the most active and widely distributed of the transaminases. The most general type of transamination in animals and plants appears to be represented by the equation:

L - amino acid + α - ketoglutaric acid

$\updownarrow$

α - keto acid + L - glutamic acid

In general, the transaminases of animal tissues and higher plants appear to be specific for L -amino acids, however, it has been noticed that certain bacteria, such as B. subtilis possess transaminases specific for both D and L - amino acids.

GOT activity of serum rises sharply following *myocardial infarction* and the rise appears to be proportional to the size of the infarcted area. Likewise, GPT activity of serum is of diagnostic value in liver disorders.

All available evidence indicates great importance of the transamination reaction in amino acid and protein metabolism. It represents a mechanism for the deamination of amino acids and also for the synthesis of amino acids from keto acids and glutamic acid. The key role of glutamic acid and α - ketoglutaric acid in amino acid and protein metabolism is obvious.

Decarboxylation

Amino acids are decarboxylated to produce amines. Such reactions are catalysed by enzymes known as decarboxylases which are found in liver, kidney and brain. These enzymes also require pyridoxal phosphate as a cofactor. Pyridoxamine phosphate is not required. The process is very important in the human body as it gives rise to important substances i.e., *biologically active amines as follows:*

Tyrosine $\xrightarrow{\text{decarboxylation}}$ tyramine

Tryptophan $\xrightarrow{\text{decarboxylation}}$ tryptamine

Histidine $\xrightarrow{\text{decarboxylation}}$ histamine

Glutamic acid $\xrightarrow{\text{decarboxylation}}$ γ – aminobutyric acid
(GABA)

5-Hydroxytryptophan

$\downarrow$ decarboxylation

hydroxytryptamine (serotonin)

Oxidative deamination

This process may be referred to as the liberation of ammonia oxidatively from amino acids, approximately two moles of NH_3 are formed for each molecule of O_2 taken up:

$$R - CH(NH_2) - COOH + 1/2O_2 \rightarrow R.CO-COOH + NH_3$$

Enzymes which bring about oxidative deamination are known as D- and L - amino acid oxidases; these act upon D - and L - amino acids respectively.

The D - amino acid oxidases are flavoproteins containing FAD, whereas L - amino acid oxidases are also flavoproteins but contain FMN (flavin mononucleotide).

The D - amino acids are not found in the tissues whereas L - amino acids are found which means that animal tissues are devoid of corresponding enzyme i.e., D - amino acid oxidases but contain L - amino acid oxidases. Both D - and L - amino acid oxidases are found in microorganisms. The function of D - oxidases is not yet known.

The mechanism of oxidative deamination may be represented by the following equations:

$$R - \underset{\substack{| \\ NH \\ \text{amino acid}}}{CH} - COOH + FP \xrightarrow[\text{enzyme}]{FP} R - \underset{\substack{\| \\ NH \\ \text{imino} \\ \text{acid}}}{C} - COOH + \underset{\substack{\text{reduced} \\ \text{enzyme}}}{FP. H_2}$$

$$R - \underset{\substack{| \\ NH \\ \text{imino acid}}}{C} - COOH + H_2O \rightleftharpoons R - \underset{\substack{\| \\ O \\ \text{keto acid}}}{C} - COOH + NH_3$$

UREA CYCLE
(Krebs - Henseleit cycle/Ornithine cycle)

Urea is the main end product of protein metabolism in the body. The deamination of amino acids produces ammonia which is toxic. By this cycle, it is converted to urea, a non-toxic compound, which is transported via blood to the kidneys and then excreted in the urine. Urea formation takes place in the liver. Two molecules of ammonia and one molecule of CO_2 are converted to urea for each turn of the cycle.

Various stages of urea cycle include:
1. Formation of carbamoyl phosphate
2. Formation of citrulline from ornithine
3. Formation of urea from arginine

1st stage: i.e. Formation of carbamoyl phosphate.

The first stage in the synthesis of urea in animals may be considered to be the formation of carbamoyl phosphate, the reaction is catalysed by the enzyme known as carbamoyl phosphate synthase (Fig. 14.1).

Carbamoyl phosphate is a reactive high energy compound. The enzyme requires an acyl glutamate such as N-acetylglutamate as a cofactor.

IInd stage i.e. Formation of citrulline from ornithine

Ornithine is converted to citrulline by the action of carbamoyl phosphate; this reaction is catalysed by the action of enzyme ornithine transcarbamoylase. **This reaction is not reversible.**

IIIrd stage i.e. Formation of arginine from citrulline

The syntheis of arginine from citrulline takes place in two stages. The first stage is the condensation of citrulline with aspartic acid to

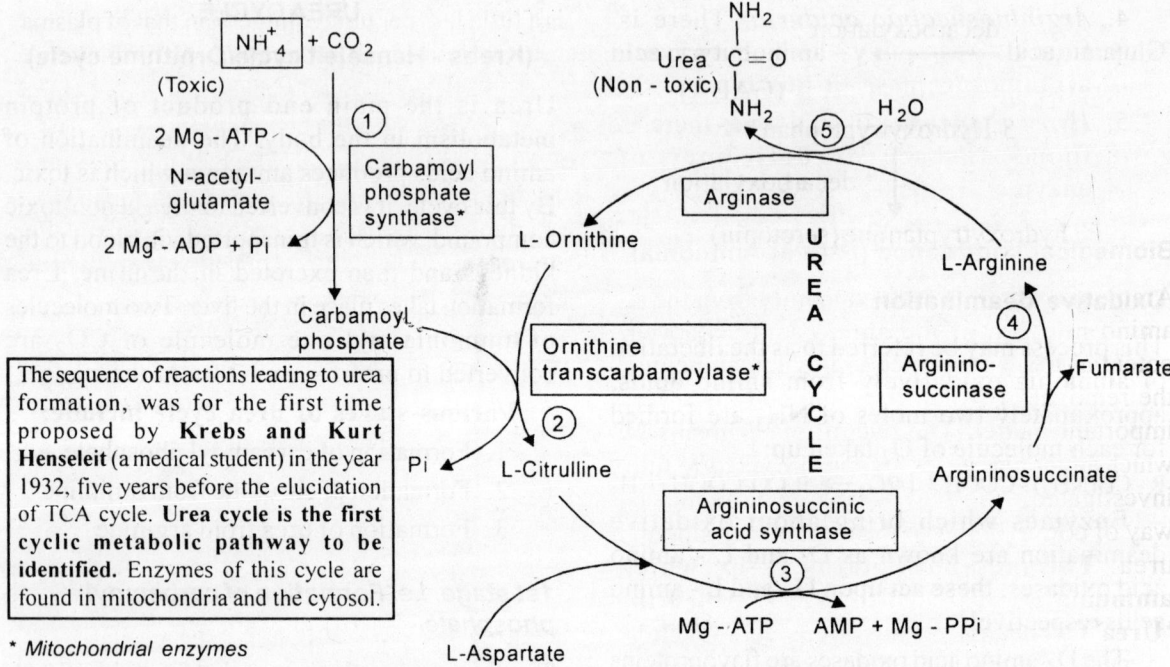

Fig. 14.1 : Reactions and intermediates of Urea Cycle

The sequence of reactions leading to urea formation, was for the first time proposed by **Krebs and Kurt Henseleit** (a medical student) in the year 1932, five years before the elucidation of TCA cycle. **Urea cycle is the first cyclic metabolic pathway to be identified.** Enzymes of this cycle are found in mitochondria and the cytosol.

* *Mitochondrial enzymes*

form argininosuccinic acid by the enzyme argininosuccinate synthetase. The argininosuccinate gets then split into arginine and fumarate by the cleavage enzyme known as argininosuccinase (Fig. 14.1).

IVth and last stage i.e. Formation of urea from arginine

Arginine is hydrolyzed to ornithine and urea by the enzyme arginase.

It has been observed that of the two N atoms in a molecule of urea, one is derived from *ammonia* through carbamoyl phosphate, and the other from *aspartic acid* through argininosuccinic acid.

$$
\begin{array}{c}
NH_2 \\
| \\
C = O \\
| \\
NH_2
\end{array}
$$
Urea
(non-toxic)

Metabolic disorders of the Urea Cycle (Krebs - Henseleit Cycle, Ornithine Cycle)

Hyperammonia or hyperammonaemic syndrome is caused due to the increased level of ammonia in the blood. Since, the formation of urea takes place from ammonia by urea cycle, therefore, any deficiency or defect of urea cycle enzyme (s) is responsible for elevated levels of ammonia.

Hyperammonaemia gives rise to mental retardation.

There are five disorders:

1. *Hyperammonaemia type I:* In this type there is found **absence of enzyme carbamoyl phosphate synthetase.**

2. *Hyperammonaemia type II:* In this type there is found **absence of enzyme ornithine transcarbamoylase.**

3. *Citrullinaemia:* There is found **absence of enzyme argininosuccinate synthetase (synthase) in this type.**

4. *Argininosuccinic aciduria:* There is found **absence of enzyme argininosuccinase in this type.**

5. *Hyperarginemia:* In this type, there is found **absence or deficiency of enzyme arginase.**

Biomedical Importance (Fate of Ammonia)

Ammonia, which is derived mainly from the α-amino nitrogen of the amino acids is a very potential toxic substance to the human beings, the removal of which from the body is a very important matter. The overall mechanisms by which ammonia causes toxicity are yet to be fully investigated. The body disposes ammonia by way of converting it to the nontoxic compound urea. **The metabolic pathway by which ammonia is converted to urea is called the 'Urea Cycle' or 'Krebs Henseleit Cycle'**

There are several diseases (disorders) in which liver functtions get seriously affected e.g., massive cirrhosis (where normal liver cells are replaced by fibroblasts and collagen) or severe hepatitis-ammonia gets accumulated in the blood causing great concern and danger to the biochemistry of body; the removal or conversion of it to a comparatively less toxic substance is very essential.

Interpretation regarding blood urea

The generally accepted range for the blood urea in normal persons on a full ordinary diet is from about 14 to 43 mg per 100 ml. It is a few mg higher in men than women, a difference rather more marked in the young and there is a slow rise with age so that the mean is in the twenties in young adults and about 40 in the old. The urea *content over a period is influenced by the amount of protein in the diet* and is found to be on lower side in people on low protein diets.

Urea diffuses readily into all the body fluids. Its concentration in the water of plasma and cells is the same but as the water content of the cells is a little less per unit volume than that of plasma, the ratio of urea in plasma to cells is about 5:4.

Blood urea is found to be lower in pregnancy than in normal non-pregnant women.

Increases in the level of blood urea may occur in a number of diseases in addition to those in which the kidneys are primarily involved. For increases, three states may be responsible, namely:

(a) **Pre-renal**

(b) **Renal and**

(c) **Post- renal**

(a) *Pre-renal* : In this state, kidneys are not involved. In this state, blood urea level gets increased in cases of dehydration due to severe and protracted vomiting **as in pyloric and intestinal obstruction;** in chronic intestinal obstruction without vomiting; in diarrhoea; etc. *Very high values* of blood urea are encountered in these conditions if they are allowed to go untreated. **Thus, in *pyloric stenosis* with severe vomiting, the blood urea may exceed 200 mg/dl,** and even occasionally be over **300** and can be quite rapidly brought down to normal with satisfactory treatment.

It may also exceed 300 mg/dl in ulcerative colitis with severe chloride loss.

In diabetic coma, it may be found in the range of 50 to 150 *mg/*dl, returning to normal as soon as the coma has been treated.

It may also be found elevated **i.e., in the range of 50 to 100 mg/dl or even higher in the cases of *Addison's disease* (hypoadrenalism).**

Other conditions in which blood urea may be found to be elevated include:

(a) Haematemesis,

(b) Shock due to severe burns,

(c) Post-operative state,

(d) Cardiac failure, etc.

(b) *Renal:* In this state, kidneys are involved as a result of which level of blood urea gets increased **in all types of kidney diseases** which include:

(i) Acute glomerulonephritis

(ii) Ellis's Type II nephritis

(iii) Malignant hypertension

(iv) Chronic pyelonephritis

(v) Mercury poisoning

(vi) Hydronephrosis

(vii) Congenital cystic kidneys

(viii) Renal tuberculosis

(ix) Hyperparathyroidism

(x) Hpervitaminosis D

(c) Post - renal: Post renal diseases lead to increased blood urea level, are those in which there is obstruction to the flow of urine. **This causes retention of urine.** If prolonged, irreversible kidney damage results. **Most important among these is** *enlargement of the prostate,* in which estimation of blood urea is an essential part of the assessment of the condition. **Besides prostate, other conditions include:**

(i) **stones in the urinary tract**

(ii) **stricture of the urethra**

(iii) **tumour of the bladder affecting the ureters, etc.**

Metabolism of Phenylalanine and Tyrosine

Both phenylalanine and tyrosine are aromatic amino acids. Tyrosine is hydroxylated

phenylalanine. The structure of these are:

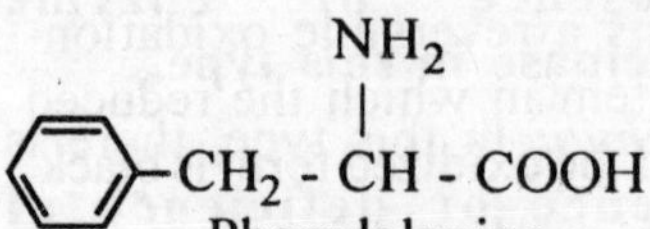

$$
\underset{\text{Phenylalanine}}{\bigcirc-CH_2-\overset{\overset{\displaystyle NH_2}{|}}{CH}-COOH}
$$

$$
HO-\bigcirc-CH_2-\overset{\overset{\displaystyle NH_2}{|}}{CH}-COOH
$$

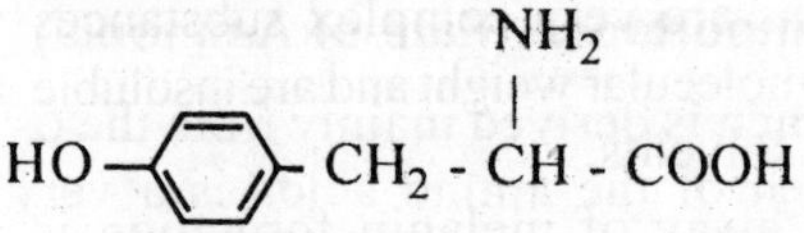

Tyrosine (p - hydroxyphenylalanine)

Phenylalanine is an essential amino acid whereas tyrosine is a non-essential amino acid. Phenylalanine can be converted to tyrosine but the reverse is not possible, hence the requirement of tyrosine can be met by the intake of adequate amount of phenylalanine in the diet. Both are *ketogenic amino acids.*

Both amino acids are involved in the synthesis of a number of important compounds in various body tissues **which include melanin pigment, epinephrine, norepinephrine, T_3 and T_4 (thyroxine) etc. as shown below:**

(a) Formation of melanin

(a) Melanins represent the dark pigments of the skin, hair and retina of the eye and are formed from 3, 4 - dihydroxyphenyl-alanine (DOPA) through a complex

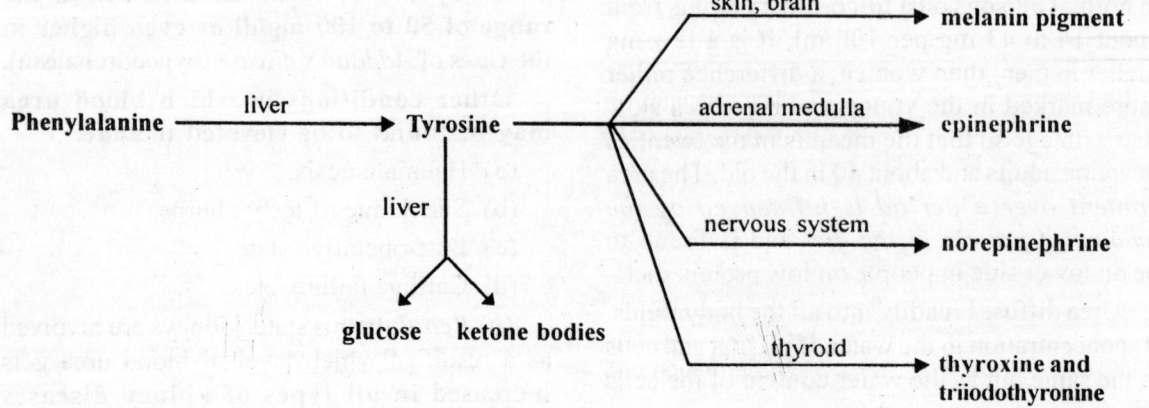

series of reactions.

(b) Melanin forms a reversible oxidation-reduction system in which the reduced form is tan and the oxidized form is black.

(c) Melanins are produced in pigment - forming cells, the *melanocytes.*

(d) Melanins are very complex substances of high molecular weight and are insoluble in most solvents.

(e) The pathway of melanin formation is given below in Fig. 14.2.

(b) Formation of epinephrine (adrenaline) and norepinephrine (arterenol)

(a) Formation of catecholamines i.e., epinephrine and norepinephrine from tyrosine in the adrenal medulla proceeds through DOPA and hydroxytryptamine.

(b) Its pathway may be represented as shown in Fig. 14.3.

(c) Formation of triiodothyronine (T_3) and thyroxine i. e. tetraiodothyronine (T_4)

(a) Synthesis of important hormones like T_3 and T_4 takes place in the thyroid gland from phenylalanine and tyrosine (Fig. 14.3).

(b) Phenylalanine is converted to tyrosine which on iodination forms monoiodotyrosine; this on further iodination gives rise to diiodotyrosine.

(c) Coupling of two molecules of diiodotyrosine yields thyroxine (Fig. 14.4).

(d) Coupling of 1 mol. of monoiodotyrosine and 1 mol. of diiodotyrosine yields triiodothyronine (Fig. 14.4).

Inborn errors of the metabolism of phenylalanine and tyrosine (hereditary defects in phenylalanine and tyrosine metabolism).

There are number of metabolic abnormalities

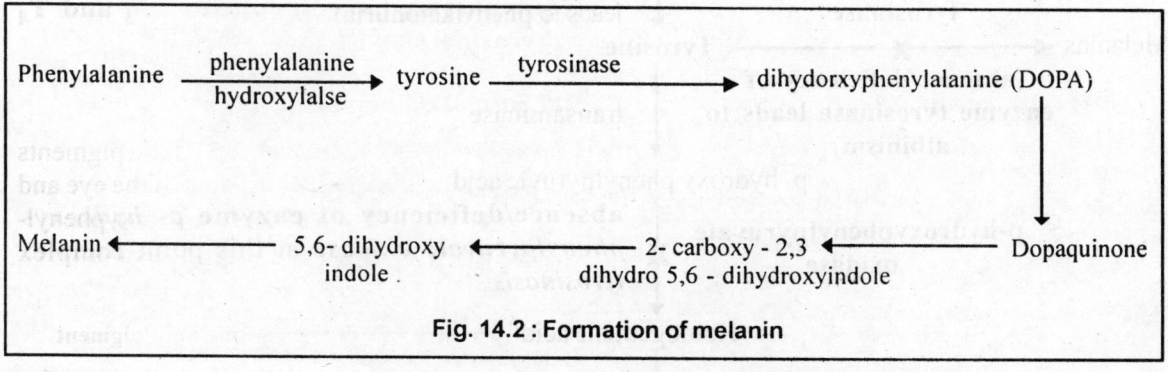

Fig. 14.2 : Formation of melanin

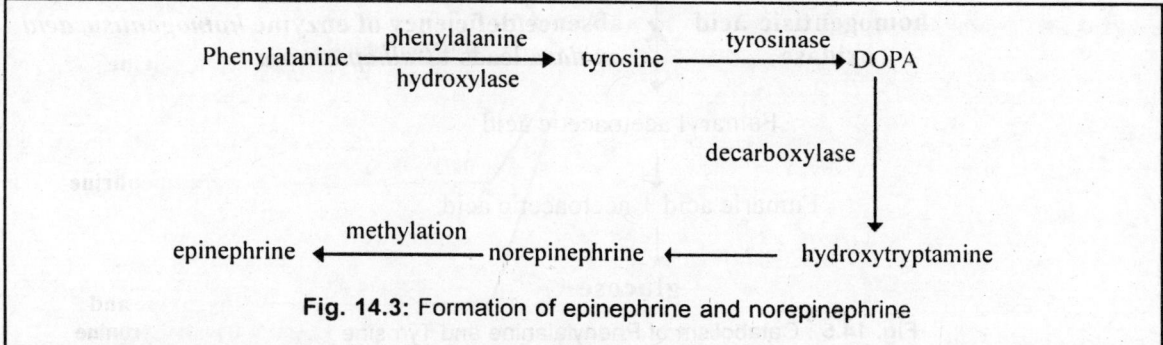

Fig. 14.3: Formation of epinephrine and norepinephrine

The steps are as shown below :

Phenylalanine

    phenylalanine   Monoiodotyrosine

    hydroxylase   +

                        Diiodotyrosine

Tyrosine

    iodination

Monoiodotyrosine   Triiodothyronine(T_3)

    iodination

Diiodotyrosine

    2 mols coupling

Thyroxine + Alanine

Fig 14.4 : Formation of T_4 and T_3

which are congenital and remain present throughout life. These disorders are hereditary (Fig. 14.5). Four well established hereditary defects in the metabolism of phenylalanine and tyrosine include **phenylketonuria (phenyl-pyruvic oligophrenia), tyrosinosis, alkaptonuria and albinism;** in each case the defect is due to hereditary absence or deficit of a specific enzyme involved in a specific reaction. These conditions belong to what **scientist Garrod called 'inborn errors of metabolism'.**

Inborn error	Enzyme defect
(i) Phenylketonuria	Phenylalanine hydroxylase
(ii) Tyrosinosis	p- Hydroxy phenylpyuvate oxidase
(iii) Alkaptonuria	Homogentisic acid oxidase
(iv) Albinism	Tyrosinase

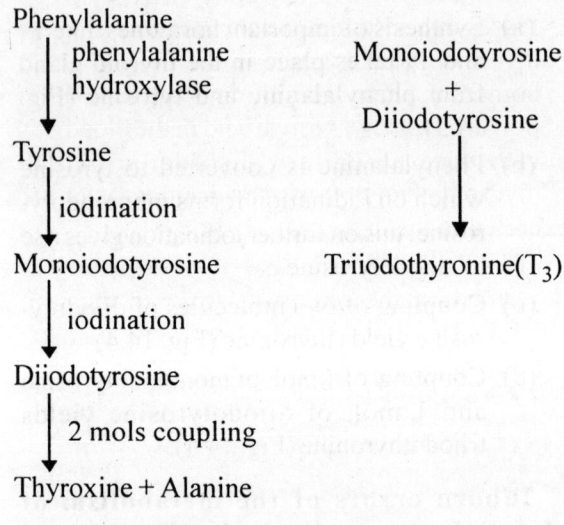

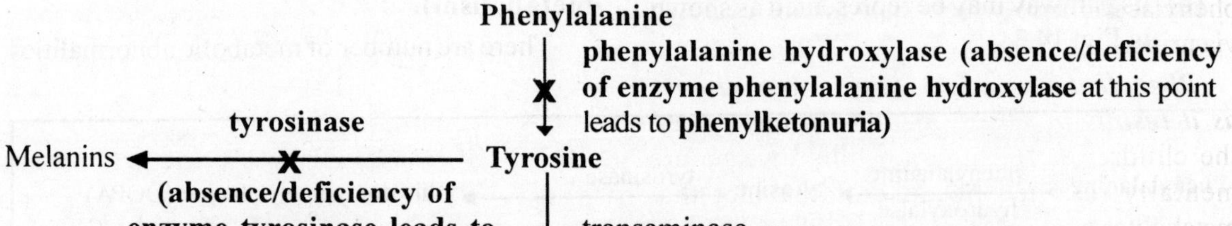

Phenylalanine

    phenylalanine hydroxylase (absence/deficiency of enzyme phenylalanine hydroxylase at this point leads to **phenylketonuria)**

Melanins ← **tyrosinase** ← **Tyrosine**

(absence/deficiency of enzyme tyrosinase leads to albinism)

    transaminase

p- hydroxy phenylpyruvic acid

p-hydroxyphenylpyruvate oxidase   **absence/deficiency of enzyme *p- hydroxy-phenylpyruvate oxidase* at this point leads to *tyrosinosis***

Homogentisic acid

homogentisic acid oxidase   **absence/deficiency of enzyme *homogentisic acid oxidase* leads to *alkaptonuria***

Fumaryl acetoacetic acid

Fumaric acid + acetoacetic acid

glucose

Fig. 14.5 : Catabolism of Phenylalanine and Tyrosine

Various blocks (checks) in the metabolism of phenylalanine and tyrosine give rise to different inborn errors of metabolism taking place either due to absence or deficiency of an enzyme which are as given in Fig. 14.5.

(i) Phenylketonuria

Phenylketonuria is an inborn error of metabolism associated with the metabolism of phenylalanine. The enzyme missing/deficient in this disease is known as *phenylalanine hydroxylase* which catalyses the conversion of phenylalanine to tyrosine. Due to the deficiency of the enzyme phenylalanine hydroxylase, the main pathway of the metabolism of phenylalanine via tyrosine (Fig. 14.5) gets blocked and the minor alternate pathway takes place as shown below . Various metabolites that accumulate in the blood are phenylpyruvic acid, phenyllactic acid and phenylacetic acid which later on are excreted via urine.

Phenylketonuria is a very serious disease as it results in severe mental deficiency and the children suffering from this disease are mentally retarded because of the fact that metabolites of phenylketonuria i.e. phenylpyruvic acid, phenyllactic acid and phenylacetic acid inhibit the formation of serotonin, a potent metabolite of brain.

(ii) Tyrosinosis

This is an inborn error of metabolism associated with the metabolism of phenylalanine and

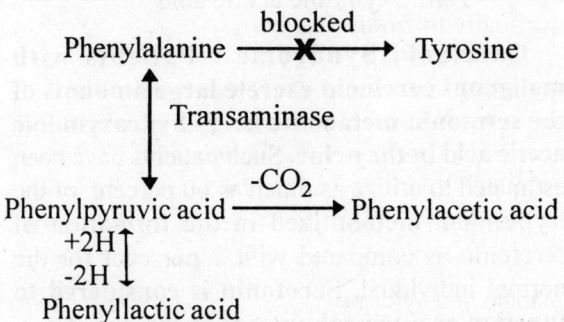

tyrosine. The enzyme missing/deficient in this disorder is known as p - hydroxyphenyl pyruvate oxidase; due to the deficiency of this enzyme p - hydroxyphenylpyruvic acid is not converted to homogentisic acid resulting in the deposition of p-hydroxyphenylpyruvic acid in the blood. It's a very rare hereditary disorder in which p - hydroxyphenylpyruvic acid and tyrosine are excreted in the urine.

The first authentic case of *tyrosinosis* was described by the scientist *Medes* in the year 1932.

(iii) Alkaptonuria

It's an inborn error of metabolism associated with the metabolism of phenylalanine and tyrosine. The enzyme missing/deficient is known as **homogentisic acid oxidase**; as a result of the deficiency of this enzyme homogentisic acid is not catalysed to form fumarylacetoacetic acid. The net result is the accumulation of homogentisic acid in the blood and other body fluids which is later on excreted via urine.

Alkaptonuria is characterized by the excretion of urine which upon standing gradually **becomes darker in colour and finally turns black.** The urine is also strongly reducing and gives a *violet colour-with* $FeCl_3$. The substance responsible **for the formation of the black pigment has been identified as homogentisic acid.**

Deposition of *homogentisic acid* in the body fluids and the cartilages and other connective tissues gives rise to a condition known as *ochronosis*.

(iv) Albinism

This is also an inborn error of the metabolism of phenylalanine and tyrosine. The enzyme missing/deficient is known as *tyrosinase,* the deficiency of which does not catalyse the formation of melanins from tyrosine. **In this disorder, the natural melanin pigments of hair, skin and**

eyes are not formed.

Total albinism is a hereditary condition in which there is complete absence of pigment in the skin, eyes and hair. It is due to absence of enzyme *tyrosinase* in the melanocytes and is transmitted as a simple recessive. **There are known various types of hereditary albinism in which pigment is only found to be lacking from certain parts of the body, such as the eye, areas of the skin and areas of the hair.**

Metabolism of Tryptophan

It's an aromatic amino acid and it is the only amino acid which contains indole ring in its structure. It is an essential amino acid. Omission of tryptophan from the diet of human beings is promptly followed by tissue wasting and negative nitrogen balance. Tryptophan has the metabolic distinction of giving rise to nicotinic acid, serotonin

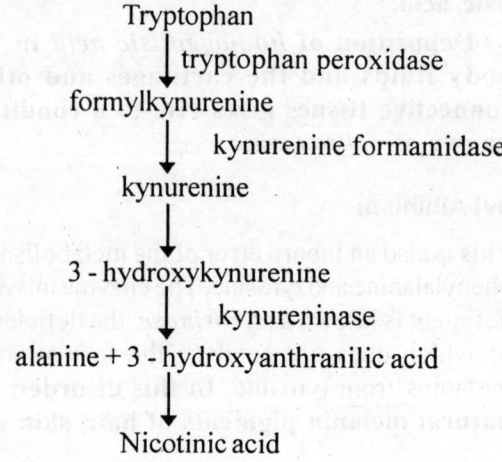

Tryptophan is metabolised in the following way:

Tryptophan
↓ tryptophan peroxidase
formylkynurenine
↓ kynurenine formamidase
kynurenine
↓
3 - hydroxykynurenine
↓ kynureninase
alanine + 3 - hydroxyanthranilic acid
↓
Nicotinic acid

and indoles on the one hand and glucose and ketone bodies on the other hand as shown below:

Salient features of this pathway are:

(i) **This pathway gives rise to the synthesis of niacin. 60 mgs of tryptophan gives rise to 1 mg of nicotinic acid in the human body.** In human diet, tryptophan is not in so much amount to meet the requirement of this vitamin.

(ii) **In the synthesis of serotonin: The vasoconstrictor substance 5 - hydroxy tryptamine or serotonin** is synthesized which remains present in the blood, particularly in the gastric mucosa, intestine, brain, mast cells and blood platelets. **It is an important substance in nerve impulse transmission (neurotransmitter). It regulates sleep, behaviour, blood pressure, etc.** This is synthesized, as mentioned below:

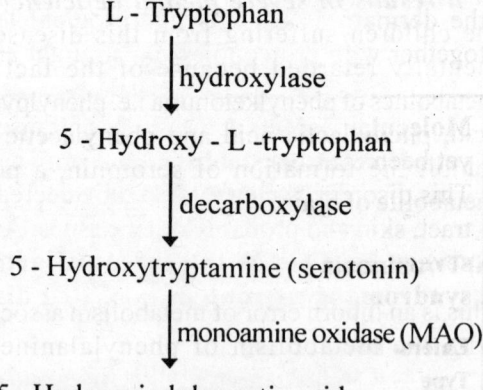

Carcinoid Syndrome : Patients with malignant carcinoid excrete large amounts of the serotonin metabolite i.e. 5- hydroxyindole acetic acid in the urine. Such patients have been estimated to utilize as much as 60 percent of the tryptophan metabolized in the formation of serotonin as compared with 1 per cent for the normal individual. **Serotonin is considered to function as a neurohumoral agent.**

(iii) In the synthesis of indole and skatole

This is the minor pathway by which tryptophan is metabolized as a result of which indole, indole acetic acid and skatole are formed in the large intestine due to action of certain bacteria. The foul smell of the faeces is due to these substances. These are excreted via urine or faeces.

Hartnup disease: This is an inborn error of metabolism associated with *tryptophan metabolism*. It has been named after the first detected family. **The enzyme deficient is** *tryptophanperoxidase.* This disease is characterized by the following three main symptoms:

(i) **Pellagra like dermatitis, the affected victims display skin lesions.**

(ii) **Sensitivity to sunlight**

(iii) **Motor ataxia characteristic of cerebellar dysfunction.**

Treatment: The treatment of patients with Hartnup disease consists in supplementing the diet with additional amount of niacin to alleviate the dermatological and neurological lesions together with protection from sunlight and the periodic sterilization of the gastrointestinal tract with antibiotics to reduce the formation of the bacterial breakdown products of tryptophan that may exert toxic effects.

The flow of information in all cells is from DNA to RNA to protein; this is known as **central dogma** of molecular biology; **it was formulated by scientist Francis Crick** shortly after the discovery of the structure of DNA. Information can also flow from DNA to DNA in both cells. Information also flows from RNA to RNA during the replication of RNA viruses such as polio virus. The final permitted information transfer is from RNA to DNA, which occurs only in the case of retroviruses such as **human immunodeficiency virus (HIV).** The only information transfer that is prohibited by the **central dogma is from protein to RNA or to DNA.** The permitted information transfers in cells (infected or uninfected) is summarized below:

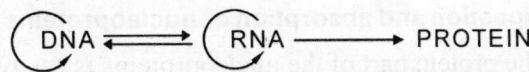

Molecular defects at the levels of transcription and translation of collagen polypeptides have not yet been clearly established but **may cause one type of Ehlers- Danlos syndrome (Type IV).** This disorder is characterized by decreased synthesis of type III collagen in the aorta, intestinal tract, skin and probably other tissues. Among the Ehlers- Danlos disorders, **Type IV is the most severe because of the threat of arterial rupture or gastrointestinal perforation. This syndrome is a group of inherited disorders as shown below:**

Ehlers- Danlos syndrome

Type	Inheritance	Biochemical defect	Collagen fibril diameter
I	AD	unknown	Increased
II	AD	"	"
III	AD	"	"
IV	AD or AR	Decreased type III collagen synthesis and its intracellular accumulation	Heterogeneous
V	XL	unknown	Heterogeneous
	XL	unknown	Increased
VI	AR	**Lysyl hydroxylase deficiency**	Decreased

AD = autosomal dominant, AR = autosomal recessive; XL = X- linked

CHAPTER 15

NUCLEIC ACIDS METABOLISM

Biosynthesis of the large complex molecules of the nucleic acids can be conveniently divided into synthesis of the monomers (mononucleotides) and the synthesis of the polymers (DNA and RNA).

Digestion and absorption of nucleoproteins

The protein part of the nucleoproteins is easily hydrolyzed by the following two types of enzymes viz:

(i)   gastric enzymes,

(ii)   intestinal enzymes

As a result of hydrolysis, the protein portion of nucleoproteins is broken down to its constituent amino acids; whereas the remaining part of nucleoproteins i.e., nucleic acids is not broken down in the stomach but is acted upon by pancreatic nucleases in the intestine. **Ribonuclease found in pancreatic juice hydrolyzes ribonucleic acid (RNA) splitting off particularly pyrimidine mononucleotides.**

Another enzyme which hydrolyzes deoxyribonucleic acid (DNA) to oligonucleotides (composed of a few mononucleotides) is a pancreatic deoxyribonuclease. Besides these two important enzymes, other enzymes found in intestinal mucosa are known as

nucleases such as phosphodiesterase which hydrolyzes the nucleic acids completely to mononucleotides which are further hydrolyzed by intestinal phosphatases **(nucleotidases)** to inorganic phosphate and nucleosides. It appears that nucleosides are not further hydrolyzed in the intestine but are absorbed as such.

Corresponding enzymes which have got the capability to further hydrolyze nucleosides to form D-ribose, D-deoxyribose, purine and pyrimidine bases are known as **nucleosidases** which are found in the extracts of various tissues of the body like liver, kidney, bone marrow etc. Some examples of them are as given below:

uracil riboside + H_2O $\xrightarrow{\text{nucleosidase}}$ uracil + ribose
(uridine)

guanine riboside+Pi $\xrightarrow[\text{phosphorylase}]{\text{nucleoside}}$ guanine+α-D-ribose-1-P
(guanosine)

Nucleoside phosphorylase found in liver and other tissues acts upon various nucleosides.

Biosynthesis of mononucleotides

Pyrimidine mononucleotides: The complete series of enzymic reaction giving rise to the parent pyrimidine mononucleotide (uridine 5'-monophosphate, UMP) is shown in Fig.15.1. **The**

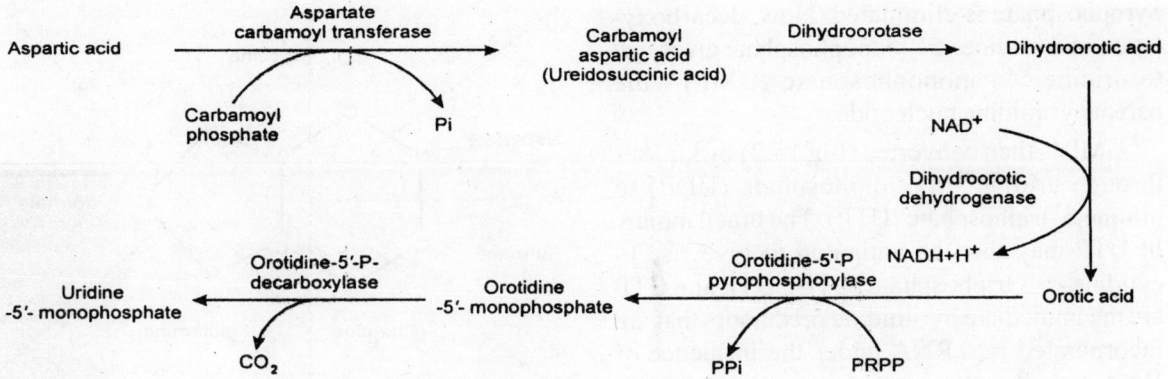

Fig. 15.1: Biosynthesis of UMP, the parent pyrimidine nucleotide

starting compounds are aspartic acid and carbamoyl phosphate (Fig.15.2) which combine to form carbamoyl - aspartate. Formation of the pyrimidine ring then takes place as a result of the action of **dihydro-orotase** forming dihydroorotic acid; dehydrogenation of which produces the important pyrimidine intermediate, orotic acid. A pyrophosphorylase reaction then follows in which orotic acid accepts a ribose - 5 - phosphate group from 5 - phosphoribosyl - 1 - pyrophosphate (PRPP). The resulting product is orotidine - 5' - monophosphate; inorganic

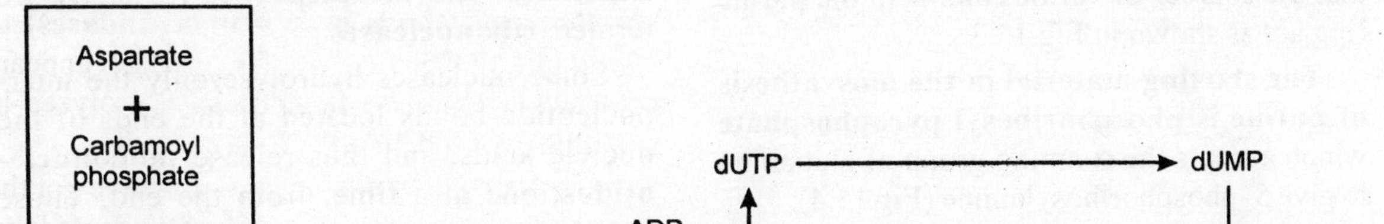

Fig15.2 : Biosynthetic pathways leading to the immediate pyrimidine precursors of DNA and RNA

pyrophosphate is eliminated. Now, decarboxylation of orotidine - 5'- monophosphate gives rise to uridine 5' - monophosphate (UMP) - the parent pyrimidine nucleotide.

UMP is then converted (Fig 15.2) by kinases through uridine - 5' - diphosphate (UDP) to uridine-5'-triphosphate (UTP). The uracil moiety of UTP may then be aminated to give rise to cytidine - 5' - triphosphate (CTP). UTP and CTP are the immediate pyrimidine precursors that are incorporated into RNA under the influence of **RNA polymerase.**

Eventually dCTP and dTTP are the immediate pyrimidine precursors that are incorporated into DNA by the action of **DNA polymerase.**

Purine mononucleotides

It is known from experiments with isotope studies that the sources of various atoms in the purine ring are as shown in Fig 15.3.

The starting material in the biosynthesis of purine is phosphoribosyl pyrophosphate which accepts the α-amino group of glutamine to give 5- phosphoribosylamine (Fig 15.4).

The ring system is completed when N-formyl-tetrahydrofolic acid donates its formyl group to the 5-amino group of the imidazole carboxamide ribonucleotide. The complete ribonucleotide is inosinic acid (inosine 5'-monophosphate, IMP).

Amination of IMP to AMP proceeds in two stages with the intermediate formation of adenylosuccinic acid (Fig 15.5).

The formation of GMP from IMP is also a two stage reaction in which xanthosine 5'-monophosphate (XMP) is initially formed and then aminated to form GMP (Fig 15.5).

The two purine mononucleotides, AMP and GMP are phosphorylated by kinases through the diphosphate stage to give ATP and GTP.

NUCLEASES

Nucleases catalyse the hydrolysis of inter-

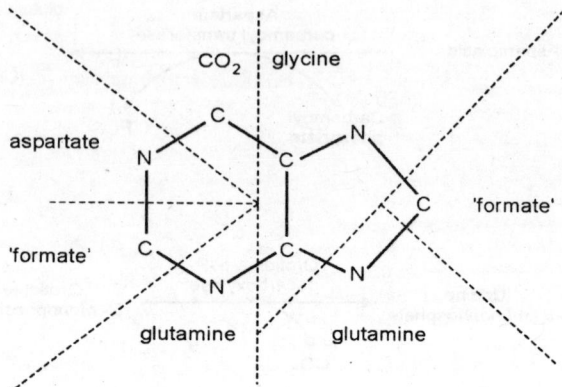

Fig 15.3 : Origin of the separate atoms in the purine ring. 'Formate' stands for the formyl derivative of tetrahydrofolic acid.

nucleotide bonds. Some are specific for DNA, and others for RNA; while some are capable of hydrolysing both types of nucleic acid. Nucleases specific for DNA are termed **deoxyribonucleases,** and those specific for RNA are termed **ribonucleases.**

Some nucleases hydrolyse only the internucleotide bonds located at the ends of the nucleic acids, and thus release **mononucleotides,** one at a time, from the end. These enzymes are known as **exonucleases.** Some of these attack the internucleotide bonds consecutively from the 5' - end of the nucleic acid, others from the 3' end. In contrast, other enzymes hydrolyse internucleotide bonds located at points throughout the length of the nucleic acid chains. These enzymes are termed **endonucleases.**

A well-known ribonuclease from bovine pancreas (pancreatic RNase) hydrolyses internucleotide bonds within RNA chains to give mono- and oligonucleotide products bearing 3'-phosphoryl groups. The specificity of this enzyme is such that bonds between purine nucleotides are not hydrolysed, bonds between adjacent pyrimidine nucleotides are hydrolysed; bonds between purine (Pu) nucleotides adjacent to pyrimidine (Py) nucleotides are hydrolysed only if the sequence in the RNA chain is 5'-Py-

glutamine → glutamate+PPi

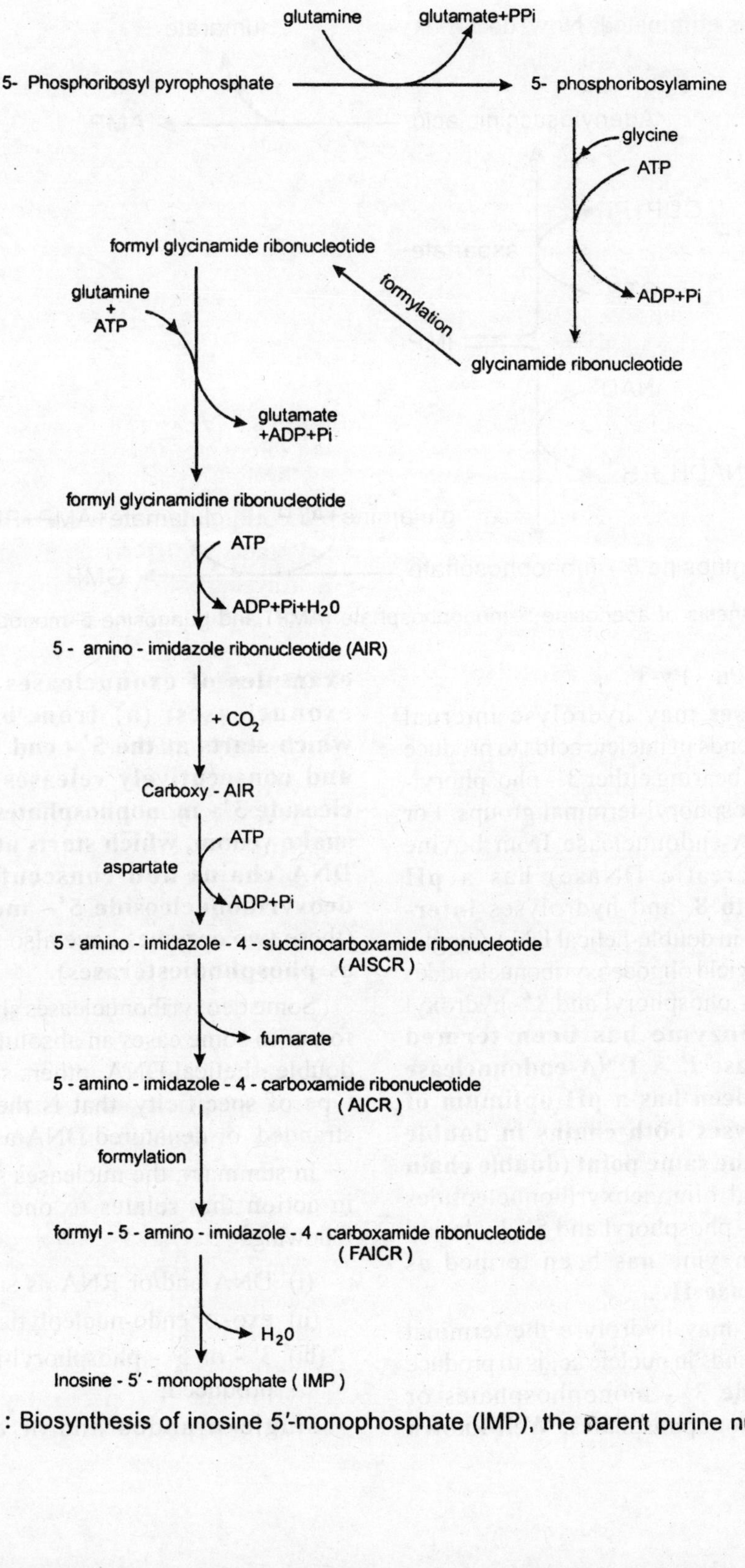

5- Phosphoribosyl pyrophosphate ⟶ 5- phosphoribosylamine

glycine
ATP
→ ADP+Pi

formyl glycinamide ribonucleotide ← formylation ← glycinamide ribonucleotide

glutamine
+
ATP
→ glutamate
+ADP+Pi

formyl glycinamidine ribonucleotide

ATP
→ ADP+Pi+H_2O

5 - amino - imidazole ribonucleotide (AIR)

+ CO_2

Carboxy - AIR

ATP
aspartate
→ ADP+Pi

5 - amino - imidazole - 4 - succinocarboxamide ribonucleotide
(AISCR)

→ fumarate

5 - amino - imidazole - 4 - carboxamide ribonucleotide
(AICR)

formylation

formyl - 5 - amino - imidazole - 4 - carboxamide ribonucleotide
(FAICR)

→ H_2O

Inosine - 5' - monophosphate (IMP)

Fig15.4 : Biosynthesis of inosine 5'-monophosphate (IMP), the parent purine nucleotide

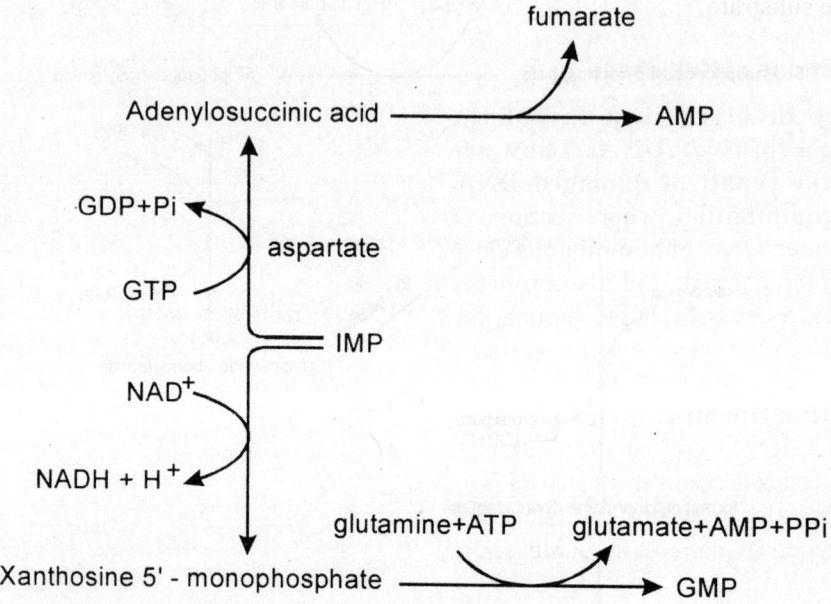

Fig15.5 : Biosynthesis of adenosine 5'-monophosphate (AMP) and guanosine 5'-monophosphate (GMP)

Pu-3' and not 5'-Pu - Py-3'.

Endonucleases may hydrolyse internal internucleotide bonds in nucleic acids to produce oligonucleotides bearing either 3'- phosphoryl-terminal or 5' phosphoryl-terminal groups. For example, a DNA-endonuclease from bovine pancreas (pancreatic DNase) has a **pH optimum of 7 to 8,** and hydrolyses **inter-nucleotide** bonds in double-helical DNA (single-chain scission) to yield oligodeoxyribonucleotides terminated by 5'- phosphoryl and 3'- hydroxyl groups. **This enzyme has been termed deoxyribonuclease I. A DNA-endonuclease from bovine spleen has a pH optimum of 4.5 and hydrolyses both chains in double helical DNA at the same point (double chain scission)** to yield oligodeoxyribonucleotides terminated by 3'- phosphoryl and 5'- hydroxyl groups. This enzyme has been termed as **deoxyribonuclease II.**

Exonucleases may hydrolyse the terminal internucleotide bonds in nucleic acids to produce either nucleoside 3'- monophosphates or nucleoside 5'- monophosphates. **Well-known**

examples of exonucleases are the DNA exonucleases, (a) from bovine spleen, which starts at the 5'- end of DNA chains and consecutively releases deoxyribonu-cleoside 3'- monophosphates, and (b) from snake venom, which starts at the 3'- end of DNA chains and consecutively releases deoxyribonucleoside 5'- monophosphates (these two enzymes have also been referred to as **phosphodiesterases).**

Some deoxyribonucleases show a preference for, or in some cases an absolute specificity for double - helical DNA, others show the reverse type of specificity, that is they prefer single stranded, or denatured DNA as substrate.

In summary, the nucleases show specificity in action that relates to one or more of the following:

(i) DNA and/or RNA as substrate;

(ii) exo- or endo-nucleolytic action;

(iii) 3' - or 5' - phosphoryl-terminal groups produced;

single-stranded and/or double-helical

condition of the substrate.

Important functions of Nucleases

Nucleases are involved in many of the important reactions of DNA. They are required for the repair of damaged DNA, for genetic recombination, where sections of the double-stranded DNA of homologous chromosomes are interchanged, and also probably for the complex process of DNA replication. Endo - and exonucleases with lower specificity also catalyse the hydrolysis of nucleic acids to nucleotides, in the living cell (for example, degradation of mRNA) and in the course of degradation of dead cells. Foodstuff derived from cellular material also contains nucleic acids which are degraded by pancreatic nucleases in the duodenum.

REPAIR OF DAMAGED DNA

Single-strand scissions in double-stranded DNA which have a 3' - hydroxyl group on one side and a 5' - phosphate group on the other (like those formed by pancreatic DNase can be repaired by the enzyme **polynucleotide ligase** (Fig 15.6).

Similar breaks are produced in DNA in vivo by X-irradiation and many of them are repaired

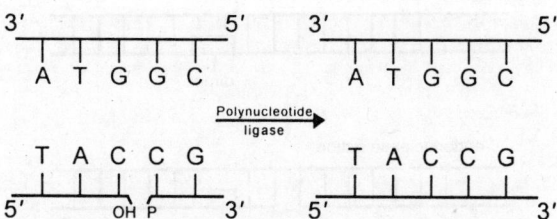

Fig 15.6: The mode of action of polynucleotide ligase.

by a polynucleotide ligase.

Ultraviolet radiation, on the other hand, gives rise to thymine dimers in DNA. Absorption of energy at 260 rim causes the 5, 6 double bonds of adjacent thymine bases in one strand of the DNA to rearrange and form dimers (Fig 15.7).

Thymine dimers locally distort the regular form of the DNA double helix and block replication. The reaction is enzymically reversible in the presence of light, but in the dark such thymine dimers are removed by a complicated series of reactions (Fig 15.8).

An endonuclease recognizes the distortion in the double helix and forms a single strand scission (3' - hydroxyl, 5' - phosphate) on the 5' side of the thymine dimer. An exonuclease, working from the scission in the 5' to 3' direction, removes nucleotides and the thymine dimer. Concurrently, a DNA polymerase (with the properties of

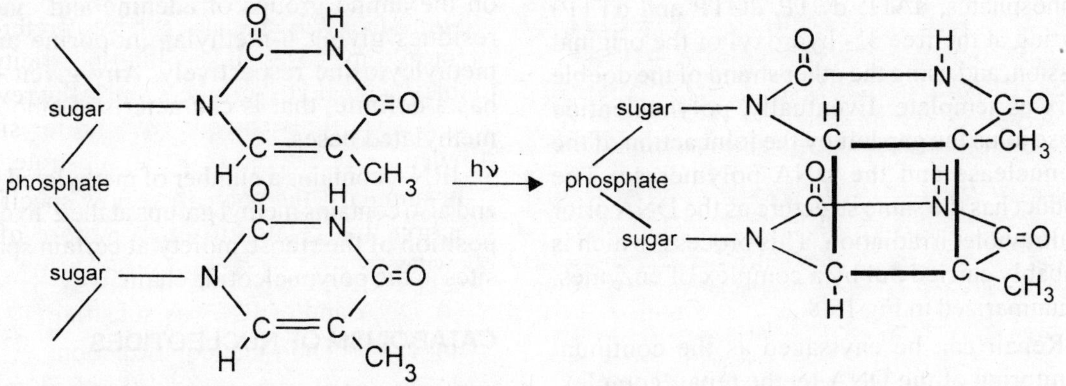

Fig. 15.7: The formation of a thymine dimer under the influence of ultraviolet light. Two adjacent thymine residues (left) in DNA become linked together as shown on the right.

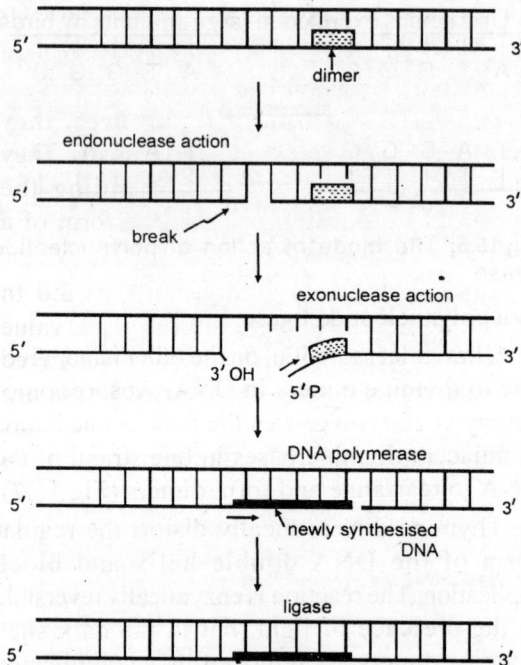

Fig. 15.8 : The repair of damaged DNA. An endonuclease cuts the affected strand on the 5' side of the dimer. An exonuclease then excises a length of the affected strand including the dimer leaving a gap which is filled in by the polymerase. The final join between the newly synthesized DNA filling the gap, and the remainder of the original strand is brought about by the ligase.

Kornberg's DNA polymerase, adds nucleotides sequentially (using the deoxyribonucleoside triphosphates, dATP, dCTP, dGTP and dTTP) starting at the free 3'- hydroxyl of the original scission, and using the other strand of the double helix as template. Eventually, polynucleotide ligase joins the gap left by the joint action of the exonuclease and the DNA polymerase. The product has the same structure as the DNA prior to ultraviolet irradiation. This process, which is probably carried out by a complex of enzymes, is summarized in Fig 15.8.

Repair can be envisaged as the continual monitoring of the DNA by the repair complex, which cuts out and replaces irregularities in the double helix. **A heritable disease in man,** **xeroderma pigmentosum, which in homozygous individuals is characterized by an extreme sensitivity to sunlight and the eventual development of multiple carcinomas on the exposed parts of the body, is caused by a defect in DNA repair.** The lesion has been identified with the absence of the specific endonuclease which forms single-strand scissions as the first step in the repair process.

ENZYMIC MODIFICATION OF NUCLEIC ACIDS

Some enzymes can modify the nucleic acids at the polynucleotide level. **Thus, after synthesis of nucleic acids, methylation, glucosylation, phosphorylation, acylation, thiolation and other alterations of the macromolecule may take place. Of these reactions, methylation is quantitatively the most important.**

Methylation of DNA and RNA is affected by specific enzymes **(methyltransferases)** which recognize not only the ribo- or deoxyribo-type of nucleic acid but also specific nucleotides at specific sites within the nucleic acid chain. Only a small proportion of the bases is methylated. The general reaction is:

nucleic acid + S-adenosylmethionine $\longrightarrow$ CH_3-nucleic acid + S-adenosylhomocysteine

The sites of methylation are predominantly on the amino groups of adenine and cytosine residues giving 6-methylaminopurine and 5-methylcytosine respectively. Any given DNA has a definite, that is characteristic amount of methylated bases.

tRNA contains a number of methylated bases and also contains methyl groups at the 2' hydroxyl position of the ribose moiety at certain specific sites in the polynucleotide chain.

CATABOLISM OF NUCLEOTIDES

Nucleotidases and nucleosidases

Some of these enzymes have very low

specificities and hydrolyse both 5' - monophosphates and 3' - monophosphates, while others display a much higher degree of specificity, degrading only the 5'- or the 3'-monophosphates. **Nucleotidases are known which hydrolyse the phosphate from one specific nucleotide only.**

The collective action of these enzymes gives rise to pentose, pentose phosphate, and to the free purine and pyrimidine bases.

Catabolism of pyrimidines. The pyrimidine bases are catabolized in mammalian tissues by preliminary reduction of uracil and thymine to the corresponding dihydro-derivatives, followed

Uric acid is excreted in large amounts by birds and reptiles, but in them it is the end product not only of purine catabolism but also of protein catabolism. **Instead of excreting urea, they excrete uric acid as a semisolid paste.** They can thus conserve water by avoiding the necessity of producing urine in the form of a dilute aqueous solution.

Human blood normally contains 3.0 to 6.0 mg of uric acid per 100 ml. This value tends to rise whenever cells are being destroyed and nucleoprotein liberated. **Raised levels are therefore encountered in such conditions as leukaemia, polycythaemia, and in**

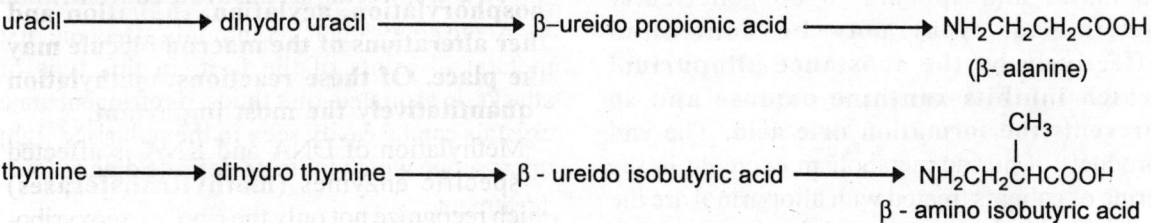

Fig 15.9 The catabolism of pyrimidine bases

by ring opening to give the appropriate ureido-acid, and removal of ammonia and carbon dioxide to give β-alanine or its methylated derivative β-aminoisobutyric acid (Fig. 15.9).

Catabolism of purines. The purine bases arising from degradation of the nucleic acids are conveyed in the blood to the liver where they are catabolized still further through a well-known series of changes resulting in the formation of uric acid (Fig.15.10). Adenine is deaminated by **adenine deaminase** (adenase) to yield hypoxanthine.Guanine is deaminated by **guanine deaminase (guanase)** to give xanthine. Further oxidation is brought about by **xanthine oxidase** in the liver. This enzyme oxidizes hypoxanthine to xanthine, and xanthine to uric acid which, in primates, is excreted by the kidney. **The amount of uric acid excreted per day in human urine varies widely from 0.1 to 2.0 g.**

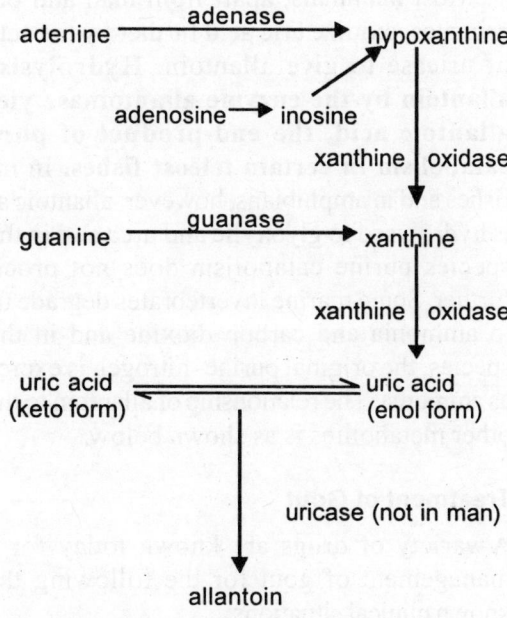

Fig. 15.10 The catabolism of purine bases

pneumonia during the process of resolution. **In chronic renal disease, the excretion of uric acid, like that of other nitrogenous compounds, is impaired and retention of uric acid occurs. Probably the highest values for uric acid in plasma are found in gout immediately before an acute attack.** In this disease, salts of uric acid are actually deposited in the tissues, causing the typical chalky swellings **(tophi)** but it is not clear why such large amounts of uric acid should be formed in gouty persons; there may be a defect in the feed-back control of the enzyme that forms 5'-phosphoribosylamine (PRA), a precursor of purine nucleotides. The disorder is found mainly in males and appears to be genetically determined. **Gout may be controlled effectively by the substance allopurinol which inhibits xanthine oxidase and so prevents the formation uric acid.** The end products of purine metabolism excreted in the urine of patients treated with allopurinol are the much less insoluble compounds i.e., hypoxanthine and xanthine.

Most mammals, apart from man and other primates, oxidize uric acid further by the action of uricase to give allantoin. **Hydrolysis of allantoin by the enzyme allantoinase yields allantoic acid, the end-product of purine catabolism in certain teleost fishes.** In most fishes and in amphibians, however, allantoic acid is hydrolysed to glyoxylic and urea and in these species purine catabolism does not proceed further. Some marine invertebrates degrade urea to ammonia and carbon dioxide and in these species, the original purine- nitrogen is excreted as ammonia. The relationship of allantoin to these other metabolites is as shown below.

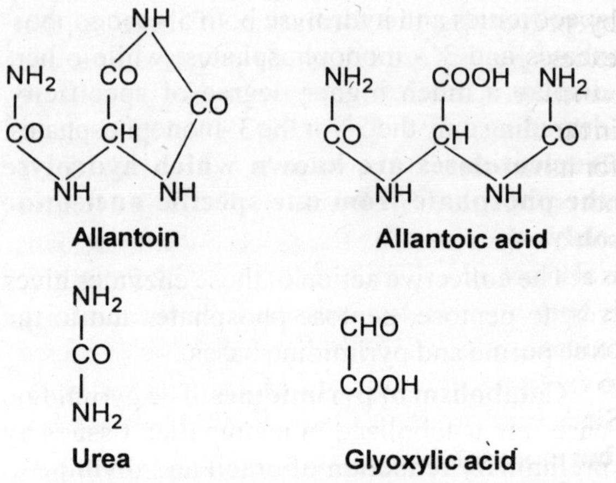

Treatment of Gout

A variety of drugs are known today for the management of gout for the following three known clinical situations:

(a) **For the treatment of acute gout arthritis**

Allantoin

Allantoic acid

Urea

Glyoxylic acid

(b) **For the prevention of acute attacks, and**

(c) **For lowering serum urate concentration**

Acute gouty attacks commonly affect the first metatarsal joints of the foot. In this type of attacks, in aspirated joint fluids, birefringent urate crystals can be easily seen in the polarised light microscope which indicate definite diagnosis.

Treatment:

(a) Administration of colchicine, nonsteroidal anti-inflammatory drugs (NSAIDs), corticosteroids, adrenocorticotropic hormone (ACTH), and analgesics. Colchicine and NSAIDS can also be used prophylactically to prevent acute attacks in patients with gout.

(b) Drugs used to lower serum urate concentrations are probenecid, sulfinpyrazone, allopurinol, etc.

Colchicine :

It depolymerizes microtubules and structures (such as mitotic spindle) consisting of microtubules. This drug is very effective in decreasing pain and the frequency of attacks but its exact mechanism of action is yet not very clear.

Allopurinol:

This is a competitive inhibitor of xanthine oxidase and has been recently developed to control gout by preventing the formation of urate so that excess purines are excreted as hypoxathine and xanthine. Allopurinol differs from hypoxanthine in the distribution of ring nitrogens. The rationale for its use is that hypoxanthine and xanthine will not precipitate in the joints. Hypoxanthine is more soluble than urate, although xanthine is not. This is also not a completely safe drug. Since xanthine is both a product and a substrate for xanthine oxidase, allopurinol therapy could be expected to cause accumulation of xanthine in the body. Since xanthine is only sparingly soluble in urine (but more soluble than uric acid), this may lead to urinary xanthine crystalluria or formation of stone.

The mechanism of action of allopurinol which is an analogue of hypoxanthine is that it inhibits xanthine oxidase enzyme and thus reduces the formation of xanthine and uric acid. It is converted by xanthine oxidase to alloxanthine,

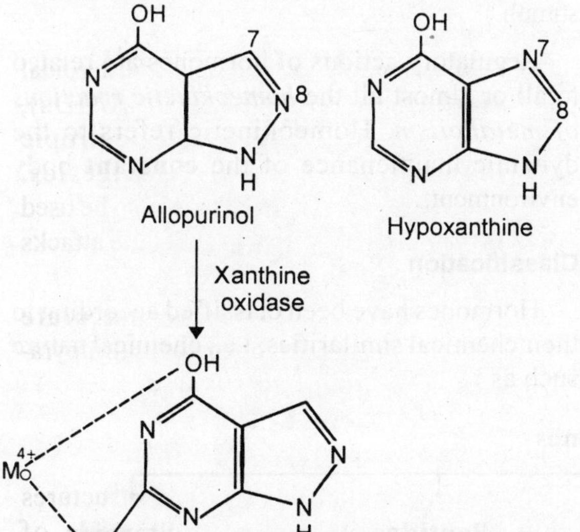

Allopurinol   **Hypoxanthine**

Xanthine oxidase

Fig. 15.11 : Inhibition of xanthine oxidase by allopurinol, an analogue of hypoxanthine. N_7 and N_8 of hypoxanthine are reversed in the structure of allopurinol. Allopurinol, a suicide enzyme inactivator, gets converted to alloxanthine, which binds tightly to the active site of the enzyme via Mo^{4+} and interrupts the reoxidation of Mo^{4+} to Mo^{6+} required to initiate the next catalytic cycle.

which binds tightly to the active site by chelation with Mo^{4+}. This greatly reduces reoxidation of Mo^{4+} to Mo^{6+} and affects catalytic activity (Fig 15.11). Such kind of inhibitor, in which a substrate analogue gets converted to an inhibitor and not released from the active site, is called as a **suicide enzyme- inactivator.**

Side by side, allopurinol may also be converted to allopurinol ribonucleotide by HPRT as shown in Fig 15.12. Uric acid formation gets decreased through depletion of PRPP.

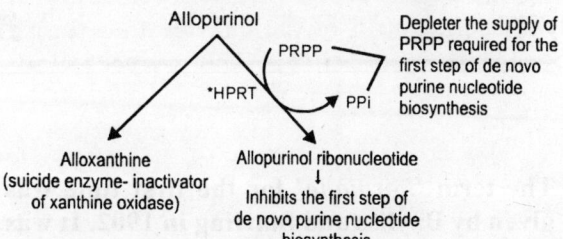

Fig.15.12 : Multiple actions of allopurinol inhibit the formation of uric acid. *HPRT/HGPRT is hypoxanthine guanine phosphoribosyl transferase.

Drugs that have a tendency to increase the excretion of uric acid in human beings include **probenecid** which is effective in the regulation of **hyperuricemia** and the resolution and prevention of tophi, and **sulfinpyrazone,** which has got the similar effects. Both the agents are weak organic acids and probably act as competitive inhibitors of tubular reabsorption of uric acid.

Dietary effect on gout: Serum urate levels may be lowered by dietary and life style changes which include:

(a) **Correction of obesity,** (b) **Avoidance of ethanol consumption i.e., alcohol, and** (c) **Avoidance of high purine foods** (e.g., organ meats).

Pseudogout: It is a disorder which is caused by the deposition of calcium pyrophosphate dihydrate usually in larger joints such as knee, wrist and ankle.

Gout and Lesch-Nyhan Syndrome: Consult Chapter 8 (Nucleic Acids).

CHAPTER 16

HORMONES

By S.P. Singh* and Anshuman Singh**

The term *'hormone'* for the first time was given by Bayliss and Starling in 1902. It was derived from the Greek word "Hormaein" which means to excite or to arouse. Hormone is a chemical substance which is produced in one part of the body, enters the circulation and is carried to distant organs and tissues to modify their structures and functions.

Hormones have three major functions in the body, namely:

1. **Integrative,**
2. **Regulative and**
3. **Morphological**

A particular hormone is involved in only one function. The integrative action is possible because hormones travel through blood from the source to the site of their action and enable the body to function accordingly in response to stimuli.

Regulatory actions of hormones are related to all or almost all the *homeokinetic reactions of metabolism.* Homeokinetic refers to the dynamic maintenance of the **constant** body environment.

Classification

Hormones have been classified according to their chemical similarities, i.e., chemical nature such as :

Hormones

Phenol derivatives	Proteins	Peptides	Steroids
■ Adrenaline	■ Anterior pituitary hormones	■ ACTH	■ Estrogens
■ Nor-adrenaline	■ Insulin	■ Vasopressin (ADH or Pitressin)	■ Androgens
■ Thyroxine	■ Human chorionic gonadotrophin	■ Oxytocin (Pitocin)	■ Progesterone
	■ Gonadotrophin, thyro-globulin and secretin		■ Adrenal corticoides

* The Author; ** Senior Medical Officer; Primary Health Centre, Phursatganj, Raibareli, U.P.

Hypothalamic releasing hormones

Hormones from the anterior pituitary is under the control of *hypothalamus* which lies in brain and forms its integral part. The stimuli are received by neuro-receptors present in hypothalamus which in turn secretes humoral substances into the *hypothalamic-hypophyseal portal circulation*. The humoral substances on reaching the adenohypophysis cause release of specific trophic hormones from the anterior pituitary gland (described under anterior pituitary gland).

ENDOCRINE ORGANS

1. Pituitary gland (or hypophysis)

It is the most important endocrine organ. This is also called as a *master gland*. This gland is divided into three functionally distinct parts as mentioned below:

(i) Anterior lobe,

(ii) Posterior lobe, and

(iii) Intermediate part

Anterior lobe

It secretes

1. Growth hormone (GH, or somatotrophin),
2. Thyroid stimulating hormone (TSH),
3. Adrenocorticotrophic hormone (ACTH),
4. Luteinizing hormone (LH),
5. Follicle stimulating hormone (FSH) and
6. Prolactin

Functions

Functions of the above mentioned hormones (known as *trophic* hormones, i.e., **nourishing hormones**) are to stimulate the growth and the functions of other endocrine organs, such as:

(i) Thyroid gland by TSH

(ii) Adrenal gland by ACTH

(iii) Gonands by LH and FSH

GH stimulates the growth of cells in general, especially those of bone and other types of connective tissue. Secretion of trophic hormones is controlled by **'releasing hormones'** (and by *'release-inhibiting* hormones), secreted by *hypothalamus.*

Posterior lobe

It secretes

1. Antidiuretic hormone (ADH or vasopressin), and
2. Oxytocin

These hormones are synthesized in the hypothalamus, and pass directly to the posterior lobe of the pituitary gland by *axonal* transport.

Functions

ADH stimulates the reabsorption of water in the kidney. Oxytocin stimulates the contraction of certain smooth muscles.

Intermediate part

It secretes melanophore stimulating hormone (MSH) only.

Functions

Its only function is in the darkening of the skin.

2. Adrenal glands

Each adrenal gland is divided into two parts as:

(i) Cortex

(ii) Medulla

Cortex

It secretes

1. Glucocorticoids and
2. Mineralocorticoids

Functions

Glucocorticoids, such as *cortisol* stimulate

the breakdown of protein into carbohydrate and have an anti-inflammatory action.

Mineralocorticoids such as *aldosterone* stimulate the reabsorption of Na^+ in the kidney, and thus control the ionic composition of plasma.

Medulla

It secretes catecholamines.

Functions

Catecholamines, such as, adrenaline (also called epinephrine) stimulate the breakdown of glycogen and triglycerides in their respective stores, and increase the blood flow. Thus, by such means, extra glucose and fatty acids are made available to the muscles and other cells for the production of ATP.

3. The Male and Female Gonads

They secrete sex hormones, which are responsible to stimulate primary and sexual characteristics.

Testes secrete androgens (such as testosterone). Ovaries secrete oestrogens (such as oestradiol and oestrone).

4. Thyroid gland

It secretes thyroid hormones as mentioned below:

(i) Thyroxine (T_4) and triiodothyronine (T_3). **They stimulate the overall metabolic rate,** i.e., the oxidation of foodstuffs throughout the body.

(ii) Caicitonin. **It has a tendency to lower plasma concentration of Ca^{2+}** by inhibiting Ca^{2+} release from the bone.

5. Parathyroid gland

It is the neighbouring gland of the thyroid gland and secretes a hormone known as parathormone which has the capability to raise Ca^{2+} levels in blood by stimulating Ca^{2+} release from bone.

6. Secretion by cells

Besides glands, hormones are also secreted by specific cells present in certain organs that have a predominantly non-endocrine function, for instance, **pancreas secretes insulin and glucagon.** Insulin has a tendency to stimulate an uptake of glucose from the plasma into the muscle and other cells, as a result of which blood sugar level gets reduced, whereas the role of *glucagon* is just opposite to insulin which means that glucagon has a tendency to stimulate release of glucose from liver glycogen into the bloodstream.

Kidney secretes *renin,* which through another hormone stimulates the secretion of aldosterone from the adrenal cortex. Likewise, *gastrointestinal tract* also secretes a number of hormones which have a tendency to stimulate the secretion of *hydrochloric acid* and digestive enzymes.

Types of hormones

1. GH, TSH, LH, FSH, ACTH, prolactin, insulin, glucagon, calcitonin, parathormone, renin, MSH, ADH, and oxytocin are **polypeptides.**

   Catecholamines and thyroid hormones are amino acid derivatives. All these hormones are stored in the cells in which they are synthesized in the form of small vesicles. Release of hormones, by stimulation of the cells in which they are stored, is by **'exocytosis'** of the vesicular contents.

2. *Prostaglandins,* a class of **'local hormones'** not produced by specific cells, are in fact *derivatives of polyunsaturated fatty acids* which control smooth muscle contraction.

3. Glucocorticoids, mineralocorticoids, androgens and oestrogens are steroids in nature and are derived from cholesterol.

Mechanism of Action (Principles of hormone action)

Hormones act in two ways, either

(i) at the cell surface, e.g., most polypeptide hormones and catecholamines. Action at the cell surface is through an activation of enzyme **adenyl cyclase** which leads to an increase in the concentration of intracellular cyclic AMP, either through increased Ca^{2+} concentration, or through increased nutrient (glucose and amino acids) entrance.

(ii) in the interior of cells, e.g., most steroidal hormones act in this fashion. Action within the cells is on *transcription* of specific genes (within the nucleus) or on *translation* of mRNA in the cytoplasm.

Disease

A decrease or increase in the synthesis of a particular hormone leads to an imbalance of metabolism for instance **diabetes mellitus, Cushing's syndrome, thyrotoxicosis, Addison's disease etc.** An increase is often due to an endocrine tumor.

Mechanism of hormone action (in detail)

The exact mechanism of a number of hormones is not yet very well understood, though, the net result is known, for instance, testosterone and oestrogens stimulate protein synthesis in target organs, but how does it happen? Thirdly, more than one biochemical action has been attributed to several hormones, for instance, insulin stimulates glucose uptake and glycolysis by muscles, glycogenesis and protein synthesis in liver, and lipogenesis in fat cells, whereas it inhibits gluconeogenesis in liver and glycolysis in fat cells. Now, the question arises, which is the action primarily concerned to its hypoglycaemic (reduction in blood glucose)function?

It has been observed that all hormones have one property in common. They interact with a specific receptor at the target cell, and as a result of that interaction, the cell responds in one or more ways. For convenience, the interactions may be easily divided into two types:

(i) interaction with a receptor at the cell surface and

(ii) interaction with a receptor inside the cells.

Interaction at the cell surface

A majority of the hormones is polypeptide in nature, such hormones are incapable of crossing the plasma membrane. This suggests that they interact with a receptor at the cell surface. It has been confirmed by several ways, that proteins, and even bigger molecules, are taken up by cells either by :

(a) **Pinocytosis or**

(b) **Phagocytosis**

But the entry of a substance by pinocytosis or phagocytosis is not the same as entry across the plasma membrane. Actually, what happens, the contents of a pinocytotic or phagocytotic vesicle become hydrolysed by lysosomal action as soon as they enter a cell, meaning to say; the molecules ingested in this manner cannot exert any specific action within the cell (viruses are an exception; their nucleocapsids (protein-RNA or protein-DNA complexes), which become exposed once they are inside a cell, are so arranged as to make them relatively resistant to the lysosomal hydrolysis).

It has been studied that not only polypeptides, but also **amino acid derived hormones such as the catecholamines and also fatty acid-derived hormones such as the prostaglandins,** act at the cell surface. In general, non-steroid hormones act at the cell surface, while the steroid hormones (and possibly thyroid hormones too) act intracellularly. Following three types of surface responses are known:

(i) Adenyl cyclase,

(ii) Calcium entry,

(iii) Other mechanisms

Role of Adenyl Cyclase

The enzyme adenyl cyclase catalyses the conversion of ATP to cyclic AMP (c-AMP). This enzyme, remains situated on the plasma membrane, 'facing inwards': in other words, reactant and product remain in the cytoplasm. Many hormones like adrenaline, glucagon, ACTH, FSH, LH, ADH,catecholamines etc., have a tendency to stimulate the enzyme, **as a result of which c-AMP has been termed as a *"second messenger"*, the first messenger being the hormone itself (cyclic GMP, which tends to be increased in situations that depress cyclic AMP, and vice versa, may be another type of second messenger).** Binding of hormone is not directly to the enzyme, but rather to a protein receptor on the plasma membrane that 'faces outwards'. Receptor and enzyme then interact, as a result of which enzyme activity is increased.

The c-AMP that is formed has several important actions, out of which the main one is to stimulate the phosphorylation of proteins. Structural proteins such as histones, and enzymes like glycogen phosphorylase, triglyceride lipase, and glycogen synthetase, exist in two forms i.e. phosphorylated and unphosphorylated. It has been studied that the phosphorylation, which is catalysed by a specific *protein kinase,* generally takes place on the hydroxyl group of a serine residue. The two forms have different activities. Histones, for instance, bind DNA less effectively in the phosphorylated form, and thus in some way 'free' DNA to enable replication and transcription to take place. Glycogen phosphorylase and triglyceride lipase are more active in the phosphorylated form, whereas glycogen synthetase is less active.

Thus, **activation of enzyme adenyl cyclase can lead to DNA replication and transcription,** to glycogen and triglycerides breakdown, and to inhibition of glycogen synthesis as well. Exactly how c-AMP that is produced near the plasma membrane reaches the nucleus to affect histone phosphorylation is not clear. There is possibility of a second type of adenyl cyclase situated at the nuclear membrane, which actually controls nuclear events. How protein hormones that do not enter cells stimulate DNA replication and transcription is also not well understood.

It has further been studied that cells possess other c-AMP-sensitive proteins, but then the cells respond to hormones in more than one way. ACTH, for example, stimulates gene activity and protein synthesis in adrenal cortex cells as well as steroidogenesis (it's a trophic hormone), and glucagon stimulates gluconeogenesis as well as glycogen breakdown in liver. In short, hormones do not stimulate one or the other metabolic event inside a cell. *Hormones* stimulate cells, the response depends upon the cell type. An endocrine cell, such as an adrenal cortex, thyroid, or gonad cell, which is programmed to grow and divide as well as to synthesize specific hormones, will respond by increasing all these activities. Side by side, a non - endocrine cell, such as a liver cell, will respond by mobilizing the pathways leading to increased glucose output namely glycogen degradation, gluconeogenesis, conversion of glucose-6-phosphate to glucose, inhibition of glycogen synthesis, and so forth.

Insulin is the main hormone responsible for a decrease of c-AMP, but how does it happen, is not yet clear; it is not by the inhibition of adenyl cyclase, as the insulin receptor does not interact with adenyl cyclase.

The effect of hormones such as adrenaline in causing an increase in intracellular c-AMP may not be as direct as one hopes. The increase may be caused by factors other than the activity of adenyl cyclase e.g., Ca^{2+}. There is ample evidence that adrenaline and other hormones stimulate cells through an increased uptake of Ca^{2+}.

Calcium Entry

The mechanism by which Ca^{2+} enters cells is not clear as yet. As the cytoplasmic concentration of Ca^{2+} is several times lower than the plasma concentration of Ca^{2+}, it is likely that the entry is positive but whether this entry is caused by opening of a Ca^{2+} 'channel', or by inhibition of the normal Ca^{2+}- exit mechanism, is not clear.

Many metabolic processes are modulated by Ca^{2+} ions e.g., degradation of glycogen. Other enzymes, such as the phosphodiesterase that degrades c-AMP to AMP, are inhibited by Ca^{2+}. Several hormones that were originally thought to act entirely by stimulating adenyl cyclase have now been shown to stimulate the *entry* of Ca^{2+} into cells. Exactly, how much of the hormonal effect is due to Ca^{2+} entry and how much due to the activation of adenyl cyclase is not clear at present.

Other mechanisms

There is a third type of mechanism, which is not yet very clear, by which interaction between hormone and the receptor at the cell surface leads to an intracellular change. This change is brought about by a stimulation of **nutrient uptake**. One hormone that acts in this manner is insulin. Muscle and fat cells are relatively impermeable to glucose and amino acids, entry of which is facilitated by diffusion, that is to say, that the specific transport proteins catalyze the entry process. The activity of the proteins is stimulated by the binding of insulin to a cell surface receptor.

Interaction with a receptor inside the cells i.e. Intracellular receptor

The theory of hormonal action at the cell surface proves to be quite satisfactory for the mechanism of action of most of the polypeptide, amino acid-derived and fatty acid-derived hormones. On the other hand steroid hormones, which readily cross the plasma membrane, act within the cells, the mechanism of entry is as follows:

The specificity of steroid hormone action is achieved through the presence of specific receptor proteins in the cytoplasm of target cells. Because there is little barrier to their permeability, steroid hormones enter all cells. In the absence of an intracellular receptor, however, the equilibrium between intracellular and extracellular hormone lies in favour of extracellular hormone (where it is bound by plasma globulins). In target cells, on the other hand, the equilibrium lies in favour of intracellular binding to the receptor proteins. These receptors readily pass into the nucleus. During passage, the size of the receptor gets altered which is evident from the fact that initially its sedimentation coefficient is approximately 9 S whereas in the nucleus it is approximately 4 S. When *steroid hormones* enter the nucleus, they become rather tightly bound to the chromatin; binding is most likely to the acidic proteins of chromatin. The receptor protein returns to the cytoplasm. Therefore, if a radioactive steroid hormone, such as oestradiol, is injected into the blood stream, the net result is that the radioactivity becomes concentrated in the nucleus of target cells.

Hormones of the anterior pituitary gland

Anterior lobe of pituitary gland is also known as adenohypophysis which secretes a number of hormones for vital importance and all are low molecular weight proteins. Secretion of most of the hormones of the anterior pituitary is under the control of the hypothalamus. Adenohypophyseal secretion is also controlled by the rate of secretion of endocrine gland through negative feed back mechanism (Fig. 16.1).

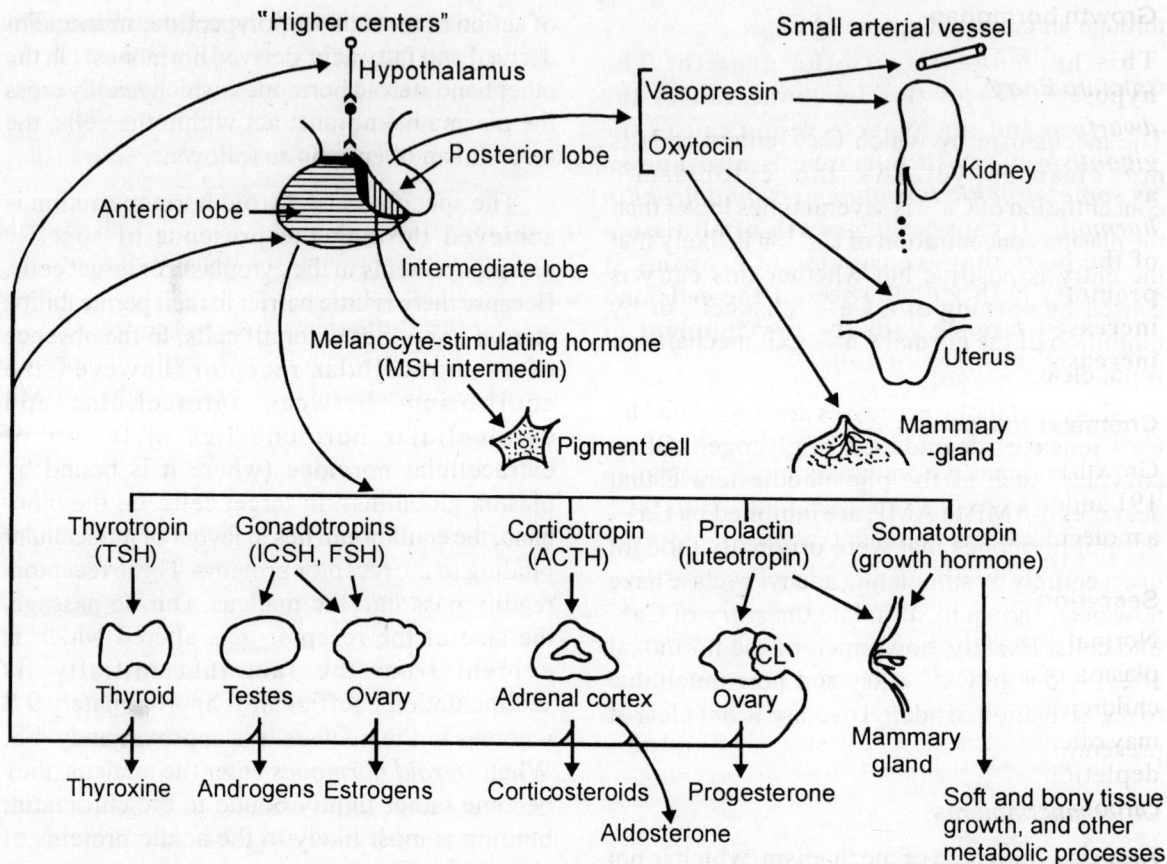

Fig. 16.1 : Scheme illustrating the relationships among the anterior and posterior pituitary glands and their target structures.

Anterior pituitary hormones

Hormones	Structure	Approx. M. Wt.	No. of Amino Acids
1. GH	Single chain polypeptide	21,500	191
2. Prolactin	Single chain polypeptide		
3. TSH (Thyroid stimulating hormone)	Double chain glycoprotein	28,000	209
4. FSH (follicle stimulating hormone)	Double chain glycoprotein	28,000	-
5. ACTH	Single chain polypeptide	4,500	39
6. LH	Double chain glycoprotein	28,000	-
7. MSH	α-Single chain	1,820	13
	β-(Polypeptide)	2,730	22

Growth hormones

This hormone affects the growth. The hyposecretion of this hormone causes the *dwarfism* and the hypersecretion causes the *gigantism*. Growth hormone is also known as *somatotrophic hormone* or *somatotrophin hormone*. It causes the growth of all tissues of the body that are capable of growing. It promotes both, i.e., the size of the cells and increased mitosis with the development of increased number of cells.

Chemical nature

Growth hormone is a protein-molecule containing 191 amino acids in a single chain and possesses a molecular weight of about 22,005.

Secretion

Normal concentration of growth hormone in plasma of an adult is about 3 mμg/ml and in children about 5 mμg/ml. However, these values may often increase to as high as 50 mμg/ml after depletion of the body stores of proteins or carbohydrates.

Biochemical functions of growth hormone

1. Growth hormone does not affect directly the cartilages and the bones. However, growth hormone indirectly stimulates their growth with the help of several small proteins, collectively known as *somatomedin* which is mainly synthesized in liver and perhaps in the muscles, kidneys and placenta as well.

   Somatomedin acts directly on cartilages and bones to promote their growth.

   Somatomedin is required for the deposition of chondroitin sulphates and collagen, both of which are necessary for the growth of cartilages and bones.

2. GH increases protein synthesis of all cells of the body by increasing the amino acids transport through the cell membrane. This increases the concentration of amino acids in the cells (this control of amino acids transport is similar to the effect of insulin in controlling glucose transport through the membrane) .

3. GH increases the formation of RNA. GH also stimulates the transcription process in the nucleus for a longer time, causing the formation of increased quantity of RNA. This in turn promotes the protein synthesis and thus, promotes the growth. Sufficient amino acids, energy, vitamins and other necessary factors for growth are, thus, available.

4. GH is also responsible to increase fat utilization for energy purposes. It increases the fatty acids concentration in body fluids by releasing them from adipose tissue. In addition, in tissues it enhances the conversion of fatty acids to acetyl CoA with subsequent utilization. Thus, under the influence of GH, fat is utilized for energy in preference to both the carbohydrates and the proteins.

5. GH has got a tendency to convert more glucose into glycogen which is stored in the tissues for emergency period.

6. GH reduces the uptake of glucose by the cells and thus increases blood glucose concentration.

7. GH fails to cause growth in an animal lacking pancreas and it also fails to cause growth if the carbohydrates are excluded from the diet.

Thyroid stimulating hormone : TSH

Chemical nature

TSH is a glycoprotein secreted by basophilic staining cells of the anterior-pituitary (Fig. 16.2). It has a molecular weight of about 30,000.

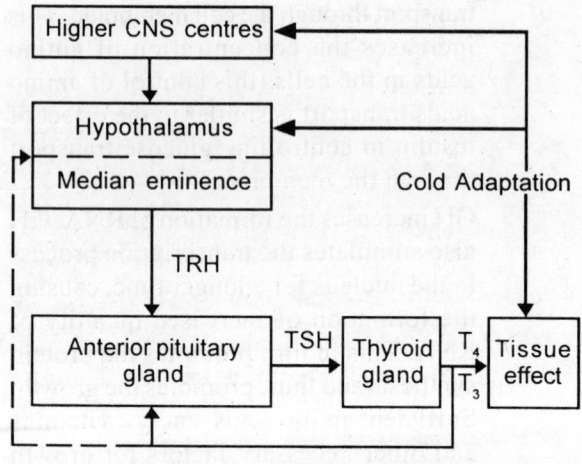

Fig. 16.2 : Scheme showing major regulatory influences on thyroid glands i.e., CNS, TRH & TSH

Actions.

(i) TSH stimulates the secretion of thyroxine and other iodothyronines.

(ii) TSH increases oxygen utilization, glucose uptake and oxidation processes. Nicotinamide adenine dinucleotide phosphate levels also rise in association with stimulus to glucose oxidation.

(iii) TSH stimulates adenyl cyclase activity in isolated thyroid cell membrane and also increases the tissue levels of c-AMP.

ADRENOCORTICOTROPIC HORMONE (ACTH)

Chemical nature

This hormone is also known as Corneotropin. The hormone ACTH is a polypeptide consisting of 39 amino acids. It is secreted from the anterior pituitary gland under the control of the corticotrophin releasing hormone of the hypothalamus (Fig 16.3).

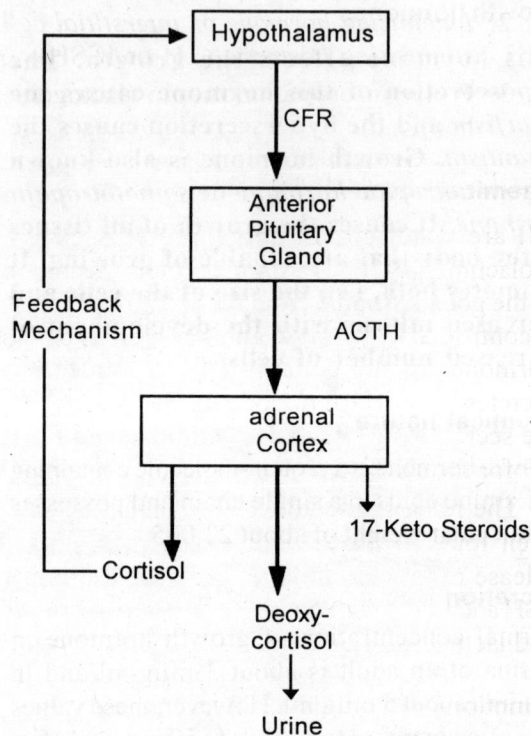

Fig 16.3 : A diagram of the normal hypothalamic pituitary adrenal axis showing regulation of adrenal cortex.

Actions

(i) It stimulates the synthesis of cortisol and 17-ketosteroids by the adrenal cortex. It has little or no effect on aldosterone secretion.

(ii) ACTH is also necessary to maintain adrenocortical size, structure, and vascularity.

(iii) The action of ACTH is mediated by c-AMP.

(iv) ACTH promotes insulin secretion from β– cells of pancreas.

Gonadotrophic hormones

Anterior pituitary secretes three gonadotrophic hormones.

1. Follicle stimulating hormone, i.e. FSH - (follicle stimulator thylokentin)

2. *Luteinizing hormone or interstitial cell stimulating hormone* (LH or ICSH).

3. Prolactin or mammotropin (lactogenic hormone).

Chemical nature

All are water soluble glycoproteins except prolactin. Prolactin is a simple protein. Secretion of the gonadotrophin from the anterior pituitary is controlled by hypothalamus as well as by the hormones of the gonads. The hypothalamus secretes luteinizing hormone releasing factor for the secretion of luteinizing hormone and FSH-RF for the FSH hormone.

The releasing factor for FSH and LH have been found to exert inhibitory effects on the release of prolactin, therefore, decrease in the FSH and LH tends to increase prolactin secretion and lactogenesis as well.

Functions of Gonadotrophins

(A) Luteinizing hormone

Both LH and FSH are required for the spermatogenesis. It is currently held that all the effects of LH are mediated by way of testosterone. Testosterone and FSH are hormones which act directly on the seminiferous tubular epithelium. In the immature animal, initiation of spermatogenesis requires both testosterone (or LH) and FSH.

(B) Follicle stimulating hormone : FSH

The early work of Smithzohndek and Aschhiem indicated that the sex functions are controlled by the secretion of pituitary gland. **FSH was shown to cause spermatogenic activity in testes.**

Purified preparations of FSH have been made but the actual structure of this hormone is still not known.

— In mammals FSH stimulates the maturation and growth of ovarian follicles. Cyclic

AMP formation in target tissues is also found to be increased.

— In males it causes the growth of testes and induces spermatogenesis. **Girls have significantly higher FSH in comparison to the boys at the age of 5,10, and 12 years.**

(C) Prolactin and testicular functions

In females prolactin hormone stimulates milk production and is required for establishing a functional corpus luteum in some species. It was only with the knowledge of specific radioimmunoassays that it was realized that prolactin circulated in the plasma of males was observed to be somewhat on lower side than their counterparts, i.e., females. *Plasma level of prolactin in males increases with puberty and decreases following castration and can be restored by treatment with gonadal steroids.*

Hyperprolactinemia : Considerable number of studies suggest that prolactin synergizes with LH and testosterone to increase the reproductive functions in males. The prolactin producing tumors result in testicular involution and decreased testosterone levels. All men with small prolactin producing pituitary tumors are impotent regardless of their plasma testosterone levels.

In addition, sexual function is restored by lowering prolactin level with *Bromergocryptine* or by surgical removal of the pituitary tumor. The later observation suggests that prolactin can produce impotence independent of its action on testosterone secretion. **Although the mechanism by which prolactin influences sexual desire is not known.**

Hormones of the middle lobe of the pituitary gland

Middle lobe of pituitary secretes MSH (melanocyte stimulating hormone). This is also known as *intermedin*.

Chemical nature

Two forms of MSH have been reported, i.e. α-MSH and β-MSH (Fig 16.4):

α-MSH is a single chain having a molecular weight of about 1,820 and contains 13 amino acids.

β-MSH is a polypeptide having 22 amino acids and a molecular weight of about 2,730. Its structure is as shown below. MSH secretion is inhibited by corticosteroids and its activity is inhibited by catecholamines.

Actions

1. Both α- and β-MSH increase melanin biosynthesis by stimulating melanocytes present in dermis and epidermis of the skin.

2. MSH promotes the dispersion of the melanin pigment in entire cells making them dark in appearance.

3. 30-60 mg cortisone is given orally to prevent excess deposition of melanin in the skin.

4. Importance of MSH in man has not been fully evaluated but increase in its production accounts for the increase in pigmentation as seen in Addison's disease, some cases of thyrotoxicosis and pregnancy as well.

1. α-MSH

(pig, beef, horse)

CH₃CO - Ser - Tyr - Ser - Met - Glu - His - Phe - Arg - Trp - Gly - Lys - Pro - Val - NH₂
1   2   3   4   5   6   7   8   9   10   11   12   13

2. β-MSH

Ala - Glu - Lys - Lys - Asp - Glu - Gly - Pro - Tyr - Arg - Met - Glu - His - Phe -
1   2   3   4   5   6   7   8   9   10   11   12   13   14

Arg - Trp - Gly - Ser - Pro - Pro - Lys - Asp.
15   16   17   18   19   20   21   22

Fig. 16.4: Structures of α-MSH and β-MSH

NEUROHYPOPHYSIS (HORMONES OF THE POSTERIOR LOBE OF PITUITARY)

(Please refer to Figure 16.1)

Posterior lobe of pituitary gland secretes following two important hormones:

(a) Vasopressin (Pitressin, Antidiuretic hormone i.e., ADH) and

(b) Oxytocin (Pitocin)

Vasopressin (Antidiuretic hormone i.e. ADH)

Chemical nature

This hormone is a cyclic octapeptide (nonapeptide if cystine is considered as *two* cysteines). The sequence of amino acids in different preparations of vasopressin has been found to be the same except one amino acid. Vasopressin isolated from most of the mammals, i.e. human, beef, sheep etc., possesses arginine amino acid (hence, called arginine vasopressin) whereas vasopressin isolated from pigs contains amino acid lysine in place of arginine, hence, called as lysine vasopressin. Chemical structures are as given below:

Regulation

Volume receptors (**"stretch receptors"**) are believed to be involved in the regulation of its secretion.

Physiological and biochemical functions

(i) Principal physiological action of ADH is

```
      S ────────────────────────── S
      |                            |
  H – Cys – Tyr – Phe – Glu (NH₂) – Asp – (NH₂) – Cys – Pro – Arg – Gly – NH₂
      1     2     3      4          5            6     7     8     9
```

$$H - Cys - Tyr - Phe - Glu(NH_2) - Asp - (NH_2) - Cys - Pro - Arg - Gly - NH_2$$

Arginine Vasopressin (most mammals)

```
      S ────────────────────────── S
      |                            |
  H – Cys – Tyr – Phe – Glu (NH₂) – Asp – (NH₂) – Cys – Pro – Lys – Gly – NH₂
      1     2     3      4          5            6     7     8     9
```

Lysine Vasopressin (pigs)

the regulation of water balance by promoting reabsorption of water in the cells of the distal tubules. **Failure of hypothalamus to produce enough ADH or prevention of release by damage of the nerve tracts causes an important disorder known as 'diabetes insipidus', in which volume of urine increases to as much as 20 litres per day. Therefore, in this disorder, the specific gravity of urine, decreases to very low (1.001). Normal secretion and the release of ADH are regulated by the osmoreceptors in the diencephalon of the brain.**

(ii) The specific biochemical action of ADH is probably by the stimulation of the synthesis of cyclic 3', 5'- AMP, which promotes reabsorption of water through the membranes of epithelial cells constituting the distal tubules.

(iii) Its powerful action is in raising blood pressure.

Oxytocin (Pitocin)

Chemical nature

Oxytocin is also a octapeptide - (nonapeptide if cystine is considered as two cysteines). Its secretion from the posterior hypophysis is under the control of hypothalamus. The structure of oxytocin is as shown on the next page.

Physiological and biochemical functions

(i) **This hormone is a powerful stimulant of uterine contraction. The pregnant uterus is more susceptible to it than the virgin uterus; this effect is utilized in obstetrics to stimulate inert uterus, and to provoke quick delivery as well as to stop uterine bleeding. Due to this very property, its name has been derived (Greek word, oxytocin = rapid birth).**

(ii) **Oxytocin appears to be the natural (physiological) initiator of labour.** It has been observed that even the minute dose of it induces the labour.

(iii) **It also facilitates upward movement of spermatozoa in the vagina and the fallopian tubes, even non-motile sperms ascend the female genital tract.**

(iv) It also stimulates the contraction of the myoepithelial tissue around the ducts of the lactating mammary gland, thereby, stimulates the ejection of milk **(milk "let-down" action).**

$$S \text{———————} S$$
$$| \qquad\qquad\qquad\qquad\qquad |$$

H – Cys – Tyr – Phe – Glu (NH$_2$) – Asp – (NH$_2$) – Cys – Pro – Leu – Gly – NH$_2$
   1   2   3   4   5   6   7   8   9

Oxytocin (mammals, birds)

THYROID HORMONES

Iodine has long been known to be associated with thyroid gland. Bauman in 1895 observed that iodine was 10 times more abundant in thyroid gland than any other tissue and that it was in organic combinations.

Kendall succeeded in isolating the substance in a state of purity. The constitution of the hormone was established by Harington in 1926 and confirmed by synthesis in 1927 by Harington and Berger. Principal hormones of the thyroid gland are thyroxine and triiodothyronine.

Chemistry

Natural form is L-thyroxine which is twice as active as D-thyroxine. Thyroxine is an iodo-derivative of hydroxyphenyl tyrosine. A part of iodine present in thyroid gland remains present as diiodotyrosine.

If a solution of di-iodotyrosine is kept at pH 8.8 at 70°C for several days, thyroxine is formed. **Human thyroid gland weighs about 20-25 g and contains about 25mg thyroxine and 40mg diiodothyronine.** The triiodothyronine is also formed in the peripheral tissues by the deiodination of thyroxine. Structures of thyroxine and triiodothyronine are as given below:

Biosynthesis of Hormones

Biosynthesis of thyroid hormones involves several fairly well defined steps, the first of which is the "trapping" of iodide in the thyroid gland. Now, synthesis of L-thyroxine (3, 5, 3', 5' i.e. tetraiodothyronine) begins with the iodination of tyrosine as shown below in the schematic diagram resulting in the formation of L-monoiodotyrosine. Now, further iodination of L-monoiodotyrosine takes place forming L-diiodotyrosine, which in the presence of one molecule of L-diiodotyrosine gives rise to L-thyroxine.

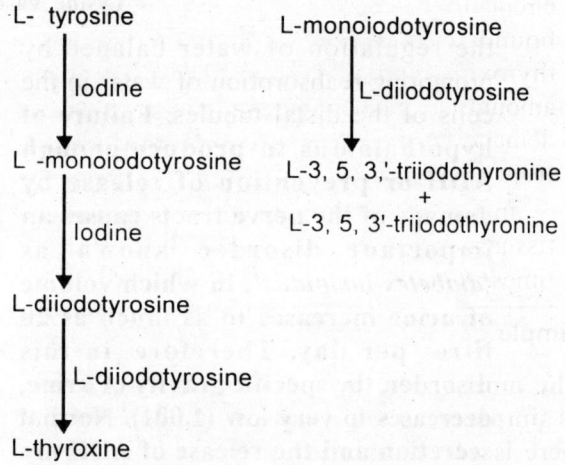

If a molecule of monoiodotyrosine condenses with a molecule of diiodotyrosine, then, two molecules of triiodothyronine are formed as shown above.

Thyroxine synthesized in the chemical laboratory has the same physiological properties as that obtained from thyroid gland. **Thyroxine remains present in the thyroid gland in a protein called thyroglobulin, which is the principal "colloid" of the gland.**

Iodine metabolism

Iodine is a raw material essential for the synthesis of thyroid hormones. Ingested iodine is converted into iodide and is absorbed.

HO—⬡—O—⬡—CH$_2$-CH(NH$_2$)-COOH

Thyroxine (T$_4$)

HO—⬡—O—⬡—CH$_2$-CH(NH$_2$)-COOH

3, 5, 3'-Triiodothyronine (T$_3$)

Thyroglobulin is the storage form in the follicles and the principal form in the circulating blood is thyroxine or a derivative bound to an *alpha-globulin* known as thyroxine-binding protein (TBP). Small amounts are also bound to albumin. As the demand for the hormone arises, it is freed from the protein carriers.

In addition to thyroxine, the blood and tissues also contain T$_3$, which is 4 to 10 times as potent as T$_4$.

Simple goiter (goitre)

The most common type of goiter is known as simple or endemic goiter. In this condition there is an enlargement of the thyroid gland, which is very clear by a swelling in the neck (Fig. 16.5). In simple goiter, the basal metabolic rate (BMR) is normal or below normal. **Simple**

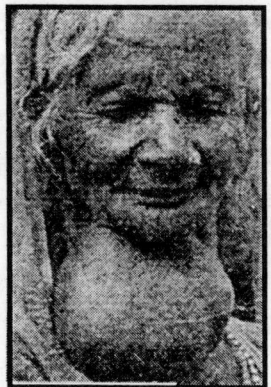

Figures 16.5 : Sufferers of 'goitre'

- **Control of iodine deficiency disorders i.e., I.D.D. is one of the National Health Programme,** planned and implemented with a view to ensure that real benefits reach the people at large in the community through community measures aimed at prevention and control of IDD.

- In India IDD is responsible for many physical and mental abnormalities with various motor disfunction problems.

- In India, it is estimated that nearly 167 million persons are prone to the risk of IDD.

- Out of the persons at the risk of IDD, 54 millions are having *Goitre,* 2.2 millions are *cretins,* and 6.6 millions have mild *neurological disorders.*

- It is estimated that every passing hour, 10 children are being born in this country who will not attain their optimum mental and physical potential due to neonatal hypothyroidism caused by iodine deficiency.

- With continuous depletion of *Iodine* from natural resources, the situation is expected to worsen in the coming years unless measures are taken to control the situation.

- IDD are highly prevalent in the sub-himalayan belt as well as in the plains of **Uttar Pradesh.** The deficiency presents wide spectrum of disabilities which includes *Goitre, deaf-mutism, mental retardation, retardation of physical growth* and various degrees of impairment of intellectual and motor functions. Because of the magnitude of the problem, IDD **control programme** has been given *National Priority* and has been included in the *Prime Minister's* **20 Point Programme** in our country.

- Lack of iodine in the environment has serious consequences for both human and animals.

  The wide spectrum of disorders by inadequate iodine consumption are known collectively as iodine deficiency disorders (IDD), which include:

  (i) Lowering of IQ and impaired learning.

  (ii) Energy loss.

  (iii) Reproductive losses e.g. increased miscarriages, increased still births.

  (iv) Cretinism
    - Mental retardation,
    - Deaf-mutism, squint,
    - Dysplegia (spastic paralysis of the lower limbs),
    - Dwarfism, coordination abnormalities.

  (v) Goitre - the most visible manifestation but it is less dangerous than the above mentioned losses.

  (vi) Reduced milk, egg, meat and wool *yields* in animals.

  (vii) Reproduction failure in animals.

- Deficiency of iodine in pregnant women can cause irreversible brain damage in the unborn baby.

- The world's single most significant cause of preventable brain damage and mental retardation is deficiency of iodine.

- Current research indicates that iodine deficiency results in lowering the average intelligence of entire school age population by as much as 10 to 15 I.Q. points.

- The number of primary school age children in endemic areas is estimated to be 40 millions. The total I.Q. points lost in these children amount to be 400 millions.

- No state in India is free trom IDD. In India, out of the 216 districts surveyed (in 29 states and union territories), 186 districts have goitre prevalence rate ranging trom 10% to over 65%.

- With every passing hour, 10 children are being born in India who will not attain their optimum physical and mental potential due to iodine deficiency.

goiter is a condition of hypofunction rather than hyperfunction of the thyroid gland. In fact, the enlargement of the thyroid may be looked upon as a compensatory attempt to produce the required amount of thyroid hormones. The increase in the size of the gland results from an increase in the amount of colloid present; therefore, this type of goiter is sometimes called as **"colloid goiter"**. The administration of iodine in the form of iodides is beneficial and the right choice of treatment but it should be carried out in consultation with some physician. **Simple goiter may be treated as the first stage of exophthalmic goiter.**

Prevention

- Preventing iodine deficiency raises the learning capacity of school children and improves   school performance.

- IDD is preventable.

- Daily consumption of iodised salt prevents the spectrum of disorders caused due to the deficiency of iodine.

- Consumption of iodised salt is safe.

- Iodisation of salt is a low cost, highly effective mean of preventing iodine deficiency.

- The cost of iodising salt is only about 30 paise per person per year.

■ Within just 12 months of iodised salt becoming available and used in a community, no more *cretins* will be born, **no more babies will suffer from retarded mental and physical development** attributed to iodine deficiency.

Deficiency of iodine in diet sometimes occurs in the areas where the water supply and the soil are poor in iodine and produces a condition known as *simple* or *endemic goiter* or *colloid goiter*. In this type of goiter, there is enlargement of thyroid gland, the obvious sign of which is swelling in neck. This condition is relieved by ensuring adequate supply of *inorganic iodides* in the diet.

Goitrogenic foods (in raw state harmful otherwise not)

1. **Cauliflower,**
2. **Broccoli (a variety of cauliflower with greenish flower head)** and
3. **Cabbage, etc.**

Iodine is essential not only for the human beings but also for the animals.

Hypothyroidism

It is a state in which there is not sufficient development of thyroid gland, in the embryonic life, the child becomes a *dwarf* or *cretin*. A *cretin* grows slowly (stunted growth) and has a low mentality and low I.Q. ; his hair is scanty and coarse, and his skin is thick and dry. His BMR is also low. If such a child is given thyroid extract or thyroxine, he or she does not remain a *cretin* but develops normally. This treatment, however, must be continued indefinitely in consultation with a physician in order to prevent the child from developing into a *cretin*.

If the gland is removed or if it becomes subnormal in activity in an adult, myxoedema develops (Fig. 16.6) in which the skin becomes thick and dry, the hair coarsen and fall out, and there is a disinclination towards work, either physically or mentally. There becomes a tendency to *put on weight*. The metabolic rate is reduced, nitrogen metabolism gets lowered, and the body's temperature is subnormal. Further, ossification of the bones is delayed; density of the carpals in the wrist is often used as a criterion of thyroid activity or physiological age in a prepubertal child. Stimulation of ossification by T_4 and T_3 may be offset by thyrocalcitonin, which has a tendency to decrease blood Ca^{++} level.

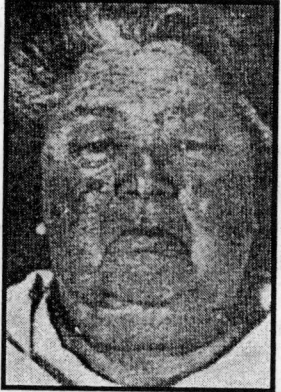

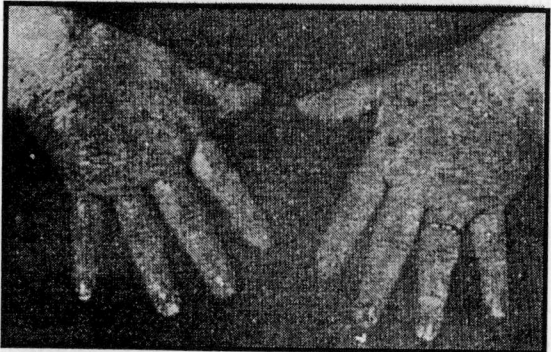

Fig. 16.6 : Photographs of the face and hands of a woman, aged 70, suffering from myxoedema. Note the dull expression, scanty eyebrows and dilated vessels on the cheeks. The face and hands are puffy and the skin of the hands is dry and wrinkled.

IODINE-CONTENT OF COMMONLY CONSUMED FOODS

Iodine is an important trace element, the deficiency of which in food and water leads to iodine deficiency disorders including goiter.

Green leafy vegetables have relatively higher concentration of iodine if compared to fruits, spices and beverages. Fruits like apple and sweet lime have almost negligible amount of iodine.

Among pulses like lentil, bengal gram, green gram (Moong), red gram (Arhar), black gram (Urad) and horse gram (Chana), **the iodine content in horse gram is the highest** (58 μg/kg) and that of red gram is the lowest (30 μg/kg).

Hyperthyroidism

It is a state in which thyroid gland is too active, as a result of which a condition known as **exophthalmic goiter occurs.** A common symptom of this disease is the bulging of the eyes; hence the name. The disease is also known as **'Graves'** or **'Basedow's disease.** The symptoms of exophthalmic goiter are just the opposite of myxoedema which mean that the basal metabolic rate (BMR) is high instead of low, nitrogen metabolism is increased instead of low, the hair is fine instead of coarse, the body temperature is above instead of below normal. The patient is nervous and irritable instead of sluggish; his mentality is above rather than below normal and he or she is underweight. His/her heart beat is generally fast and irregular.

Usually, but not always, the thyroid gland is enlarged in exophthalmic goiter. **Such a condition**

Normally, **PBI content** is found to be in the range of 4 to 8 μg/100ml of blood; however, **in myxoedema** it is found to be in the range of 0.2 to 2.5 μg/100ml of blood.

$$
\begin{array}{cc}
NH_2 & NH-C=O \\
| & | \quad\quad | \\
C=S & S=C \quad CH \\
| & | \quad\quad ||| \\
NH_2 & HN-CH \\
\text{Thiourea} & \text{Thiouracil}
\end{array}
$$

can be easily treated by removing part of the thyroid gland; the improvement produced in the patient by this method is wonderful. Radioactive I^{131} sometimes is efficacious in decreasing the secretion of the thyroid gland.

Hyperparathyroidism may also be treated by the use of drugs such as thiourea, thiouracil, propylthiouracil, and the sulfa drugs. These are thought to act by inhibiting either the uptake of iodine by the thyroid gland or the formation of thyroxine from diiodotyrosine.

In **'Graves' disease,** there is hyperfunction of the gland and increased BMR is seen. In this disease; PBI content is found in the range of 8-18 μg/100ml of blood which is a good index of hyperthyroidism.

HORMONES OF THE ADRENAL CORTEX

Adrenal cortex, in fact, **synthesizes dozens of different types of steroid molecules,** but only a few of them have got biological activity. For convenience, they have been classified into three categories. viz:

(i) Glucocorticoids,

(ii) Mineralocorticoids and

(iii) Androgens (sex hormones)

These hormones initiate their actions by combining with specific intracellular receptors, and this complex binds to specific regions of DNA to regulate gene expression.

Biomedical Importance

1. The hormones of the adrenal cortex, particularly the glucocorticoids, give the body capacity to adjust to stress, such as

In the human the *adrenal,* or *suprarenal* glands are a pair of flattened, triangular bodies located adjacent to the superior pole of each kidney. They measure approximately 5 x 3 x 1 cm and have a combined weight of about 10 to 15 g. Each gland is enclosed in a thick, connective tissue capsule.

The glands are composed of two distinct parts, a central one which is known as *medulla* and an outer *cortex.* In the adult, medulla represents about 10 percent of the total weight of the adrenal gland.

Most of the parenchymal cells of the adrenal cortex are under partial control of the adenohypophysis and function in regulating metabolism and maintaining normal electrolyte balance.

prolonged exposure to cold or shock.

2. **Mineralocorticoids are required for normal Na$^+$ and K$^+$ balance.**

3. Synthetic analogs of both classes i.e., glucocorticoids and mineralocorticoids are used therapeutically. Many glucocorticoid analogs are potent anti-inflammatory agents.

4. Excessive or deficient plasma levels of any of the above mentioned three classes of the hormones, whether due to disease or therapeutic use, result in severe complications leading even to death.

5. Increase blood glucose level and liver glycogen content as well, chiefly by stimulating gluconeogenesis but also by decreasing sensitivity to insulin. Synthesis of necessary enzymes gets induced.

6. Decrease synthesis of acid-sulfated mucopolysaccharides in bone and connective tissues.

7. Increase release of fatty acids from adipose tissue, and side by side, decrease

In young animals, deprivation of cortical hormones delays growth and maturation.

The most potent and physiologically important glucocorticoid is hydrocortisone, 17- hydroxycorticosterone or cortisol (also known as compound 'F' because, it was the sixth compound to be isolated by Kendall as pure crystals from cortical extracts).

Glucocorticoids such as cortisone and cortisol have an anti-inflammatory action, possibly by inhibiting proliferation of fibrous, connective tissue by fibroblasts.

Cortisone has proved of value in many diseases other than rheumatoid arthritis and rheumatic fever. Among these may be mentioned as asthma, hay fever, inflammatory eye diseases and Addison's disease, etc.

synthesis of fat from glucose.

8. They accelerate the rate of catabolism, in general.

9. They inhibit the anabolism of proteins.

Zones of the Adrenal Cortex:

The adult cortex has 3 distinct zones/layers as mentioned (Fig 16.7):

   (i) Zona glomerulosa (responsible for the production of mineralocorticoids).

   (ii) Zona fasciculata ⎤ responsible for the
   (iii) Zona reticularis ⎦ production of glucocorticoids and androgens

Biosynthesis of Adrenal Corticosteroids

The adrenal cortex synthesizes three classes of hormones as described above i.e., **glucocorticoid, mineralocorticoid and sex hormones.** Although, **nearly 50 hormones are synthesized from the adrenal cortex,** out of which only a small number are secreted in

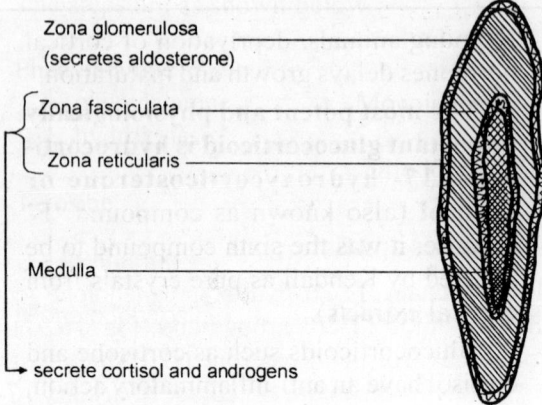

Zona glomerulosa
(secretes aldosterone)

Zona fasciculata

Zona reticularis

Medulla

secrete cortisol and androgens

Fig 16.7 : Secretion of adrenocortical hormones by different zones of the adrenal cortex.

significant amounts and out of these secreted, only few possess significant hormonal activity. The most important steroids secreted by the normal adult human adrenal cortex are: (Fig. 16.8).

(a) the glucocorticoid, named as cortisol, and

Parenchymal cells of the adrenal cortex secrete a variety of hormones collectively referred to as corticosteroids. Functions of the adrenal cortex are essential for life in contrast to the adrenal medulla which are not so essential. Although, numerous steroids have been extracted from the adrenal, only a few are normally secreted, by the gland. The parenchymal cells of the **zona glomerulosa** secrete a class of steroid hormones known as **mineralocorticoids,** the function of which is in the maintenance of normal electrolyte balance. **Aldosterone** is the most potent mineralocorticoid and accounts for approximately 95% of the activity of this class.

The parenchymal cells of **zona fasciculata,** and to a lesser extent those of *zona* reticularis, secrete a class of steroid hormones known as

---

glucocorticoids, which influence carbohydrate metabolism the most. *Hydrocortisone,* or *cortisol* is the most important member of this class and accounts for most of the glucocorticoid activity.

The secretory activity of the cortical parenchymal cells of the inner two layers (Zona fasciculata and Zona reticularis) is regulated by the adenohypophysis through the secretion of adrenocorticotrophic hormone (ACTH). ACTH stimulates secretion and release of corticosteroids, promotes growth of the adrenal cortex, and also increases blood flow through the adrenal gland. The release of ACTH is regulated by a feedback system which involves the adenohypophysis, the hypothalamus, and higher brain centres. The hypothalamus produces corticotropin-releasing factor (CRF) which stimulates cells in the adenohypophysis to release ACTH. The circulating levels of corticosteroids influence the release of both CRF and ACTH. High plasma levels of corticosteroids inhibit CRF and ACTH release; whereas *low levels* of *it trigger the* hypothalamus to release CRF which causes the adenohypophysis to release ACTH. Target cells within the adrenal cortex respond to ACTH and release additional corticosteroids.

Aldosterone secretion by the cells of the *zona glomerulosa* is regulated by the renin-angiotensin system and the plasma levels of sodium and the potassium. ACTH has little or no direct effect on the secretion of aldosterone. The renin-angiotensin system is believed to be the major controlling system involved in the release of aldosterone.

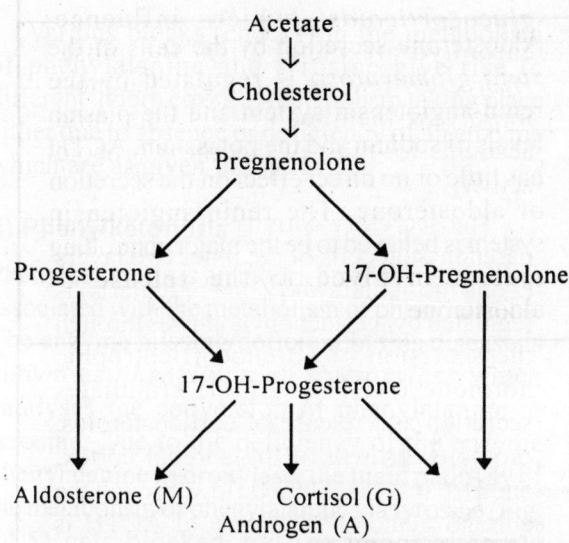

Acetate
↓
Cholesterol
↓
Pregnenolone

Progesterone   17-OH-Pregnenolone

17-OH-Progesterone

Aldosterone (M)   Cortisol (G)
Androgen (A)

Fig. 16.8: Major steps in the synthesis of the three principal steroids where M denotes mineralocorticoid effect; G for glucocorticoid effect, and A for androgenic effect.

(b) the mineralocorticoid, named as aldosterone.In addition, small quantities of estrogens and steroid precursors, including progesterone are released into the circulation. Adrenal androgens, although secreted in large amount, are of less physiological significance.

Mineralocorticoid (Aldosterone)

Since 17 α-hydroxylase remains absent in the zona glomerulosa, progesterone is converted on the smooth endoplasmic reticulum of the glomerulosa first to 11-deoxycorticosterone (DOC) by 21-hydroxylation (Fig. 16.9) and then by 11 β-hydroxylation, within the mitochondrion, to corticosterone, "substance B". Then the mitochondrial enzyme, 18-hydroxylase, catalyzes its conversion to 18-hydroxycorticosterone, which in turn, is later on dehydrogenated to form aldosterone in the presence of an enzyme which is found only in the mitochondria of the zona glomerulosa. It is secreted at a rate of 50 to 200μg per day.

Androgens and Estrogens

The side chain of 17 α-hydroxypregnenolone gets cleaved at the 17-20 carbon bond (Fig. 16.9) to form dehydroisoandrosterone (D) which, with its sulfate, is the major precursor of urinary 17-ketosteroids. Minor quantities of 17-hydroxyprogesterone are converted by a similar reaction to another 17-ketosteroid, Δ^4-androstenedione, which can be further converted to *testosterone* by the reduction of the 17-ketone. Estrogens apparently can be synthesized by adrenal tissue, as evidenced by estradiol and estrone production *in vitro* by feminizing adrenal tumor tissue. The amounts normally produced, if any, are very small, however, and the biosynthetic pathways are not very clear. It is likelihood, they may involve 19-oxidation of testosterone, followed by 19-demethylation and aromatization of the A ring to yield estradiol-17 β. A similar series of reactions might produce *estrone* from Δ^4-androstenedione.

The role of the foetal adrenal cortex in the production of maternal estrogen is of special interest. Be it known that the placenta can form large amount of pregnenolone and progesterone, but lacks the enzyme 17-hydroxylase which is required for further metabolism. These substances are released into the umbilical vein and are carried to the foetal adrenal cortex where progesterone is used to form DOC, corticosterone, and cortisol. The pregnenolone is sulfated, 17-hydroxylated, and converted to DHA sulfate. Now, DHA sulfate is metabolized to form 16 α-hydroxy-DHA by the foetal liver. When the blood returning from the foetus reaches the placenta, very active enzymes known as sulfatases split the ester linkages. Oxidation of

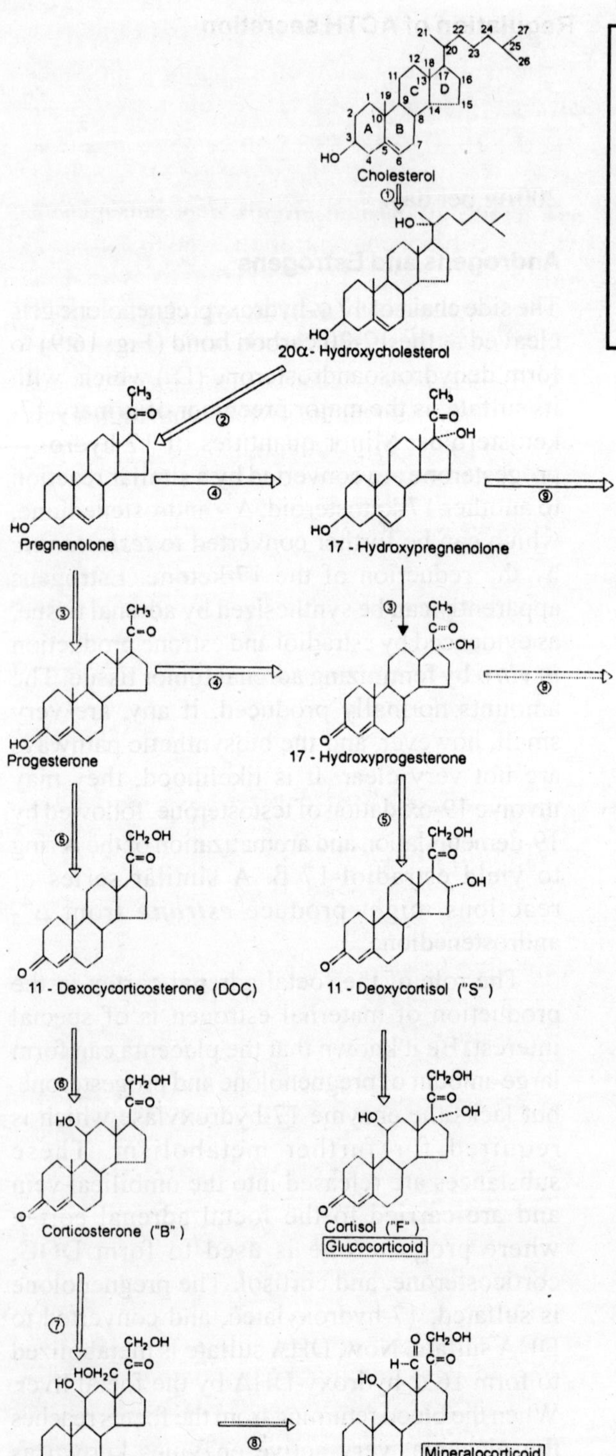

Aldosterone secretion by the cells of the *zona glomerulosa* is regulated by the renin-angiotensin system and the plasma levels of sodium and the potassium. ACTH has little or no direct effect on the secretion of aldosterone. The renin-angiotensin system is believed to be the major controlling system involved in the release of aldosterone.

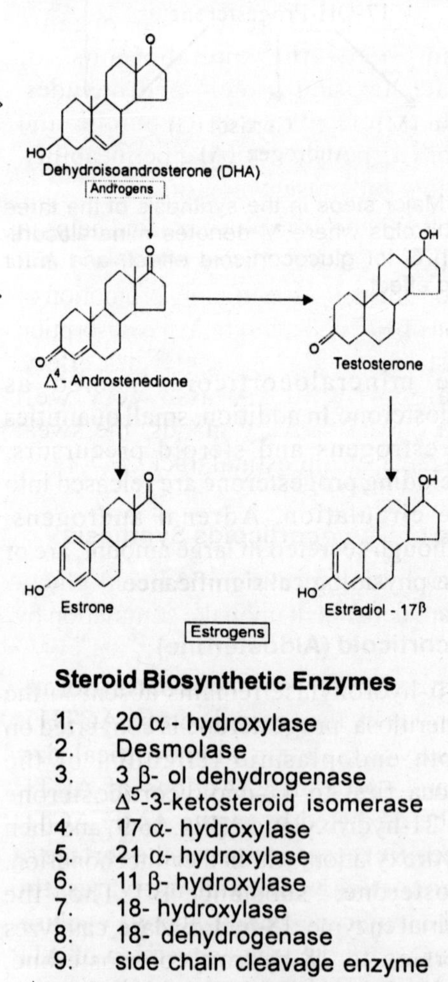

Steroid Biosynthetic Enzymes

1. 20 α - hydroxylase
2. Desmolase
3. 3 β- ol dehydrogenase
   Δ⁵-3-ketosteroid isomerase
4. 17 α- hydroxylase
5. 21 α- hydroxylase
6. 11 β- hydroxylase
7. 18- hydroxylase
8. 18- dehydrogenase
9. side chain cleavage enzyme

Fig. 16.9: A simplified scheme showing the pathways in adrenocortical steroid biosynthesis after formation of cholesterol. The probable major reactions are indicated by heavy arrows.

DHA gives rise to androstenedione and testosterone, which are rapidly converted to *estrone* and *estradiol.* The 16 α-hydroxy-DHA, which remains present in higher concentration, is also converted to *estriol.* These steps are solely responsible for the presence of large amounts of estriol in the maternal urine during the third trimester of pregnancy.

Physiological effects of adrenal corticosteroids:

The term, *glucocorticoid,* refers to the sum of a wide range of influences on organic metabolism i.e., the metabolisms of carbohydrate, fat, and protein and includes, among others, effects on the immune and inflammatory responses, vascular permeability, wound healing and muscle integrity.

On the other hand, mineralocorticoid helps in the regulation of balance between $[Na^+]$ and $[K^+]$ in blood and cells, specifically promotion of reabsorption of Na^+ and inhibition of reabsorption of K^+ by distal tubules of kidney. Besides, effects of mineralocorticoid are also very well understood on the salivary glands, the sweat glands and the gastrointestinal tract.

Regulation of Glucocorticoids Synthesis

The synthesis and secretion of adrenal gluco-corticoids are dependent upon the stimulation by ACTH.

ACTH stimulates the synthesis of cortisol and 17-ketosteroids by the adrenal cortex. ACTH is also necessary to maintain adrenocortical size, structure and vascularity. Actions of ACTH appear to be mediated by cyclic AMP. ACTH binds to specific receptor sites on the surface of the adrenocortical cell and activates the associated membrane-bound adenyl cyclase, which in turn promotes the conversion of ATP to cyclic AMP. ACTH and cyclic AMP stimula-te new protein synthesis and that this new protein is required for increased *steroidogenesis.*

Regulation of ACTH secretion

Following three factors are of major importance in the regulation of ACTH secretion:

1. Firstly, there is homeostatic negative feedback inhibition of ACTH secretion by circulating cortisol. Decreased plasma cortisol concentrations lead to increased pituitary ACTH release; whereas, increased levels of plasma cortisol inhibit ACTH secretion.

2. Secondly, plasma cortisol concentrations show a circadian rhythm, with high levels (15 to 25 µg/100 ml) in the early morning and low levels (less than 7 µg/100ml) late in the evening.

3. **Thirdly, the most important factor which governs the ACTH secretion is "stress".** Thus, plasma ACTH levels get increased during fever, laparotomy or acute severe depression, resulting into increased secretion of cortisol.

THE ADRENAL MEDULLA

The central portion of the adrenal gland, the *medulla,* is composed of endocrine parenchymal cells (called as *chromaffin cells),* connective tissue, and numerous blood vessels and nerves. Chromaffin cells of the adrenal medulla are relatively large, rounded cells.

Biosynthesis of Catecholamines

The synthesis of epinephrine which is the most important catecholamine secreted by the adrenal medulla, is outlined in Fig. 16.10.

Tyrosine, the precursor, is derived primarily from dietary sources. The first step in the biosynthetic pathway, i.e. the conversion of tyrosine to DOPA, is the rate-limiting reaction; this reaction is catalyzed by the enzyme tyrosine hydroxylase which is found only in neuroectodermal tissues.

Chromaffin cells (**named because they react with chromate salts**) of the adrenal medulla are a part of the APUD (Amine Precursor uptake and Decarboxylation) system of cells. The chromaffin reaction is thought to involve oxidation and polymerization of the catecholamines contained within the secretory granules of the cells. These cells are capable of synthesizing and secreting **catecholamines.**

Histochemical studies have demonstrated that there are two types of cells, out of which one contains **epinephrine** and the other **norepinephrine**.

The release of the catecholamines by the chromaffin cells of the adrenal medulla is initiated by the impulses conveyed in the preganglionic sympathetic fibres which end on the chromaffin cells. In response to these signals, the chromaffin cells release the catecholamines into the adjacent blood vessels.

In the next reaction, DOPA is converted to dopamine by L-aromatic amino acid decarboxylase. Now, dopamine is acted upon by the enzyme dopamine β-hydroxylase forming norepinephrine which later on by the action of enzyme phenylethanolamine-N-methyl transferase gets converted to the main substance i.e. **epinephrine.**

Storage and Release of Catecholamines

Unlike the adrenocortical steroids, which are released almost as soon as they are synthesized, **catecholamines** are stored in the adrenal medullary cells. They remain present in membrane-enclosed secretory vesicles and are complexed with adenosine triphosphate (1 mole of ATP for 4 molecules of catecholamines) and a specific protein of the molecular weight of 40,000. Besides, the vesicles also contain a Ca^{2+}

and Mg^{2+}- dependent ATPase. These subcellular vesicles take up epinephrine and norepinephrine by a transport process. The vesicle uptake mechanism is blocked potently by reserpine, an antihypertensive drug. The free catecholamine which is not taken up immediately by the vesicles is metabolized by monoamine oxidase (**MAO**) located within the mitochondria.

The hormone contained within the secretory vesicle can be released in response to an appropriate stimulus which, in the case of adrenal pheochromocyte, is acetylcholine secreted by the preganglionic nerve fibres that terminate in the medulla. Other agents include histamine and glucagon which can also stimulate the release of epinephrine.

Metabolism of Catecholamines

Norepinephrine and epinephrine are metabolized by two enzymes, primarily MAO, which remains present in the mitochondria of cells of most organs, the richer sources include liver, kidney, intestine, and stomach. MAO deaminates the α–carbon of norepinephrine, epinephrine and other catecholamines, such as serotonin and dopamine.

The other enzyme is catechol - o-methyl transferase (**COMT**) which is a soluble enzyme and is found in many tissues. This enzyme catalyzes the transfer of the methyl group from S-adenosylmethionine to the catechol 3-hydroxyl radical and also requires Mg^{2+} as a cofactor. The major metabolites of epinephrine and norepinephrine are given in Fig. 16.11.

Free or conjugated catecholamines, vanillyl-mandelic acid (VMA), or total metanephrines (normetanephrine plus metanephrine) can be found in the urine. Free epinephrine is excreted in the amount of 20 μg or less per day; whereas the excretion of free norepinephrine, the greater amount of which is released by the sympathetic nerve endings, is nearly 80 μg or less per day. The upper normal limits for total metanephrines and VMA are 1.3 mg and 6.5 mg/day,

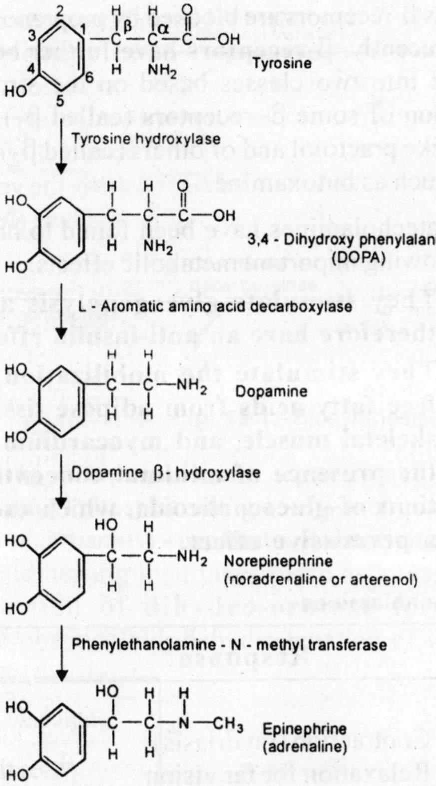

Fig. 16.10: Biosynthetic pathway for the conversion of tyrosine to norepinephrine and epinephrine

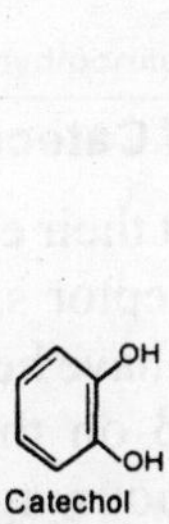

Dopa readily crosses the blood brain barrier, promoting the catecholamine synthesis. Thus, in disorders involving deficiency of catecholamine synthesis, administration of dopa may have some beneficial effects. In Parkinson's disease in which deficiency of dopamine synthesis affects nerve transmission in the substantia nigra of the upper brain system, administration of dopa leads to some symptomatic relief. Parkinsonism is a chronic, progressive disorder characterised by involuntary tremor, decreased motor power and control, postural instability and muscular rigidity.

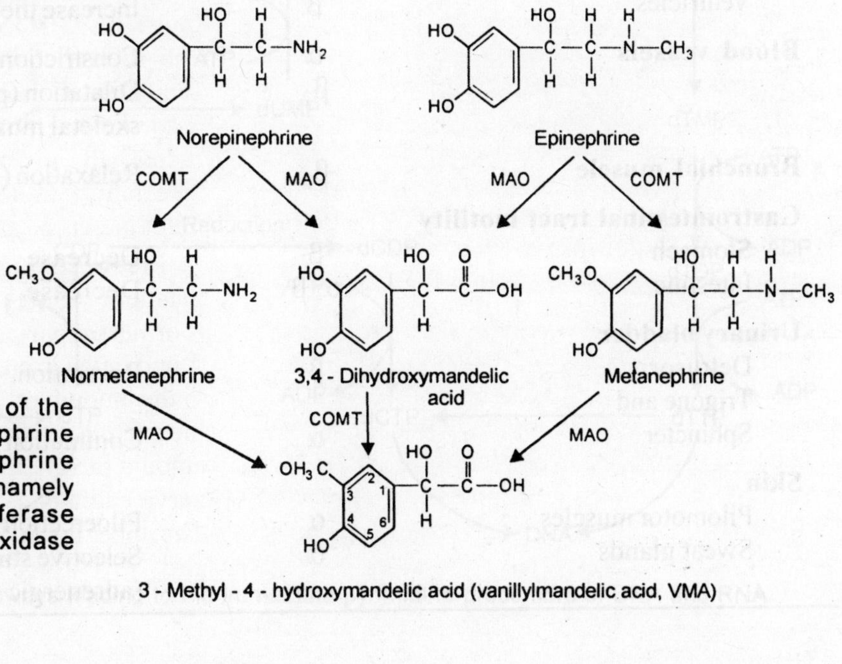

Fig. 16.11: Major pathways of the metabolism of norepinephrine (noradrenaline) and epinephrine (adrenaline). Two enzymes namely catechol-o-methyl transferase (COMT), and monoamine oxidase (MAO) are involved.

3 - Methyl - 4 - hydroxymandelic acid (vanillylmandelic acid, VMA)

respectively.

Physiological effects of Catecholamines

The catecholamines exert their effects on target tissues by binding to receptor sites on the cell membrane. The receptors have been divided into two categories, α and β on the basis of the relative potency of various agonists, which activate the receptors, and of various antagonists, which block them (Table 16.1).

β-receptors are most sensitive to stimulation by isoproterenol (isopropylnorepinephrine) and least to norepinephrine, whereas with α-receptors, the reverse is the case. It has been studied that α- receptors are selectively blocked by phenoxybenzamine and phentolamine whereas β-receptors are blocked by propranolol. More recently, β-receptors have further been divided into two classes based on the strong inhibition of some β–receptors (called β_1) by drugs like practolol and of others (called β_2) by drugs such as butoxamine.

Catecholamines have been found to have the following important metabolic effects.

(a) **They stimulate glycogenolysis and therefore have an anti-insulin effect.**

(b) **They stimulate the mobilization of free fatty acids from adipose tissue, skeletal muscle, and myocardium in the presence of minimal concentrations of glucocorticoids, which exert a permissive effect.**

Table 16.1: Some effects of catecholamines

Effector Organ	Type of Receptor	Response
Eye		
Radial muscle, Iris	α	Contraction (mydriasis)
Ciliary muscle	β	Relaxation for far vision
Heart		
Atria	β_1	Increase the contractility
Ventricles	β	Increase the contractility and irritability
Blood vessels	α	Constriction
	β_2	Dilatation (predominates in skeletal muscle)
Bronchial muscle	β_2	Relaxation (bronchodilatation)
Gastrointestinal tract motility		
Stomach	β	Decrease
Intestine	α, β	Decrease
Urinary bladder		
Detrusor	β	Relaxation
Trigone and Sphincter	α	Contraction
Skin		
Pilomotor muscles	α	Piloerection
Sweat glands	α	Selective stimulation (adrenergic sweating)

Epinephrine has been found to be more potent than norepinephrine in producing these effects.

Comparable effects of L-adrenaline and L-noradrenaline in man are given in Table 16.2.

Table 16.2 Comparison of the effects of L-adrenaline and L-noradrenaline in man

	Effect of L-adrenaline	Effect of L-noradrenaline
Blood pressure	Rise	Much rise
Blood sugar	Increase	Slight increase
Bronchus	Dilatation	Less dilatation
Cardiac output	Increase	Variable
Central nervous system	Anxiety	No effect
Eosinophil count	Increase	No effect
Heart rate	Increase	Decrease
Kidney	Vasoconstriction	Vasoconstriction
Muscle vessels	Dilatation	Constriction
Metabolism	Increase	Slight increase
Oxygen consumption	Increase	No effect
Respiration	Stimulates	Stimulates
Skin Vessels	Constriction	Constriction
Uterus in vivo in late pregnancy	Inhibits	Stimulates

Normal adrenal tissue from man and many other animals contains noradrenaline (norepinephrine) as well as adrenaline (epinephrine) and they are often together referred to as *catecholamines*. The ratio of adrenaline to noradrenaline in fresh human adrenals is 4:1

Excretion

Urinary excretion of catecholamines in man varies significantly within 24 hours from time to time as shown in Table 16.3.

Table 16.3 Urinary excretion of catecholamines in man

Condition	Urinary excretion in ng/min Adrenaline	Noradrenaline
After adrenalectomy	0	8-15
Chromaffin cell tumors	Slightly increased	100 times or more
Insulin hypogly- caemia	10 times	No effect
Mild exercise	2 times	2 times
Mental stress	Increased	No effect
Myocardial infarction	Upto 35 times	Upto 8 times
Rest	2-5	16-27
Strenuous exercise	10 times	10 times
Tilt, recumbent to head up	Little change	Increased

Adrenalectomized animals adjust to stress, such as prolonged exposure to cold or shock, much more slowly and less effectively than normal ones do, meaning to say, **the hormones secreted by adrenal cortex act as buffering agents against cold or shock.**

Adrenalectomized rats have decreased urea nitrogen excretion, blood glucose concentration, and liver glycogen storage, indicating decreased protein catabolism and decreased gluconeogenesis.

The role of cortisol in lipid metabolism is not well understood. Total body fat gets increased by glucocorticoid administration but the synthesis of fatty acids gets inhibited in liver.

Hypofunction of the adrenal medulla has not yet been recognized to produce any pathology. However, actively secreting tumors (pheochromocytoma) of the chromaffin cells of the adrenal medulla or of the organs of Zuckerkandl are known to produce large quantities of noradrenaline with a small amount of adrenaline, and their discharge at intervals into the blood may produce elevation of arterial pressure. As much as 2 mg of catecholamines may then appear in the urine per day.

The amount of catecholamines in the blood can be assessed by either fluorimetry or other more recent sophisticated techniques like radioimmunoassay, etc. Human blood plasma contains about 0.3 µg of noradrenaline per litre and 0.06 µg of adrenaline per litre. **Healthy man excretes not more than 50 µg/24 hours of catecholamines and adrenaline is less than 15 per cent of this.**

Adrenaline by producing vasoconstriction in the skin and vasodilatation in the muscles, moves blood from the skin to the muscles; it stimulates the metabolism and mobilizes glycogen as glucose.

Noradrenaline, on the other hand produces a general vasoconstriction (except in the coronary arteries) but its effects on the metabolism are not very well understood. **This may be regarded as a pressor hormone required for the maintenance of blood pressure.**

Bad Hormones ('bad' in the sense that their hypersecretion comparatively is very bad than others)

1. **Cortisol :** The major natural glucocorticoid elaborated by the adrenal cortex; it affects the metabolism of glucose, protein and lipids and has mineralocorticoid activity.

2. **ACTH (i) Glucocorticoids :** That are chiefly involved in glucose, protein and fat metabolism, and

    Overproduction of adrenal adrogens, with high 17-ketosteroid excretion, leads to the adrenogenital syndrome (virilism, hirsutism and precocious masculinization) with enhanced protein synthesis and muscularity.

    (ii) Mineralocorticoids : That are involved in the regulation of electrolyte and water balance.

    Overproduction of aldosterone is responsible for **hypertension, cardiac, hepatic** and **renal diseases**.

    These are used clinically for hormonal replacement therapy, for suppression of ACTH secretion, as anti-inflammatory agents and to suppress the immune response.

3. **Prolactin :** A hormone of the anterior pituitary that stimulates and sustains lactation in postpartum mammals and shows luteotropic activity in certain mammals.

4. Many others

Good Hormones (Impart soothing effect)

1. **Endorphins** (α, β and γ) : These are **neuropeptides** which are amino acid residues of β-lipoprotein that bind to opiate receptors in various areas of the brain **and have potent analgesic effect.**

2. Others

CHAPTER 17

VITAMINS

FAT-SOLUBLE VITAMINS

1. Vitamin A
2. Vitamin D
3. Vitamin E
4. Vitamin K

WATER-SOLUBLE VITAMINS

5. Thiamine (B_1)
6. Riboflavin (B_2)
7. Niacin, Nicotinic acid, Niacinamide, B_3
8. Pantothenic acid, B_5
9. Pyridoxine, Pyridoxal, Pyridoxamine, B_6
10. Biotin (Vitamin H)
11. Folic Acid (Pteroylglutamic acid), B_9
12. Vitamin B_{12}, Cyanocobalamine
13. Ascorbic acid (Vitamin C)
14. Lipoic acid

VITAMINS

INTRODUCTION

It will not be wrong to say that **'necessity is the mother of invention'**. In the **Japanese Navy** a high proportion of the sailors suffered for many years from **beriberi,** a condition now known as a vitamin B_1 deficiency disease.

Scientist Takaki, after many attempts was finally able in the 1880s to arrange certain reforms in the diet of the Japanese navy. Meat and vegetable allowances were increased and evaporated milk was added to the diet. The effects on the health of the men were so dramatic that extension of the reforms was undertaken and thereafter only few cases of **'beriberi'** were detected in Japanese navy.

Scurvy, another deficiency disease, was so widespread among various early sailing crews that long voyages were usually either victims of a high incidence of sickness or loss of life. It were the English who early introduced limes or lemons into the diet of their sailing men to help protect against Scurvy. The English sailors are still called as **'limeys';** the term supposedly originated from the fact that they carried crates of limes aboard the vessels.

Today, a number of vitamins are known to exist which have been studied thoroughly from every angle.

What are Vitamins?

Vitamins are chemical entities which are essential for maintaining the metabolic processes at a normal level in animals and some have important roles in the plant metabolism also. With some exceptions, all animal species require the major vitamins preformed in the diet for the obvious reason that they are unable to synthesize them from other food constituents. A large number of vitamins have been isolated, characterized and then synthesized.

Plants and various microorganisms synthesize vitamins; animals eat the plants and store certain vitamins and the animal tissues also serve as vitamin sources for other species.

Vitamins, on the basis of solubility, have been divided into two categories as shown below:

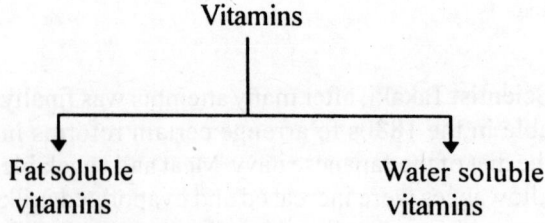

FAT SOLUBLE VITAMINS

These include vitamins A, D, E and K and are fat soluble as is evident from the name itself.

VITAMIN A

The discovery of vitamin A resulted from feeding experiments with rats and mice using purified rations. **McCollum is generally credited with the discovery of this vitamin.**

Vitamin A occurs in animal tissues only, but many plant tissues contain substances that, when fed to rats suffering from xerophthalmia, for instance, will relieve the condition. Thus, one must distinguish between vitamin A content and vitamin A activity. A number of carotenoid pigments of plants act as precursors of vitamin A. In other words, the animals can consume these pigments and bring about chemical alterations in them to produce vitamin A. **Remember, carrots and yellow corn contain no vitamin A, but since carotenes are present, they afford vitamin A activity to**

animals that eat them.

Chemistry of vitamin A

A number of naturally occurring pigments can be converted into vitamin A (retinol) by animal tissues. These pigments known as the carotenoid pigments, are found primarily in green leafy plants and yellow vegetables. They are important sources of vitamin A for man and some animals.

Kuhn and Karrer showed that β-carotene is a symmetrical molecule containing two β-ionone rings connected by a carbon chain. It has the structure as given on next page.

Because of the marked chemical similarity of the carotenoid pigments, it is practical to show their differences without setting down the entire formulae. The two rings in β-ionone are marked A and B. The formula of α-carotene, for instance, can be indicated by showing the difference in the B ring of this pigment compared to the B ring of β-carotene. The remainder of the molecules are identical.

Since, the A ring in these pigments is a β-ionone ring, these compounds are vitamin A precursors. In **xanthophyll** (found in nature with the carotenes), each ring contains a hydroxyl group and thus this pigment does not yield vitamin A. **Licopene** has two open rings (as the B ring in γ-carotene) and hence, no activity is found in it.

The manner in which animals convert various precursor pigments into vitamin A is not understood; presumably it is an enzymatic process.

The relationship of insulin to vitamin A metabolism is not clear. It has been felt by various workers that diabetic individuals have impaired efficiency of carotene conversion to vitamin A.

Vitamin A_1 (retinol), $C_{20}H_{29}OH$ and vitamin A_2 (retinol$_2$), $C_{20}H_{27}OH$ are alcohols with the structures as given on the next page.

Vitamin A_2 contains one more double bond

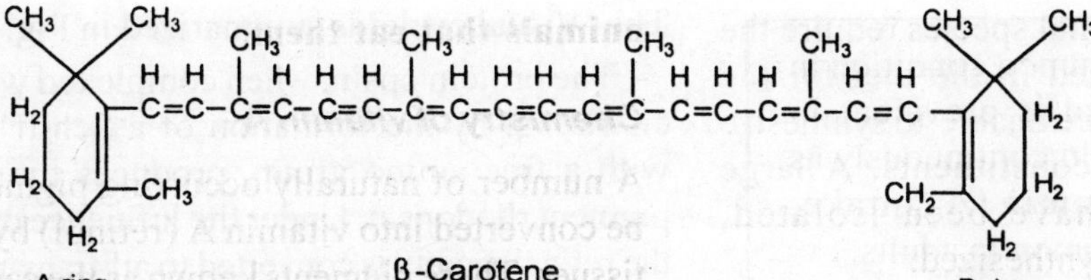

β-Carotene

A ring

B ring

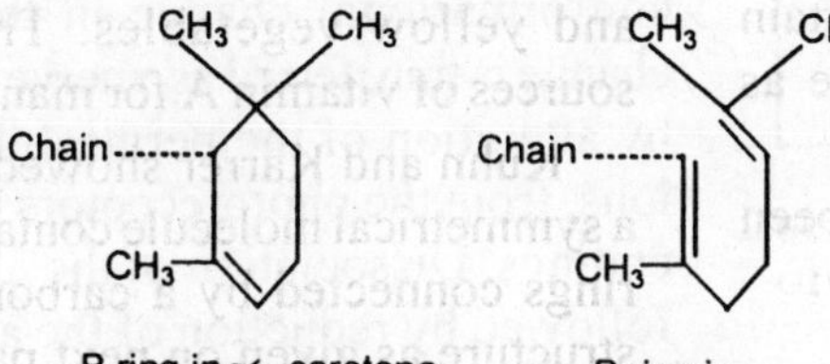

B ring in ∝- carotene
shift in double bond

B ring in
γ - carotene
open ring

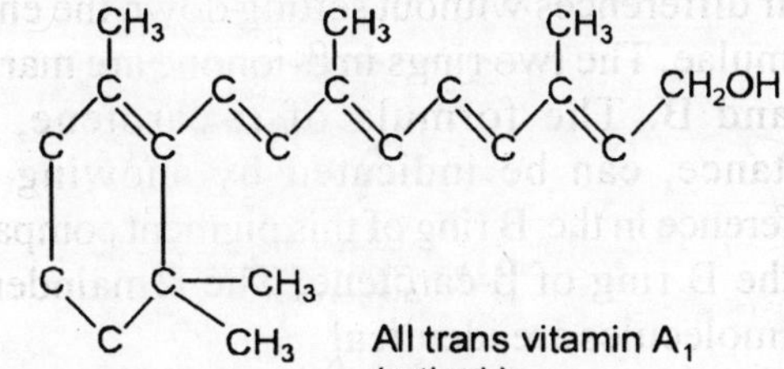

Chain--------

Chain--------

All trans vitamin A₁
(retinol₁)

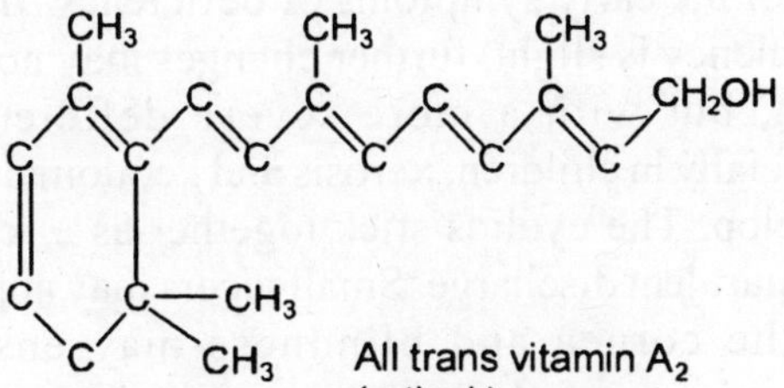

All trans vitamin A₂
(retinol₂)

in the ring. It is a dehydrovitamin A_1 formed by the loss of two H atoms in the body. No carotenes are known from which the animal body can form directly.

Absorption of vitamin A

In the small intestine, the vitamin A esters of foods are hydrolyzed to fatty acids and the free vitamin. The vitamin is absorbed here mainly by the lymphatic system and appears in blood plasma as the ester, indicating reesterification in the intestinal wall. Carotene is absorbed in the small intestine. Bile salts help in the absorption of carotene and vitamin A but may not be essential for the latter.

Physiological functions of vitamin A

1. **Growth.** In the absence of a vitamin A source, animals fail to grow and may die before body stores are completely exhausted, and often before typical deficiency symptoms develop. The mechanism of vitamin A in the growth processes is not understood.

2. **Epithelial tissue.** The epithelium of a wide variety of organs in the body under goes changes in vitamin A deficiency. The changes have been demonstrated in the salivary glands, tongue and pharynx in the mouth, the respiratory tract, the genitourinary tract, the eyes and certain glands of internal secretion. The chemical and physiological functions of these lining tissues are thus altered.

3. **Eyes.** There are various eye conditions resulting from vitamin A deficiency. Early symptoms in rats (and other species) are enlargement of the eyelids and

---

Nightblindness is a common condition in man during famine and is prevalent in certain parts of the world continuously as a result of low vitamin A intake. **Xeroderma** is also common in adults.

In children one finds poor dark adaptation, xerosis, keratomalacia, growth failure and death.

---

inflammation of the conjuctiva. This is followed by corneal changes leading to blindness.

In man, **night blindness or nyctalopia,** is one of the early symptoms of deficiency. If the deficiency is slight, further changes may not be seen, but with a more severe deficiency, especially in children, xerosis and keratomalacia develop. The eyelids stick together as a result of a purulent discharge. Small ulcers may appear on the cornea and blindness may ensue. Metaplasia of the corneal epithelium and vascularization of the **substantia propria** are typical findings and generally lead to infection and obstruction of the ducts of the ocular glands.

The basis for the relationship of the dark adaptation test to vitamin A status lies in the work of scientists Hecht and Wald. The latter investigator pointed out a functional role of vitamin A in vision. As early as 1935, he indicated a mechanism, called as **visual cycle (Rhodopsin cycle),** involving vitamin A in the vision as mentioned below.

Visual cycle (Rhodopsin cycle)

The biochemistry of vitamin A in the visual process involves both types of photoreceptor cells in the retina. The rods provide black and white vision and respond to dim light. The cones provide colour vision and respond to bright light. Both these cells require vitamin A, also called retinol, for the formation of the visual pigments.

The 'Visual cycle' is summarized in Fig. 17.1.

The protein opsin, when complexed with 11-cis-retinal by the formation of a Schiff's base with a free amino group, produces the visual pigment rhodopsin. Under the influence of light, the retinal moiety is converted to all-trans-retinal. This isomerization is associated with a conformational change in the opsin. Such a change is transferred as a nerve impulse, possibly by alteration of the permeability to Na^+ or K^+ ions, from the photoreceptors to the optic nerve endings. Dissociation of the all-trans- retinal is followed by reduction of the aldehyde group to the primary alcohol to give all-trans-retinol. Retinol returns to the circulating blood pool of vitamin A that is stored in the liver.

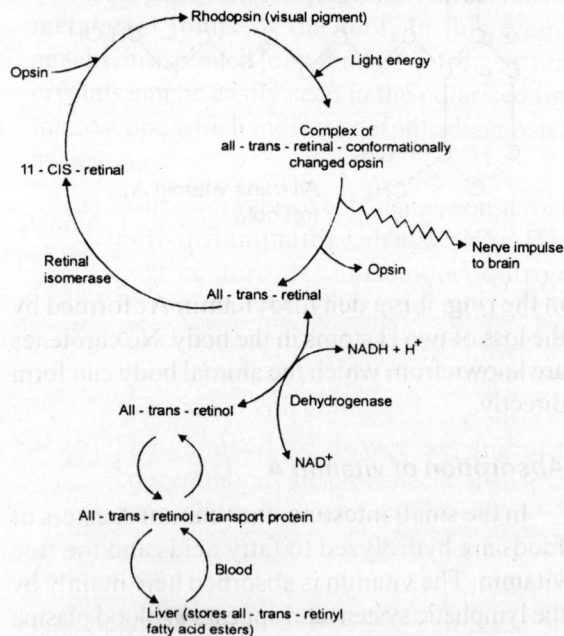

Fig. 17.1 : The Rhodopsin cycle (Visual cycle) and storage of Vitamin A

The retinol is then converted back to all-trans retinal in the retina where it is also isomerized back to 11-cis-retinal. The cycle is completed when 11-cis-retinal reacts with opsin to produce rhodopsin.

Colour vision

Similar photochemical events occur in both the rod and the cone cells. Each cone cell has one of three different colour sensitive pigments, blue (430 mμ), green (540 mμ), or red (575 mμ). The three pigments contain the same 11-cis-retinal moiety, but their opsins are different. Each pigment has a different wavelength of maximum absorbance, as noted above in parentheses and its photochemical reaction responds to one of the three primary colour components of the incident light. In each case the visual cycle is the same as that noted for rhodopsin.

4. *Reproduction.* In rats, reproduction fails in vitamin A deficiency. Males develop rather rapidly an atrophy of the germinal epithelium; this is reversed after the administration of the vitamin. In females, the normal estrous cycle is not maintained. Cattles are also known to show poor reproduction in vitamin A deficiency. Practically no data are available regarding human reproduction in relation to vitamin A deficiency.

5. *Skin.* Only comparatively recently has a vitamin A deficiency been associated with specific lesions of the skin in man. The lesions vary considerably in different individuals. The general features of the deficiency involve dryness and roughness of the skin. This appears early in the deficiency and is due to a suppression of the sweat glands. A keratosis, especially of hair follicles is a prominent feature. Papules, masses of keratinized epithelium develop, which may be readily felt by rubbing a finger over the involved area.

6. *Bones and teeth.* Bone growth is markedly impaired in vitamin A deficiency.

Teeth are derived from epithelial tissue, so, it is logical to expect a correlation between   dietary vitamin A and tooth development.

7. *Urolithiasis.* In a long-standing vitamin A deficiency in rats, Higgins found that a high percentage of animals developed this condition.

8. *Infection.* **Vitamin A has been called the anti-infective vitamin.** The vitamin does help to establish and maintain a resistance to infection in the body.

9. *Carbohydrate metabolism.* A more specific function of vitamin A in metabolism involves its role in glucose synthesis from triose molecules.

Hypervitaminosis A

Excess vitamin A intake in humans leads to a number of untoward symptoms including in the acute phase, headache, nausea and vomiting, and drowsiness. In the chronic disease the findings include anorexia, dry itchy skin, alopecia, cracking of the lips and painful areas over various bones. **Often the serum alkaline phosphatase level is found to be elevated.**

Sources of Vitamin A

Many marine fish oils, especially the liver oils, have high concentrations of the vitamin. **Soupfin shark, ling cod, halibut and swordfish are among the species whose liver oils contain very high concentrations at certain seasons.**

Synthetic vitamin A preparations such as vitamin A palmitate, are now used in great quantity. Such products have no fishy taste and are preferred by many than the natural concentrates. .

Eggs, milk, cheese and the green leafy vegetables are good sources and many of the yellow crops such as corn and carrots are fair vitamin A sources for human beings.

Units and requirements of vitamin A

The USP (United States Pharmacopoeia) unit

There is some evidence that Vitamin A and retinoids protect an individual against cancer. The evidence appears to be strongest for lung cancer, but an inverse relationship between vitamin A intake and cancers of bladder, upper gastrointestinal tract and breast has also been proposed.

Vitamin A deficiency

1. Eye changes
   (a) **Bitot's spot**
   (b) Corneal ulcer
   (c) Keratomalacia
2. Blindness

1. Cell differentiation
2. Epithelial metaplasia
3. **Keratin debris→ kidney stones**
4. **Increased Cancer?**

and the international unit (I.U.) of vitamin A are identical. The international standard is a specially prepared vitamin A acetate; and one unit of vitamin A is equal to the activity of 0.344 μg of this ester. This is equivalent to 0.3 μg of vitamin A and to 0.6 μg of β-carotene.

Recommended daily vitamin A intake for different categories is as follows:

1. For average men and women (age 18-75 years) : 5000 I.U./day (600 mcg)
2. Boys (9-18 years) : 4500-5000 I.U./day
3. Girls (9-18 years) : 4500-5000 I.U./day
4. Children:
   1-3 years : 2000 I.U./day
   3-6 years : 2500 I.U./day
   6-9 years : 3500 I.U./day
5. Infants:
   0-1 year : 1500 I.U./day

Storage of vitamin A

Vitamin A is stored in the liver in large amounts ranging from 0.2 to 2.0 μmoles/g. Clinical problems do not arise so easily unless deprivation is extreme and is continued for relatively long periods i.e. for several months.

VITAMIN D

The disease rachitis (Figures 17.2, 17.6, 17.7 & 17.8), now popularly known as 'Rickets' is prevalent since ancient times.

HYPOVITAMINOSIS D : RICKETS AND OSTEOMALACIA

Both of these chronic conditions are basically same and characterised by a deficient calcification of bones caused by insufficient saturation of body fluids with calcium and phosphate, usually due to hypovitaminosis D. The age at which this occurs makes all the difference in their clinical, biochemical and pathological features. **Rickets occurs in the growing and osteomalacia in grown bones.**

CLINICAL FEATURES

A. Rickets

The name given by Ell is after an English bone setter named Rickets who around 1620 became famous for the diagnosis and treatment of the vitamin D deficiency. The affected infant may not look severely malnourished but is restless and irritable and has flabby toneless muscles. A 'pithed frog' position is usually adopted and abdomen is distended. There are also craniotabes, visible enlargement of epiphysis of lower end of radius and beading of ribs (Figs. 17.2, 17.7 and 17.8). There may be accompanying diarrhoea, respiratory infection and delayed milestones. In somewhat later stage there are frontal and parietal 'bossings' and chest deformities like Harrison's sulcus in untreated cases. By the age of 2-3 years, these signs become exaggerated and more severe deformities like **kyphosis** or **lordosis** of spine and low legs develop. Still later, the pelvic deformities develop which lead to serious obstetrical complications in women who had rickets in childhood. In more severe cases, infantile tetany may follow closely.

B. Osteomalacia

The patient suffering from osteomalacia is almost always a young mother, having been burdened with a rapid succession of pregnancies and lactations. Depending upon the severity of the condition she may present with anorexia, weight loss, bone pains, bony deformities (Fig. 17.6, 17.7 & 17.8), muscular weakness (myopathy), urinary tract infections, renal stones, chronic pyelonephritis and tetany. The gait is typically waddling. The sequence of postures adopted on trying to rise from squatting is also characteristic. The patient cannot suddenly rise, there is first extension of knees with hips remaining flexed. The trunk is straightened by the help of arms.

Chemistry of vitamin 'D'

This is a fat soluble vitamin. Two following anti-rachitic substances are active when taken by mouth:

(a) D_3 (cholecalciferol, Fig. 17.3), a derivative of cholesterol, and

(b) D_2 (ergocalciferol) (Fig 17.5), a synthetic derivative of plant sterol.

There is no vitamin D_1 but vitamin D_2 and D_3 are of great importance to human beings. Vitamin D_4 is activated 22-dehydroergosterol; whereas vitamin D_5 is activated 7-dehydrosi-tosterol. A number of other products have been found to have some degree of antirachitic activity. Ergosterol and lumisterol are not antirachitic; however, tachysterol after reduction to dihydrotachysterol is used especially in the treatment of some types of 'tetany' in human beings. The vitamins are not strictly sterols since ring B is open. The immediate precursor of D_3 is 7- dehydrocholesterol, which is found in the skin and sebum, and the agent promoting the change is ultraviolet light (Figs. 17.3 & 17.4). **If**

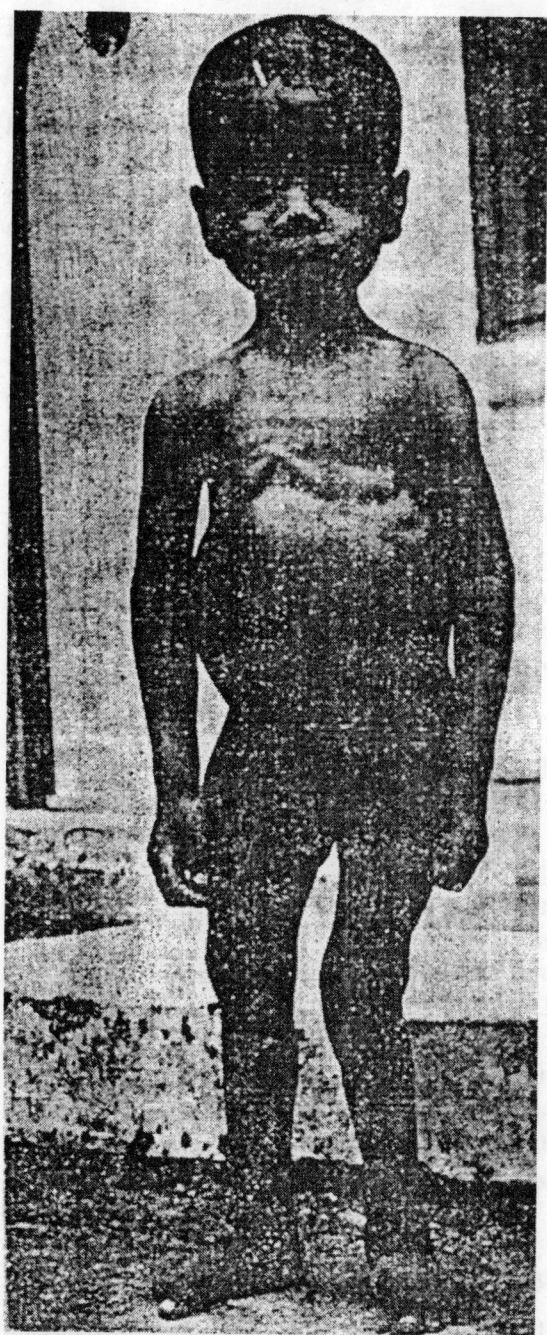

Fig. 17.2 : Rickets and osteomalacia, the puzzling quiz: Indians seem to be peculiarly susceptible to hypovitaminosis D (and calcium deficiency). This child from Darjeeling exhibits all the classical signs of rickets; big forehead, bent legs and swollen wrists ('cuffs'). (Picture by courtesy of WHO.)

the skin is exposed sufficiently to direct sunlight; sufficient vitamin will be formed, its intake in food is then unnecessary. There is indeed evidence that endogenously produced cholecalciferol derivatives are retained more efficiently in the body than those formed from ingested vitamin D. This evidence is based on the measurement of plasma levels of 25-OH-cholecalciferol, where it is associated with a specific vitamin-D-binding protein. Prolonged exposure of the whole body to ultra-violet light does not cause the 25-OH-D$_3$ levels to rise to more than double the normal level, whereas high doses of oral vitamin D may cause it to rise 10 fold. As 25-OH-D$_3$ is the metabolite most closely associated with toxic effects of hypervitaminosis D, it is now being suggested that supplementation of foodstuffs should not be regarded as adequate prophylactic, by comparison with UV irradiation of the skin.

The most important of the active substances, so far as the present knowledge goes is dihydroxycholecalciferol, which is formed from calciferol by two successive hydroxylations. (Fig 17.3). The first of these takes place in liver and the second in kidney. Thus cholecalciferol is taken up by liver from plasma, although it is not stored there, and 25-OH-D$_3$ is resecreted into plasma. The product of the second hydroxylation, 1,25-di-OH-D$_3$ has a short half-life. **It is now clear that production of 1,25-di-OH-D$_3$ is under hormonal control.** It is found that its concentration in plasma rises when the body's demand for Ca is high, as in

(a) Pregnancy, and

(b) Lactation

Regulation of Vitamin 'D'

It appears that its regulation is monitored through the action of parathyroid hormone on the renal cells, and not through direct feedback by plasma Ca^{++} or by calcitonin.

Owing to the regulatory action of the parathyroid gland, the serum Ca level in rickets is rarely low, even when the rickets is directly due to Ca deficiency in the diet. Instead, the inorganic phosphate level in serum is usually diminished.

PROVITAMINS:

(i) Ergosterol (plants, yeast)

(ii) 7-dehydrocholesterol (skin)
Vitamin D$_2$ is known as ergocalciferol
Vitamin D$_3$ is known as cholecalciferol

Physiological functions

Vitamin D is associated with a number of physiological processes in the body. Following are the established actions of vitamin D in the body:

(1) **Vitamin D is required for normal growth in mammals.** This is probably related to calcium and phosphorus absorption and their utilization, vis-a-vis it promotes minerals (mainly Ca and P) deposition in the skeleton.

(2) **It increases calcium and phosphorus absorption from the intestine.**

(3) It is antirachitic. Its deficiency causes rickets (Figure 17.6) which is a disease of young ones. The disease may involve a low blood calcium level or a low blood phosphorus level. In humans, the latter type is generally seen. **In infancy, the inorganic phosphorus level of blood is normally 4 to 6 mg per cent but in rickets this may be decreased to 1 to 2 mg percent.**

(4) Vitamin D has got a specific function on kidney tubular reabsorption of calcium and phosphate, thus inhibits their excretion via urine.

(5) It has got a general effect on the metabolism of citric acid which is a normal

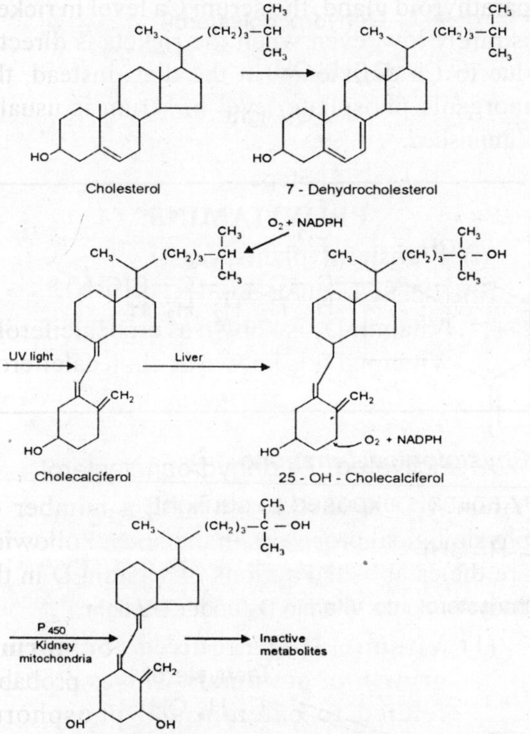

Fig 17.3 : The transformation of cholesterol into the major active metabolite 1,25-di-OH cholecalciferol.

constituent of many body tissues, including bone. Rachitic rats given vitamin D show increased urinary excretion of citric acid and increased levels in blood, bone, kidney, heart and small intestine with no elevation in liver.

Hypervitaminosis

In human beings, it mainly causes:

  (i) Hypercalcaemia,
 (ii) Hypercalcinuria, and
 (iii) Nephrocalcinosis

Daily requirements

Daily requirements for different categories of human beings are as follows:

  (a) For infants and   : 200 IU/day
      children   (5.0 mcg)

In infants and children clinical symptoms of severe deficiency are readily seen on gross examination. Enlargement of the ankle, knee and wrist joints are noted. Other prominent features are bowed legs, delayed closure of the frontanelle, beading of the ribs at the costochondral junction (**"rachitic rosary"**), and delayed tooth eruption.

The mineral content of the bone decreases as the severity of the rickets progresses.

In adults osteomalacia occurs.

Absence of vitamin D causes rickets, a disease of infants. The bones become soft, the legs unable to support the weight, the flat bones deformed. The rib cage may become so deformed that death from respiratory failure occurs. The skeleton of the newborn child is always deficient in calcium and any derangement of Ca metabolism quickly makes the bones soft.

In adults, vitamin D deficiency causes osteomalacia, but the calcium reservoir in the adult is so large that the deficiency must be present for several years before the softening of the bones is present (it is usually only seen associated with pregnancy and lactation).

  (b) During pregnancy   : 400 IU/day
      and lactation   (10.0 mcg)
  (c) Adults   : 100 IU/day
                       (2.5 mcg)

Serious overdosage is toxic which may cause calcification of the renal tubules. **Several deaths, mostly of children from vitamin D overdosage have been reported in last few years in several countries.**

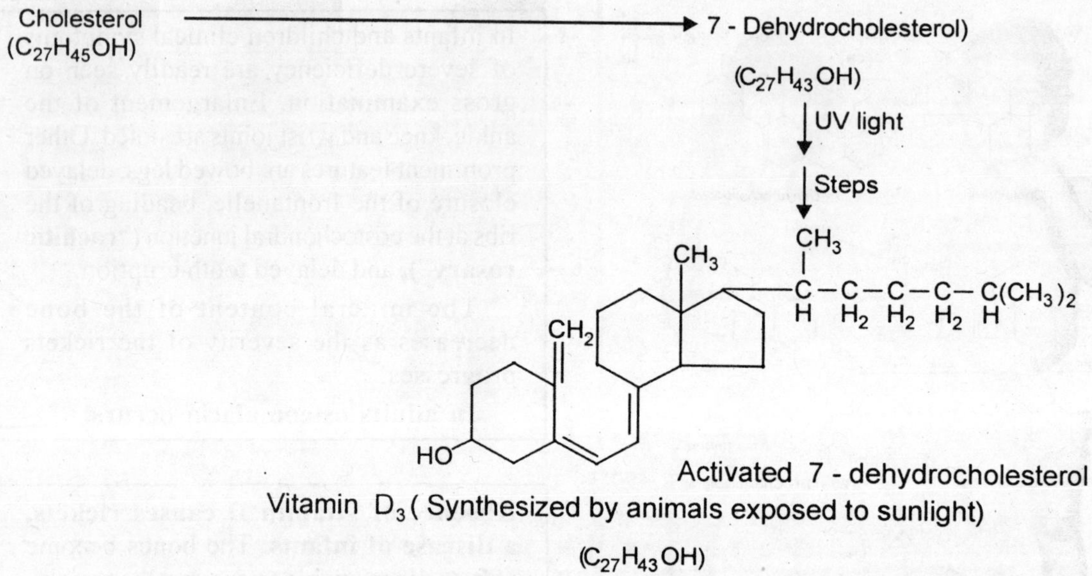

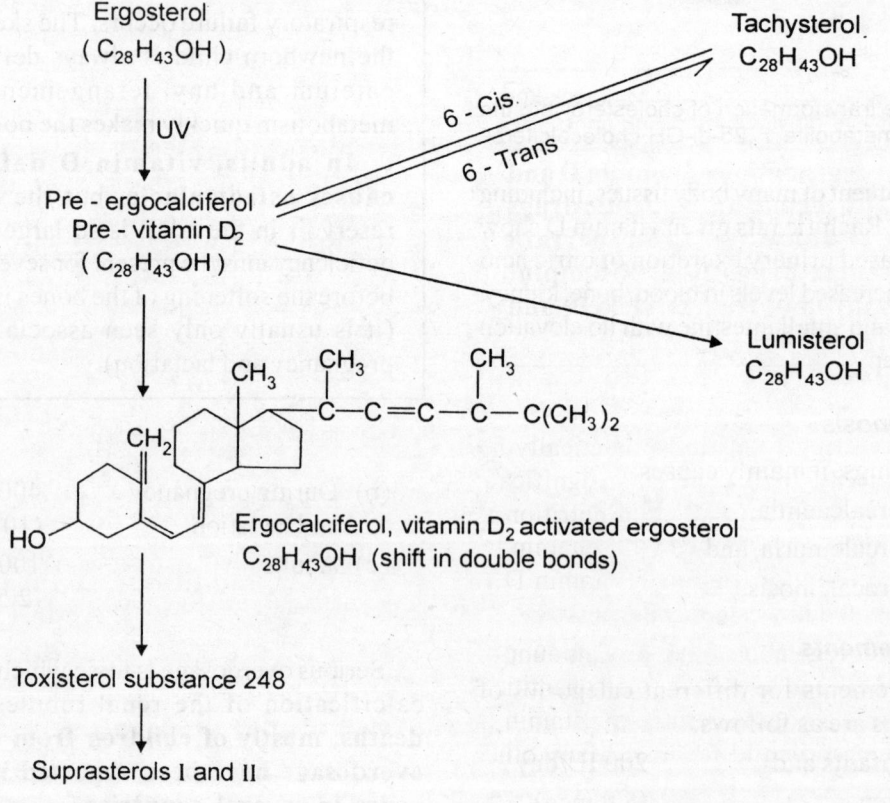

Cholesterol
$(C_{27}H_{45}OH)$ ⟶ 7 - Dehydrocholesterol)

$(C_{27}H_{43}OH)$

↓ UV light

↓ Steps

Activated 7 - dehydrocholesterol

Vitamin D_3 (Synthesized by animals exposed to sunlight)

$(C_{27}H_{43}OH)$

Fig 17.4 : Scheme to show the conversion of cholesterol into Vitamin D_3 under UV light

Ergosterol
($C_{28}H_{43}OH$)

Tachysterol
$C_{28}H_{43}OH$

↓ UV

6 - Cis

6 - Trans

Pre - ergocalciferol
Pre - vitamin D_2
($C_{28}H_{43}OH$)

Lumisterol
$C_{28}H_{43}OH$

Ergocalciferol, vitamin D_2 activated ergosterol
$C_{28}H_{43}OH$ (shift in double bonds)

Toxisterol substance 248

Suprasterols I and II

Fig 17.5 Scheme to show the conversion of erogosterol into Vitamin D_2 under UV light

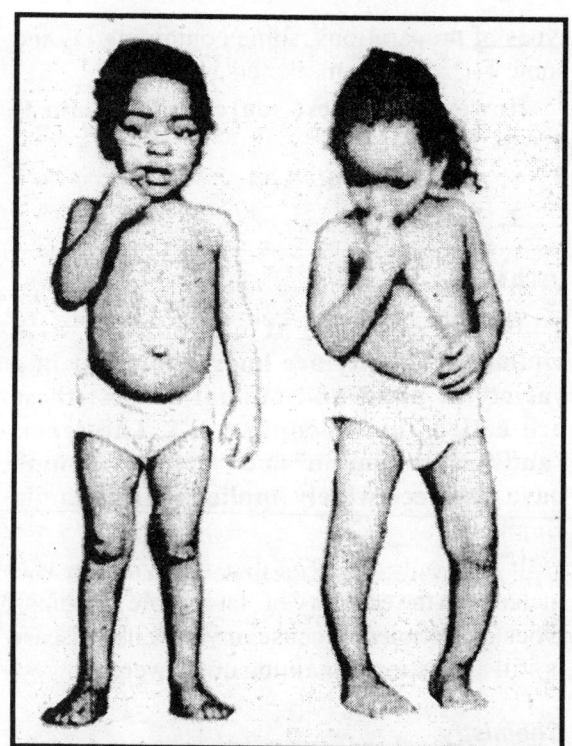

Fig 17.6 : Rachitic children, showing knock-knees in child on left and bowlegs in one on right.

Enhanced degradation of vitamin D and 25(OH) D by certain antiepileptic drugs such as 'Phenytoin' and certain antitubercular drugs like 'Rifampin' (Rifampicin) may lead to rickets and osteomalacia.

Sources

Naturally occurring foods have practically no vitamin D activity. Milk contains insignificant amounts as far as infant and child nutrition is concerned unless it is fortified with vitamin D. That is why, milk , fortified with vitamin D is widely distributed in western countries.

Grains and vegetables have less amount of vitamin D. Butter and liver have small quantities. Cod liver oil is a popular source of vitamin D (D_3) for infant and child feeding. Many other

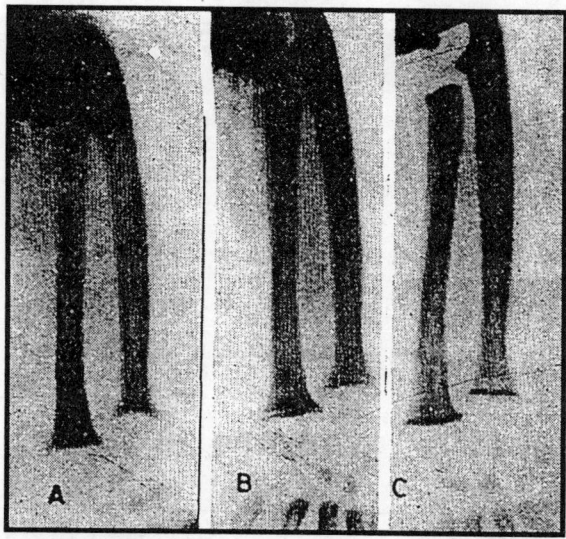

Fig 17.7 : X-ray films of forearm of a rachitic child, showing the effect of treatment A to C, views of the forearm. A, Before treatment: marked trabeculation of the radius and ulna is apparent, particularly in the cortical portion of the bone, with slight periosteal thickening. The *end* of the bone is slightly mushroomed *and* cupped and shows distinct fringing; the cartilage is swollen. The distal epiphyses of the radius are absent. There are two small centers of ossification in the wrists. B, One month after the treatment: a new centre of ossification has appeared in the distal epiphysis of the humerus. The centres of ossification at the wrists are still two in number but are larger *and* more distinct in outline. There is a fresh line of calcium deposition at the ends if the radius *and* the ulna, in the *zone* of provisional cartilage (line test). A clear area is present between this new calcification and the shaft (submetaphyseal rarefaction). Cupping, fringing *and* stippling are present; spur formation is also *noted,* outlining the swollen cartilage at the distal epiphysis of the ulna (beginning healing). C, *One* & a half months after the treatment. Healing is *now* advanced. The shaft shows calcification of subperiosteal osteoid at the outer aspect of the radius, giving the bone a greater width. Calcification of the provisional zone in the metaphyses is much more distinct *and* the submetaphyseal area is filling in.

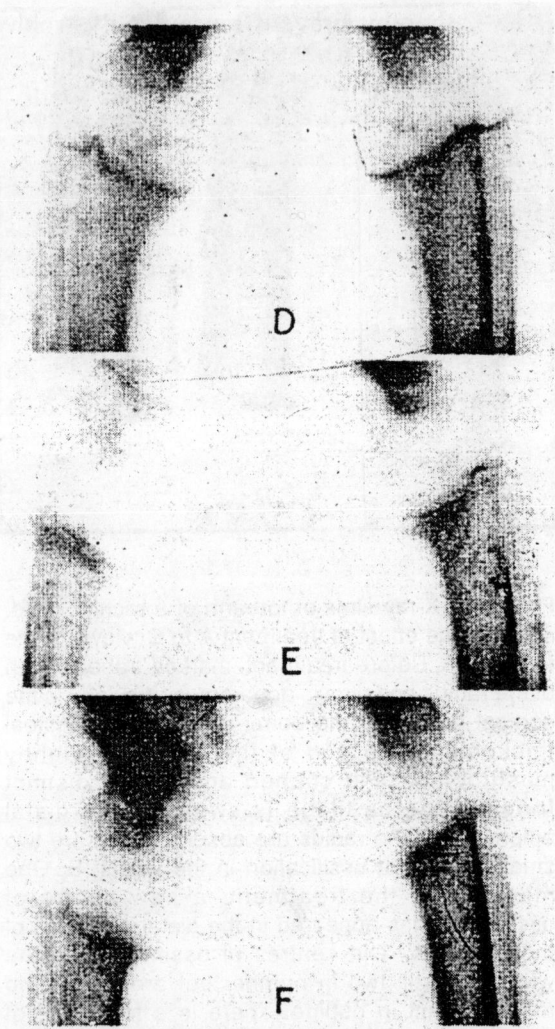

Fig 17.8 X-ray films of legs of a rachitic child A. Before treatment: cupping of the distal ends of both tibias and fibulas with compression and widening of the end of the shaft. B. One month after treatment: beginning healing of the distal ends of both bones (tibia and fibula) (line test). Submetaphyseal rarefaction. Periosteal hyperplasia at the distal third of both tibias. C. One and a half months after treatment: advanced healing. Submetaphyseal rarefaction is now well filled in. The ends of the bones are well calcified with marked stippling in the distal cartilage of the tibia and the beginnings of a centre of ossification in the distal epiphyseal cartilage of the tibia.

types of preparations, some containing D_2 and some D_3, are also marketed.

However, the best sources of vitamin D are as follows:

1. Fish liver oils and
2. Margarine

VITAMIN E

Today, at least eight compounds with vitamin E activity are known to occur in a variety of plant and animal tissues; these are called the "tocopherols". The terms "antisterility vitamin" and "fertility vitamin" have also been widely applied to the vitamin E.

It was only in 1977 that this vitamin was included in the category of 'fat soluble vitamins'. Does its deficiency cause any specific disease is still a question remaining unanswered?

Chemistry

Evans and co-workers prepared three crystalline derivatives of compounds from the nonsaponifiable fraction of wheat germ oil and showed that the original alcohol obtained by hydrolysis of one of them had high vitamin E activity. These workers gave the active alcohol the name "α-tocopherol".

There are eight naturally occurring tocopherol derivatives known. Six are toco derivatives and two are tocotrienol derivatives as given below:

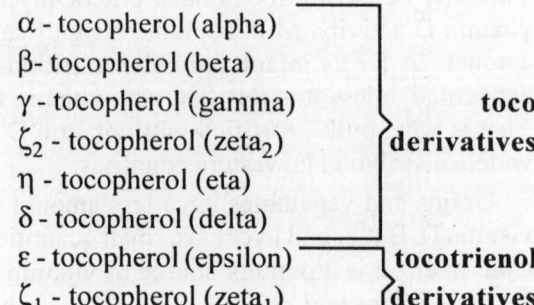

α - tocopherol (alpha)
β- tocopherol (beta)
γ - tocopherol (gamma)
ζ_2 - tocopherol (zeta$_2$)   toco
η - tocopherol (eta)   derivatives
δ - tocopherol (delta)
ε - tocopherol (epsilon)   tocotrienol
ζ_1 - tocopherol (zeta$_1$)   derivatives

Pure tocopherols are oils and are fat-soluble.

The tocopherols are extraordinarily stable to heat in the absence of oxygen and they withstand acids at elevated temperatures. Ultraviolet light destroys the vitamin activity as does oxidation. **The tocopherols are excellent antioxidants.** This property is assuming great importance from a physiological standpoint. **α-tocopherol is biologically more potent than any other form,** the structure of which is as shown below:

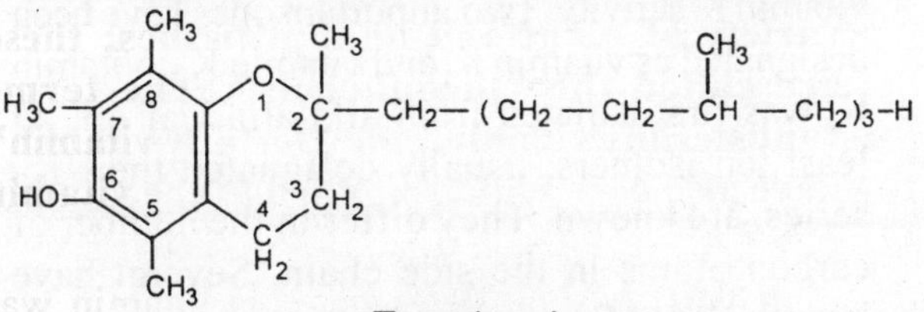

α - Tocopherol

(5,7, 8-Trimethyltocol)

> There is no evidence that large doses (mega doses i.e. in grams) of this vitamin provide any benefit to the human beings in the form of the maintenance of muscular activity or sexual vigour or the youthfulness of the skin.

Functions

Tocopherols act as antioxidants to prevent many undesirable oxidations in the body out of which some important ones are the following:

1. Scavenger of free radicals: By their antioxidant actions, tocopherols, function as scavengers of free radicals like free OH radical, superoxide anion (O_2), free halogen radicals (Cl), etc. to prevent their peroxidative effects on unsaturated lipids present in membranes, and thus are responsible for stabilizing the membranes.

   By reducing free radicals in this way, tocopherols preserve the integrities of membrane-bound organelles and thereby prevent muscular dystrophy, hepatic necrosis or increased erythrocyte fragility. E-deficiency promotes peroxidation of polyunsaturated fatty acids in lysosomal membrane.

2. Antioxidant action of tocopherols is very helpful in preventing the peroxidative effects of atmospheric pollutants like O_3, H_2O_2 and NO_2 on lipids of respiratory membranes.

3. Antioxidant action of tocopherol is also helpful in protecting selenide at the active sites of membrane selenoproteins against the harmful effects of free radicals.

4. Since, the tocopherols are responsible for preventing peroxidative changes in the mitochondrial membranes, therefore they maintain the translocation of phosphate ions into mitochondria; in this way, **they may increase the rate of oxidative phosphorylation.**

5. Antisterility factor: It has been proved that tocopherols prevent sterility in lower animals like rodents etc. but it has yet to be established in human beings.

Vitamin E deficiency

In man, deficiency symptoms are not well established, primarily because known cases of deficiency are rare. It is agreed that man requires vitamin E. **Red blood cells are subject to hemolysis by hydrogen peroxide or dialuric acid to a greater degree in vitamin E deficiency.** In some newborn infants, the red

> **Deficiency of vitamin E causes anaemia in premature infants.**
> Hypervitaminosis has been reported to induce blurred vision, headache, dizziness, fatigue, acne, vasodilation, gastrointestinal symptoms, prolonged clotting time and rise in serum cholesterol and fats.

blood cells are readily hemolyzed by hydrogen peroxide. Gyorgy found that administration of vitamin E by mouth prevents this hemolysis.

Sources

The most potent natural sources of tocopherols are the vegetable oils; of these, wheat germ oil has the highest concentration. Corn oil, cottonseed oil and safflower oil contain considerable amount. Fish oils are poor sources. Lettuce and alfa-alfa are good sources of the vitamin. Other foods have little activity. Of the animal tissues, liver is usually the highest in vitamin E although the level is generally low in other animal tissues.

Requirement of Vitamin E

Although animal requirements for vitamin E are fairly well established, there are no acceptable experimental data on human requirements.

It has been opined that the adult human requirement may vary from 10 to 30 mg per day; whereas for infants an intake of 0.5 mg per kg body weight has been suggested.

VITAMIN K

History

In 1929, Dam reported that chicks developed a hemorrhagic condition and prolonged blood clotting time when grown on specific synthetic rations. In 1935, he proposed the term vitamin K (Koagulation-vitamin) for a factor in certain foods which protected chicks against this haemorrhagic syndrome. Many foods were tested by Dam for vitamin K activity, who later on concluded that hog liver was very high, cod liver oil practically devoid of activity, whereas egg yolk as a poor source. **Among the vegetable material tested, hemp seed was found to be an excellent source.** The factor was found to be fat soluble.

Dam, Karrer and their co-workers isolated the vitamin from alfa-alfa in 1939. In the same year Doisy and associates isolated the principle from both alfa-alfa and fish meal. It was evident that the vitamin from alfa-alfa was clinically different from the product obtained from fish meal. Vitamin K_1 was used to designate the former one and K_2 the latter one.

Chemistry

There are several compounds that exhibit vitamin K activity. Two important ones have been designated as vitamin K_1 and vitamin K_2. Vitamin K_1 was first isolated from alfa-alfa leaf oil. At least ten isomers, usually designated the K_2 series, are known. They differ in the number of carbon atoms in the side chain. Several have been isolated from natural sources.

Vitamin K_1 is 2-methyl-3-phytyl -l, 4-naphtho-quinone. The original K_2 contains two farnesyl units in the side chain at position 3 which is equivalent to 6 isoprene unit or 30 carbon atoms. Other K_2 molecules contain 7 isoprene units and 9 isoprene units in the side chains (35 and 45 carbon atoms). To simplify naming of these compounds, it was suggested that they be designated as vitamin $K_{2(30)}$, vitamin $K_{2(35)}$ and $K_{2(45)}$.

Vitamin K₁
(2 - methyl - 3 - phytyl - 1, 4 - naphthoquinone)

Vitamin K₂ in which n can be 6, 7, 9,

Menadione (Vitamin K₃)

A number of vitamins of both the K_1 and K_2 series have been synthesized. A simple molecule,

2 - methyl - 1, 4 - naphthoquinone, is known as vitamin K_3 or menadione and is readily obtainable in pure form.

Physiological Aspects

1. The specific function of vitamin K is to stimulate the production of prothrombin by the liver. Since the clotting process depends on the conversion of fibrinogen to fibrin by the action of thrombin, a deficiency of prothrombin prolongs the clotting time of the blood by slowing the rate of formation of fibrin threads. The action of thrombin is enzymic; prothrombin is, therefore, a zymogen or inactive form.

2. It is also involved in the manufacture or preservation of other blood-clotting factors, including proconvertin, Christmas factor and Stuart factor.

3. The newborn infant is subject to an alimentary vitamin K deficiency because of the fact that vitamin K is not readily passed from the mother to the foetus. The disease is characterized by low prothrombin levels and consequently, a tendency to haemorrhage. Many common intestinal flora synthesize the vitamin, and a part of it becomes available to the host. In order to avoid tendency of haemorrhage in infants, this vitamin is either administered to women just previous to delivery or to the newborn infant; such kind of practice is now common.

4. It is believed that it also plays role in mitochondrial electron transport and oxidative phosphorylation.

Therapeutic uses; toxicity

This vitamin is required in small doses by the human beings. Since, it is found in abundance in the foods which a man commonly consumes daily, hence dietary supplementation is rarely necessary in adult humans. It is of value, however, in treating cases of congenital hypoprothrombinemia or in minimizing the decrease in prothrombin concentration, often seen in newborn infants.

Vitamin K_1 is also administered to patients where prothrombin time has been deliberately increased (clotting slowed) by the use of vitamin K antagonists such as **dicumarol.** When a thrombus (blood clot) is formed in a coronary artery, the portion of the heart muscle being supplied by that artery becomes necrotic and the person usually has symptoms of **'heart attack'.** The rationale of administering an antagonist of vitamin K is to slow the clotting time of the blood to minimize the possibility of the formation of additional clots; since an excessive amount of such antagonists will cause spontaneous haemorrhages by inhibiting the clotting mechanisms, the dosage must be carefully controlled and vitamin K_1 administered if the prothrombin time becomes too long.

Requirements and sources

Official requirements for human beings have not yet been set, but the minimal amount for adults has been estimated as 2 mg of menadione, injected intravenously. Microgram quantities are required to prevent the decrease in prothrombin concentration that usually takes place in the blood of infants a few days after birth; **this can be administered either to the new born infant**

Green leafy vegetables, such as alfa-alfa, spinach, cabbage are the best sources of vitamin K. Roots, tubers, seeds and fruits contain only small amounts.

Certain microorganisms found in the intestinal tract are able to synthesize vitamin K_2 and undoubtedly provide an important source of this vitamin for the human beings.

or to the mother shortly before delivery. Because of the termination of supply from the maternal circulation with the cutting of the umbilical cord, the concentration of the several blood-clotting factors are low in the circulatory system of newborn infants; supplements of vitamin K often prevent haemorrhage by stimulating synthesis of prothrombin in the liver.

As regards sources of this vitamin; they include both plants and animals, a list of which is as shown in Table 17.1.

Table 17.1: Major sources of vitamin K

Sl. No.	Source	Vitamin K (mg/100g edible portion)
1.	Alfa-alfa	425-850
2.	Spinach	334
3.	Cauliflower	275
4.	Cabbage	250
5.	Soyabean	190
6.	Wheat bran	80
7.	Wheat germ	37
8.	Wheat, whole	36
9.	Liver, pork	115-230

Vitamin K activates blood clotting factors II, VII, IX and X

Its deficiency causes in:

Infants : haemorrhagic disease of newborn

Adults : defective blood clotting

WATER SOLUBLE VITAMINS

As is evident from the title itself, vitamins included in this group are soluble in water which include well established members of the B complex group i.e. thiamine (B_1), riboflavin (B_2), niacin, pantothenic acid, pyridoxine (B_6), biotin, folic acid, cyanocobalamine (B_{12}), choline, inositol, lipoic acid and p-aminobenzoic acid have also been included in this category. Ascorbic acid (Vitamin C) and compounds with related activity, such as citrin (**Vitamin "P"**), are also water-soluble vitamins.

Since the vitamins of this category are soluble in water, therefore, their absorption remains unaffected by malabsorption states except severe diarrhoea in which it certainly gets affected. Various members of this group function as coenzymes in intermediary metabolism and thus play very important roles in the human body, particularly in energy-releasing mechanisms and haematopoiesis (formation of erythrocytes and other blood cells).

THIAMINE (VITAMIN B_1) (ANTI-BERIBERI OR ANTI-NEURITIC VITAMIN)

History

The term **'deficiency disease'** was first applied to a condition known as beriberi, which was found to be common in south-eastern Asia and the islands of the Pacific Ocean. The similarity in pathology between this disease and polyneuritis noticed in chickens given a restricted diet of polished rice only, both of which could be cured by feeding the **"silver skin" (i.e., pericarp and germ) of the grain,** prompted scientist Eijkman to investigate the subject thoroughly from the nutritional standpoint. Eijkman, then was able to produce beriberi by feeding a diet of polished rice and prevented the syndrome by dietary means. He reported his classic studies in 1896-97. Besides those oriental countries where polished rice is the main item of diet, **other places in which beriberi has been observed include prisons or asylums, localities where the diet is faulty, war-stricken countries, etc.**

The vitamin was finally crystallized from rice polishings by Jansen and Donath in 1926 in the same laboratory where Eijkman conducted his original studies. **Eijkman was able, after thirty years, to confirm the antineuritic activity of the crystalline vitamin hydrochloride. A**

A deficiency of this vitamin primarily involves the following two important systems of the human body namely:

(i) **Nervous system, and**

(ii) **Circulatory system**

In the absence of thiamine, peripheral neuritis develops, resulting in paralysis (Fig. 8.9). Cardiovascular symptoms like edema and loss of appetite also appear.

Its deficiency in man leads to the condition known as **beriberi;** in animals the syndrome is referred to as polyneuritis.

Beriberi is widespread amongst low-socioeconomic groups of South-East Asia, where due to poverty B_1-deficient polished rice forms the main food item of their diet.

Nausea, vomiting, anorexia, loss of body weight, lassitude and rise in blood pyruvate level are found in all types of 'beriberi'.

decade later the structure and synthesis of the vitamin were announced by R.R. Williams and his co-workers.

The cause of Beriberi was proved beyond doubt to be in the finding that the highest concentration of hitherto unknown nutrient in cereals was in the germ and pericarp and high milling and polishing removed the same with resultant deficiency. **A discovery that won Nobel Prize for Eijkman.**

Clinical cases of thiamine deficiency in the western hemisphere are rare today. In the United States, U.K. and other advanced countries, foods are readily available to provide an adequate dietary intake of thiamine for all ages. Prior to the distribution of enriched foods of this vitamin, the neuritis in chronic alcoholics was shown to be the result of insufficient thiamine. **However, these days, it is difficult to find the cases of the deficiency of this vitamin even among alcoholics.**

Physiological and Clinical Aspects of Thiamine

This vitamin is essential for the growth and metabolism of all animals as well as of many plants and microorganisms. Deficiencies are characterized by a variety of symptoms and clinically are often complicated by the effects of lack of other nutrients.

In thiamine deficiency (avitaminosis B_1), a form of peripheral neuritis is manifested affecting both the sensory and motor nerves. During the early stages, neuralgia and cramps of the calf muscles are common; as the condition advances, the thigh muscles become weak and toe and foot-drop develop with hyperthesia. **The acute disease, beriberi, may be of following five types:**

(i) **Dry beriberi**

(ii) **Wet beriberi**

(iii) **Acute cardiac beriberi**

(iv) **Infantile beriberi and**

(v) **Wernicke-Korsakoff encephalopathy**

Onset of Beriberi

Both dry and wet beriberi have a similar, usually insidious onset in the form of anorexia, lassitude and weakness in the legs making walking difficult. Some patients may have a little pain in the pericardium, palpitation and edema, usually of face or legs. There is associated paresthesia and/or anaesthesia of limbs. **Such patients, mostly belonging to labourer class usually ignore such symptoms and keep working.** A bout of undue exertion or fever may precede the above symptoms, or if they are already present, may drag the patient into more severe stages as described below.

(i) Dry Beriberi

This is usually a chronic condition and the patient is markedly wasted or bedridden with some superadded infections like tuberculosis or dysentery which overshadow the basic nutritional disorder. The diagnostic feature is polyneuropathy and the history is characteristic of progressively increasing weakness and wasting of muscles leading to correspondingly deteriorating walking capacity. Flaccid paresis, wrist drop and foot drop also are present.

In this type cachexia, numbness, and paralysis are the primary symptoms.

(ii) Wet Beriberi

As the name implies, this condition is marked by presence of **anasarca (generalized edema)**. In contrast to dry beriberi, onset is marked by pain and tenderness in leg muscles after walking. **There are also palpitation, dyspnoea and congestive heart failure and a risk of passing into acute cardiac failure and death.**

It is associated with marked edema ('pitting') and paresthesia of the extremities.

(iii) Acute Cardiac Beriberi

The patients of acute cardiac beriberi present with suddenly appearing, fulminating cardiac failure, which if untreated results in death within a few hours.

(iv) Infantile Beriberi

This presents as a syndrome and is at times quickly fatal. **It affects infants within the first six months (mostly between one to four months and babies on breast).** Of the two forms, viz., acute and chronic, the former is more lethal and less likely to be correctly recorded because of the abrupt onset of cardiac failure leading to cyanosis and dyspnoea associated with convulsions, coma and death within 24-48 hours. **The whole thing may be over just in a few days.** The infants affected are pale, oedematous and ill tempered; have loss of appetite, **vomiting and green coloured diarrhoeic stools.** There

is a characteristic thin whining cry, at times even aphonia (loss of voice). The involvement of cranial nerves predominates in contrast to that of the spinal in adults. The picture may be confused with encephalitis due to convulsion and coma. The other form, the chronic, is less common and presents a picture resembling marasmus, due to general poor nutrition associated with anorexia, vomiting and diarrhoea, and is less likely, to end fatally.

(v) Wernicke-Korsakoff Encephalopathy

This extremely rare presentation in India is found more in the Western countries and is usually superimposed upon conditions like alcoholism, chronic gastrointestinal disease, carcinoma of stomach, prolonged diarrhoea, hyperemesis gravidarum or, irregularly controlled diabetes. The patient presents with an acute picture of a psychiatric nature- the **Korsakoff's psychosis**, and may progress rapidly to coma and death.

This is characterized by lesions and haemorrhages near the third cerebral ventricle, paralysis of eye movements, depression, severe loss of memory and mental confusion, etc.

In animals, the symptoms are loss of muscular coordination, spastic movements, retraction of the head (opisthotonos), and paralysis (Fig. 17.9). Recovery from the symptoms of **'polyneuritis'** is very rapid when this vitamin is administered, especially by injection.

Debility and progressive decline in weight are observed early in thiamine deficiency due to **anorexia** (loss of appetite). This is one of the most striking symptoms of this deficiency which is due to reduced food intake, ultimately leading to failure of growth. The depression of appetite is related to the failure to metabolize carbohydrate at the point of pyruvic acid decarboxylation (see carbohydrate metabolism, glycolysis - TCA cycle).

In polyneuritis pathological changes in the

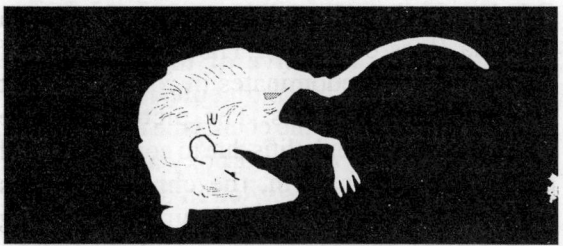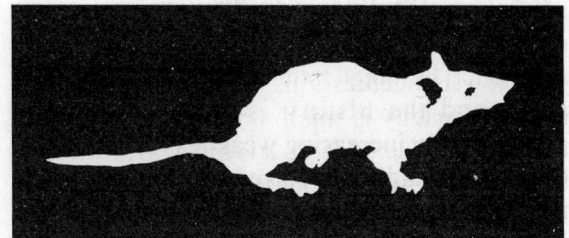

Fig. 17.9 Effect of thiamine deficiency and subsequent change after an adequate diet.

Thiamine deficiency in man leads to the condition known as beriberi, in animals the syndrome is referred to as **polyneuritis.**

Beriberi is not found in advanced countries but is widespread amongst low socioeconomic groups of South-East Asia, where due to poverty B_1 deficient polished rice forms the main food item of their diet.

Nausea, vomiting, anorexia, loss of body weight, lassitude (weariness, heaviness) and rise in blood pyruvate level are found in all types of 'beriberi'.

The vitamin has a characteristic yeasty odour and taste. It is a basic substance and forms insoluble compounds with picric, phosphotungstic and tannic acids. As the pH increases beyond neutrality, thiamine becomes unstable, especially at elevated temperatures. In foods, this is stable at cooking temperatures, though a considerable function gets extracted into the cooking water and may be lost if this is discarded.

The principal ester of thiamine is the pyrophosphate, known as cocarboxylase or diphosphothiamine.

tissues and organs of the body include cardiovascular and neural disturbances, atrophy of the endocrine glands and other vital organs and hypertrophy of the adrenals. **Prolonged deficiency leads to cardiac failure and death.**

Free thiamine is phosphorylated in vivo to a coenzyme known as cocarboxylase i.e., thiamine pyrophosphate by liver and kidney; the phospho-rylating agent is ATP i.e., adenosine-5'-triphosphate. In animal tissues, **cocarboxylase** plays a role in various reactions involving principally the decarboxylation of pyruvic and other keto acids. In erythrocytes, transketolase, an enzyme of HMP shunt of glucose metabolism, requires the participation of cocarboxylase. In the brain, cocarboxylase plays a role in the reduction of pyruvate to lactate and the dismutation to CO_2 and acetate, and their subsequent oxidation to carbon dioxide and water. In liver and other tissue cells, cocarboxylase is involved in the conversion of pyruvate to oxalacetate which combines oxidatively and irreversibly with another molecule of pyruvate to enter the citric acid cycle. The oxidative decarboxylation of ketoglutarate to succinate and of pyruvate to acetoacetate, and the conversion of pyruvate to the acetyl group of acetyl coenzyme-A are additional examples of the reactions found to be mediated by cocarboxylase.

It has been shown by controlled studies in a number of experimental animals, and in man, that the activity of erythrocyte transketolase gets progressively decreased as the thiamine deficiency develops. In man, the addition of cocarboxylase to haemolyzed red cells which were obtained from a thiamine deficient person, restores the transketolase activity towards normal. **Therefore, thiamine occupies a key position in carbohydrate metabolism.** In advanced thiamine deficiency both pyruvate and lactate accumulate in the blood whereas glycogen concentration increases in the liver and heart muscle.

Storage and synthesis of thiamine

It is found to be stored in animal tissues in a very low concentration, meaning to say, it's storage capacity is small. It occurs both in free and phosphorylated form. It is found to be present in somewhat higher concentration in the heart, liver, and kidneys than in muscles and brain. It is possible to increase the thiamine content of the tissues by dietary means, however, total storage capacity is so limited that even under these circumstances only a few weeks' reserve can be maintained. It is, therefore, important that the daily diet should include an adequate supply of thiamine. **In man, this is synthesized by intestinal form, the nutritional importance of this contribution is not known.**

Chemistry

For the first time, it was isolated in crystalline form by Williams. Its structure was elucidated by Williams, Clarke and their co-workers. It consists of a pyrimidine and a thiazole ring system joined by a methylene bridge as shown below:

In acidic medium it may withstand prolonged heating at 120°C; whereas it is rapidly destroyed in alkaline medium. It is not oxidized by atmospheric oxygen under ordinary conditions. Mild oxidizing agents convert it to a pigment known as thiochrome which has got no vitamin activity.

Physiological actions of this vitamin are due to its pyrophosphoric ester, popularly known as cocarboxylase (TPP), which is formed by the phosphorylation of the vitamin under the influence of ATP and magnesium ions.

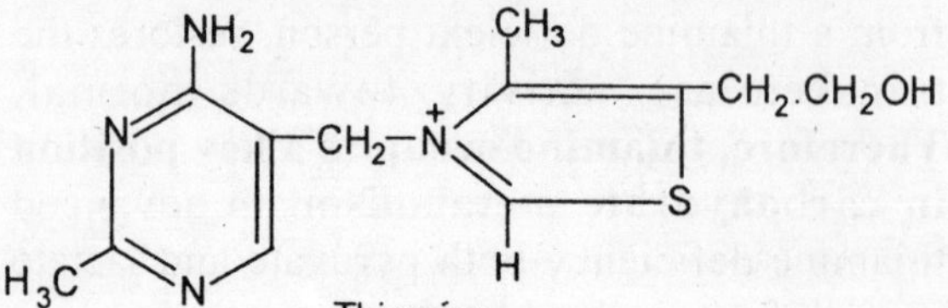

Thiamine

Coenzyme activity of thiamine

An important derivative of thiamine is the pyrophosphate. This molecule is known as cocarboxylase and is the coenzyme or prosthetic group of the enzyme decarboxylase, which is involved in the decarboxylation of α-ketoacids in the body. The structure of thiamine pyrophosphate is shown below.

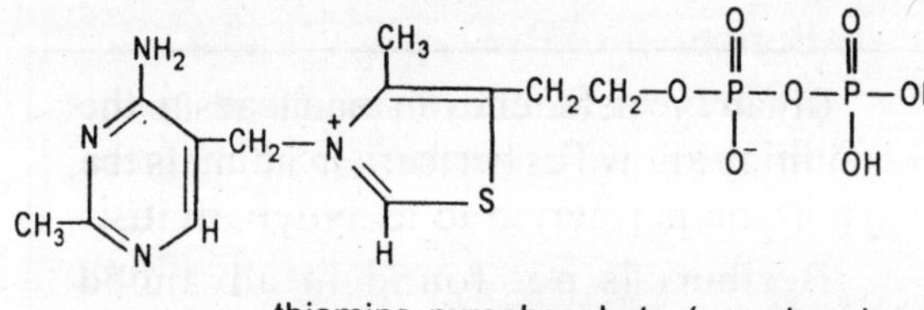

thiamine pyrophosphate (cocarboxylase)

$$CH_3COCOO^- + Pi \longrightarrow CH_3COCOOP + HCOO^-$$

pyruvate   inorganic   acetylphos-   formate
        phosphate   phate

TPP is also involved as a coenzyme in a phosphoroclastic cleavage of α-keto acids.

In such a reaction the acyl of the acid is converted through acyl CoA to acylphosphate and the carboxyl group may become formate.

Deficiency

In humans its deficiency causes a disease called as **'beriberi'**. This disease is rare in the Western world because of food habits and food enrichment. Initially, in this disease, anorexia (loss of appetite), weight loss, fatigue and gastrointestinal-disturbances are noted; whereas in the later stage, cardiac impairment is seen. Administration of the vitamin or foods rich in it is the quick answer of the disease. Most thiamine deficiency states in human beings get aggravated by the deficiency of other B vitamins.

Daily Requirement

The recommended daily requirement is nearly 1 mg (333 IU), but it increases as the intake of carbohydrate increases.

- Its deficiency is generally encountered amongst 'chronic alcoholics' because alcohol interferes with the absorption of thiamine by intestine.
- Principal tissues which are affected by its deficiency include the heart, central nervous system and the peripheral nerves.
- Beriberi is of five types; viz.,
  (a) **Dry or neuritic beriberi:** In this type, inflammation of peripheral nerves may lead to hyperaesthesia, pain, paralysis and wasting of limb muscles, enlarged heart, inflammation of ophthalmic nerve leading to blindness, etc.
  (b) **Wet or edematous beriberi:** Extensive edema in the extremities and heart, congestive heart failure and cardiac enlargement are encountered.
  (c) Acute cardiac beriberi
  (d) Infantile beriberi
  (e) **Wernicke-Korsakoff syndrome:** Characterized by lesions and haemorrhages near the third cerebral ventricle, paralysis of eye movements, abnormal gait, depression, insomnia, disorientation, extreme anxiety, severe loss of memory and mental confusions etc. **This syndrome is produced by B_1-deficiency in patients genetically deficient in transketolase activity.**

Sources

The vitamin is widely distributed in both plant and animal tissues. In plants, the seeds generally contain the highest concentration.

Dry peas, beans and soyabeans are excellent sources. This vitamin is concentrated in the outer layers of the grain kernels. Bran and rice polishings are, thus, good sources. Whole wheat bread and white bread made from enriched flour contain a good supply of thiamine. Yeast is an outstanding source of thiamine and of certain other members of the B complex. Many nuts have a high concentration of the vitamin. Peanuts contain a good supply, whereas Brazil nuts have still more.

Thiamine deficiency causes 'Beriberi' in human beings. Symptoms are anorexia, weight loss, fatigue and GIT disturbances.

Good sources are:
1. Dry peas, beans, soyabeans
2. Bran and rice polishings
3. Whole wheat flour
4. Nuts, yeast
5. Gooseberries and dried prunes, oranges
6. Pork chops and fat ham

Milk contains only one tenth, the amount of thiamine that is found in peanuts, but because the milk is consumed in larger quantity by an individual, therefore, milk is by far considered to be a very good source. Cheese also contains this vitamin.

Among fruits, gooseberries and dried prunes are the richest source of B_1. Oranges have around half the quantity found in figs or prunes.

Many animal tissues are also excellent sources of this vitamin for example pork chops, fat ham, beef cuts, etc.

RIBOFLAVIN (B_2)

Lactoflavin (name rarely used)

This vitamin is also called as B_2 or vitamin G. Pure riboflavin was isolated from milk and other foods in 1933 by scientist Kuhn and his co-workers. Lactoflavin (milk), hepatoflavin (liver), ovoflavin (eggs) and verdoflavin (grass) proved to be chemically identical with riboflavin. In nature, this vitamin is synthesized by all green plants and by most microorganisms.

Chemistry

The flavins are widely distributed in nature. Many derivatives have been studied. Structure of vitamin B_2 is as given below:

Riboflavin

(6,7 - dimethyl - 9 - (D - 1′ - ribityl) - isoalloxazine)

> Secondary deficiency of vitamin B_2 may occur with diffuse intestinal disease or by the prolonged use of psychotropic drugs that interfere with the production of FMN and FAD or by chronic alcoholism; extensive injuries (trauma, burns) and severe chronic debilitating (weakening) diseases. If the deficiency is of very severe nature then, the bone-marrow may become hypoplastic which induces a marked normocytic, normochromic anaemia.

The D in the chemical name of riboflavin indicates that the ribityl group is related to the D series of sugars. The one prime (1′) indicates attachment of the ribityl group at the first carbon atom, and the 9 that this attachment is to position 9 of the isoalloxazine ring system.

Deficiency

In human beings, the deficiency is generally associated with abnormal ectodermal tissue maintenance, the usual signs of which are:

(i) In human beings, the deficiency affects primarily the ectodermal tissues, producing lesion of the skin, eye and nervous system. One of the earliest symptoms is **cheilosis,** manifested at first by transverse fissures at the corners of the mouth, raw and scaly lips, and finally by many vertical, deep fissures.

(ii) Inflammation of the tongue (**glossitis**) : The tongue assumes a purplish or magenta tinge and glossitis (flattening of the papillae) is observed.

(iii) A seborrheic dermatitis: It occurs at the body folds e.g., at the alae nasi, and in the scrotal and vulvar regions.

(iv) The ocular manifestations i.e., corneal vascularization: They include dryness, burning and itching, photophobia and lacrimation, and vascular invasion particularly at the scleral junction of the cornea.

Coenzyme activity

The enzymes containing riboflavin are called flavoproteins. Two coenzymes viz; riboflavin phosphate, or flavin mononucleotide (**FMN**) and flavin adenine dinucleotide (**FAD**). The first flavoprotein isolated was **Warburg's yellow enzyme** which is composed of FMN and apoenzyme (specific protein). The enzyme can be separated into protein and FMN by dialyzing against dilute HCl. No enzyme activity resides in the individual constituents, but upon recombining them activity reappears.

FAD and FMN combine with different apoenzymes to form a large number of oxidation-reduction enzymes. FAD, for instance, is found in xanthine oxidase, D-aminoacid oxidase, aldehyde oxidase and fumaric dehydrogenase. FMN is associated with Warburg's yellow enzyme, cytochrome C reductase, L-amino acid reductase and others. **These enzymes operate in electron transport system.**

The structures of FMN and FAD are shown herewith.

Sources

It is found both in plant and animal sources. Plant seeds synthesize the vitamin during germination, hence germinating seeds are rich in this vitamin. **A few bacteria and the yeasts are very good sources. Other good sources are liver, kidney, eggs, cheese, peanuts, milk, ham, soyabean flour, white bread, dry peas, dry beans, etc.**

Polished rice, cereal foods and potatoes are not good sources but daily consumption of potatoes in the refreshment preparations and lunch or dinner contributes a lot and thus, potatoes are considered to be a very good source of this vitamin.

Daily requirement

Daily requirement ranges from 1.0 to 2.0 mg. During pregnancy and lactation, this allowance should be increased a little.

NIACIN - NICOTINIC ACID, NIACINAMIDE (B₃)
(Pellagra-Preventing (P-P) factor)

The terms niacin and niacinamide have replaced the older terms nicotinic acid and nicotine acid amide (nicotinamide). The latter

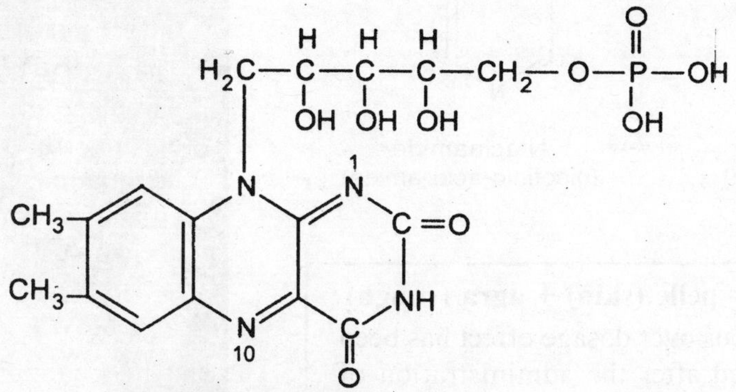

Riboflavin phosphate,
Flavin mononucleotide, FMN

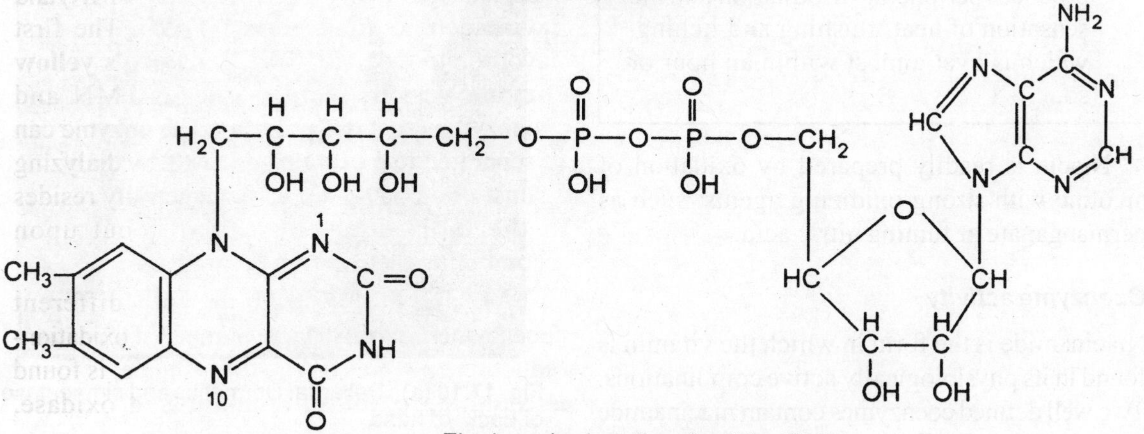

Flavin adenine dinucleotide, FAD

names were found to be undesirable because of the confusion and the unwarranted belief by many that they were physiologically related to nicotine.

The deficiency of this vitamin in human beings causes a disease named as **pellagra** {Fig 17.10 (a & b)} (from the Italian **pelle agra, rough skin**). Funk was the first to isolate the vitamin from rice polishings in 1914.

Chemistry

Niacin or nicotinic acid is pyridine 3-carboxylic acid. Niacinamide or nicotinic acid amide is the acid amide; the structure of these are given below.

Niacin
(nicotinic acid)

Niacinamide
(nicotinic acid amide)

Pellagra = pelle (skin) + agra (rough)

No serious over dosage effect has been identified after the administration of niacin. Parenterally (not orally) it produces peripheral vasodilation and the sensation of heat, flushing and itching, which is over almost within an hour or so.

Niacin is readily prepared by oxidation of nicotine with strong oxidizing agents, such as permanganate or fuming nitric acid.

Coenzyme activity

Niacinamide is the form in which the vitamin is found in its physiologically active combinations. Two well defined coenzymes contain niacinamide

which act with a large group of hydrogen-transport enzymes (oxidation-reduction system).

The first is **NAD** (nicotinamide adenine dinucleotide, coenzyme I (Co I), or diphosphopyridine nucleotide **(DPN)**. It contains nicotinamide-ribose-phosphate-phosphate-ribose-adenine.

The other coenzyme containing niacin is triphosphopyridine nucleotide **(TPN)**, also called as coenzyme II (Co II) or **NADP** (nicotinamide adenine dinucleotide phosphate). This is composed of nicotinamide- ribose-phosphate-phosphate-ribose-2'-phosphate-adenine. It

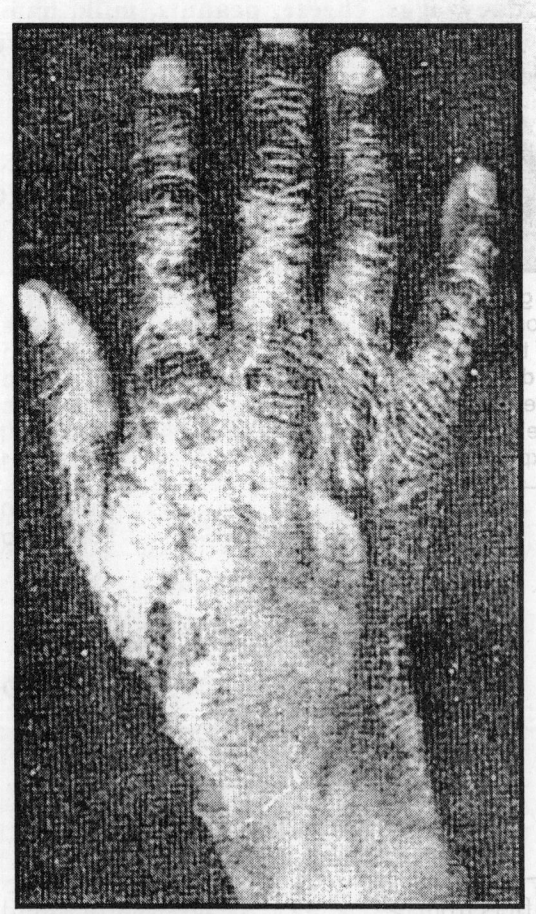

Fig. 17.10 (a) : Pellagra. Dermatitis and pigmentation of back of hand

attached to adenine. It is synthesized from NAD and ATP.

The primary action of the two coenzymes is to remove hydrogen from substrates as part of dehydrogenase enzymes and transfer hydrogen and/or electrons to the next coenzyme in the chain or to another substrate which then becomes reduced. These enzymes are, thus, alternatively oxidized and reduced. NADH represents the reduced form. Many metabolic processes utilize one or other of these coenzymes. The structures of NAD and NADP are as shown below.

Deficiency

Pellagra is especially frequent among people eating corn as a large part of the diet. In some degree this may be explained by low tryptophan content of corn.

The flushing syndrome is well known in human beings taking nicotinic acid either by

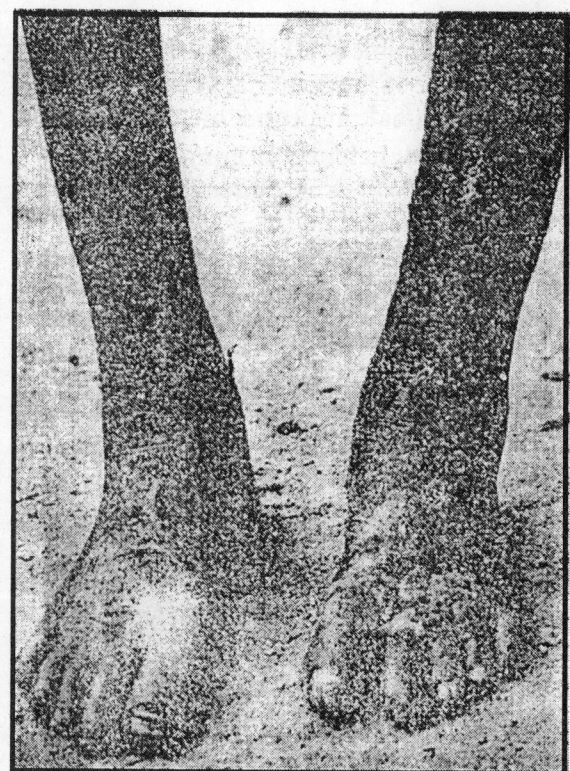

Fig. 17.10 (b): Pellagra, a changed concept: Considered a maize eaters' disease in other parts of the world, **it has been found in jowar eaters in India,** a finding that has almost radically changed the concept of its pathogenesis. This patient shows well marked skin lesions sharply limited to the areas exposed to sun.

> The prevalence of pellagra is high in areas of the world where the diet is limited to maize (corn), molasses and salt pork, with very little lean meat or other sources of animal protein.
>
> In body, niacin may be synthesized in sufficient quantities by tryptophan, therefore, sufficient intake of tryptophan will never allow the deficiency symptoms of niacin to develop.

differs from NAD only in the presence of a third phosphate group on carbon 2 of the ribose

NAD or DPN or CoI

NAD or DPN or Co I where R = H
NADP or TPN or Co II where R = PO (OH)$_2$

mouth or parenterally. The amide does not produce these symptoms. It is the niacinamide which is found in natural sources of the vitamin. Some individuals flush with only a few milligrams of niacin, while others are able to take 100 mg without untoward effects. Many people flush on the intravenous administration of 5 or 10 mg of niacin.

Serum cholesterol is lowered in human beings after the ingestion of large doses of nicotinic acid. In young adults the basal metabolism is also increased. The mechanism by which blood cholesterol is lowered has not yet been resolved.

Sources

In natural sources the vitamin occurs as free nicotinic acid, bound nicotinic acid, or nicotinamide in coenzyme form.

The vitamin is found to be present both in plant and animal tissues. Certain animal organs, e.g. liver, kidney, heart, lean meat and some fish flesh are outstanding sources.

As regards plant sources, peanuts, wheat germ, dried legumes and yeasts are also outstanding sources. Fresh legumes and a few green vegetables are good sources whereas milk, eggs and most fruits are poor sources. Niacin, like other B vitamins resides in wheat primarily in the bran and middling fraction.

Requirement

A diet providing 60g of mixed protein contains around 600 mg of tryptophan or 10 niacin equivalents from the amino acid. Recommended daily allowance for an average adult weighing 70 kg is 19 mg niacin equivalents and upto 22 for boys of the age group of 15-18 years (68 kg).

Role of Diet

It is a disease of those whose staple diet is maize. Maize actually contains more nicotinic acid than

Niacin (nicotinic acid) is a vitamin used as a precursor of the nicotinamide moiety of the nicotinamide nucleotides.

Niacin deficiency in humans causes 'Pellagra' which is characterized by 3D's i.e.

(a) Dermatitis

(b) Diarrhoea and

(c) Dementia

In 1926, Goldberger and co-workers demonstrated that foods rich in 'water soluble B' were effective curing the symptoms of pellagra in man and black tongue in dogs. In 1937, Elvehjem and co-workers were able to isolate nicotinic acid amide from liver, which they found to be a cure for black tongue in dogs and pellagra in man.

Both nicotinic acid and its amide are active, the latter being preferred in medical practice because of its better tolerance than the former. In order not to confuse these compounds with nicotine they have been given the names niacin and niacinamide.

Pellagra is generally common in low-socioeconomic group. The disease starts with inflammation of the skin on the back of the hands {Fig 17.10 (a)}, forearms and neck. The skin becomes brown and scaly and finally open sores develop. The tongue becomes red and swollen and ulcers develop beneath it. Gastrointestinal disturbances, nausea, diarrhoea, intestinal ulcers are common. Nervous symptoms like insomnia and headache appear and in advanced stage, mental deterioration is also seen.

60 mg of tryptophan = 1 mg of niacin

oats, rye and white wheaten bread. Pellagra is not found in those who consume besides maize, wheat and rice also. Maize has 6.7 niacin equivalents per 1000 Kcal and levels less than 4.4 are needed to produce pellagra.

Besides occurring primarily in maize eaters, pellagra **has been reported in India in jowar eaters though,** there is no deficiency of nicotinic acid in that cereal.

Milk administration cures pellagra, though it contains very little nicotinic acid.

Pellagra is not encountered in populations who consume appreciable quantities or proteins of animal origin with nicotinic acid content not necessarily high.

The curative value of milk (and other animal proteins) has been found to be in its tryptophan content. Body can evidently synthesise nicotinic acid from tryptophan

Pellagra is not found in people who treat maize with lime (Mexico and Central America). This has been explained on the basis of the fact that in maize, niacin is found in a bound form and lime treatment releases it.

PANTOTHENIC ACID (B$_5$)

[Filtrate factor; chick antidermatitis factor (name rarely used)]

In 1933, Williams and co-workers demonstrated the widespread distribution of a substance that acted as a growth factor for yeast and other microorganisms. At that time these workers gave the name as pantothenic acid (Greek, from every where) to the active principle.

Chemistry

Chemically, pantothenic acid is α, γ-dihydroxy-β, β-dimethylbutyryl-β'-alanide. Its structure is as shown below:

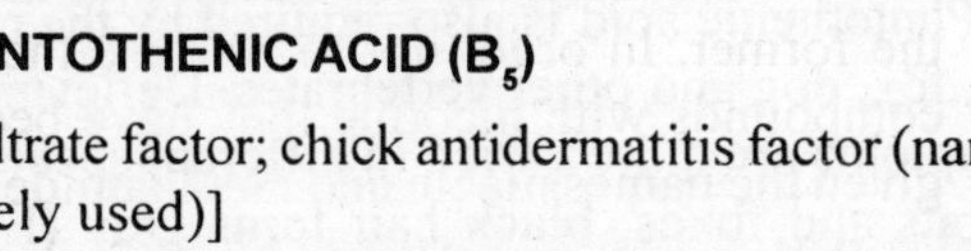

$$
\begin{array}{cccccccc}
H_2 & CH_3 & OH & O & H & & H_2 & H_2 \\
| & | & | & \| & | & & | & | \\
C & - C & - C & - C & - N & - C & - C & - COOH \\
| & | & | & & & & & \\
OH & CH_3 & H & & & & &
\end{array}
$$

Pantothenic acid

It is a condensation product of β-alanine and a hydroxyl-and methylsubstituted butyric acid. It is a pale yellow, unstable, viscous oil. The natural or vitamin active form of pantothenic acid is the dextrorotatory isomer. Commercially, it is synthesized as the calcium and sodium salts, in either dextrorotatory or racemic form, the latter having half the potency of the former. Pantothenic acid is soluble in water, ethyl acetate, dioxane and glacial acetic acid and is slightly soluble in ether and amyl alcohol and insoluble in chloroform and benzene. Being water-soluble, much of the pantothenic acid of a food may be lost in cooking if the cooking water is poured off.

Biochemical functions of pantothenic acid

Identification of pantothenic acid as part of the coenzyme A molecule has given this vitamin tremendous value in biochemistry i.e., biochemical reactions. **Scientist Lipmann and associates studied in depth about the role of coenzyme A vis-a-vis pantothenic acid.** Coenzyme A is the only known functional form of pantothenic acid in plant tissues, animal tissues and microorganisms, meaning by this vitamin is component of coenzyme A, the cofactor required for the metabolism of two-carbon compounds, notably acetyl groups. **In addition to the main contribution in acetylation reactions, it is also required for adrenocortical activity i.e., for the biosynthesis of cortical hormones.**

The physiologically active form of pantothenic acid in the animal organism appears to be coenzyme A (CoA) whose molecule contains pantothenic acid, mercaptoethylamine, adenine, ribose and phosphoric acid. CoA is readily synthesized by animal tissues provided pantothenic acid is supplied in the diet. **CoA participates in a wide variety of reactions involved in:**

(a) **Carbohydrate metabolism,**

(b) **Fatty acid synthesis and metabolism,**

(c) Propionate metabolism, and

(d) Branched chain fatty acids metabolism

Coenzyme A is found in larger quantities in liver if compared to the adrenals and other tissues where it is found in lesser quantities. There may be as much as 400 mg of CoA per kg. of liver. Lipmann has summarized many reactions in which CoA gets involved:

Acetyl Transfer

1. ATP - CoA - acetate:
   $ATP+CoA+Ac \rightarrow Ac-CoA+AMP+PP$
2. Phosphotransacetylation:
   $Ac - P + CoA \rightarrow Ac - CoA + P$
3. Formotransacetylation
   $Pyruvate + CoA \rightarrow Ac - CoA + formate$
4. Transacetylation
   $Ac-CoA+butyrate \rightarrow butyryl\ CoA+Ac$
5. Acetoacetate
6. Citrate
7. $Acetaldehyde+CoA+NAD \rightarrow Ac-COA$
8. $Pyruvate + CoA + NAD \rightarrow Ac - CoA + NADH + CO_2$

These reactions are examples of donor systems. The examples of acceptor systems may be: acetokinases (for aromatic amines, choline, histamine, amino acids and glucosamine) and condensation reactions (for acetoacetate, citrate and pyruvate).

Succinyl Transfer

As a donor system,

$\alpha\text{-Ketoglutarate}+NAD+CoA \rightarrow Succinyl\ CoA + NADH$

and as an acceptor system, the example may be the role of succinyl CoA in the synthesis of heme.

Benzoyl Transfer

Hippuric acid synthesis is an example.

Complex Synthesis

CoA is also involved in complex systems like fatty acid synthesis, butyrate and fatty acid oxidation, fat synthesis, steroid synthesis, etc.

Effects of Deficiency

The effects of deficiency are:

- growth failure in chick,
- dermatitis in chick,
- graying of the hair in rats and other animals,
- adrenal necrosis in the rat, and
- haemorrhage in the rat.

Pantothenic acid is essential in the diet of poultry. If it is deficient in the diet of hens, they produce eggs of low hatchability. If it is deficient in the diet of chicks, they develop dermatitis. Scales appear at the corners of the mouth and the neighbouring skin becomes inflamed. The chick dies in two or three weeks. Feeding calcium pantothenate cures this condition.

Pantothenic acid is also required by the rat, pig, fox, dog and other vertebrates. Deficiency symptoms are quite varied in different species. In rats and foxes, black hair turns gray (Fig. 17.11) when their diet is devoid of pantothenic acid. The gray hair turns black again when calcium pantothenate is fed to them. In dogs, the symptoms include respiratory disturbances, degeneration of kidneys and liver, and inflammation of the digestive tract.

Besides being widely distributed in plant and animal sources, this vitamin is also synthesized by intestinal microorganisms in humans, therefore, deficiency symptoms in them are rarely met with. However, its deficiency symptoms may include neuromotor disorders.

Cardiovascular instability, gastrointestinal distress, susceptibility to infections and mental depression - all these signs of deficiency disappear when pantothenic acid or its salts are added to the diet.

Distribution

It is widely distributed, and remains present in all living tissues whether of plant or animal origin. Excellent sources include:

(a) liver   (b) kidney

(c) egg yolk   (d) peas

(e) peanuts   (f) rice bran

(g) molasses   (h) yeast

(i) skimmed milk   (j) butter milk

(k) cabbage   (l) cauliflower etc.

It is also found in appreciable amount in sweet potatoes, wheat, barley, oats, rye and broccoli. Wheat germ is a rich source, but the content of milled white flour is rather low.

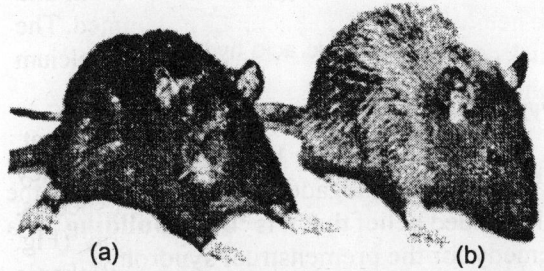

(a)   (b)

Fig. 17.11 Pantothenic acid deficiency in a rat. These rats were litter mates, both originally black. Their diet, after weaning contained no pantothenic acid but the one on the left side (a) received 100 micrograms of this vitamin daily. After three weeks on this diet, the animal (b) on the right side showed evidence of graying which gradually became more pronounced. Other deficiency symptoms included scaly dermatitis, inflammation of the nasal mucosa and hemorrhages in various organs, particularly in the adrenal cortex.

Its poor sources include beets, turnips, egg white, prunes, raisins, canned peaches, canned peas, beans and apples.

> **Tea contains significant amount of vitamin B$_3$ (Pantothenic acid).**

Daily Requirement

For human beings, the daily requirement is generally accepted as 10 mg, which is the amount usually consumed daily by an individual with approximately 2,500 calories of an adequate diet.

PYRIDOXINE GROUP (B$_6$)

Vitamin B$_6$ includes pyridoxine (which was the first one to be isolated), as well as pyridoxal and pyridoxamine, which were discovered later on by microbiological assay. The structures of them are as given below:

Pyridoxine   Pyridoxal

Pyridoxamine

Any of the three members of this group are active biologically.

Biosynthesis

A limited amount of pyridoxine can be synthesized by the bacterial flora of the gut.

Biochemical functions

1. It plays a very important role as a coenzyme in the intermediary metabolism of amino acids and complex glycolipids.

2. The active coenzyme form of vitamin B$_6$ is known as pyridoxal phosphate.

3. The enzymes which require pyridoxal phosphate as a coenzyme are:

   (a) **Amino acid decarboxylases.**

   (b) **Transaminases.** Among the several transaminase reactions, only those between glutamate and pyruvate to form alanine and between glutamate and oxaloacetate to form aspartate are reversible. In the deficiency of B_6, naturally, the activity of transaminase becomes slow.

(c) **Racemases.** These are the enzymes that catalyze the formation of an equilibrium mixture of DL-alanine from either D-or L-alanine.

(d) **Enzymes** involved in tryptophan metabolism e.g. tryptophanase, which converts tryptophan to indole, pyruvate and ammonia.

(e) **Cystathionase.** This enzyme is involved in the conversion of cystathionine to serine and homocysteine.

- Pyridoxine exists in the form of pyridoxal phosphate in the cells and functions as a coenzyme for a variety of chemical reactions concerned with the amino acids and protein metabolism.
- Its important role is that of coenzyme in the transamination process for the synthesis of amino acids.
- It is also believed to facilitate the transport of some amino acids across the cell membranes.

Distribution

It is widely distributed in vegetables, fruits, grains, meats and other foodstuffs; therefore its dietary deficiency is not at all common.

Deficiency States:

However, secondary deficiency states may be produced by long-term use of a variety of drugs such as isoniazid (**used in the treatment of tuberculosis**).

Alcoholism may also lead to its deficiency. In addition, there is a group of uncommon inborn errors of metabolism known as pyridoxine-dependency syndromes, which require massive doses of this vitamin.

However, a lack of vitamin B_6 has been associated with dermatitis, glossitis, cheilosis, and in infants and children diarrhoea, anaemia, peripheral neuropathy and sometimes convulsions. In rats several symptoms are observed as shown in Figure 17.12.

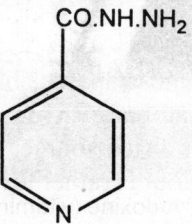

Isonicotinic acid hydrazide

Hypervitaminosis

A severe neuropathy has been described in patients taking megadoses of pyridoxine in the ill-founded belief that it is '**body building**' or a remedy for the premenstrual syndrome.

Antagonist

Isonicotinic acid hydrazide is a potent antagonist of B_6 which is extensively used as a potent antitubercular drug.

BIOTIN (VITAMIN H, NAME RARELY USED)

Biotin is known by a variety of names i.e. bios, vitamin H, coenzyme R and **the antiegg-white injury factor.**

As early as 1916, the toxicity of diets rich in egg white was observed. Later on, scientist Boas described egg white injury in those rats which were fed a diet containing raw egg white as the source of protein. She described muscle incoordination, dermatitis, loss of hair and

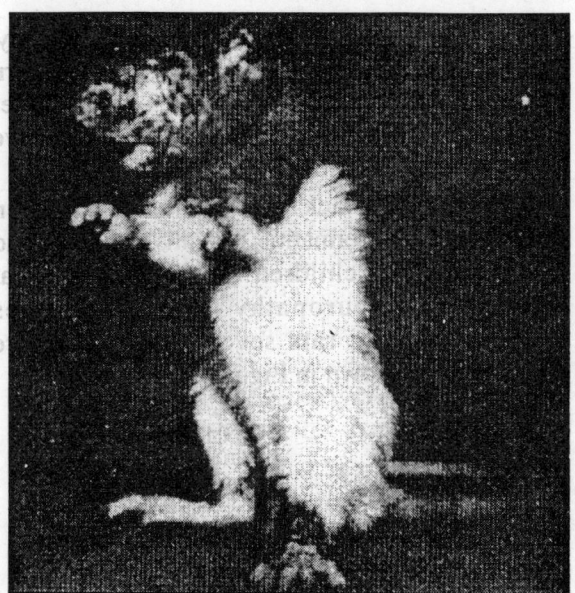

Fig. 17.12 : Pyridoxine (vitamin B deficiency in a rat, characterized by dermatitis of the extremities, beginning with swelling of the ears, nasal region, and paws and followed by crust formation on these areas.

nervous manifestations as the symptoms of this syndrome. She observed that cooked egg white was not toxic and that liver, yeast and certain other foods apparently contained a substance that protected rats against the toxicity of the raw egg protein; this protective substance was called vitamin H by Gyorgy. Lease and Parsons showed that chicks were subject to egg white injury. Williams and co-workers some six years later demonstrated that egg white injury in rats and chicks was actually due to an antivitamin in egg white; this substance is a basic protein and is known as **avidin**, and its ability to inactivate biotin was later on confirmed in 1941.

Biotin was isolated as crystalline methyl ester from egg yolk, yeast, liver and milk. Its structure was established by du Vigneaud and his associates as 2-keto-3, 4-imidazolido-2-tetrahydrothiophene-n-valeric acid.

Chemistry

1. Biotin is a monocarboxylic acid, only slightly soluble in water and alcohol.

2. Its colourless crystalline needles melt between 231° - 232°C.

3. The vitamin is destroyed by acids and alkalies only on rigorous treatment and by oxidizing agents such as peroxide and permanganate.

4. It is soluble in dilute alkali and hot water and practically insoluble in organic solvents.

5. In natural products it occurs mainly in bound form. One of the simple biotin compounds isolated is: **biocytin which can be hydrolyzed by an enzyme known as biotinidase.**

6. It is a cyclic compound containing two rings, i.e., a cyclic ureid and the other a reduced thiophene ring. A valeric acid side chain remains attached to the reduced thiophene ring.

It structure is as shown below:

$$
\begin{array}{c}
O \\
\parallel \\
C \\
HN \qquad NH \\
| \qquad\qquad | \\
HC \qquad CH \\
| \qquad\qquad | \;\diagup H \\
H_2C \qquad C - CH_2 - CH_2 - CH_2 - CH_2 - COOH \\
\diagdown \;\;\; \diagup \\
S
\end{array}
$$

Biotin

Physiological and biochemical properties of Biotin

It appears to be necessary for certain biochemical reactions. It may serve as a coenzyme. It may also be necessary for enzyme synthesis. Its main roles are as mentioned below:

1. The role in carboxylation and decarboxylation reactions.

It plays a key role in carboxylation reactions involving CO_2, fatty acids and various dicarboxylic acids. Thus, it participates in such reactions as the interconversion of pyruvic and oxaloacetic acids, of propionic and succinic acids and of oxalosuccinic and α-ketoglutaric acids; in the synthesis of citrulline from ornithine, of serine from CO_2 and of fatty acids from acetyl CoA.

In 1958, Wakil and Gibson provided the

— Deficiencies of this vitamin are difficult to produce experimentally because it is synthesized by intestinal flora in higher animals.

— Biotin is an essential food factor and is coenzyme for carboxylation.

— Biotin is the prosthetic group in a number of carboxylation reactions, and functions as a carrier of CO_2

— **The protein material from egg white, avidin is denatured and inactivated by heating, therefore, egg should not be taken in raw state.**

— Avidin, if not denatured by heating, then forms a stable complex with biotin, resulting in inactivation of the biotin.

CH$_2$COS.CoA + CO$_2$ + ATP
Acetyl CoA

Mn++
Acetyl CoA
Carboxylase

HOOC. CH$_2$COS.CoA + ADP + Pi
Malonyl CoA

---

evidence that biotin is required for carboxylation reactions by first observing that CO_2 was required for fatty acid synthesis and that use of the enzymes of fatty acid synthesis contained large amount of biotin. Biotin remains tightly bound to the enzyme. The biotin-enzyme catalyzes the carboxylation of acetyl CoA to malonyl CoA according to the following reaction:

Now a days, several biotin-enzymes that are involved in carboxylation reactions have been isolated and characterized, the examples of which are propionyl CoA carboxylase, pyruvic acid carboxylase, β-methylcrotonyl CoA carboxylase, etc.

2. It plays a role in the deamination of certain amino acids, and

3. It also plays a role in the synthesis of oleic acid by certain lactic acid-producing bacteria.

Deficiency

1. Deficiencies of this vitamin are difficult to produce experimentally because it is synthesized by intestinal flora in higher animals. However, deficiency symptoms may be induced by feeding either materials (such as avidin) which combine with the biotin to form non absorbable complexes or sulfa drugs which interfere a lot with bacterial synthesis of this vitamin in the intestines.

2. One of the first symptoms of biotin deficiency in young animals is cessation i.e. check of growth which is followed by a typical dermatitis (Fig. 17.13). Scales develop around the mouth and between the toes and the eyelids may become granular and stick together.

3. Rats, chicks and human beings develop a dermatitis as mentioned above when fed large quantities of raw egg white. This so-called **'egg white injury'** may be

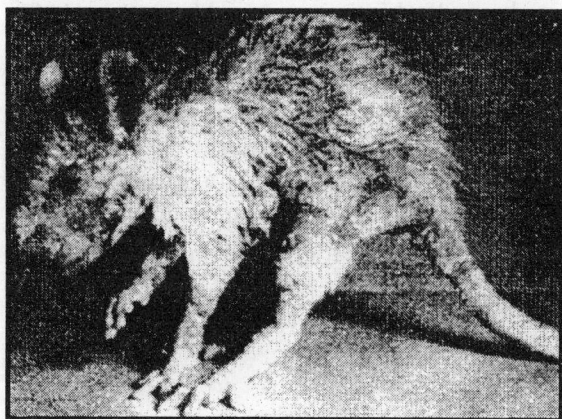

Fig. 17.13 : Biotin deficiency in a rat. This animal had been on a diet containing 35% uncooked dried egg white as the sole source of protein. Alcoholic extract of yeast supplied vitamin B complex. Although not biotin-free, the uncooked egg white combines with the biotin, making this unavailable to the animal. This deficiency is characterized by swelling and redness of the lips, denuded areas and brown scaliness of the skin with extensive dermatitis. Later, the eyes become gummed shut, the edema of the paws increases and nerve involvement is shown by progressive spasticity. In advanced cases, the rat exhibits the so-called "kangaroo posture" as seen here.

easily prevented by boiling the egg before feeding. Raw egg white contains a protein called **'avidin',** which combines with biotin and thus prevents its absorption, as a result of which symptoms of biotin deficiency develop.

4. In human volunteers, raw egg-white feeding leads to low urinary biotin level, depression, nausea, easy fatigue, incoordination of movements, dermatitis, etc.

5. Clinical cases of its deficiency in man are very rare. **In a rare genetic deficiency of holocarboxylase synthase** which makes helpful the utilization of biotin in several metabolic roles, the affected child is unable to utilize biotin, as a result of which he/she suffers from dermatitis, loss

of hair, incoordination of movements, poor growth and high urinary lactate, β-hydroxypropionate and β-methylcrotonate.

Sources

Biotin remains present in a variety of foodstuffs. It is found in abundance in liver, kidney, peas, yeast, cauliflower, egg yolk, milk etc. It is found in lesser amount in other foodstuffs i.e. a variety of vegetables, cereals and nuts.

For man and some other animals, synthesis by bacteria in the intestinal tract is an important source.

Requirement

150 to 300 μg per day for man.

FOLIC ACID (PTEROYLGLUTAMIC ACID), VITAMIN B₉ OR VITAMIN M (NAME RARELY USED)

Sources

Folic acid is found abundantly in nearly all natural foods which include fresh or fresh-frozen, uncooked vegetables and fruits. Good sources are green leafy vegetables and yeast. Grain also, contains this vitamin. Sufficient amounts may also be obtained through bacterial synthesis in the intestine or the rumen.

Daily requirement

Adult man or woman: 0.1 mg; pregnant women: 0.3 mg; lactating women: 0.15 mg; infants and children: 0.05 - 0.1 mg.

Chemistry

Folacin or folic acid or pteroylglutamic acid (PGA) is composed of one molecule each of p-aminobenzoic acid, glutamic acid and the pigment pteridine. It is a yellow crystalline substance and is slightly soluble in water. It is soluble in dilute alcohol. Its structure is as shown below:

Functions

1. **Folic acid helps in the transfer and metabolism of one-carbon compounds.** It is firstly reduced to H_4 folate (5, 6, 7, 8-tetrahydrofolate) by the enzyme dihydrofolate reductase in the presence of NADPH. H_4 folate is the active form of folic acid which may receive C_1 groups such as the formyl, methyl, methenyl, methylene and formimino groups on its N^5 and/or N^{10} from different substrates during their catabolism: H_4 folate then acts as a carrier and donor of these C_1 groups to other substrates as the coenzyme for many one-carbon group transferases.

2. Role as a coenzyme: Various coenzyme

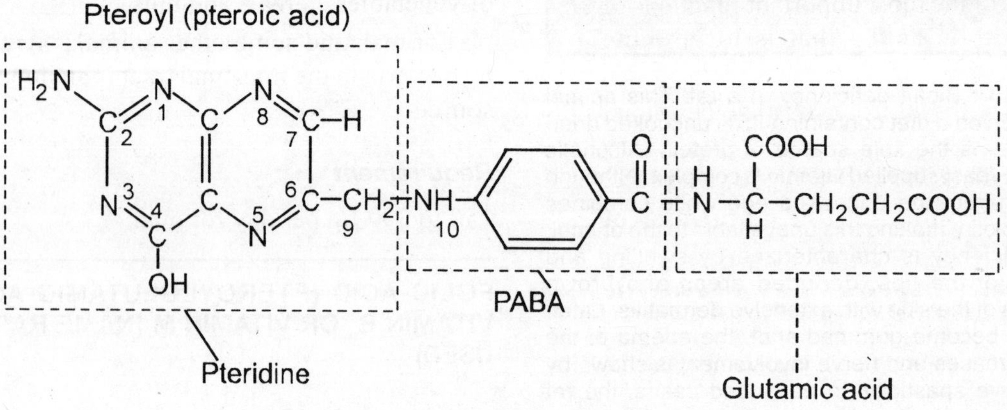

Pteroyl (pteroic acid)

Folic acid, pteroylglutamic acid (PGA)

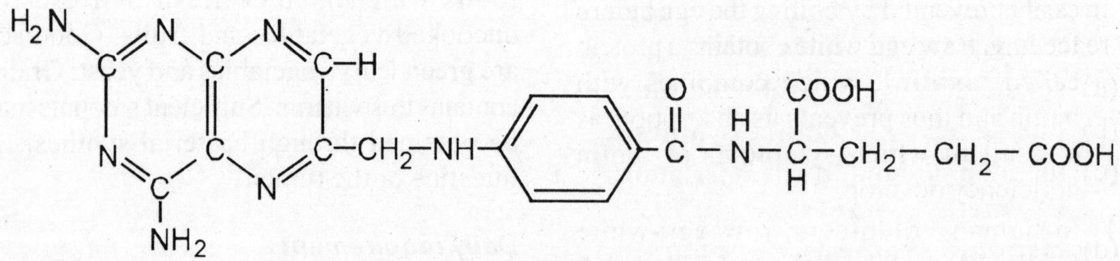

Aminopterin (4 - Amino PGA)

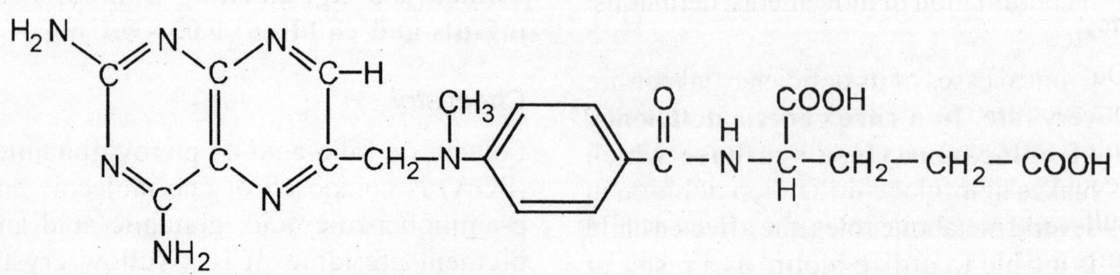

Amethopterin

— It functions as a carrier of hydroxymethyl and formyl groups.

— **Perhaps its most important use in the body is in the synthesis of purines and thymine,** which are required for the formation of deoxyribonucleic acid i.e. DNA. Therefore, this vitamin i.e., folic acid, like vitamin B_{12} is also required for the replication of cellular genes. This, probably explains one of the most important functions of the folic acid - that is to promote growth.

— If it is absent from the diet, the animal shall not grow properly i.e., very unsatisfactory growth will take place.

— **It is required for the maturation of red blood cells.**

— **Its deficiency causes macrocytic anaemia.**

— **Its deficiency also causes megaloblastic anaemia.**

forms of folic acid play an important role in a variety of important metabolic reactions as shown below:

(a) **serine-glycine interconversion,**

(b) **purine acid pyrimidine synthesis,**

(c) **methionine-homocysteine relations i.e., methyl synthesis,**

(d) **histidine synthesis,**

(e) **formiminoglutamate formation, etc.**

Deficiency

1. Deficiency of folic acid is difficult to produce in most of the animals unless intestinal bacterial growth is inhibited by feeding certain types of drugs, such as sulfonamide drug or antibiotics. Folic acid antagonists like aminopterin and amethopterin have also got a tendency to produce its deficiency.

2. In man, its deficiency causes macrocytic anaemia, which resembles pernicious anaemia except that the nervous involvement of the latter condition is absent.

3. Folic acid deficiency occurs most commonly among pregnant women because of their increased need for this nutrient.

4. Its deficiency symptoms have also been observed in chronic alcoholics and drug addicts; such people generally belong to the affluent society and do not believe in the consumption of green fresh vegetables and fruits.

5. Its deficiency also causes megaloblastic anaemia.

6. Its deficiency is also responsible for diarrhoea, gastrointestinal lesions and other related symptoms.

7. Folic acid is also effective in treating pernicious anaemia, although it is without effect on the nervous symptoms, which respond to vitamin B_{12}.

8. The **sprue syndrome** and some other types of anaemia in humans also respond to folic acid therapy.

Determination of the absorption of folic acid

For determining the absorption of folic acid-folic acid labelled with tritium is given by mouth to the patient and then the radioactivity is determined in the serum three hours later.

Folic acid antagonists

There are two well known antagonists of folic acid named as **aminopterin and amethopterin** whose structures are as given on page 258.

Folic acid antagonists namely aminopterin and amethopterin bear a striking resemblance to folic acid.

> *Aminopterin* has been used with some success to obtain temporary relief in some cases of **acute leukaemia** in children.

These antagonists inhibit the enzymatic reduction of folic acid to tetrahydrofolic acid (FH_4) by binding very tightly to the enzyme. Such kind of inhibition results in blocking a number of reactions involving FH_4 and its derivatives - e.g.

(a) amino acid synthesis

(b) methyl group synthesis and

(c) purine synthesis from formate

VITAMIN B$_{12}$ (COBALAMINE)

(**Cyanocobalamine**, cobamide, antipernicious **anaemia factor, 'extrinsic factor' of Castle**)

Antipernicious anaemia factor from liver extract was isolated in 1948 by Rickes and co-workers and by Smith. This factor is known as '**animal protein factor**' and has got the capability to cure pernicious anaemia and is now termed as vitamin B_{12}. It is found in animal tissues in the form of a conjugate with a polypeptide.

For the first time, **pernicious anaemia** was treated successfully by Minot and Murphy in 1926. In 1929, Castle suggested that gastric mucosa forms a carbohydrate-rich protein known as **intrinsic factor** which, together with a factor present in the food (**extrinsic factor**), forms a system responsible for the proper maturation of the erythrocytes. **People with pernicious anaemia do not make this protein. Pernicious anaemia turned out to be a genetic defect of the stomach, rather than a dietary deficiency disease.** With the isolation of vitamin B_{12} and its dramatic action in cases of pernicious anaemia, the extrinsic factor has been identified. Vitamin B_{12}, when injected, restores the red cell count to normal and also improves the functioning of central

nervous system as well.

It has been suggested that the commercial vitamin cyanocobalamine does not normally occur in nature, but is an artifact of the isolation procedure.

Chemistry

1. **Vitamin B$_{12}$ is a dark red compound containing one atom of cobalt which remains linked to four reduced pyrrole rings, forming a macro ring. The structure of vitamin B$_{12}$ is given in Fig. 17.14.**

The central portion of the molecule is composed of four reduced and highly substituted pyrrole rings namely A, B, C and D around cobalt atom; this structure bears a close, but not complete resemblance to the porphyrins. The

> — B_{12} is known to act as a coenzyme in the methylation of homocysteine, and in a reaction in which methyl malonyl CoA is converted to succinyl CoA. Both of these reactions involve methyl group transfer.
> — In pernicious anaemia, the maturation of erythrocytes is greatly delayed.
> — Intramuscular injection of B_{12} induces a rapid increase of peripheral blood.
> — Biochemical action of the B_{12} in the process of red blood cell production is unknown.
> — **Plant tissues are devoid of B$_{12}$**
> — It is abundant in animal tissues, especially in the liver, kidney, pancreas, adrenal and pituitary and as well as in fish and oysters. **Milk and eggs are also good sources.**
> — Microorganisms in the digestive tracts of ruminants have got the capability to synthesize vitamin B_{12}

central structure is referred to as a 'Corrin' ring system. Below the corrin ring system, there is a 5, 6-dimethylbenzimidazole riboside, which remains connected at one end to the central cobalt atom and at the other end from the ribose moiety (Fig. 17.14).

Addition of cyanide forms 'cyanocobala-

mine' which is identical with the originally isolated vitamin B_{12} and the removal of cyanide group results in the formation of the compound known as **'cobalamine'. Cyanide group if substituted by a hydroxy group forms** 'hydroxycobalamine'; replacement by a nitro group accordingly forms 'nitrocobalamine' and

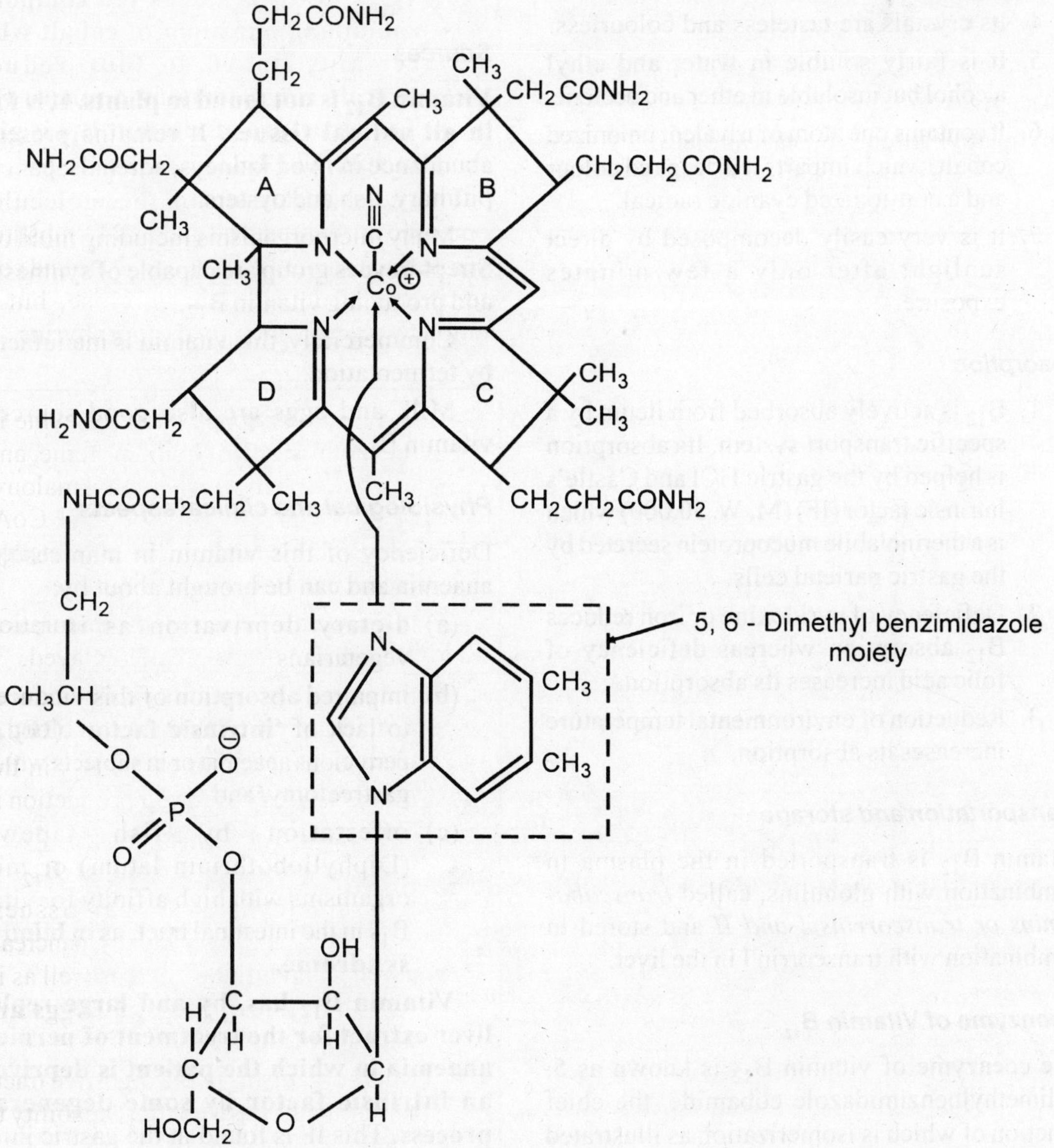

5, 6 - Dimethyl benzimidazole moiety

Fig. 17.14 : Vitamin B_{12}, $C_{63}H_{88}N_{14}O_{14}PCo$

by a methyl group forms 'methylcobalamine'. It contains nearly 4.35 per cent cobalt in its molecule.

2. Cyanocobalamine has a net charge of one.

3. Its molecular weight is 1490 ± 150 and its empirical formula is $C_{63}H_{88}N_{14}O_{14}PCo$.

4. Its crystals are tasteless and colourless.

5. It is fairly soluble in water and ethyl alcohol but insoluble in ether and acetone.

6. It contains one atom of trivalent unionized cobalt, which imparts it a deep red colour and a non-ionized cyanide radical.

7. It is very easily decomposed by direct sunlight after only a few minutes exposure.

Absorption

1. B_{12} is actively absorbed from ileum by a specific transport system. Its absorption is helped by the gastric HCl and Castle's intrinsic factor (IF) (M. W. 50,000) which is a thermolabile mucoprotein secreted by the gastric parietal cells.

2. Deficiency of pyridoxine or iron reduces B_{12} absorption whereas deficiency of folic acid increases its absorption.

3. Reduction of environmental temperature increases its absorption.

Transportation and storage

Vitamin B_{12} is transported in the plasma in combination with globulins, called *transcobalamins or transcorrins I and II* and stored in combination with transcorrin I in the liver.

Coenzyme of Vitamin B_{12}

The coenzyme of vitamin B_{12} is known as 5, 6-dimethylbenzimidazole cobamide, the chief function of which is isomerization as illustrated by the following equation:

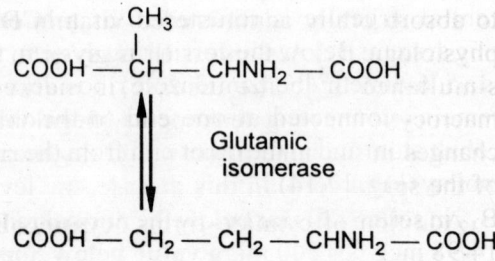

Sources

Vitamin B_{12} is not found in plants. It is found in all animal tissues. It remains present in abundance in liver, kidneys, adrenals, pancreas, pituitary, fish and oysters.

Many microorganisms including mold of the Streptomyces group are capable of synthesizing and producing vitamin B_{12}.

Commercially, this vitamin is manufactured by fermentation.

Milk and eggs are also good sources of vitamin B_{12}.

Physiological and clinical aspects

Deficiency of this vitamin in man results in anaemia and can be brought about by:

(a) dietary deprivation as in case of vegetarians

(b) impaired absorption of this vitamin due to lack of **'intrinsic factor' (IF)** as in pernicious anaemia or in subjects with total gastrectomy, and

(c) infestation by fish tapeworm (Diphyllobothrium latum) or micro-organisms with high affinity for vitamin B_{12} in the intestinal tract, **as in blind loop syndrome.**

Vitamin B_{12} has, by and large replaced liver extract for the treatment of pernicious anaemia in which the patient is deprived of an intrinsic factor by some degenerative process. This IF is found in the gastric juice of healthy subjects. Patients devoid of IF are unable to absorb orally administered vitamin B_{12} in physiological doses unless IF is given to them simultaneously. The disease is marked by macrocytic anaemia, leukopenia, megaloblastic changes in the bone marrow and degeneration of the spinal cord. In this disease, the level of B_{12} in serum falls far below the normal range of 14-98 mcg per 100 ml, **a value below 8 mcg is considered diagnostic of pernicious anaemia.** The symptoms are reversed by the parenteral administration i.e. intramuscular injection of cyanocobalamine. A daily dose of one or two micrograms given intramuscularly for one week produces a therapeutic response, whereas 5 mcg daily by mouth with intrinsic factor (gastric mucopolysaccharide) or a single dose of 5,000 mcg orally without IF will be effective.

Metabolic functions

This vitamin participates in a number of metabolic functions as described below:

1. Purine biosynthesis: **It plays a role in the formation and synthesis of nucleic acid.**
2. Synthesis of labelled methyl group: Vitamin B_{12} increases the biosynthesis of the methyl group from precursors such as the α-carbon of glycine and β-carbon of serine. The α-carbon of glycine and the β-carbon of serine or formate are utilized less efficiently in the absence of vitamin B_{12}.
3. Its deficiency impairs transmethylation.
4. It plays an important role in the stimulation of protein synthesis, especially incorporation of amino acids into proteins.
5. **Vitamin B_{12} plays a role in the conversion of carbohydrate to lipid.** Vitamin B_{12} deficiency can be corrected by the parenteral administration of glutathione (GSH) or by the injection of vitamin B_{12}. Dietary deprivation of vitamin B_{12} results in a decrease in the

reduced glutathione content and in the enzyme which degrades glucose to ribose, in the red blood cells and in the hepatic $NADH_2$ and in the increase of CoA. Be it known that hepatic $NADH_2$ is necessary for the maintenance of the activity of enzymes involved in lipid metabolism.

Effects of deficiency

Symptoms of vitamin B_{12} deficiency are those of pernicious anaemia as mentioned below:

1. **achlorhydria (no HCl in gastric juice)**
2. **severe macrocytic and megaloblastic anaemia**
3. **neurological degeneration and**
4. **glossitis**

> **Animal proteins are the sole source of this vitamin.** The animals, in turn, acquire the vitamin from microorganisms growing in soil, water and their intestinal tract.

Requirement

Daily requirement is as follows:

(a) Adult man/ woman: 1 μg
(b) Pregnant or lactating woman: 1.5 μg
(c) Infants and children: 0.2-1 μg

ASCORBIC ACID (VITAMIN C)

(The Antiscorbutic Vitamin)

This is one of the water-soluble vitamins. This is also known as Vitamin C, whose absence gives rise to **scurvy.** At one time 'scurvy' was supposed to be the most common disease amongst sailors whose foods were found to be devoid of green fresh vegetables and citrus fruits because of the fact of their nonavailability during such long voyages. **This disease is characterized by a tendency of bleeding and pathological changes in the teeth and gums. Supplementation of their diets by lime and**

lemon juice cured all the symptoms of 'scurvy'.

Dietary deficiencies of this vitamin are sometimes encountered in chronic alcoholics, the very elderly people who live on a 'tea and toast' diet and the neglected underprivileged poor of the world who are generally unable to afford citrus fruits and fresh green vegetables.

Chemistry

In its chemical properties, it is quite strongly acidic, owing to the ionization of the two hydroxyl groups separated by the double bond. **Szent-Gyorgi** isolated the crystalline compound from paprika plant and named it hexuronic acid. It was later on isolated by **King** from lemon juice. The true configuration of the molecule was established by **Haworth** in his laboratory in 1933 in England.

The pure substance is optically active and is soluble in water. It is a very strong reducing agent. It is easily oxidized by air, especially in the presence of traces of metal ions like Cu^{++} or Fe^{+++}.

It is also oxidized even by dissolved oxygen at room temperature, particularly if Cu^{2+} ions are present. **The first oxidation product is dehydroascorbic acid.**

It melts at 190 - 192°C and is stable for years in crystalline form. Its taste is sour. It is insoluble in most organic solvents. It readily forms salts of several metals. It takes up iodine at the double bond and can be reduced by hydrogenation.

Synthesis

Plants and all animals except pigs, man and other primates have an ability to synthesize ascorbic acid. The rat, for instance, is resistant to scurvy. In animals, probably the main sites for its synthesis are the liver and adrenals (cortex). In plants, all tissues contain vitamin C except woody tissues or seeds, although it remains present in the early stages of germination.

On the basis of many studies in recent years, the following scheme is presented for the biosynthesis of ascorbic acid in non-primates, which probably is also applicable to plants:

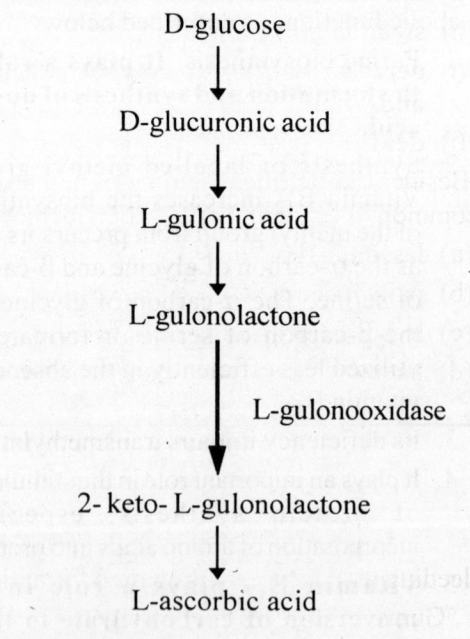

D-glucose
↓
D-glucuronic acid
↓
L-gulonic acid
↓
L-gulonolactone
↓ L-gulonooxidase
2- keto- L-gulonolactone
↓
L-ascorbic acid

The defect in man that prevents the synthesis of ascorbic acid is the absence of the enzyme L-gulonooxidase.

O = C ———
| |
HO — C |
|| |
HO — C   O
| |
H — C ——— |
|
HO — C — H
|
CH₂OH

L-Ascorbic acid, $C_6H_8O_6$

Ascorbic acid can also be synthesized from another sugar i.e. D-galactose via D-galacturonic acid, L-galactonic acid, L-galactono-γ-lactone, and 2-keto-L-galactonolactone.

Deficiency Symptoms

Deficiency of this vitamin causes a disease named 'Scurvy' (Fig. 17.15). In its extreme form it is characterized by:

(a) **weakness**

(b) **loss of teeth and shrinkage of gums**

(c) **weakened blood vessels, particularly microvessels** having the least muscular support

(d) **peripheral haemorrhages**

(e) **defective synthesis of osteoid (a derivative of collagen)**

(f) **failure of wounds to heal**

(g) **failure of fractures to heal**

(h) **swollen and painful joints**

(i) **decreased ability to combat infections and often**

(j) **death**

Besides, **'subclinical scurvy'** is perhaps not uncommon; the symptoms of which include:

(a) lassitude (heaviness)

(b) pain in back

(c) hyperkeratosis of the hair follicle

(d) haemorrhage around the hair follicles

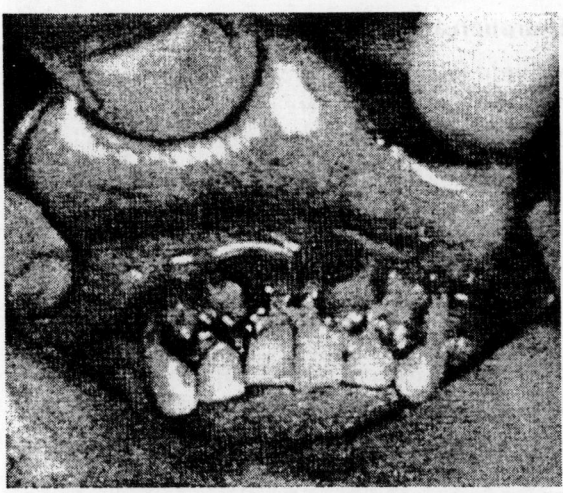

Fig 17.15 : Scurvy. Gingival swelling and petechiae

Diagnosis

Diagnosis of scurvy is made by X-rays which reveal skeletal abnormalities and sometimes microfractures, low plasma levels of vitamin C, urinary excretion measurements following administration of vitamin C (saturation test) and increased capillary fragility test (positive tourniquet test). Bleeding time (BT) and coagulation time (CT) are usually normal.

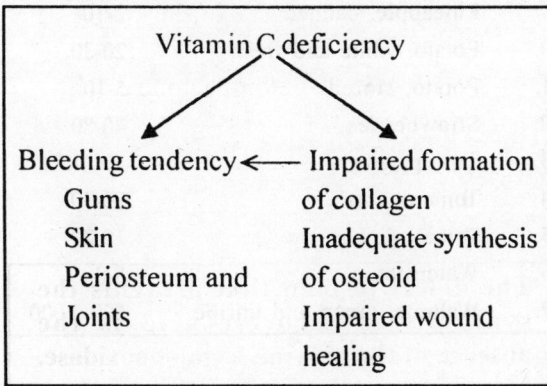

Test for Ascorbic acid deficiency

Inflate a blood pressure cuff over the upper arm and observe the red blotches (eruptions upon the skin) in the skin of forearm which is due to severe deficiency of ascorbic acid.

Cause. On inflating the cuff, venous return of blood gets occluded as a result of which, the capillary pressure rises which leads to the rupture of capillaries because of the fact that blood vessels become fragile in 'scurvy' and as a result many small petechial haemorrhages beneath the skin cause purpuric (pertaining to skin disease) blotches which may be seen easily in the forearm.

Excretion and storage

Vitamin C is not excreted by the kidneys until the body tissues are saturated and the concentration in the blood exceeds a certain level. Vitamin C is not stored, as are vitamins A and D in the body fat. Deprivation of this vitamin results in a gradual decrease of the tissue levels. The decrease in vitamin C levels is reflected in the blood, particularly in the leucocytes. Replacement of vitamin C in the diet brings the patient back to health quite rapidly. Saturation, shown by excretion of the vitamin in the urine occurs in less than two weeks.

Biochemical functions

1. **The major function of vitamin C appears** to be in the formation of normal collagen.
2. In the formation of hydroxyproline from proline.
3. In the formation of hydroxylysine from lysine.
4. In the oxidation-reduction reactions. This property is concerned with the hydroxylation of aromatic compounds and thus in the metabolism of tyrosine and is also possibly involved in the hydroxylation of the steroid nucleus.
5. Absorption and utilization of iron: Vitamin 'C' helps in the intestinal absorption of iron by reducing Fe^{3+} to Fe^{2+} and by forming water soluble iron-ascorbate chelates. Besides this, it also increases the utilization of iron by reducing Fe^{3+} of tissue ferritin to Fe^{2+} for its release into plasma.
6. Hydroxylation of dopamine to norepinephrine: In adrenergic neurons and chromaffin cells of adrenal medulla, a Cu^{2+}-protein known as dopamine β-hydroxylase utilizes L-ascorbate as an electron donor in hydroxylating dopamine to norepinephrine.

Daily requirement

1. It is established that the minimum amount of ascorbic acid required to prevent or cure scurvy in an otherwise healthy adult is about 10 mg daily or less. It has been argued, however, that the daily intake should be sufficient to saturate the body tissues. This amount is 60 to 100 mg daily depending upon the age, size and associated stressful conditions, such as wound healing or whether a woman is pregnant or lactating.
2. Studies of Hodges and associates have indicated that in **a healthy, normal adult, 45 mg daily is quite satisfactory.**

Ascorbic acid content of various routine food items are as mentioned in Table 17.2.

Table 17.2 : Ascorbic acid content of some routine food items

Sl. No.	Food	Ascorbic acid (mg per 100 g)
1.	Apple	3-10
2.	Beans, green (canned)	2-5
3.	Cabbage, fresh	40-70
4.	Cabbage, cooked	15-20
5.	Lemon juice	40-60
6.	Lettuce, head	5-10
7.	Orange juice	40-70
8.	Pineapple, fresh	20-30
9.	Pineapple, canned	2-10
10.	Potato, white and fresh	20-30
11.	Potato, stored	5-10
12.	Strawberries	40-80
13.	Turnip, green	100-150
14;	Tomato, fresh	20-30
15.	Tomato juice	10-20
16.	Watermelon	5-8
17.	Walnuts, green and unripe	500-2,000

MAIN PHYSIOLOGICAL/BIOCHEMICAL FUNCTIONS OF VITAMIN C

1. Collagen biosynthesis
2. Antioxidant property
3. Formation of hydroxyproline
4. Formation of hydroxylysine
5. Absorption and utilization of iron
6. Synthesis of chondroitin sulfates
7. Maintenance of the folate pool
8. Synthesis of neurotransmitters

MAJOR SOURCES

1. Fresh fruits (especially citrus)
2. Vegetables

MEGADOSE CONTROVERSY OF VITAMIN C

Some physicians are of the opinion that the intake of Vitamin C in large doses (nonphysiologic quantity of Vitamin C) helps in curing the attack of common colds and as well as advanced cancers, but the controlled scientific studies do not prove these above myths. An occasional individual may experience some slight alleviation of symptoms, probably because large doses of vitamin C have got a mild antihistaminic effect. In cases of metastatic cancer, megadose of vitamin C has been proved to be of no value in either way.

Contrarily, in large doses it predisposes to oxalate and urate urinary tract stones, may be responsible for aspirin-induced gastric erosions, interacts with the metabolism of some drugs, **unnecessarily increases intestinal absorption of iron and may lead to iron overload and may be responsible for various other side-effects.**

LIPOIC ACID (THIOCTIC ACID)

This vitamin for the first time was isolated from yeast and later from various animal tissues like liver, etc. This is treated to be an essential growth factor for various microorganisms but not for mammals.

It is a cyclic disulfide containing a carboxyl group which is attached to a protein by means of an amide linkage, probably to lysine. Its structure is as shown below:

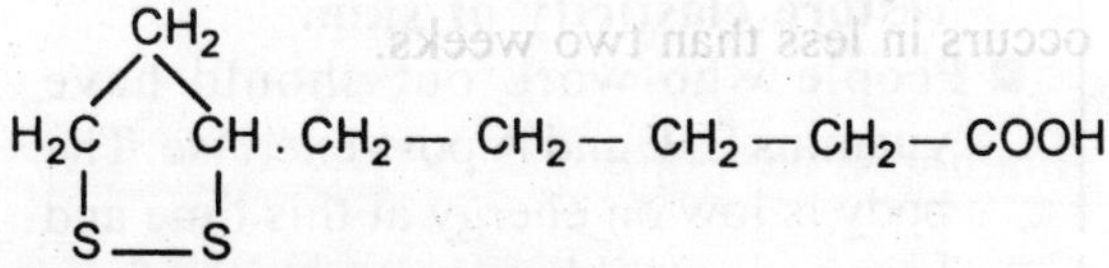

$$CH_2$$
$$H_2C \quad CH . CH_2 - CH_2 - CH_2 - CH_2 - COOH$$
$$S - S$$

Lipoic acid or thioctic acid

Main biochemical function of this vitamin is that it participates in the enzymatic oxidative decarboxylation of α-keto acids at a stage between thiamine pyrophosphate and coenzyme A. In oxidative decarboxylation, loss of CO_2 is accompanied by oxidation of an aldehyde to an acid. Important examples of the oxidative decarboxylation reactions are the ones involving enzymes like pyruvate dehydrogenase, oxoglutarate dehydrogenase, etc. as shown below:

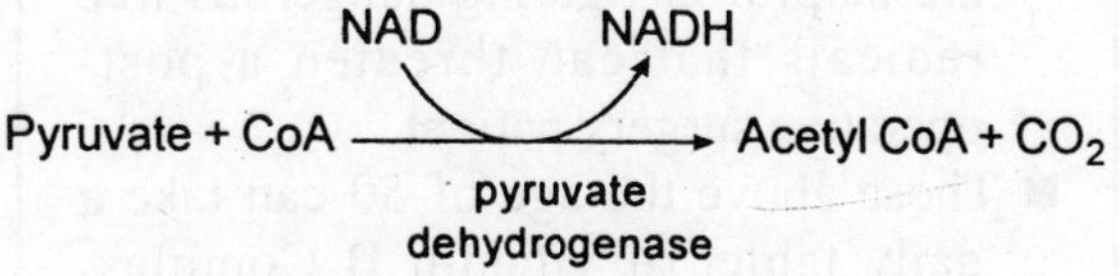

$$\text{NAD} \quad \text{NADH}$$
$$\text{Pyruvate + CoA} \longrightarrow \text{Acetyl CoA + CO}_2$$
$$\text{pyruvate}$$
$$\text{dehydrogenase}$$

The pyruvate dehydrogenase enzyme has a complex mechanism, which involves binding sites for pyruvate, NAD^+, thiamine pyrophosphate and lipoic acid. Acetyl Co A thus formed now enters the tricarboxylic acid cycle as discussed in the chapter of carbohydrate metabolism.

MAKE VITAMINS WORK FOR YOU

- Children between eight and 16 years should have adequate vitamin A which helps in vision improvement and boosts the immune system.
- **Pregnant women should take vitamin B Complex with folic acid, which is good for foetal growth.**
- **Menopausal women should have vitamins C, E and B Complex. These will check excessive bleeding and restore elasticity of skin.**
- People who work out should have vitamins C, E and A post-exercise. The body is low on energy at this time and hence susceptible to easy attacks from the free radicals that are deadly for our constitution.
- People who are constantly on the computer are exposed to the danger of **Carpel Tunnel Syndrome,** which affects the region between the elbow and the index finger, which is active while using the mouse. Vitamin B Complex works as both, a preventive as well as a curative device.
- During PMS syndrome, vitamin B_6 reduces irritability.
- Vitamin B_{12} helps in depression.
- Vitamins C, E and A are antioxidants and are helpful in fighting dangerous free radicals that can threaten a post-operative surgery patient.
- Those above the age of 50 can take a daily tablet of vitamin B Complex, containing vitamin B_{12} and folic acid.
- Vegetarians, who do not consume milk and milk products, should take vitamin B_{12} daily.

WAYS TO MAXIMISE VITAMIN ABSORPTION

- Do not refrigerate vegetables and fruits (raw and uncut) **for more than two days.**
- Don't go by the advertisements that show refrigeration not slowing down loss of nutrients from fruits. It can't stop the process altogether and fruits certainly do not get any fresher by refrigerating them for a long time.
- **Eat your fruits whole rather than cutting them into pieces.** When exposed to air (oxygen), vital vitamins are lost. **By that logic, raw fruits are better than fruit juices and pies.**
- Take a sunbathe around 9 A.M. for 15-20 minutes and you do not need to pop any vitamin D supplements, except if otherwise advised by a medical practitioner.
- Give full attention to food while eating rather than sharing the meal with your favourite soap on TV, so that your parasympathetic nervous system is dominant and the digestive system works to its optimum level.

DANGER: OUR DAILY DIET DECONSTRUCTED

Today there are more reasons why one should have vitamin tablets/ tonics daily. The increased consumption of processed foods like **pizza, pastries, fried chips and burgers** (basically foods that do not have any nutrients) make it essential to supplement the diet with pills. Caffeinated products like tea, coffee, all types of aerated drinks and chocolates should be minimised, if not abstained from, as they prohibit the absorption of vitamins. Alcohol and tobacco products are even worse.

CHAPTER 18

COMPOSITION AND METABOLISM OF MUSCLE

> Muscles play the same role especially for the males (men) which lipstick, powder, face creams, hair etc. play for the females (women) in increasing their beauty and look (appearance). These days, even the females are becoming more fond of muscles but the craze for the same is manifold more in male youngsters. That is why a good number of males are joining 'gym' and this joining gets enhanced by several folds during summer vacation of the students. Males are rather more crazy and concerned for their `biceps' and `triceps' rather than their counterparts.

STRUCTURE OF SKELETAL MUSCLE

Even the smallest skeletal muscle is made up of very large numbers of muscle cells, sometimes called muscle fibres. The individual cells, from 1 to 120 mm long or more in man, and from 10 to 100 μm in diameter have a tough outer membrane, the sarcolemma about 10 nm thick. Most of the space within each cell is occupied by numerous myofibrils about 1 μm in diameter, and the remainder by sarcoplasm (cytoplasm) containing several nuclei together with a network of tubules known as the sarcoplasmic reticulum. **The size of the cells and the amount of tissue lying between them increases with age; exercises which strengthen muscles and increase their bulk produce an increase in the cross-sectional area of the muscle cell.** At the end of the muscle cells, the myofibrils are in contact with the sarcolemma which at this position shows complex folds into which the collagen fibres of the tendon are fitted.

When examined by the ordinary light microscope, muscle fibres appear to be transversely striated and these striations are due to alternating zones of different refractive index within the myofibrils. The A (anisotropic) bands are birefringent having a high refractive index, whereas the I (isotropic) bands have a lower refractive index. In most preparations of striated muscle tissue, the A bands show up more deeply coloured. In the centre of each I band is a Z line (Fig. 18.1) which is, in fact, a disc of material running across the whole muscle fibre and joining the myofibrils to each other. The central region of the A band is paler and is known as the H (Hensen's) band (Fig.18.1). The region between one Z line and the next is known as a sarcomere. The length of a sarcomere varies between 1.5

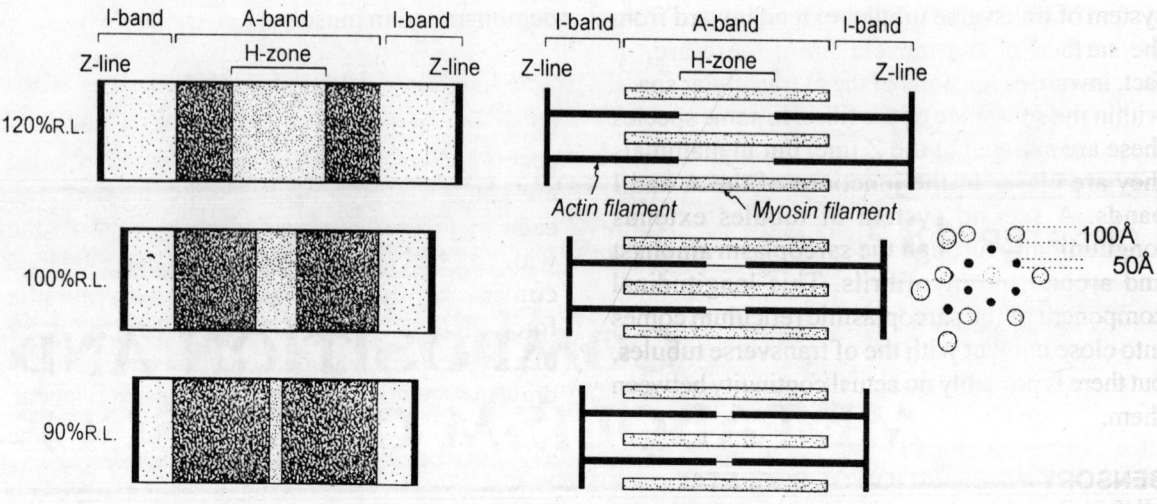

Fig. 18.1: Diagrammatic representation of the structure of skeletal muscle. The three diagrams on the left show the appearances as seen with the phase contrast or interference microscope at various percentages of the resting length (R.L.). Note that the A band remains constant in length, about 1.5 μm in the rabbit muscles. The diagrams on the right show the arrangement of the filaments in muscle in both longitudinal and transverse section.

and 3.0 μm depending upon the state of extension of the muscle fibres.

Electron microscope photographs (Fig. 18.1) give more information about the structure of myofibrils. Each myofibril contains a system of longitudinal filaments arranged in a regular pattern (Fig.18.1). In the I bands thin filaments consisting mainly of the protein actin are attached to the Z line (or Z disc as it may more appropriately be called). In a transverse section of the myofibril, these thin filaments are seen to be arranged in a hexagonal pattern. The thin filaments extend into the A band where they interdigitate (interlocking of parts by finger - like processes) with a system of thicker filaments consisting mainly of the proteIn myosin. Here, too, there is a regular arrangement of filaments; the thick filaments are about 45 nm apart, and each thick filament is surrounded by six thin filaments (Fig.18.1).

As the muscle changes in length, the thick

and thin filaments slide over each other; during shortening, the thin filaments move progressively further in between the thick filaments, and the I band becomes correspondingly narrower, though the A band remains of the same width. At the shortest muscle lengths, there is a region in the centre of the A band into which the thin filaments do not extend; this is the paler H zone, which becomes wider as the muscle fibre length increases.

Each thick (myosin) filament carries a series of side chains which project outward toward the six adjacent actin filaments; six such side chains occur in a helical arrangement over a distance of 40 nm. These side chains play an important part in the mechanism of muscle contraction. The central part of the thick filament does not have them.

Amongst the myofibrils is a system of fine tubules, the sarcoplasmic reticulum, which is important in activating muscle contraction. A system of transverse tubules extend inward from the surface of the muscle fibre; these are, in fact, inward extensions of the extracellular space within the substance of the fibre. In some species these are situated at the Z line, but in mammals they are closer to the junctions of the A and I bands. A second system of tubules extends longitudinally through the sarcoplasm amongst and around the myofibrils. This longitudinal component of the sarcoplasmic reticulum comes into close contact with the of transverse tubules, but there is probably no actual continuity between them.

SENSORY INNERVATION OF SKELETAL MUSCLE

Skeletal muscle contains many sense endings; some of these give rise to sensations of discomfort or pain when the muscle is fatigued.

Myasthenia gravis:

In myasthenia gravis in man, the quanta of acetylcholine are only about one fifth of the normal size and although the normal number of quanta may be discharged on the arrival of a nerve impulse, the muscle fibres may fail to contract. In this condition there is severe muscular weakness going on to paralysis. It can usually be corrected by an anticholinesterase such as neostigmine. A hormone from the thymus may be responsible for reducing the size of the quanta. **Excess of acetylcholine at a neuromuscular junction (cholinergic crisis) also causes muscular weakness.** This condition may be mitigated by cholinesterase reactivators which are used as antidotes to **'nerve gases'.**

It has long been known that in tissues innervated either with adrenergic or with cholinergic endings, the effect of denervation is to increase their sensitivity to the direct application of noradrenaline or of acetylcholine respectively, and this change can readily be

demonstrated in muscle.

THE CONTRACTILE MECHANISM:

Changes in the length of a muscle fibre are accompanied by movements of the thin (actin) and the thick (myosin) filaments in relation to each other with corresponding changes in the width of the I bands. A. F. Huxley has produced convincing evidence for the view that the forceful contraction of a muscle fibre is the result of a sequence of chemical reactions that actively draw the actin filament along the myosin filament.

A cyclical reaction is postulated in the course of which links form between the thin filaments and side chains of the thick filaments; the formation of such a link, however, is accompanied by a change in the mechanical properties of the thick filament, the side chains of which now tend to flex, taking the thin filaments along with them in a shortening movement. Having shortened, the cross-link now becomes within the orbit of an enzyme system which tends to break it down. The side chain then resumes its original position and the cycle can begin again with the formation of a new cross link at another point on the thin filament, The sequence of events is illustrated in Figure 18.2.

Fortunately, the behaviour of contracting myofibrils can be examined after destruction of the membranes of the muscle fibre by immersion in glycerol at low temperatures. In such a preparation, chemical agents can be applied directly to the myofibrils. Contraction occurs when ATP is added to glycerinated muscle fibres in the presence of free calcium ions and some magnesium ions; during the course of this contraction ATP is converted to ADP and it is this conversion that provides the energy necessary for the mechanical work done during shortening. If, in such a preparation, the available supply of ATP becomes exhausted, the reaction ceases but the fibres remain stiff; **a state that is analogous to the 'rigor mortis' that**

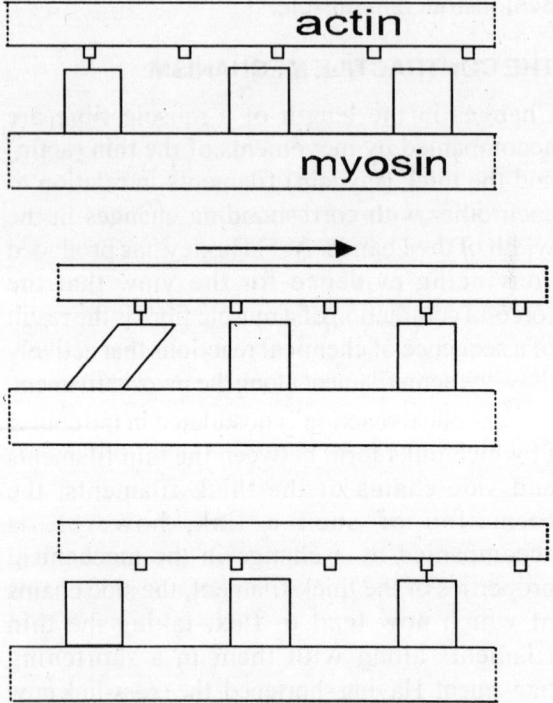

Fig. 18.2: Diagram showing, very schematically, the possible mode of action of cross-bridges. A cross-bridge attaches to a specific site on the actin filament, then undergoes some configurational change which causes the point of attachment to move closer to the centre of the A band pulling the actin filament along in the required manner. At the end of its working stroke, the bridge detaches and returns to its starting configuration, in preparation for another cycle. During each cycle, probably one molecule of ATP is dephosphorylated. Asynchronous attachment of other bridges maintains steady force.

occurs when ATP disappears after death. This stiffness in the absence of ATP implies that the reaction has ceased with the filaments linked together, that is the ATP is used in the stage of uncoupling the thin filaments from the myosin side chains.

Calcium ions play a crucial part in the contractile process; in the absence of calcium ions, the myofibrils remain inactive, and evidently no links are formed between the thick and thin filaments. But, on the other hand, an intracellular microinjection of calcium ions can initiate a local contraction of the myofibrils. Indeed, it is now becoming clear that a release of calcium within the muscle fibre is the physiological method of initiating a muscle contraction, and the removal of this free calcium brings the contraction to an end.

In addition to actin and myosin, muscle contains the 'modulating' proteins tropomyosin and troponin which remain present in the thin filaments. They seem in some way to control the onset and end of contraction by providing a receptor mechanism for Ca^{2+}. In the absence of Ca^{2+}, these proteins allow relaxation by inhibiting the primary actin-myosin interaction. It has been suggested that Ca^{2+} is bound to troponin, and tropomyosin exerts a predominantly stimulating effect on the Mg^{2+} activated interaction between actin and myosin. In some such manner the presence of Ca^{2+} abolishes the inhibitory effect of these modulating proteins and permits the ATPase-stimulating and physicochemical interactions between actin and myosin to proceed.

Chemistry of skeletal muscle (Muscle proteins, etc.) (Figures 18.3 A, B, C & D)

Skeletal muscle contains about 75 percent of water, 20 percent of protein, and 5 percent of other materials. Of the structural proteins in muscle, the most important are the contractile substances myosin, actin and tropomyosin B, which together comprise more than half the total protein content. The remaining proteins include albumin, globulin X and stroma protein. All the enzymes which catalyse the various steps in the process of glycolysis are included in the protein fraction.

Muscle also contains in the sarcoplasm of the cell, the respiratory pigments, myoglobin and cytochrome which function in the transport of oxygen from the blood to the oxidising systems.

Fig. 18.3 A

Proteins of muscle

Muscle consists of fibres, which in turn are composed of fibrils. It is at the level of fibrils that the molecular level is approached.

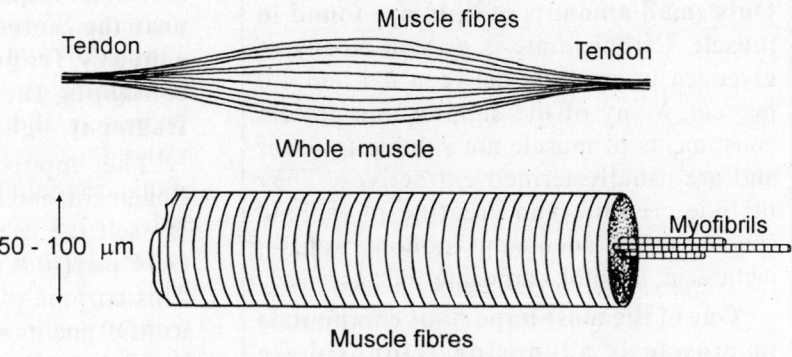

Fig. 18.3 B.

Within the muscle fibre, the fibrils are closely associated with the sarcoplasmic reticulum.

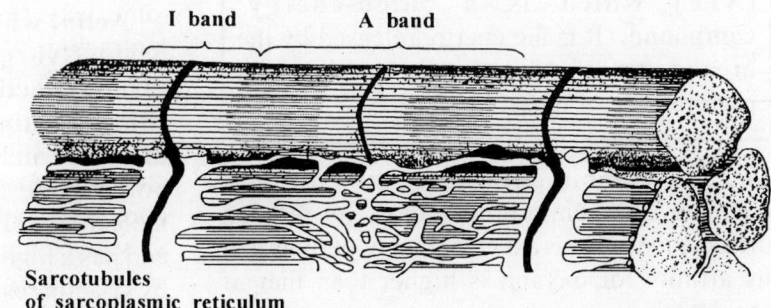

The sarcoplasmic reticulum contains one major protein, a Ca²⁺ stimulated ATPase. When the muscle is stimulated, the sarcoplasmic reticulum releases Ca²⁺, which is needed for the contractile process. The Ca²⁺ is then pumped back into the sarcoplasmic reticulum by the Ca²± stimulated ATPase.

Fig. 18.3 C.

The myofibrils contain the protein myosin, and an assembly of the proteins actin, troponin and tropomyosin.

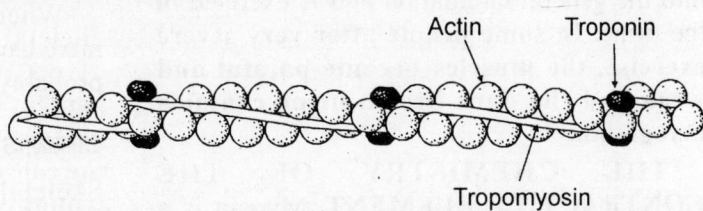

These assemblies of actin, troponin and tropomyosin are termed as the thin filaments. These slide against the thick filaments of myosin during contraction.

Fig. 18.3 D.

The thick filaments are bundles of myosin molecules, with the myosin headpieces protruding from the side of the bundle.

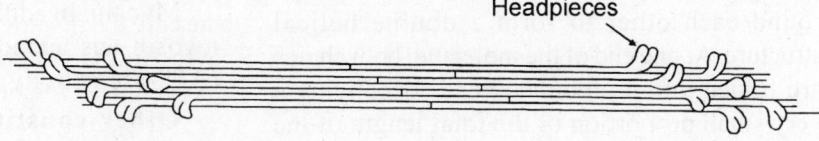

Only small amounts of lipid are found in muscle. Carbohydrate is present mostly as glycogen in amounts between 0.5 and 1.0 percent. Many of the simpler non-protein constituents of muscle are soluble in water and are usually termed extractives. They include creatine and creatine phosphate (phosphagen), adenosine monophosphate, lactic acid, inositol, carnosine and anserine.

One of the most important compounds in muscle is adenosine triphosphate (ATP) which is a 'high-energy' compound. It is the energy released by the breakdown of ATP that is used in the performance of muscular work.

Since myoglobin does not show allosteric changes, as haemoglobin does., its oxygen dissociation curve is a rectangular hyperbola and its affinity for oxygen is higher than that of haemoglobin.

After certain forms of injury such as automobile accidents, there may be prolonged crushing of muscle which reduces its blood supply and finally brings about the death of the tissue. In such circumstances myoglobin diffuses into the general circulation and is excreted in the urine. **In some people after very severe exercise, the muscles become painful and weak and the dark brown urine contains myoglobin.**

THE CHEMISTRY OF THE CONTRACTILE ELEMENT. Myosin is a fibrous protein of molecular weight 4,70,000. Its rod shaped molecule, about 160 nm in length consists of two identical very long polypeptide chains (mol. wt. 2,25,000); each containing about 1800 amino acids. Each chain is in the α-helical configuration and the two chains are wound round each other to form a double helical structure. At one end of the molecule, both chains are folded into a globular 'head' occupying a very small proportion of the total length of the molecule. **Exposure to trypsin splits myosin near the centre of the tail into two portions, a heavy fragment, heavy meromyosin containing the globular 'head', and a light fragment, light meromyosin.**

The important discovery was made by Engelhardt and Ljubimowa in 1939 that myosin is itself the enzyme adenosine triphosphatase (ATPase) (or is inseparably associated with it). This enzyme catalyses the breakdown of ATP to ADP and its activity has now been located in the globular 'head' of the myosin molecule.

Actin, which was discovered in 1941 by Szent-Gyorgyi in Hungary, exists in two forms, G-actin (globular actin) and F -actin (fibrous actin). G-actin has a molecular weight of 46,000 and its molecule consists of a single polypeptide chain, globular in shape. Each molecule can bind one calcium ion very strongly and has a high affinity for ATP. Binding of ATP by G-actin results in polymerisation to F -actin, one molecule of ATP being split to ADP and inorganic phosphate for each G-actin unit added to the F -actin chain. The ADP so formed remains attached to the G-actin units.

F -actin is made up of two long strands of G-actin units coiled round each other.

When solutions of myosin and actin are mixed, myosin binds actin at two specific sites, probably in the 'heads', to form **actomyosin.**

CHEMISTRY OF MUSCULAR CONTRACTION

Skeletal muscle contains specific proteins involved in muscular contraction. These are known as (1) actin and (2) myosin. In 1941 Szent Gyorgi discovered two types of actins. Actin has a strong affinity for myosin and combines with it in the ratio of 1:3 to form the contractile substance, actomyosin.

Myosin: In addition to its role in contraction, myosin has adenosine triphosphatase activity (ATP-ase activity).

Other constituents of muscle include

glycogen, ATP and creatine phosphate.

Main events in Muscular Contraction

The main events in muscular contraction can be discussed under the following heads: (i) Contractile process, (ii) ATP as source of energy for contraction; (iii) Role of creatine phosphate in maintaining ATP reserves; (iv) Glycolysis as a source of ATP; (v) Oxygen debt in working muscle and (vi) Synthesis of ATP and creatine phosphate during aerobic oxidation of lactic acid to CO_2 and water.

Contractile Process: Studies by various workers have shown that myosin and actin can combine in solution to form the protein complex actomyosin, The protein complex forms threads which actually contract in vitro upon the addition of ATP. Simultaneously, ATP is hydrolysed by the myosin because of its high ATPase activity.

Role of ATP in Muscular Contraction: Muscle contains about 0.1 percent ATP and 0.5 percent creatine phosphate. ATP initiates muscular contraction. In vitro studies have shown that when ATP is added to muscle fibre, the muscle contracts. At the same time, ATP is hydrolysed to ADP and inorganic phosphate by myosin which has ATPase activity. If ATP is added in the presence of an inhibitor mersalyl which inhibits the breakdown of ATP in muscle, no contraction occurs. On the other hand, the fibre is extended to the original length. ATP acts as a plasticizer restoring the original length in contracted muscle fibres. There is also evidence that endoplasmic reticulum of muscle cells causes relaxation of contracted myofibrils by removing Ca^{++} ions from them. The calcium uptake by the muscle requires energy and is dependent on ATP-Mg.

Repletion of ATP Content of Muscle

The ATP present in muscle is required continuously for muscular contraction. During muscular contraction, ATP is constantly being broken down to ADP and inorganic phosphate. There are three mechanisms operating in muscle for repleting the ATP reserves in muscle; (i) **Formation of ATP from ADP and creatine phosphate (Lohmann reaction);** (ii) Synthesis of ATP from two molecules of ADP by the enzyme myokinase; and (iii) Synthesis of ATP from ADP during glycolysis of glucose and during aerobic oxidation of lactic acid in muscle.

(i) **Formation of ATP from ADP and Creatine Phosphate (Lohmann Reaction):** Muscle contains 0.5 percent creatine phosphate which is an energy rich compound. This converts ADP to ATP in the presence of an enzyme creatine kinase (creatine phosphotransferase).

$$ADP + \text{Creatine phosphate (CP)}$$

$$\downarrow \text{Creatine kinase}$$

$$ATP + \text{Creatine (C)}$$

As the equilibrium constant of

$$\frac{(ATP)\,(C)}{(ADP)\,(CP)}$$

is 20, about 99 percent ADP formed is converted into ATP.

(ii) **Synthesis of ATP from 2 mols of ADP**: A further source of ATP in muscle is due to the presence of another enzyme, **myokinase (adenylate kinase)** which catalyses the transfer of high-energy phosphate from one mole of ADP to another molecule of ADP forming ATP and AMP.

$$\text{ADP} + \text{ADP} \xrightarrow{\text{Myokinase}} \text{ATP} + \text{AMP}$$

(iii) **Formation of ATP during Glycolysis**: When muscle contracts under anaerobic conditions, glycogen present in muscle is broken down to lactic acid by a series of reactions known as glycolysis. Two of the initial reactions (hexokinase and phosphofructokinase reactions) requires two mols of ATP while two of the latter reactions (phosphoglycerate kinase and pyruvate kinase) synthesises 4 mols of ATP. The net result is a gain of 2 mols of ATP which can be used for muscular contraction.

(iv) **ATP formation during Aerobic Oxidation of Lactic Acid**: During the aerobic phase of carbohydrate metabolism in muscle, lactic acid is oxidised to CO_2 and water according to the TCA cycle. During this process, about 36 mols of ATP are synthesised by oxidative phosphorylation.

Repletion of Creatine Phosphate in Muscle

As mentioned earlier, creatine phosphate converts ADP to ATP in the presence of an enzyme creatine kinase and this reaction helps to maintain ATP level during the initial stages of muscular contraction. At some stage, all the creatine phosphate is brokendown to creatine to form ATP. This reaction is reversible. When the ATP production in muscle increases enormously during the aerobic phase of carbohydrate metabolism, the reverse reaction takes place leading to the resynthesis of creatine phosphate originally present.

Creatine + ATP

↓ Creatine kinase

Creatine phosphate + ADP

In this way, the repletion of creatine phosphate content of muscle is achieved.

Heat production in Muscle during Contraction

When oxygen is excluded, muscle produces heat under anaerobic conditions in two phases (a) initial heat at the time of contraction and (b) anaerobic delayed heat which is evolved during relaxation and afterwards. During the anaerobic contraction, lactic acid is produced from glycogen or glucose. When oxygen is admitted, lactic acid disappears and more heat is evolved. This is called, **'Aerobic delayed heat'**. Usually only 1/5th of the lactic acid produced is oxidised to CO_2 and water and the remaining 4/5th escapes into circulation and is reconverted into glucose in liver. The explanation for the different types of heat production is given below:

(a) **Initial Heat**: This is the heat produced by the breakdown of ATP to ADP (7,600 cal. per mol of ATP broken down).

(b) **Anaerobic Delayed Heat:** This is the heat produced during the breakdown of glycogen to lactic acid. This amounts to 56,000 calories per 2 mols of lactic acid formed.

(c) **Aerobic Delayed Heat:** This is the heat produced during the oxidation of lactic acid to CO_2 and water. This is very large and amounts to 1,26,000 Cal. per 2/5 mols of lactic acid oxidised to CO_2 and water (only 1/5th of the two mols of lactic acid produced is oxidised).

Oxygen debt

The oxygen consumption and heat output during exercise are given in Table 18.1. During severe exercise, the circulation cannot provide adequate amounts of oxygen for oxidising all the metabolites produced from the oxidation of carbohydrates. Due to inadequate oxygen supply, the metabolites accumulate in the tissues and are slowly oxidised after the exercise is over. This oxidation of accumulated metabolites requires more oxygen than normal resting individuals. This excess O_2 consumed by the individual after severe exercise, is called **'Oxygen debt'**. For example, the level of lactic acid in blood during mild exercise like slow-walking is about 15 mg/100 ml. This means lactic acid is oxidised as soon as it is formed. In severe exercise, it rises to about 100 to 150 mg per 100 ml blood. The level again comes down to the normal level of 10 to 15 mg/100 ml blood after one hour of exercise. During the post exercise

Table 18.1 : Effect of exercise on cardiac output, oxygen consumption and heat output in an adult

Exercise	Cardiac output litres/min	O_2 consumed litres/min	Heat output Kcal/min
Sitting in a chair	5	0.25	1.25
Walking 2 mph	10	0.8	4.0
Walking 5 mph	20	2.5	12.5
Running 7.5 mph	25	3.0	15.0
Very severe exercise	34	4.0	20.0

rest period, the subject consumes much more oxygen than normal to wipe out the **'Oxygen debt'** required for oxidising accumulated metabolites. In the example given in Table 18.2, a subject at rest (sitting) consumed 0.25 liters of O_2/min. while during severe exercise he consumed 3.0 litres of O_2/min. During the 10 min. rest period after exercise, he consumed 10 litres of O_2 while a resting person will need only 2.5 litres in 10 minutes. The extra O_2 (10-2.5 = 7.5 litres) consumed is the oxygen debt in the body.

Cori Cycle

Cori and Cori discovered that a greater part of the lactic acid produced in muscle during severe exercise escaped into the general circulation and was converted into glucose in liver. They found that muscle can convert glucose into glycogen but cannot convert lactic acid to glucose due to the absence of certain enzymes (glucose-6-phosphatase and fructose 1, 6 diphosphatase) required for this process. According to Cori (1)

muscle lactic acid is transported to liver by blood and converted into glucose and glycogen in liver and (2) glucose produced from muscle lactic acid in liver is transported from liver to muscle by blood for the glycolytic process. **This process is known as Cori cycle.** (Fig 18.4).

Metabolism in Muscle

The fibres of a muscle can be classified into types according to their content of different enzymes, and this is related to their function.

The muscle fibres can be classed as Type I or Type II fibres according to their content of certain enzymes, such as the enzymes of the glycolytic pathway. Fibres containing high levels of these enzymes are classed as Type II fibres, or fast twitch fibres. These fibres contain relatively few mitochondria. Other fibres that contain lower levels of glycolytic enzymes, but higher levels of citric acid cycle enzymes and cytochromes are classed as slow twitch or Type

Table 18.2 : Oxygen consumption before, during and after exercise

	Oxygen consumed litres/min	litres/10 min
Sitting at rest	0.25	2.5
Severe exercise (one minute)	3.00	--
Rest after severe exercise (10 minutes)	1.00	10.0
Oxygen debt during one minute severe exercise =	10 - 2.5 =	7.5

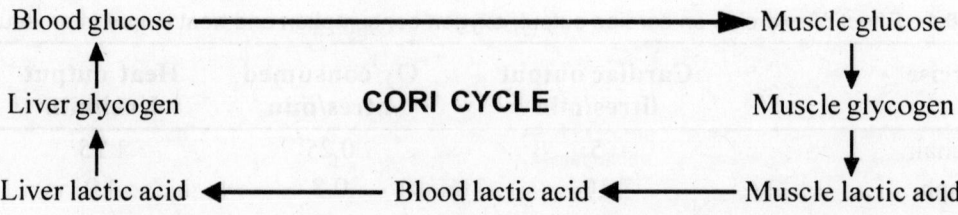

Fig. 18.4 : Cori cycle (Conversion of muscle lactic acid to blood glucose)

I fibres. Formerly, muscles containing large numbers of Type I or Type II fibres were referred to as red and white muscles respectively (red muscles containing high amounts of myoglobin and cytochromes). Type II fibres can contract very rapidly, but for short-periods of time only (lobster abdominal muscle, responsible for the tail flick escape reaction, is an example). Type I fibres on the other hand are capable of more sustained, slower contraction.

Hormonal changes during exercise

The adrenal cortex is activated in exercise. A day's skiing produces a fall of up to 80 per cent in the circulating eosinophils; this could be described as beneficial and strengthening exercise. In long-distance swimmers, the eosinophils may disappear almost entirely from the circulation while the output of 17-hydroxysteroids in the urine may increase eight fold-an increase comparable to that occurring after major surgery. The serum growth hormone (HGH) rises in exercise. The raised HGH level falls quickly after the end of exercise in fit persons but in unfit persons HGH only slowly returns to the basal value. HGH probably initiates and maintains the mobilisation of depot fat during exercise. The fall of plasma insulin during exercise allows the mobilisation of fat and prevents the blood glucose falling too low.

Muscle Energy

The overall energy for muscle activity is provided as ATP and is formed by (a) anaerobic glycolysis taking place in the soluble sarcoplasm, leading to the breakdown of glucose and glycogen to pyruvic and lactic acids, and (b) oxidation of lactic acid to pyruvic acid and further oxidation of pyruvate via acetyl-CoA in the tricarboxylic acid cycle by the mitochondria. Oxidation of fatty acids (β–oxidation and oxidation of acetyl-S-CoA by the TCA cycle in mitochondria) also contributes to the ATP supply of muscle.

ATP in excess of immediate needs reacts with creatine under the catalytic action of creatine phosphokinase to form creatine phosphate:

Creatine + ATP $\rightleftharpoons$ Creatine - P + ADP

The reaction is freely reversible, and during activity the ATP concentration is maintained at the expense of the creatine phosphate store.

Thus, all of the muscle ATP is formed in the sarcoplasm, but it provides energy for both myofibrillar and sarcoplasmic processes.

Figure 18.5 shows the overall metabolic processes by which muscle obtains energy as ATP for the performance of work.

Processes that lead to the breakdown of ATP in muscle with the liberation of energy are (a) the contraction-relaxation cycle; (b) numerous synthetic reactions, such as synthesis of peptides and proteins, CO_2 fixation, formation of glycogen, and various key metabolic intermediates; (c) secretory processes of the cell, active transport, and polarisation of the sarcolemma; (d) hydrolysis by myosin ATPase in the myofibril and by granular ATPase in the sarcoplasm.

Muscle Contraction

The proteins previously discussed provide the basic machinery for muscle contraction and

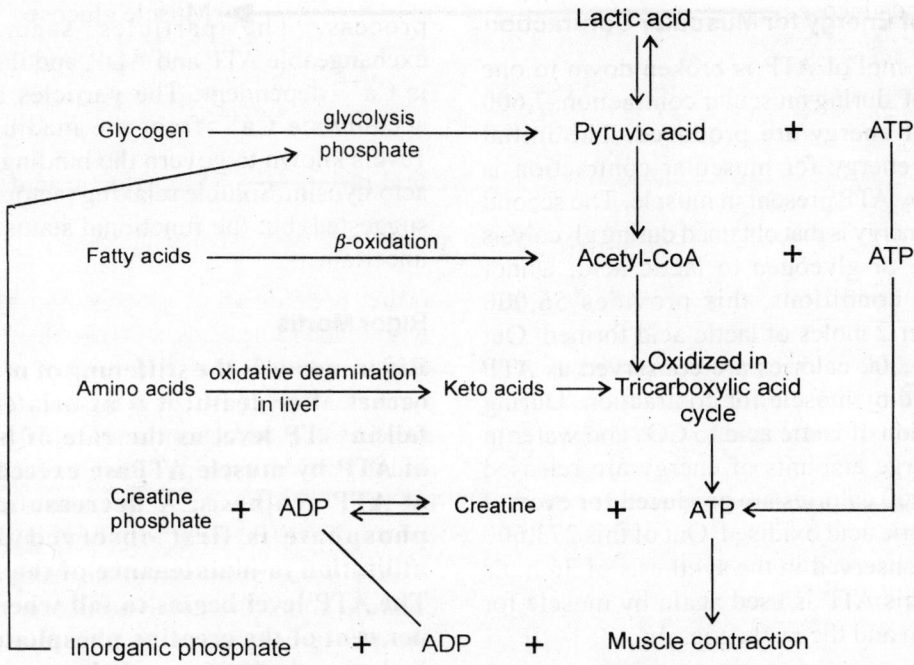

Figure18.5 : Energy production in muscle.

serve to convert chemical energy into mechanical work. Although none of the specific molecular events associated with muscle contraction are established with certainty, a general view of the process may be summarised as follows. Within the interrelated protein structure, the release of energy at active sites affects the movement of some small element of structure. The contractile elements inside the fiber are the myofibrils. Each fibril consists of overlapping arrays of filaments. When a muscle contracts, the arrays of actin and myosin filaments slide past each other, and thus a fibril shortens. If such movement occurs, the chemical events must produce a relative or driving force between the two filaments. H. E. Huxley states that this force is produced by a cyclic process occurring at cross bridges perhaps at the sites of actin-binding and ATPase activity. As contraction continues, each cross bridge attaches to a succession of sites along the filament. It would appear that the breakdown of one

molecule of substrate (ATP?) by enzyme action (myosin ATPase?) constitutes one cycle of events. When contraction is over, enzymatic action is brought to a halt, possibly by intervention of the relaxing system; then the cross bridges detach and the muscle can be re-extended by a small force. It is generally stated that the direct source of energy for muscle contraction is provided by the hydrolysis of the terminal phosphate group of ATP with the formation of ADP:

$$ATP + H_2O \xrightarrow{\text{ATPase}} ADP + Pi$$

It is also generally assumed that creatine phosphate ($CrPO_4$), the high- energy reserve in muscle, rapidly regenerates ATP:

$$CrPO_4 + ADP \longleftrightarrow Creatine + ATP$$

Creatine is again phosphorylated by ATP, newly formed metabolically, and so the cycle is completed.

Sources of Energy for Muscular Contraction

When one mol of ATP is broken down to one mol of ADP during muscular contraction, 7,600 calories of energy are produced. The initial source of energy for muscular contraction is provided by ATP present in muscle. The second source of energy is that obtained during glycolysis of glucose or glycogen to lactic acid. Under anaerobic conditions, this provides 56,000 calories per 2 moles of lactic acid formed. Out of this, 15,200 calories are conserved as ATP and re-used by muscle for contraction. During the oxidation of lactic acid to CO_2 and water in muscle, large amounts of energy are released i.e., 6,30,000 calories are produced for every 2 mols of lactic acid oxidised. Out of this 273,600 cals. are conserved in the synthesis of 36 mols of ATP. This ATP is used again by muscle for contraction and the cycle goes on.

Muscle Relaxation

It is generally assumed that muscle relaxation is the reversal of contraction and that it represents a dissociation of actin and myosin and a decrease in the cross-linking between these elements. Several components have been implicated in relaxation, including sarcoplasmic microsomes, ATP, Ca^{++}, and a transphosphorylating enzyme. Kelley in reviewing this field states that it is now well established that a particulate fraction of muscle is a relaxing agent for the actomyosin system. This particulate material is probably a portion of the sarcoplasmic reticulum and is not just microsomes. Some 85 per cent of the relaxing factor appears to be associated with vesicles or bubbles present as closed structures bound by a continuous smooth-surfaced membrane. Activity is also associated with ribosomes and glycogen granules. Relaxing factor has a strong affinity for Ca^{++}. The Ca^{++}-binding ability is dependent on ATP, and vesicles can accumulate impressive amounts of Ca^{++}. Such accumulation is likely an active transport process. The particles seem to bind exchangeable ATP and ADP, and the exchange is Ca^{++} dependent. The particles are able to accumulate Ca^{++} from the medium at Ca^{++} levels known to govern the binding of Ca^{++} to actomyosin. Soluble relaxing factors have been suggested, but the functional status of these is uncertain.

Rigor Mortis

Rigor mortis is the stiffening of muscles that occurs after death; it is associated with the fall in ATP level as the rate of breakdown of ATP by muscle ATPase exceeds the rate of ATP synthesis. A decrease in creatine phosphate is first observed due to its utilisation in maintenance of the ATP level. The ATP level begins to fall when about 70 per cent of the creatine phosphate has been hydrolysed, the signs of rigor appear when the ATP level has fallen to 85 percent of its initial value and it is practically complete when the ATP has fallen to 15 per cent of this value.

Rigor is associated with a decrease in extractability of myosin by KCl and phosphate solutions, undoubtedly due to combination of actin and myosin into the less soluble complex actomyosin. ATP breaks the linkages between actin and myosin and permits relaxation. In the absence of sufficient ATP, the actin and myosin filaments (I and A filaments) become locked together by interaction of the active groups of the proteins resulting in a partially contracted state, the state of rigor. It appears that factors other than decreased ATP levels may be involved in rigor, but these are imperfectly understood.

It is of interest that the muscles of an animal subjected to severe exercise just prior to death go into rigor much more quickly than the muscles of an unexercised animal. This is due to depletion of ATP reserves in the exercised muscles.

bind
oxchange
be exchange
able to
of Ca
of these
plete
of
crease in

CHAPTER 19

CHEMISTRY OF CONNECTIVE TISSUE, BONE AND MINERALS

The term connective tissue is very broad in its meaning and is used to denote the material which joins up the other three primary tissues, namely the epithelial, muscle and the nervous tissues. Some kinds of connective tissue cells secrete solid intercellular substances-cartilage and bone-which provide protection and support. Other kinds form loose or dense fibrous tissue, tendons, blood vessels, adipose tissues and possibly also the blood cells. Apart from cells most connective tissues also contain extracellular proteins such as collagen and elastin, mucopolysaccharides and, in the case of bone and teeth, inorganic salts.

CONNECTIVE TISSUE

Distribution. Connective tissue is distributed throughout the body and, as its name implies, literally connects the body together. It makes up the capsules and frameworks of organs and the sheaths of tendons and muscles. The skin is attached to the rest of the body by connective tissue (dermis), and connective tissue forms the supporting framework of blood and lymph vessels and nerves. It keeps organs in position.

Connective tissues provide barriers against infective agents and are of primary importance in wound healing. **They are involved in the so-called collagen diseases.**

Composition. Connective tissue is made up of three parts-namely, ground substance, fibers, and cells, which are composed of fibroblasts (osteocytes in bone and chondrocytes in

cartilage), mast cells, and reticuloendothelial cells. The fibers which constitute the supporting mechanism of connective tissue, are embedded in the ground substance along with the cells, which ultimately are the source of both ground substance and fibers.

Ground Substance

Ground substance is found distributed throughout the extracellular space. It is a gel of varying consistency and contains water, salts, proteins, and large polysaccharides in solution. The macropolysaccharide molecules (Table 19.1) may be free or attached to protein. The mucilaginous or slippery feeling of macromolecule preparations has given to these substances the general prefix of **"muco-"**, but it has been suggested that the use of this prefix be dropped.

Table 19.1 : Polysaccharides of ground substance

Polysaccharide	Hexosamine	Hexuronate	Hexose
Hyaluronate	Glucosamine	Glucuronate	—
Chondroitin-4-sulfate	Galactosamine	Glucuronate	—
Chondroitin-6-sulfate	Galactosamine	Glucuronate	—
Dermatan-4-sulfate	Galactosamine	Iduronate	—
Heparin	Glucosamine	Glucuronate	—
Heparitin sulfate	Glucosamine	Glucuronate	—
Keratin sulfate	Glucosamine	—	Galactose

Table19.1 lists the chief complex polysaccharides of connective tissue. Each polysaccharide is composed of two different units which alternate along the straight chain of the saccharide. These units arc joined by C-1-C-4 and C-1-C-3 linkages as is illustrated. In all cases, one of the units is a hexosamine and the other a uronic acid. The amino group of the hexosamine is either acctylated or sulfated. Since the amino group is not free, it does not become cationic by

the association of a proton. With the large number of groups such as carboxylate, ester sulfate, or amide sulfate, the polysaccharides are strongly polyanionic. The association of cations with these negative groups may have important physiological implications.

The repeating hexosamine and uronic acid units joined by alternate C-1-C-4 and C-1-C-3 bonds are as follows:

Section of sodium hyaluronate

Section of sodium chondroitin sulfate

These polysaccharides are formed by the mast cells of connective tissues, and the UDP and UTP derivatives of glucose, glucuronic acid, and acetyl glycosamine are involved. The origins and interconversions of a number of these intermediates are summarized as follows :

UDP-glucose $\rightleftharpoons$ (epimerase) UDP - galactose

UDP-glucose → +2DPN → UDP-glucuronic acid

UDP - galactose → + 2DPN → UDP-galacturonic acid

Similarly, the hexosamine components are formed from the UDP-derivatives as follows:

D-glucose-6-P + glutamine

$\uparrow\downarrow$

glucosamine-6-P + glutamic acid

glucosamine-6-P + acetyl-S-CoA

$\uparrow\downarrow$

N-acetyl-glucosamine-6-P

$\uparrow\downarrow$ mutase

N-acetyl-glucosamine-1 -P + UTP

↓

UDP-N-acetylglucosamine

$\uparrow\downarrow$ epimerese

UDP-N-acetylgalactosamine

Hyaluronic acid synthesis appears to proceed as follows:

UDP-glucuronic acid + UDP-N-acetylglucosamine

↓

hyaluronic acid

Chondroitin sulfate formation involves sulfation by **"active sulfate"** as follows :

UDP-glucuronic acid + UDP-N-acetylgalactosamine + active sulfate

↓

chondroitin sulfate

Hyaluronic acid is broken down by hyaluronidases found in microorganisms, snake venom, and mammalian tissues, the testis being particularly rich in hyaluronidase. Hyaluronidases in general hydrolyze the bond between carbon 1 of glucosamine and carbon 4 of glucuronic acid.

Chondroitin sulfates A and C are hydrolyzed by exhaustive action of testicular hyaluronidase chiefly to sulfated tetrasaccharides, while chondroitin sulfate B is not hydrolyzed by the enzyme.

Rheumatic joints show proliferation of connective tissue with partially depolymerized or incompletely polymerized hyaluronic acid in the synovial fluid. Growth hormone stimulates production of the acid mucopolysaccharides. The turnover rate of skin mucopolysaccharides is decreased in the diabetic animal and restored toward normal by insulin administration. **The increased susceptibility to infections, slow wound healing and tendency to atherosclerosis seen in diabetics is probably, in part, related to deficiency in synthesis of mucopolysaccharides caused by insulin deficiency.**

Fibers of Connective Tissue

Connective. tissue contains collagen, reticulin, and elastic fibers.

Collagen : It derives its name from the fact that when boiled in water it yields gelatin or glue. It is a protein of unusual amino acid composition. One third is glycine and another third is proline and hydroxyproline. It contains alanine but no tryptophan or cysteine. Hydroxyproline and hydroxylysine are found only in collagen and elastin. **Vitamin C is required for their formation and in its absence collagen formation is defective.** Since collagen contains 14 percent hydroxyproline, the collagen content of a tissue can be deduced from the estimation of its hydroxyproline content. Similarly the urinary excretion of hydroxyproline provides a measure of the rate of collagen turnover in the body; **high values are found in growing children and in some patients with bone diseases.**

Collagen is the major fibrous protein of extracellular connective tissues, and it is also the most existing and plentiful protein in the animal kingdom. Some 25-35 per cent of total body protein is collagen. The high glycine content of collagen (32-35 percent) is very constant throughout the animal kingdom. The imino acids, proline and hydroxyproline, make up another 25 per cent of the amino acids present. Formation of collagen fibers takes place as shown in { Fig 19.1 (a)}.

The collagen molecule is a rigid rod 2900 Å by 15 Å. The major portion consists of three polypeptide chains, each in a left-handed helical conformation. The three helixes are wound about each other to form a three-stranded rope like structure. The three chains are cross-linked by covalent, ester, and special γ-glutamyl and β-aspartyl linkages. Collagen is synthesized by mesenchymal cells such as the fibroblast, but the protein is found subsequently in the extracellular spaces. Aggregation of secreted molecules {tropocollagen Fig. 19.1 (b)} results in the formation of the cross-striated fibrils seen in collagen preparations. Tropocollagen units {Fig 19.1(b)} are reported to come together in an overlapping or staggered array of about one quarter of their length, giving rise to a collagen fibril with a repeating period of about 700Å. The collagen fibrils also laminate in plywood- like sheets.

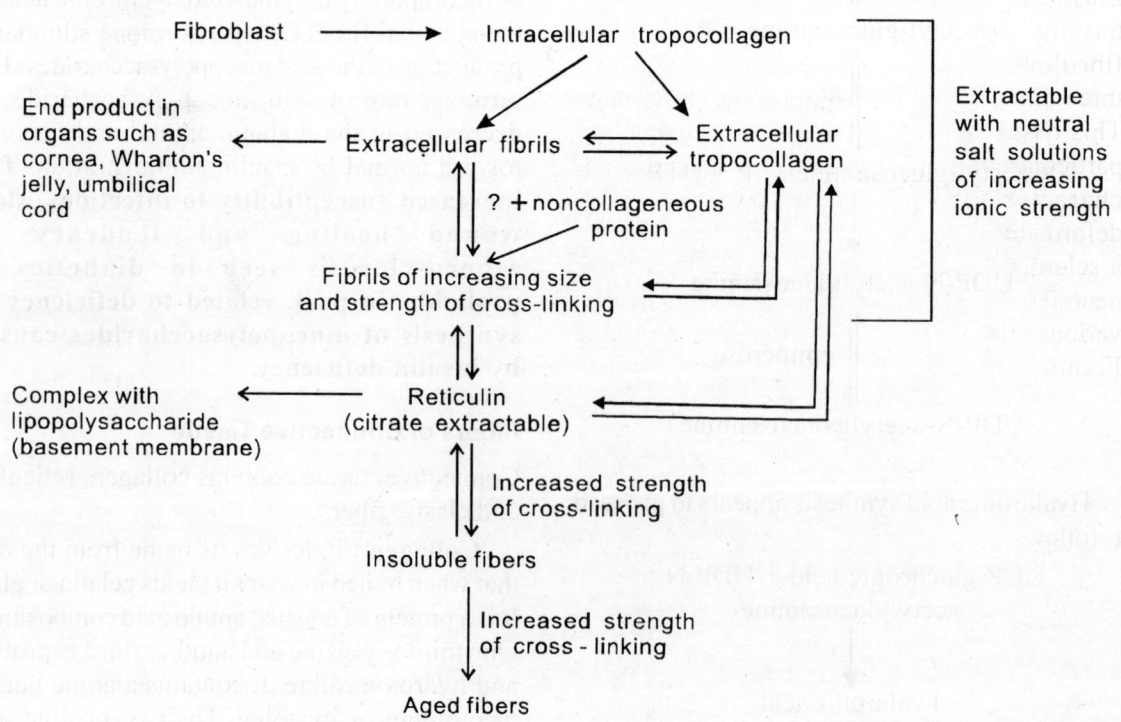

Fif. 19.1a: Formation of Collagen fibers.

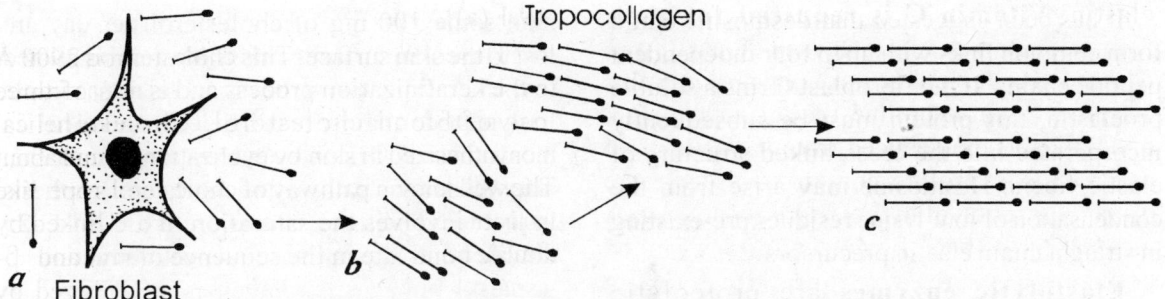

Fif. 19.1b: Tropocollagen molecules are extruded from fibroblast (or osteoblast) and aggregate extracellularly to give collagen fibres with the regular banding which may be detected by electron- microscopy.

Hydroxyproline of collagen has been reported to be formed from proline at the time when an unhydroxylated, microsomal bound polypeptide is converted to collagen. This conversion requires an H donor and another nonenzymatic factor of the soluble protein fraction.

Elastin: Another component of the supportive tissues of the body is elastic tissue. Elastic tissue is a yellow refractile material having a fibrillar, membranous, or fibrillomembranous structure arranged as a three-dimensional meshwork without free ends. This tissue is found in aorta, skin, lungs, and particularly ligamentum nuchae. An important characteristic is its long-range reversible deformability similar to that of rubber. Elastin is a scleroprotein and complete solubilization in neutral solvents is difficult. Exposure to alkali or various acids will render much of elastin soluble. Formic acid treatment appears to disaggregate the fibrils of elastin without causing other fundamental change. Collagen is usually the most difficult contaminant to remove from elastic tissue.

The amino acid composition of elastin is different from that of collagen. Glycine, alanine, valine, proline, and leucine are the chief amino acids present; glycine being present in highest concentration (23-26 percent). The exact chemical structure of elastin is unknown. The elastic properties of the wet fiber are due to the inherent elastic nature brought about by its cross-linked structure. The cross-links are not S-S bridges but may be covalent in character.

The discovery of new amino acid structures in elastin may help explain some of its unique properties Desmosine and isodesmosine, tetracarboxylic, tetra-amino acids, have been isolated from hydrolyzed bovine elastin, and their labelling by tracer lysine has been followed.

desmosine, side chains at 1,3,4,5
isodesmosine, side chains
at 1,2,3,5

desmosine

It has been suggested that desmosine could form common links with up to four independent peptide chains. If the fibroblast forms a soluble proelastin, this protein must be subsequently incorporated into the cross-linked structure of elastic fibers. Desmosine may arise from the condensation of four lysine residues pre-existing in straight chain elastin precursors.

Elastolytic enzymes are proteolytic enzymes found in pancreas and other tissues that have wide peptide bond specificity.

Reticulin. There appear to be two types of reticulin in connective tissue. One type is present in developing connective tissue and represents thin collagen fibers, soluble in acid citrate buffer, which precede the thicker collagen fibers. The other is associated with basement membranes of parenchymatous organs and is present around nerve and muscle fibers and between connective tissue and epithelium. This reticulin is very insoluble and appears to be a complex of collagen, lipid, and a polysaccharide. This reticulin, under normal physiological conditions, does not develop into typical collagen fibers.

EPITHELIAL TISSUES

These tissues compose the purely cellular, nonvascular layer covering all the free surfaces of the body, and include such structures as the epidermis, hair, nails, horns, hoofs, and feathers. Most of these structures are biologically inert and are the products of underlying living tissue.

Keratins are highly insoluble proteins of the albuminoid type and consist of the amino acids i.e., alanine, ammonia, arginine, aspartic acid, half- cystine, glutamic acid, glycine, histidine, isoleucine, leucine, lysine, methionine, phenylalanine, proline, serene, threonine, tyrosine and valine.

Lipid found on the surface of the skin is a complex mixture of almost all known lipid classes. Cholesterol of surface lipid is of particular interest. It has been estimated that in man some 100 mg of cholesterol per day are lost to the skin surface. This cholesterol is related to the keratinization process and is not a simple loss of blood cholesterol. Cholesterol is biosynthesized in skin by cyclization of squalene. The well known pathway of cholesterol synthesis in liver involves the saturation of a C-24-C-25 double bond late in the sequence of reactions.

LIVER

The liver is composed of units called "lobules" in the centre of which are branches of the hepatic vein, the hepatic artery, and the portal vein. **The major role played by the liver is in the metabolism of sugars, fats and amino acids, in detoxication processes, and in the synthesis of many substances.**

In order to accomplish these functions, the liver has a high rate of energy production and utilization. Its protein is very labile, with a high rate of turnover. Liver protein very rapidly decreases during starvation, along with decreases in cytoplasm, mitochondria, microsomes, and enzymes. RNA levels are lowered, but the DNA content is not affected. Glycogen and phospholipid levels are greatly decreased. However, upon resumption of food intake, the liver rapidly recoups its losses and returns to normal.

MAMMARY GLAND

The mammary gland is unique as a tissue. The lactose of milk is formed largely from blood glucose. It has been estimated that about 80 percent of lactose carbon originates from plasma glucose or from compounds rapidly converted to glucose. Glucose may be converted to lactose by reactions involving UDPG as follows:

1. glucose → glucose-6-P → glucose-1-P → UDP-glucose → UDP-galactose

2. UDP-galactose + glucose-1-P → lactose-1-P → lactose

3. UDP galactose + glucose → lactose

CARTILAGE

Cartilage consists of cells (chondroblasts), connective tissue fibers (predominantly collagen), and an organic matrix secreted by the cells. Cartilage is the chief constituent of the internal skeletons of cartilaginous fish and forms parts of the skeletal structures of higher animals.

When cartilage is heated with water under pressure, the organic matrix and collagen fibers are disrupted to yield gelatin (from collagen) and chondromucoid. Chondromucoid is a mucoprotein made up of the mucopolysaccharide, chondroitin sulfuric acid, united to protein. Chondroalbuminoid, the insoluble protein remaining after extraction of the other proteins, resembles elastin in properties. Cartilage contains relatively small quantities of chondroalbuminoid.

The blood and interstitial fluid supply to cartilage is very limited, and food is supplied to it and waste products eliminated from it largely by slow diffusion. **This results in cartilage being one of the less metabolically active tissues.**

BONE

Bone, like cartilage, consists of cells (osteoblasts and osteoblasts) and an organic matrix, formed by the osteoclasts, in which characteristic bone mineral is deposited in orderly arrangement. Some bones are formed by mineral deposition in cartilage, while others arise by ossification of fibrous tissue. Hollow bones may contain much marrow, which is high in lipid content (up to 25 per cent). All bones contain more or less lipid, most of which is fat. The water content of marrow-free bones generally amounts to 20 to 25 per cent. Both the lipid and water contents of bones vary with age and the nutritive state of the animal.

Dry lipid-free bone is composed of about one-third organic matrix and two-thirds bone mineral. The great strength of bone is due to the hardness of the mineral component and the toughness of the protein matrix in which the mineral is embedded.

The organic matrix of bone is composed chiefly of a mixture of the three proteins ossein, osseoalbuminoid, and osseomucoid. **Ossein remains present in greatest amount.** It is apparently identical with collagen, since it yields gelatin. Osseoalbuminoid is present as a very tough elastic and fibrous substance and resembles the elastin of connective tissue and tendons. Osseoalbuminoid contains more nitrogen and less sulfur than chondroabluminoid of cartilage.

Osseomucoid, like chondromucoid, is a mucoprotein and contains chondroitin sulfuric acid as the prosthetic group. Osseomucoid closely resembles tendomucoid in properties.

While the proteins of bone are of the same type as those found in cartilage, it is apparent that in the ossification of cartilage to form bone some changes in the cartilage proteins do take place.

The composition of bone mineral is relatively constant. Average values for the chief components are as shown in Table 19.2.

Table 19.2 : composition of dry fat-free bovine cortical bone

	Percent	meq/g
Cations		
Calcium	27.24	13.6
Magnesium	0.44	0.36
Sodium	0.73	0.32
Potassium	0.06	0.01
Anions		
Phosphate	12.5 (as P)	12.1 (as PO_4^{---})
Carbonate	3.5 (as CO_2)	1.6 (as CO_3^{--})
Citric acid	0.87	0.14 (as Cit^{---})
Chloride	0.08	0.02
Fluoride	0.07	0.04

It is well established that the mineral of bone consists chiefly of microcrystals of a compound of calcium and phosphate with the structure of the mineral apatite. The apatites have their constituent ions arranged in a three-dimensional symmetry. Generally the apatites are (a) divalent cations (Ca^{++}, Pb^{++}, Sr^{++}), (b) tetrahedral anions (PO_4^{--}, SiO_4^{--}) and (c) electronegative anions (OH^-, F^-), all in a hexagonal symmetry. Some cations and anions can be substituted without disturbmg the symmetry.

Chemical analysis and x-ray diffraction ndicate that the basic structure of bone mineral is some form of hydroxyapatite-e.g., $Ca_{10}(PO_4)_6(OH)_2$.

Calcium ions in bone mineral are replaced by lead ions in cases of chronic lead poisoning and are mobilized into the blood under conditions that cause bone calcium to be mobilized (diets low in calcium and phosphorus, excessive doses of vitamin D, parathyroid hormone, acidosis). Similarly, ionic exchange causes the deposition of strontium, radium, beryllium, potassium, and various other elements in bone.

The dynamic state of bone mineral is also strikingly evident in conditions imposing large demands upon blood calcium and phosphorus, such as heavy lactation and pregnancy, when dietary calcium and phosphorus are inadequate. Under these conditions much calcium and phosphorus may pass from bone mineral into the blood to serve for the production of milk or bone mineral of the fetus.

The breakdown or resorption of bone mineral is brought about by the osteoclasts through mechanisms not well explained. It appears that the initial process may involve depolymerization of the mucopolysaccharides.

Formation of bone: Osteoblasts are the cells primarily concerned with bone formation and produce the proteins and mucopolysaccharides making up the connective tissue fibers and the cementing gel in which the fibers and mineral components are embedded. This organic matrix of fibers and cementing substance is first formed, and then deposition of bone mineral takes place. This mineral deposition in orderly arrangement appears to be related to the association of chondroitin sulfate with the collagen fibers, the chondroitin sulfate serving as a cation exchanger which binds Ca^{++} and other cations for deposition with phosphate and other anions as bone mineral between the collagen fibers. Little is known about the finer details of this deposition. It appears that mineral deposition takes place concomitantly with the process of glycolysis and the production of organic phosphates in the osteoblasts. **The osteoblasts generally contain much alkaline phosphatase, and it may be that this enzyme hydrolyzes an organic phosphate at the site of mineralization to provide PO_4^{---} ions for the process.**

The metabolic processes of the bone lead to the synthesis of citrate, presumably via the tricarboxylic acid cycle, which is probably retained in the bone largely through adsorption to the mineral crystal lattice, from which it may be released to the circulation.

TEETH

Teeth represent complex calcified structures in which calcification is differentiated in three district anatomical regions: enamel, dentine, and cementum. Dentine is the major tooth component into which extends the pulp cavity containing the blood vessels and nerves. The dentine is covered with a layer of cementum in the the root and a layer of enamel in the exposed part of the tooth. Enamel is the most highly calcified and also the hardest tissue of the body. Dentine is softer than enamel but harder than bone and shows an intermediate degree of calcification. Cementum and bone represent comparable degrees of calcification and hardness. The mineral phase constitutes about 98 per cent of enamel, 77 per cent of dentine, and 70 percent of cementum. The general composition of cementum is analogous to that of bone.

The protein matrix of dry enamel amounts to about 1 per cent (0.49-1.95 percent) of the tissue and is composed chiefly of a protein that in some respects resembles keratin. The protein of enamel is of epidermal origin. Dry dentine contains, on an average, 22 per cent of protein matrix, which is largely collagen and is of mesodermal origin. All phases of tooth structure contain some lipid material.

In addition to the common constituents of teeth, spectroscopic analysis has indicated the presence of traces of barium, strontium, tin, zinc, manganese, titanium, nickel, vanadium, aluminium, silicon, boron, iron, chromium, platinum and silver.

The mineral of enamel is more basic than that of dentine. The small amount of F^- in teeth exchanges with OH^-, as it does in bone. Similarly, traces of many elements may be present in teeth as in bone through ionic exchange without appreciable alteration of the crystal lattice. However, exchange reactions proceed more slowly in teeth than in bone.

Although the amount of fluorine in teeth is very small, it appears to be highly important. **The ingestion of small amounts of fluorides has been shown to have a definite effect in the prevention of caries. Excessive amounts are harmful and may cause mottled teeth.** The proper number of F^- ions in the enamel crystal structure appears to make it more resistant to solution in acids. It is claimed that the topical application of fluoride solutions to teeth renders them less soluble in acids and reduces the incidence of caries.

Development of teeth. For an appreciation of normal tooth development, it is necessary to consider four phases: (1) origin and differentiation of cellular elements, (2) organic matrix formation, (3) inorganic crystal growth, and (4) structural aspects of development. Enamel is of ectodermal origin and is formed by the ameloblast derived from epithelial cells of the enamel organ. Dentine and cementum are of mesenchymal origin being formed by odontoblast and cementoblast, respectively. These cells involved in tooth formation have been studied extensively, and cell organelles have been implicated in various steps of tooth formation. Frank and Nalbandian state that the first step of dentine, enamel, and cementum formation is characterized by extracellular deposition of an organic matrix. The matrices are fibrous protein embedded in a ground substance. The fibrous protein of dentine and cementum is collagen; the protein of enamel is a modified α-keratin called δ-keratin. The collagen fibrils of dentine show typical periodic bandings of 640 Å. Just prior to the formation of bone mineral, there is an increase in the density of the amorphous phase.

Calcification is the process of deposition within the soft organic matrix of a difficulty soluble salt of calcium resembling hydroxyapatite. Hydroxyapatite, $Ca_{10}(PO_4)_6(OH)_2$, is present as microcrystals in the shape of plates and needles 25-75 Å thick, 40-75 Å wide, and 50-500 Å long. Each crystal is composed of thousands of unit cells with some of the positions being capable of substitution by sodium, potassium, magnesium, carbonate, citrate, sulfate, fluoride, and other trace materials. It is estimated that the crystals in the calcified tissues of a 70 kg man have a surface area of as much as 100 acres, and these crystals compose 60 percent of the solid phase of mature cortical bone.

JOINTS

Movements between adjacent long bones take place at their appropriate cartilagenous ends. The scanning electron microscope has shown that the apparently smooth surface of articular cartilage remains in fact in motion like a wave and is many times 'rougher' than engineering bearings. The peak to peak distance of the wave like motions is about 25μm and the valleys are about 2.5μm deep. The superficial zone of the cartilage matrix contains tightly packed small collagen fibers lying parallel to the surface forming a 'skin'; the deeper fibers are longer and form an open meshwork; the fibers next to the bone are disposed radially towards the joint surface. A fibrous capsule lined internally by synovial membrane passes from one bone to the other forming a closed cavity which contains a small quantity of lubricating fluid; this synovial fluid in the human knee joint amounts to only 0.2 ml. It is a clear yellow fluid containing only a few cells; **its viscous, elastic and thixotropic (the property of certain gels of becoming fluid when shaken and then again becoming semisolid)** properties depend upon its content of hyaluronic acid linked to a protein.

Calcium Metabolism

The skeleton contains at least 99 percent of the total body calcium which in a young adult is about 1 kg (2600 m-equiv.). As mentioned earlier skeletal calcium is constantly exchanging with the calcium of the extracellular fluid. In an adult in balance, the rate of bone mineral deposition is about 400 mg/day or 10 to 15 percent of the total skeletal calcium per year. The rate of bone resorption is similar. In older subjects, especially in women, bone resorption exceeds bone accretion (the growing of separate things into one) and there is a progressive loss of calcium from the skeleton. This process of **'osteoporosis'** appears to be universal, at least in Western communities, but the cause is not known.

Dietary calcium: In Europe and U.S.A., the average daily calcium intake in adults is 800 to 1000 mg. In developing countries the intake is often considerably lower (200 to 400 mg/day). The main sources of calcium are milk and cheese, green vegetable and (in Britain and the United States) artificially enriched bread. Drinking water is seldom a significant source of calcium but very hard water may provide up to 200 mg per day.

At one time it was thought that dietary lack of calcium was a factor contributing to poor development of bone and teeth. This may be true in some very underprivileged communities but the body has a remarkable facility for adapting to a low calcium intake and it is unlikely that calcium intakes of as little as 200 mg/day have any harmful effects in otherwise normal subjects. More calcium than usual is needed during periods of rapid growth, and during pregnancy and lactation. While it is reasonable to ensure an adequate diet at these times the healthy subject readily adapts by increasing the proportion of calcium absorbed from the diet.

INTESTINAL ABSORPTION: In an adult in calcium balance, and on a diet containing 1000 mg/day, the faeces contain about 900 mg/day and the urine about 100 mg/day. Thus the absorption from the diet appears to be 100 mg/day or one tenth of the dietary calcium. In fact the true intestinal absorption is about 350 mg/day but about 250 mg/day is secreted into the gut with the intestinal secretions.

Calcium can be absorbed from all parts of the small intestine by an active transport mechanism. In normal subjects the proportion of dietary calcium absorbed is greatly increased after a period on a low calcium diet. This 'adaptation' which becomes evident within a week of the change in diet is not seen in the absence of vitamin D. **Nicolaysen in 1943 suggested that there was an 'endogenous factor', a hormone, which was responsible for regulating Calcium absorption, in relation to calcium needs. This factor is probably 1, 25- dihydroxy-cholecalciferol, a recently-discovered metabolite of vitamin D.** Parathyroid hormone in excess also stimulates calcium absorption, but not in the absence of vitamin D.

THE PLASMA CALCIUM: The total plasma calcium in man is normally between 8.8 and 10.3 mg/100 ml (4.4 to 5.2 m-equiv./litre). Just under half of this amount is bound to plasma proteins, particularly albumin, a small proportion (less than

0.5 mg/100 ml) is complexed with citrate, and the remainder (about 5 mg/ 100 ml) circulates as ionized calcium. The complexed and the ionized calcium are together known as the **'diffusible' calcium.** A constant concentration of ionized calcium is necessary for the normal function of muscles and nerves, and a later section will deal with the control of the level of ionized calcium.

URINARY EXCRETION OF CALCIUM:
About 15 g calcium daily passes into the glomerular filtrate from the diffusible fractions of the plasma calcium. All but 50 to 200 mg is reabsorbed in the tubules but the exact site is not yet known. Calcium reabsorption is diminished in vitamin D deficiency and in the presence of a sodium dieresis (division).

The calcium lost in the sweat is very variable, between 20 and 350 mg/ day. This limits the accuracy of calcium balance experiments.

FACTORS AFFECTING THE PLASMA CALCIUM

A constant and normal concentration of ionized calcium in the extracellular fluid is of great importance in, among other things, muscular contraction, neural and neuromuscular transmission and the activity of several enzymes.

If the ionized calcium is low tetanic spasms may occur and may be fatal. **If the plasma calcium is high, cardiac function is disturbed and calcium may be deposited in the kidney or other tissues.**

PHYSICO-CHEMICAL FACTORS: If EDTA (ethylene-diamine tetra-acetate, a calcium-complexing agent) is injected intravenously into man or the dog, the plasma calcium falls rapidly but returns to a normal value (10 mg/100 ml) within a few hours. If EDTA is given after removal of the parathyroid glands, the plasma calcium again returns to the preinfusion value (7 to 8 mg/ 1 00 ml) but not so rapidly. Thus chemical equilibrium between the labile part of the bone mineral and the interstitial fluid, quite independent of the parathyroid glands, keeps the plasma calcium up to 7 to 8 mg/100 ml. In intact animals parathyroid hormone is responsible for maintaining the normal serum calcium level of around 10 mg/100 ml.

PARATHYROID HORMONE (PTH) (Fig 19.2): The parathyroid glands develop from the third and fourth pharyngeal pouches of the embryo. They lie in the neck immediately adjacent to the posterior surface of the thyroid gland with which, however, they have no physiological relationship. **As a rule they consist of four oval bodies about 6 mm long each weighing 20 to 50**

```
        1                                                    13
H₂N—Ala—Val—Ser—Glu—Ile—Gln—Phe—Met—His—Asn—Leu—Gly—Lys—

   15                    20   21   22   23   24   25   26   27   28
His—Leu—Ser—Ser—Met—Glu—Arg—Val—Glu—Trp—Leu—Arg—Lys—Lys—Leu—

   29   30                                                   42
Gln—Asp—Val—His—Asn—Phe—Val—Ala—Leu—Gly—Ala—Ser—Ile—Ala—

      44   45              50                                57
Tyr—Arg—Asp—Gly—Ser—Ser—Gln—Arg—Pro—Arg—Lys—Lys—Glu—Asp—Asn—

      60                              70
Val—Leu—Val—Glu—Ser—His—Gin—Lys—Ser—Leu—Gly—Glu—Ala—Asp—Lys—

      75              80              84
Ala—Asp—Val—Asp—Val—Leu—Ile—Lys—Ala—Lys—Pro—Gln—COOH
```

Fig. 19.2: Amino acid sequence of bovine PTH. The fragment 1 to 44 (heavy type) is biologically active, in vivo and in vitro, on both bone and kidney receptors

mg; but they are variable in number, size and position; accessory parathyroid tissue is not uncommon lower in the neck or even in the thorax.

Bovine PTH is a single-chain polypeptide, containing 84 amino acids (Fig 19.2); it has a molecular weight of 8,500. PTH secretion apparently ceases when the plasma calcium exceeds 12 mg/100 ml. Plasma calcium appears to be the sole stimulus for PTH secretion. Since the half-life of the hormone in the blood is about twenty minutes, changes in hormone secretion may play an important part in the minute to minute regulation of the plasma calcium.

Quite independent of its action on blood calcium PTH has effects on bone and kidney, and probably also on the gastrointestinal tract and on the mammary gland in lactation. The effects on the bone and intestine, but not on the kidney, require the presence of vitamin D. PTH exerts its action on bone by stimulating osteoclasts to mobilize bone. PTH decreases the reabsorption of phosphate by the kidney tubules, and so increases phosphate excretion. It also increases the urinary excretion of sodium, potassium and bicarbonate, and decreases the excretion of hydrogen ions. In the intestine, PTH enhances calcium absorption. The exact mechanism of action of PTH is not known but recent evidence suggests that cyclic 3': 5'-AMP may be involved.

Clinical disorders of both excess and deficiency of parathyroid activity are recognized. Actively secreting tumours of the parathyroid glands produce excessive amounts of PTH, and the resulting disturbance of phosphorus and calcium metabolism leads to withdrawal of large amounts of these elements from the bones which therefore become weak and deformed and liable to fracture (Fig. 19.3). The absorption of calcium from the gut is increased. The serum calcium may be 16 mg

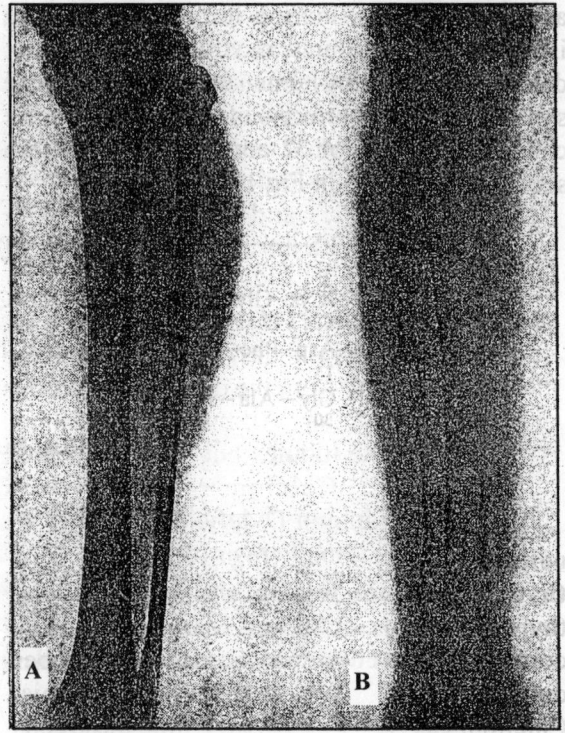

Fig.19.3: X-ray photograph of the right lower legs of the two women, aged 25. A is from a normal subject, B from a patient with a parathyroid tumour. In B the fibula is deformed and both bones cast a poor shadow because of extensive resorption of calcium salts.

per 100 ml or more and the urinary excretion may be greatly raised so that stones may form in the kidneys.

Parathyroid deficiency sometimes occurs after accidental removal of parathyroid glands during thyroidectomy. Neuromuscular excitability and muscular spasm (tetany) are the four main symptoms. The condition improves with the administration of PTH but large doses of vitamin D are also given in longterm management.

CALCITONIN: In 1962 Copp and his colleagues produced evidence for the existence of a hormone which lowered the plasma calcium. He called it **calcitonin.** Subsequent work has amply confirmed this the hormone has been isolated and its chemical structure has been determined. Recently human calcitonin has been synthesized. The hormone is a lipophilic single chain polypeptide of **32** amino acids with the sequence as shown in Fig 19.4.

has some actions on the kidney and bone. It seems mainly to be concerned with the long-term control of calcium balance and the adaptation to chronic dietary lack of calcium.

OTHER HORMONES AFFECTING CALCIUM METABOLISM: An adequate

$$S\text{-----------------------------}S$$

$$\overset{1|}{NH_2}-Cys-\overset{2}{Gly}-\overset{3}{Asn}-leu-\overset{5}{Ser}-Thr-Cys-Met-Leu-\overset{10}{Gly}-Thr-Tyr-Thr-$$

$$Gln-Asp-\overset{15}{Phe}-Asn-Lys-Phe-\overset{20}{His}-Thr-Phe-Pro-Gln-\overset{25}{Thr}-Ala-Leu-Gly-$$

$$\overset{30}{Val}-Gly-Ala-\overset{32}{Pro}-CONH_2$$

Fig 19.4: Human Calcitonin

In man calcitonin is secreted by the C cells of the thyroid, parathyroids and thymus. The parafollicular (C cells) of the thyroid have been known since 1932. They contain granules which increase in number during a period of prolonged hypocalcaemia. Calcitonin has been identified within these cells by the immuno-fluorescent antibody technique.

Calcitonin secretion is stimulated by hyper-calcaemia and its best documented action is the inhibition of parathormone-induced bone resorption. Calcitonin also reduces bone resorption even in the absence of parathormone and promotes phosphate and sodium excretion in the kidney. Recently calcitonin release has also been shown to be stimulated by gastrin, pancreozymin and glucagon. Therefore, as calcium is absorbed from a meal, there is little or no rise in serum calcium.

Calcitonin excess has been described in patients with medullary-cell carcinomas of the thyroid. Surprisingly, these patients seldom have hypocalcaemia. There is as yet no convincing evidence of a syndrome due to calcitonin deficiency.

1,25-DIHYDROXYCHOLECALCIFEROL: This hormone, a metabolite of vitamin D is produced by the kidney. It promotes the absorption of calcium in the intestine and probably

supply of growth hormone from the anterior pituitary is necessary for proliferation of the cells of the epiphyseal cartilage and, therefore, for the growth in length of a long bone.

THE PLASMA CALCIUM IN DISEASE: Hypercalcaemia of hyperparathyroidism, has already been mentioned. Hypercalcaemia may also be caused by tumours which cause rapid bone destruction, by tumours secreting a PTH-like substance, by vitamin D poisoning and the excessive ingestion of milk and alkali by patients with peptic ulcer. Signs of hypercalcaemia include thirst, tiredness, weakness, mental disturbances and, if severe, coma and death. **Untreated hypercalcaemia causes renal damage.**

Hypocalcaemia is found in hypoparathyroidism, osteomalacia, rickets, and renal failure. Tetany is a prominent feature. The outstanding feature of tetany is neuromuscular irritability which manifests itself first as hypertonicity of muscles and then as fibrillary twitching of muscle fasciculi, leading finally, especially in children, to generalized clonic movements. The muscle hypertonic produces the characteristic attitude of the hand in tetany, **the main d' accoucheur.** Simultaneously the feet are held firmly flexed at the ankles with all the toes plantar- flexed. The condition, called carpopedal spasm may be accompanied in infants by spasm of the glottis (laryngismus stridulus), which can be severe enough to cause alarming cyanosis.

PHOSPHORUS

The mean phosphorus content of an adult man is 800 g; four-fifths of this is in the bones, the remainder being in the cells as phosphates or nucleic acids. The inorganic phosphorus concentration in the plasma in fasting adults is between, 2.5 and 4.5 mg/100 ml. Higher values are found in infants. Almost all the inorganic phosphate is dialysable, only 12 percent being protein-bound. At normal blood pH (7.4) 85 percent of the ionized inorganic phosphate is present as HPO_4^{2-} and 15 percent as $H_2PO_4^-$. Small amounts of the phosphate may be bound to calcium and magnesium. It has been stated that the amount of non-ionized phosphate may be 50 percent of the dialysable phosphate.

Phosphorus is excreted by the kidney, and in the steady state the amount excreted is equal to that which the gut absorbs. Ninety percent of the phosphorus filtered at the glomerulus is reabsorbed in the tubule and there is no good evidence for tubular secretion of phosphorus. Phosphate depletion may occur with tubular defects and a **high plasma phosphate may be a consequence of renal (glomerular) failure.**

OTHER MINERALS

Magnesium: The adult human body contains only 25 g (2000 meq) of magnesium, about half being in the bones and half. in the cells. The cells contain 30 to 40 meq per litre where it is an essential part of many enzymes, including phosphoglucomutase in the mitochondria. The plasma and the gastrointestinal secretions contain only 1.7 to 2.3 meq per litre; about 55 percent of the plasma magnesium is ionized. The average urinary secretion is usually over 100 mg or 10 meq per day; the amount depends very much on the intake, which may lie between 17 and 34 meq. per day. **Since green vegetables and cereals contain much magnesium, a dietary deficiency is unlikely unless there is intestinal loss of magnesium, because of diarrhoea or some form of malabsorption.** If the serum level falls epileptic fits, tetany and muscular weakness are seen in man these disturbances may in fact be due to an accompanying hypocalcaemia.

Copper: The daily intake of copper is about 2 mg. If copper is absorbed, it is rapidly removed from the blood by the liver and excreted in the bile. About 15 μg of copper are excreted per day in the urine. When absorbed from the upper small intestine copper is at first loosely attached to albumin but within 12 to 18 hours it becomes firmly bound to a non-dialysable α_2-globulin (ceruloplasmin) which has weak oxidase activity. Human liver contains about 40 μg Cu per g dry matter; **in cirrhosis or Wilson's disease there may be up to ten times as much.**

Copper is an essential trace element. Its most important role is as a component of cytochrome oxidase, which is involved in the final step for the reduction of molecular oxygen. It is concerned also in phospholipid synthesis and in the copper protein enzymes, tyrosinase, ascorbic acid oxidase and monoamine oxidase. **Deficiency in domestic animals produces anaemia and damage to the central nervous system.**

Zinc. The daily intake of zinc is between 10 and 15 mg, almost all of which is excreted in the faeces. Urinary excretion is 0.4 mg daily. Blood contains about 0.75 mg per 100 ml, nearly all of which is present in the red cells in the enzyme carbonic anhydrase; blood plasma contains about 90 μg of zinc per 100 ml. Zinc is also present in carboxypeptidase, alcohol dehydrogenase, liver glutamic dehydrogenase and alkaline phosphatase. Zinc deficiency is common in domestic animals and may retard growth and development of the gonads. The plasma zinc is lowered in man in many conditions including disorders of the skin and liver; in some patients administration of zinc has produced improvement. **Zinc deficiency may not be uncommon in man.**

Manganese: The intake of manganese is about 5 mg daily, mainly derived from cereals and tea. Plasma contains 2.5 µg per litre carried by β_1-globulin; whole blood contains about 12 µg per litre. Manganese is accumulated in both mitochondria and microsomes. It is excreted mainly in the faeces; the urine contains negligible amounts. The effects, if any, of deficiency in man are not known but overdoses of manganese produce effects in man resembling **Parkinsonism.**

Cobalt: The body contains about 80 µg of cobalt in cyanocobalamin. A deficiency syndrome has not been encountered in man but lack of cobalt in ruminants causes wasting.

Strontium: The body contains about 350 mg of strontium in the skeleton where it behaves much like calcium. Strontium has no known physiological function, but is of possible clinical importance because ^{90}Sr is radioactive and is produced as a result of atomic fission. This isotope has a long half-life (25 years) and accumulates in the skeleton. Fortunately the amount of ^{90}Sr in human bone has declined since a peak figure was reached in 1964.

Fluorine: Fluorine is present in animal soft tissues in amounts ranging from 0.2 to 1.5 mg per 100 g of the dry material. Bones and teeth contain larger amounts (20 to 30 mg per 100 g ash) and dentine may contain more than the enamel of teeth. The incidence of caries tends to be lower in geographical areas where the drinking water contains one part per million of fluorine than in places where the fluorine content is much less. In districts where the water contains three parts per million or over of fluorine the enamel of the teeth may show bands of brown pigmentation between chalkish white patches but they are still resistant to caries; the bones may be thickened but without any functional disability. In districts where the water supply is not fluoridated the intake of fluorine lies between 0.6 and 1.8 mg per day. Deliberate fluoridation of the water supply may double these figures but this dose is well below the level known to cause toxic effects. **Tea and sea-fish are the only other significant sources of fluorine in the diet.**

Iron metabolism and **iodine metabolism** have been discussed in the chapter of mineral metabolism.

CHAPTER 20

NERVOUS TISSUE

The marvellous and unimaginable development you are visualizing all around whether missiles, supersonic jets, aeroplanes, rockets, in space technology, in telecommunication- information technology and other fields is due to *me*. Thanks to the `CREATOR' who has made mine biochemistry quite developed and not like those of animals in whom *me* is underdeveloped. I have a very complicated structure along with its chemistry. Answer of many hurdles (especially neurological and geriatric problems) is hidden in me. I work faster than computer which has brought revolution in present era.

Nervous tissue constitutes about 2.4 per cent of the body weight of man, the brain representing the major portion of this amount. The following distribution of nervous tissue is given for an adult man.

	Grams
Brain	1400
Spinal nerves	151
Spinal cord	27
Cranial nerves	12

Nervous tissue is highly specialised in function and composition. Although information is available about nervous tissue metabolism and nerve conduction, **very little is known about the biochemistry of brain functions such as memory and behaviour.**

The passage of substances to the brain from the blood is restricted and regulated by the blood-cerebrospinal fluid barrier and the blood-brain barrier, which appears to consist of an extra layer of glial cells surrounding the capillaries. These barriers in particular limit the passage of negatively and positively charged ions, both organic and inorganic, from the blood to the brain, as well as the passage of large organic molecules, such as lipids, polypeptides, and polysaccharides.

It is of importance that the blood-brain barrier of persons with brain tumors permits the passage of the dye iodofluoroscein labelled with I^{131}, which accumulates in the tumors and thus permits localization of the tumors through radioactivity measurements.

The most striking fact about the composition of brain (and nerves) is the large amount of lipid material relative to protein in the brain solids. Brain contains more lipid by far than any other tissue except adipose tissue. The composition of the different parts of the brain may vary within wide limits. For example, the water content of the gray matter of adult human brain is about 85 percent, while that of the white matter is only 70 per cent. The white matter thus contains about twice as much solids as the gray matter (30: 15 per cent). The water content of brain also varies with age, being highest in young brains. The high solid content of the white matter of brain is largely due to its great content of lipids.

The lipids of brain (and nerves) are chiefly composed of cholesterol, phospholipids, glycolipids (cerebrosides), and sulfolipids or sulfatides. Relatively little neutral fat is present.

The composition of brain varies widely with age. Adult brain contains less water, much more lipid, less protein, less organic extractives, and less mineral material than the brain of a child.

Brain lipids

The lipids of brain have received considerable study and our knowledge of them has increased greatly in recent years with the development of elegant chromatography techniques. With such methods, it is possible to determine the lipid composition to a high degree of precision and to detect minor components that were previously unrecognized. **Various types of lipids found in brain include cholesterol, ethanolamine glycerophosphatides, serine glycerophosphatides, choline glycerophosphatides, sphingomyelin, cerebroside, cerebroside sulphate, ceramide, etc.** Out of these, cholesterol is found in maximum concentration followed by ethamolamine glycerophosphatides and choline glycerophos-phatides respectively.

The myelin sheath. Myelin is a sheath-like structure which consists of a series of tightly packed wrapping of the external membrane of the Schwann cell around the nerve axon. By electron microscopy, a single membrane of this unit can be shown to be bound by two dense lines and a thinner line with a clear zone between the lines. Electron microscopy combined with x-ray diffraction studies and precise chemical determinations suggest a pattern for the organisational structure of the myelin membrane. **The peripheral regions of the membrane are considered to be occupied by polar groups of lipids and associated proteins, while the central region is occupied by the hydrocarbon portions of lipid molecules.** The central region consists of two lipid molecules packed tail-to-tail with an overall separation of about 51 Å. The lipids of the myelin membrane are metabolically inert. Models of this membrane have been prepared by Finean and Vandenheuvel. From a study of such models, it is concluded that the lipids in myelin are held together by three major forces and not by covalent bonds. These forces are (1) electrostatic interactions between polar groups of lipids and oppositely charged adjacent proteins; (2) hydrogen bonding between oxygen and nitrogen atoms of lipids and proteins; and (3) London-van der Waals dispersion forces between $-CH_2-$ pairs in hydrocarbon tails of adjacent lipid molecules. The major force may well be the latter. **There are many implications of the proposed structure to the relation of membrane stability and the problem of disease associated with demyelinization.**

Roberts and Baxter point out that the development of ultramicroanalytical procedures has made it possible to study the distribution of biochemical processes in specialised portions of the nervous system. Rapid weighings of amounts of tissue as small as a single dried red blood cell and the determination of as little as 10^{-19} mols of certain coenzymes are possible.

Brain Proteins

Proteins make up about 40 percent of the dry weight of whole brain and 8 percent of the weight of whole fresh brain.

The association of brain proteins with much lipid material and the presence of protein-lipid complexes have made the extraction and separation of relatively pure brain proteins a difficult task. Brain proteins have been separated into groups by extraction with different solvents, and six or more apparently distinct proteins have been identified by electrophoresis in extracts which include mainly albumin, globulins (α_1, α_2, β_1, β_2 and γ), fibrinogen, etc.

> The brain synthesizes proteins. Most of this synthesis takes place in the microsomes.
>
> It has been found that conditions of severe stress cause marked decreases in the cytoplasmic proteins and nucleic acids of the brain cells of guinea pigs, with restoration in 48 hours.

The young unipolar neuroblast, which consists of about two thirds nucleus, contains much DNA and little RNA. As the cell develops through the various stages to the adult nerve cell, the DNA content remains unchanged while the contents of RNA and protein show parallel increases. These processes agree with the concept that DNA is the primary genetic material which controls the synthesis of RNA, which, in turn, controls protein synthesis.

Wilson's disease or hepatolenticular degeneration is a hereditary disease which shows pathological changes of the liver, kidneys, and central nervous system, the latter being localized especially in the lenticular bodies. The disease is associated with excessive absorption of copper from the intestine, increased urinary excretion of copper, and low levels of plasma copper combined with an α-globulin known as **"ceruloplasmin"**. The level of uncombined plasma copper is high, which apparently permits the observed deposition of excessive amounts of copper in the kidneys, liver, and brain. Presumably the intellectual

deterioration associated with Wilson's disease is related to this excess brain copper, and probably to increased protein-bound copper.

Amino acids of brain: The total free amino acid concentration of brain is high relative to that of plasma, being some six times higher in rat brain and eight times higher in human than in plasma. Ten amino acids present in highest concentration in brain include glutamic acid, N-acetylaspartic acid, glutamine, cystathionine, ethanolamine, aspartic acid, glutathione, taurine, γ-aminobutyric acid and asparagine.

The brain contains compared to plasma, very large amounts of the following amino compounds: γ-aminobutyric acid, aspartic acid, N-acetylaspartic acid, taurine and glutathione.

Marked increases in plasma amino acid concentration due to administering amino acids may cause severalfold increases in the amino acids of muscle, liver and kidney with no appreciable effect upon brain amino acid concentration.

Metabolism of Brain

Carbohydrate and oxygen. Brain exhibits a very high rate of oxygen metabolism, which accounts for some 25 per cent of the total oxygen utilized by the body at rest. The brain tissue of children (mean age 6.2 years) uses about 5 ml O_2 per 100 g per minute, while brain tissue of adult subjects at rest uses about 3.5 ml O_2 per 100 g per minute, in all cases at normal blood sugar levels (about 80 mg per 100 ml). At low blood sugar levels of insulin hypoglycaemia (arterial glucose 19 mg per 100 ml), the utilization of O_2 falls to around 2.6 ml per 100 g per minute, and in insulin coma (arterial glucose 9 mg per 100 ml) to 1.9 ml per 100 g per minute.

The respiratory quotient of brain metabolism is very close to unity, indicating that carbohydrate is the predominant oxidative substrate of brain.

Brain contains very little glycogen, about 0.1 per cent, and while this glycogen is quickly broken down and metabolized upon demand, nearly all of the carbohydrate for brain metabolism is supplied by the circulating blood glucose.

Although brain tissue in vitro readily oxidize the compounds of the tricarboxylic acid cycle, and also fructose and various other compounds, these substances are relatively ineffective in restoring brain metabolism in hypoglycaemic coma, whereas glucose is highly effective. The failure of substances other than glucose to relieve hypoglycaemic coma is probably due to their failure to pass from the blood to the brain in adequate quantities.

Marked decrease in either the O_2 supply to the brain (**hypoxia**) or the glucose supply to the brain leads to greatly decreased oxidative metabolism, with decreases in high-energy compounds, such as ATP and creatine phosphate, and large increases in lactic acid and inorganic phosphate. Poisoning with cyanide, which blocks the cytochrome oxidase system, has similar effects.

Agents that produce anaesthesia or sleep cause increases in high-energy phosphates and decreases in inorganic phosphate and lactic acid, as well as a decrease in oxygen utilization. This means that the decreased utilization of high-energy compounds more than balances their rate of production, leading to a net increase.

Contrary to the effects of central nervous system depressants, greatly increased cerebral activity, such as occurs in convulsions induced by convulsive drugs, leads to quick depletion of high-energy phosphates and the accumulation of much inorganic phosphate and lactic acid.

Amino acids. It is clear that glutamic and aspartic acids and their derivatives occupy a unique position in brain metabolism, for they constitute some 70 percent of the nonnitrogenous nitrogen of brain. Glutamic and aspartic acids are related to brain metabolism in a number of different ways. In the conversion of glutamic acid to α-ketoglutaric acid, a mechanism is present for the control of oxidative metabolism by the tricarboxylic acid cycle. That this in turn may influence the all-important use of brain glucose is clear. Insulin-induced hypoglycaemia results in a fall in brain glutamate levels. If such animals are allowed access to glucose, glutamate levels do not fall. Brain glutamate (and aspartate) may provide much of the energy for cerebral functions. A second metabolic role of glutamate and aspartate is related to amidation reactions. Both glutamic and aspartic acids can be converted to the corresponding amide as :

$$\text{glutamic acid} + NH_3 \xrightarrow{\text{ATP}} \text{glutamine}$$

$$\text{aspartic acid} + NH_3 \xrightarrow{\text{ATP}} \text{aspargine}$$

The amides so formed may be related to the control of brain metabolism because glutamine passes the blood-brain barrier more easily than does glutamate. Measurement of arterial and venous levels of these compounds reveals that the concentration of glutamic acid in the blood leaving the brain is lower than that entering and that the glutamine concentration is higher. In the preceding reaction, NH_3 is utilized, this being an intracellular mechanism for the detoxication of ammonia. The transamination reactions that follow describe the dynamic interconversions that are involved in the reactions related to the Krebs cycle.

glutamic acid + oxaloacetic acid
↓
α-ketoglutaric acid + aspartic acid

While the brain contains enzymes involved in the **pentose phosphate pathway** of carbohydrate oxidation, the evidence indicates that most of the carbohydrate metabolism of brain proceeds through glycolysis and tricarboxylic acid cycle oxidation.

aspartic acid + pyruvic acid

↓

oxaloacetic acid + alanine

or, in general

glutamic acid + α-keto acid

↓

α-ketoglutaric acid + α-amino acid

An additional reaction of importance is the formation of γ-aminobutyric acid. The brain is the only tissue containing a significant concentration of glutamic decarboxylase, an enzyme that carries out the following reaction:

glutamic acid

↓

$NH_2 - CH_2CH_2 - CH_2COOH + CO_2$

γ- aminobutyric acid

The γ- aminobutyric acid is an inhibitory transmitter substance which is metabolized as follows: γ-aminobutyric acid → succinic semialdehyde → succinic acid. Pyridoxal phsophate is the coenzyme of these conversions.

Serotonin or 5-hydroxytryptamine. This substance is found in the brain and other tissues (stomach, intestine, mast cells, blood platelets, etc.) and is a constituent of various venoms. **It is a potent vasoconstrictor. Serotonin is formed in the brain and other tissues by 5-hydroxylation of tryptophan followed by decarboxylation:**

When 5-hydroxytryptophan is administered to an animal, it is followed by an increase in brain serotonin, with marked central nervous system actions, such as catatonia, rage, and fear.

Serotonin is rapidly broken down by brain amine oxidase and excites the neurones during the short interval between formation and destruction. Much of the serotonin of brain is in a bound form localized in the hypothalamus. Reserpine displaces bound serotonin from its sites in the brain and other tissues; this appears to be related to the tranquilizing effect of the drug.

Lysergic acid diethylamide in very small doses causes a schizophrenic-like condition in man, which is prevented by serotonin.

Serotonin appears to be an important transmitting agent in the sympathetic nerves of the autonomic nervous system.

It is of interest that serotonin is a potent stimulator of smooth muscle and causes contraction of the uterus and ileum.

Serotonin undoubtedly is important in regulating the activity of brain and other tissues.

Electrolytes of Brain

Table 20.1 shows the chief electrolytes of brain in comparison with those of plasma and cerebrospinal fluid.

The composition of cerebrospinal fluid is taken to approximate that of brain interstitial fluid, though these fluids originate from blood chiefly by different routes.

Nearly, all of the brain chloride, as well as most of the Na^+ appears to be present in the interstitial fluid. The intracellular concentration of Na^+ is estimated to be about 0.02 M and that of K^+ about 0.14 M. Maintenance of high intracellular K^+ and low intracellular Na^+ against the concentration gradients between the brain cells and interstitial fluid represents active transport, presumably due to the sodium pump mechanism and requires the continual expenditure of energy provided by the oxidation of glucose.

Acetylcholine and the Nerve Impulse

As pointed out in the foregoing discussion of electrolytes in nervous tissue, the concentration of K^+ is much higher inside the neurons than in the surrounding interstitial fluid, while the concentrations of Na^+ show the reverse relations. These differential ionic concentrations

Table 20.1 : Cations and anions of brain, cerebrospinal fluid and plasma
(Values represent meq per liter or kg)

Cations	Plasma	CSF**	Brain
Ca^{++}	5	2.5	2
Na^+	141	141	57
K^+	5	2.5	96
Total cations*	153	148	166
Anions			
Cl^-	101	127	37
Phosphates	2	1	16
HCO_3^-	27	18	12
N-Acetylaspartate	0.1?	-	12
Other organic acids	2	2	10
Proteins	20	0	40
Lipids	0	0	40
Total anions	152	148	167

*Mg^{++} not included; ** Cerebrospinal fluid*

are maintained by active transport across the cell membrane, probably through operation of a sodium pump mechanism.

The differential distributions of K^+ and Na^+ set up a polarization across the nerve cell membrane amounting to some 75 mv, the inner surface of the membrane being relatively negative. During transmission of an impulse, a wave of electrical negativity passes along the nerve fiber. Associated with this activity is a marked decrease in electrical resistance, with influx of Na^+ during the ascending phase of the action potential, followed by an equivalent outflow of K^+ during the descending phase. The permeability of the axonal membrane to Na^+ increases some 500 times during nerve activity. The impulse travels along the fiber as a chain process. As each local region of the fiber becomes depolarized with movement of Na^+ and K^+, it becomes refractory or inactive until energy

from metabolic processes can restore the original distributions of these ions. The impulse passes along the fiber as a succession of locally initiated depolarization currents after the initial stimulus has started the impulse.

It appears from the work of Nachmansohn and others that acetylcholine functions as a depolarizing agent of nerve membranes to facilitate the generation and propagation of nerve impulses.

Acetylcholine and acetylcholine esterase, which very rapidly hydrolyzes and inactivates acetylcholine, are present generally in nerves and are localized near the axon surface. Acetylcholine is rapidly synthesized in nervous tissue by the enzyme choline acetylase from choline and acetyl coenzyme A:

$$Choline + CH_3CO\text{-}S\text{-}CoA$$

$$\downarrow$$

$$acetylcholine + HS\text{-}CoA$$

Both the synthesis of acetylcholine to depolarize the membranes and its hydrolysis by acetylcholine esterase to stop its action appear to take place with sufficient rapidity to function in the generation and transmission of the nerve impulse.

The acetylcholine of nerve tissue in the resting state is in a bound (probably to protein) and inactive form (storage form). Upon stimulation, free acetylcholine is released from the bound or storage form and acts upon an acetylcholine receptor to cause membrane depolarization and generation of the electric potential at the site involved. The acetylcholine at this site is then hydrolyzed by acetylcholine esterase, permitting repolarization of the membrane by movement of Na^+ and K^+ ions. The reactions take place so rapidly that the whole process is accomplished in microseconds. Each local depolarization and current generation liberates free acetylcholine in the adjacent area (in the direction of impulse transmission) with repetition of the process. Thus, the impulse passes along the fiber as a succession of locally initiated depolarization currents after the initial stimulus has started the impulse.

Diisopropylfluorophosphate has also been used in the treatment of myasthenia gravis but it is a dangerous drug to use because the toxic dose is too close to the effective dose. A mechanism for detoxifying diisopropylfluorophosphate exists in kidney by the enzyme diisopropylfluoro-phosphatase, which is capable of hydrolyzing this compound to fluoride and diisopropylphosphate. This enzyme is activated by Mn^{++} or CO^{++} and specific cofactors such as imidazole and pyridine derivatives (e.g., proline or hydroxyproline)

Atropine is used as an antidote to the toxic effect of diisopropylfluorophosphate and other anticholinesterases.

ATP storage is decreased during poisoning by cyanide which blocks cytochrome oxidase system. On the other hand, agents that produce anaesthesia or sleep cause an increase in ATP storage.

Glutamic acid seems to be the only amino acid metabolised by brain tissue. However, this amino acid is of considerable importance in brain metabolism. It serves as a precursor of γ-aminobulyric acid and is a major acceptor of ammonia produced either in the metabolism of the brain or delivered to the brain when arterial blood ammonia gets elevated.

CHAPTER 21

BIOLOGICAL OXIDATION AND BIOENERGETICS

> We are the chemical reactions of paramount importance to the living matter where we supply energy for various types of works like mechanical work (muscles, locomotion, etc.), osmotic work, electric potentials, chemical synthesis, light, heat maintenance, etc.

Biological oxidation- reduction is concerned with the two main questions: (i) how does respiration support life and secondly (ii) what is the difference between the combustion taking place inside an organism and outside it. **The study of these problems, which began with the discovery of oxygen by Scheele and Priestley, has developed into the modern field of biological oxidation,** which has provided deep insights into the nature of life. We now know that oxidation and its simultaneous counterpart , i.e., reduction supply the **free energy** for all vital work and many component reactions in the metabolic network belonging to this class.

Energy is essential to every manifestation of life. Differentiation and growth involve energy requiring syntheses of vital substances, such as **proteins** and **nucleic acids.** The maintenance of temperature of warm-blooded animals, the mechanical work done by muscles and cilia, the generation of electrical impulses in nerve and brain and the transport of substances against osmotic gradients (**"active transport"**) - all require energy.

The energy for these processes is generated by the oxidation of foods and is supplied to the tissues in the form of the **chemical energy** released by reactions of specific **"energy rich"** compounds. These energy - releasing reactions, which are catalysed and controlled by specific enzyme systems, make possible the chemical, mechanical, electrical, thermal and osmotic work upon which all life depends.

In order to understand how energy can be released and utilised in the body, it is essential to understand certain principles relating to energy in general and chemical energy in particular.

Chemical Energy: Different organic compounds yield different amounts of energy when completely oxidised. Following Table 21.1 gives the calories liberated per mol by the oxidation of several compounds to carbon dioxide and water. **When the combustion takes place at constant pressure, the heat change is called the enthalpy change and is negative in sign where heat is lost from the system to the surroundings, as in a calorimeter.**

Table 21.1: Heats of combustion to CO_2 and H_2O at constant pressure **(Enthalpy)**

Substance	Calories ΔH per Mol
Acetic acid, liquid	209,400
Ethyl alcohol, liquid	327,600
Glucose, solid	673,000
n-Hexane, liquid	989,800
Pyruvic acid, liquid	279,000
Sucrose	1,349,600

Heats of combustion represent the maximum energy obtainable from substances by drastically breaking them down and oxidising their elements. The heat of combustion of a substance such as glucose, which is oxidised completely to CO_2 and H_2O in the body, represents the energy obtainable from it by the body. This oxidation, however, proceeds in many separate stages, and the energy is accordingly liberated in increments corresponding to these stages.

Chemical reactions are always associated with energy changes which finally appear as heat changes and are measured as such. Some reactions proceed with heat evolution, and these are said to be **exothermic,** whereas other reactions absorb heat from the surroundings and are known as **endothermic.**

Most of the processes concerned with the breakdown of foods in the body are exothermic and the catalysts to make them go are enzyme systems present in the tissues.

Free Energy: Living systems operate at constant temperature (isothermally) and cannot convert heat energy directly into work as an automobile or locomotive does for example.

The energy relationships in a heat engine is given to bring out the meanings of **free energy,**

enthalpy and entropy.

Free energy is the energy of a system capable of doing work.

Enthalpy is heat energy consumed or released in a system at constant pressure.

Entropy is energy associated with disorder or randomness in a system. Entropy energy is the energy of a system (mechanical or chemical) unavailable to do work.

Entropy may be considered as a measure of the degree of disorder of a system; the greater the degree of disorder, the greater the entropy of the system. The entropy of a chemical reaction is maximum at the equilibrium point. In the case of I_2 distributed between CCl_4 and H_2O at equilibrium, the work energy required to remove all of the I_2 from the water and replace it in the CCl_4 would be equivalent to the entropy increase when the system, with all of the I_2 in CCl_4 changes to the state with I_2 distributed between CCl_4 and water at equilibrium.

The energy requirements of most living cells are met by the oxidation of carbohydrates, fatty acids, glycerol and amino acids by molecular oxygen with the liberation of energy, CO_2 and H_2O. These reactions underlie the respiration of the cells and are accomplished by a highly ordered array of enzymes and coenzymes present in the cells. The oxidation of the carbon present in the metabolites to CO_2 is carried out mainly through the tricarboxylic acid (TCA cycle) (Fig. 21.1) whereas the oxidation of hydrogen to water is carried out through the electron transport system outlined in this chapter. In the course of these reactions, a part of the free energy made available is conserved as newly synthesised ATP. The different aspects are discussed under the following heads: (i) Oxidation of carbon present in carbohydrates, fats and amino acids through TCA cycle; (ii) Electron transport and the oxidation of hydrogen removed from the substrates to water, and (iii) Biochemical energetics and conservation of a

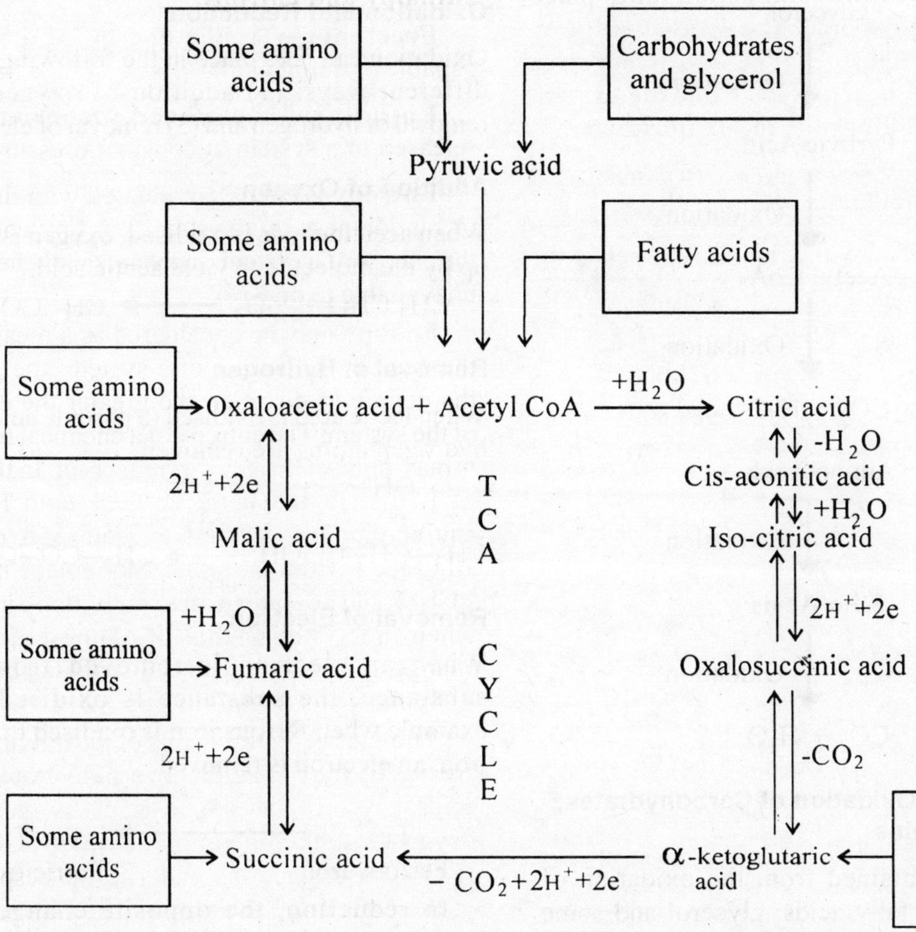

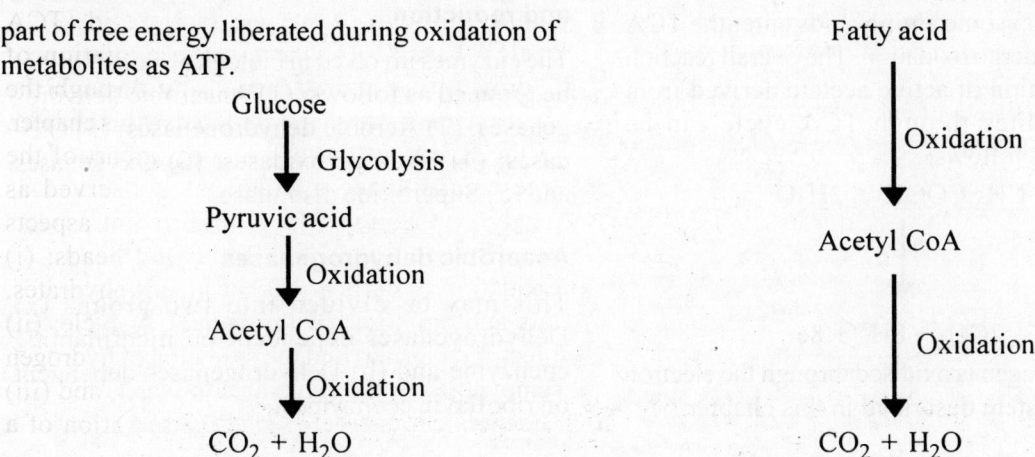

Fig. 21.1 : Oxidation of acetyl CoA and other acids obtained from carbohydrates, fats and proteins through TCA Cycle

part of free energy liberated during oxidation of metabolites as ATP.

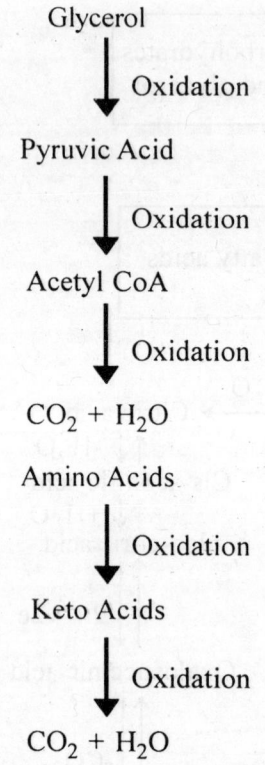

Glycerol

↓ Oxidation

Pyruvic Acid

↓ Oxidation

Acetyl CoA

↓ Oxidation

$CO_2 + H_2O$

Amino Acids

↓ Oxidation

Keto Acids

↓ Oxidation

$CO_2 + H_2O$

Integration of Oxidation of Carbohydrates, Fats and Proteins

Acetyl CoA obtained from the oxidation of carbohydrates, fatty acids, glycerol and some amino acids is oxidised through the TCA cycle as shown in Fig 21.1. Oxaloacetic acid, succinic acid, fumaric acid and α-ketoglutaric acid obtained from some amino acids enter the TCA cycle and undergo oxidation. The overall reaction in the oxidation of active acetate derived from the metabolites through TCA cycle can be expressed as follows:

$$CH_3.COOH + 2H_2O$$

↓

$$2CO_2 + 8H^+ + 8e$$

The hydrogen is oxidised through the electron transport system described in this chapter.

Oxidation and Reduction

Oxidation can take place in the following three different ways: (1) addition of oxygen; (2) removal of hydrogen and (3) removal of electron.

Addition of Oxygen

When acetaldehyde is oxidised, oxygen is taken up by the molecule to yield acetic acid.

$$CH_3.CHO + \tfrac{1}{2}O_2 \longrightarrow CH_3.COOH$$

Removal of Hydrogen

When lactic acid is oxidised to pyruvic acid, two hydrogen atoms are removed.

$$\underset{\text{CH}_3-\overset{\displaystyle\text{OH}}{\overset{|}{\text{CH}}}-\text{COOH}}{} \xrightarrow{-2H} CH_2-CO-COOH$$

Removal of Electron

When an electron is removed from the substance, the substance is oxidised. For example when ferrous iron is oxidised to ferric iron, an electron is removed.

$$Fe^{++} \xrightarrow{-e} Fe^{+++}$$

Ferrous Iron   Ferric Iron

In reduction, the opposite changes are involved.

Enzymes involved in biological oxidation and reduction

The enzymes involved in biological oxidation can be grouped as follows: (1) Anaerobic dehydrogenases; (2) Aerobic dehydrogenases; (3) Oxidases; (4) Hydroperoxidases; (5) Oxygenases and (5) Superoxide dismutase.

Anaerobic dehydrogenases

This may be divided into two groups (a) Dehydrogenases dependent on nicotinamide coenzyme and (b) Dehydrogenases dependent on riboflavin coenzymes.

Dehydrogenases dependent on Nicotinamide Coenzymes

A large number of dehydrogenases require NAD (nicotinamide adenine dinucleotide) or NADP nicotinamide adenine dinucleotide phosphate) (Table 21.2). The coenzymes are reduced by the corresponding substrate. One of the hydrogen atoms is removed from the substrate as a hydrogen nucleus (H^-) with 2 electrons (hydride ion) and is transferred to the 4 position in nicotinamide while the other hydrogen is removed from the substrate as a free hydrogen ion (H^+) which remains in solution as shown below:

$$NAD^+ + AH_2 \longrightarrow NADH + H^+ + A$$

NAD linked dehydrogenases catalyse oxidation- reduction reactions in the oxidative pathway of metabolism e.g., glycolysis, TCA cycle and respiratory chain of mitochondria. Some examples are given in Table 21.2.

NADP is also required specifically by some dehydrogenases e.g., glucose-6-P-dehydrogenase, gluconate-6-P-dehydrogenase and malate dehydrogenase.

$$NADP^+ + AH_2 \longrightarrow NADPH + H^+ + A$$

Some of these enzymes cannot use NAD in place of NADP while others can use either NAD or NADP. **Other enzymes requiring NADPH are involved in the biosynthesis of fatty acids and cholesterol from acetyl CoA.**

Anaerobic dehydrogenases containing flavoproteins

Flavoproteins contain FAD (Riboflavin adenine dinucleotide) or FMN (Riboflavin mononuleotide) (Table 21.3). Both these coenzymes are prosthetic group for several enzymes. The dimethyl isoalloxazine moiety undergoes reversible reduction and oxidation as follows:

$$FP \underset{-2H}{\overset{+2H}{\longleftrightarrow}} FPH_2$$

Some of the flavoproteins contain a metal which is essential for their activity. The flavoproteins functioning in the oxidation-reduction enzymes function in three important ways as discussed below:

1. NADH dehydrogenase: This enzyme, called NADH dehydrogenase, transfers hydrogen atom from NADH to ubiquinone and contains

Table 21.2 : Some NAD(P)-dependent dehydrogenases

Enzyme	Coenzyme	Reaction
Alcohol dehydrogenase	NAD, Zn	Alcohols → Aldehydes
Aldehyde dehydrogenase	NAD	Aldehydes → Acids
L-Glycerophosphate dehydrogenase	NAD	Glycerophosphate → Dihydroxy-acetone-P
Glyceraldehyde-3-P-dehydrogenase	NAD-SH	Glyceraldehyde-3-P → Diphosphoglycerate
Lactate dehydrogenase	NAD (NADP)	Lactate → Pyruvate
Malate dehydrogenase	NAD (NADP)	Malate → Oxalocetate
Glucose dehydrogenase	NAD (NADP)	Glucose → Gluconate
Isocitrate dehydrogenase	NAD, NADP	Isocitrate → α-Ketoglutarate
Glucose-6-P-dehydrogenase	NADP	Glucose-6-P → Gluconate-6-P
Gluconate-6-P-dehydrogenase	NADP	Gluconate-6-P → Ribulose-5-P + CO_2

Table 21.3: Some flavin-linked dehydrogenases

Enzyme	Coenzyme	Reaction
NADH dehydrogenase	FMN	NADH $\rightarrow$ NAD
Succinate dehydrogenase	FAD,Fe	Succinate $\rightarrow$ Fumarate
L-α-Glycero-P-dehydrogenase	FAD	Glycerol-P $\rightarrow$ Dihydrox-yacetone-P

non- haem iron and is firmly bound to the respiratory chain. It contains FMN as the prosthetic group.

$$NADH + H^+ + FMN \longrightarrow FMNH_2 + NAD$$

The reduced flavoprotein transfers the hydrogen to ubiquinone in the respiratory chain.

2. Anaerobic dehydrogenase {transfers electrons to Ubiquinone (CoQ)}: Some anaerobic dehydrogenases containing flavoproteins transfer electrons directly from the substrate to ubiquinone (CoQ). The prosthetic group is FAD (Table 21.3). **The important enzymes belonging to this class are NADH dehydrogenase, succinic dehydrogenase, mitochondrial α-glycerophosphate dehydrogenase, etc.** (Table 21.3).

3. Electron transferring flavoproteins (ETF): Some flavoprotein dependent dehydrogenases transfer hydrogen to another flavoprotein (instead of transferring to respiratory chain) called electron-transferring flavoprotein (ETF). The ETF then transfers

hydrogen to the ubiquinone in the respiratory chain. Fatty acid CoA dehydrogenases require ETF.

$$AH_2 + FAD \text{ enzyme} \longrightarrow A + FADH_2 \text{ enzyme}$$
$$FADH_2 \text{ enzyme} + ETF \rightarrow FAD \text{ enzyme} + ETFH_2$$
$$ETFH_2 + \text{ubiquinone} \longrightarrow ETF + \text{ubiquinone } H_2$$

Aerobic dehydrogenases containing flavoproteins

Aerobic dehydrogenases are flavin enzymes containing FMN or FAD as prosthetic group (Table 21.4). Many of them also contain a metal which is essential for their function. Hence they are known as metal flavoproteins. Enzymes belonging to this group are D-amino acid dehydrogenase, L-amino acid dehydrogenase, xanthine dehydrogenase etc. Aerobic dehydrogenases are also called oxidases as they react directly with molecular oxygen. They produce H_2O_2 instead of H_2O. The H_2O_2 produced is decomposed to H_2O and O_2 by catalase.

Table 21.4-: Some oxidases and aerobic dehydrogenases

Enzyme	Product (H_2O or H_2O_2)
Oxidases	
Cytochrome oxidase	H_2O
Ascorbate oxidase	H_2O
Aerobic dehydrogenases	
Urate oxidase (uricase)	H_2O_2
Xanthine oxidase	H_2O_2
Glucose oxidase	H_2O_2

$$\text{Xanthine} \xrightarrow[\text{dehydrogenase}]{\text{Xanthine}} \text{Hypoxanthine} + H_2O_2$$

$$2H_2O_2 \xrightarrow{\text{Catalase}} 2H_2O + O_2$$

Oxidases

Enzymes that catalyse the reaction of hydrogen removed from substrates with molecular oxygen are called oxidases. **The most important oxidase involved in the electron system is cytochrome oxidase.** It is a haem protein containing iron and copper. It is a mixture of cytochrome a and a_3. The electrons and protons (H^+) removed from substrates react as follows with molecular oxygen in the presence of cytochrome oxidase.

$$O_2 + 4e^- \longrightarrow 2O^{--}$$
$$2O^{--} + 4 H^+ \longrightarrow 2H_2O$$

The other oxidases present in tissues are phenol oxidase and ascorbic acid oxidase.

Oxygenases (Oxygen transferase or dioxygenases)

These enzymes catalyse the direct transfer and incorporation of oxygen into a substrate molecule.

$$A + O_2 \longrightarrow AO_2$$

These enzymes cause the cleavage of aromatic ring through the formation of cyclic peroxide. Important examples of this type of enzymes include homogentisate dioxygenase, 3-hydroxyanthranilate dioxygenase and L-tryptophan dioxygenase (tryptophan pyrrolase). They are listed in Table 21.5.

Hydroxylases (Monooxygenases)

These enzymes catalyse the incorporation of one oxygen atom as hydroxyl group into a substrate molecule, the other oxygen atom being reduced to water. These enzymes require an additional electron donor. Some of the important enzymes belonging to this group are listed in Table 21.5.

Table 21.5: Oxygenases and hydroxylases

Enzyme	Co-substrate (reducing agent)	Reaction
Oxygenases		
Homogentisate oxygenase	-	Homogentisate → Maleylace-toacetate
Tryptophan oxygenase	-	Tryptophan → Formylkynurenine
Lipooxygenase	-	Polyunsaturated fatty acid → Peroxide
Hydroxylases		
Tyrosinase	DOPA	Tyrosine → DOPA → Melanin
Tyrosine hydroxylase	Reduced pteridine	Tyrosine → DOPA
Tryptophan 5-hydroxylase	-	Tryptophan → 5-Hydroxy-tryptophan
Phenylalanine hydroxylase	Reduced pteridine	Phenylalanine → Tyrosine

$$AH + O_2 + ZH_2 \longrightarrow A\text{-}OH + H_2O + Z$$

The important enzymes belonging to this group are tyrosinase, tryptophan-5-hydroxylase and phenylalanine hydroxylase.

Hydroperoxidases

These enzymes catalyse oxidation in which oxygen is obtained from hydrogen peroxide. **They include peroxidases and catalase.** Peroxidases found in milk and plants bring about the following reactions using H_2O_2.

$$AH_2 + H_2O_2 \longrightarrow A + 2H_2O$$
$$A + H_2O_2 \longrightarrow AO + H_2O$$

Catalase found in animal tissues and plants help to decompose H_2O_2 formed as it is toxic to tissues.

$$2H_2O_2 \xrightarrow{\text{Catalase}} 2H_2O + O_2$$

Peroxidase catalyses the following reactions in plants.

$$\text{Para-diphenols} + H_2O_2$$
$$\downarrow$$
$$\text{Paraquinone} + 2H_2O$$

Superoxide dismutase

Oxygen in the form of H_2O_2 or superoxide radical (O_2^-) is toxic to tissues. H_2O_2 is decomposed by catalase to H_2O and O_2. superoxide is formed when reduced flavin enzymes e.g., reduced xanthine dehydrogenase are oxidised univalently by molecular oxygen. It is also formed during univalent oxidations with molecular oxygen in the respiratory chain.

$$EnZH_2 + O_2 \longrightarrow EnZH + O_2^- + H^+$$

Superoxide (O_2^-) ion can reduce cytochrome C.

$$O_2^- + Fe_3^+ \longrightarrow O_2 + Fe_2^+$$

It can be removed by the specific enzyme superoxide dismutase in the presence of protons as indicated below:

$$O_2^- + O_2^- + 2H^+ \xrightarrow[\text{dismutase}]{\text{Superoxide}} H_2O_2 + O_2$$

This enzyme is present in all the tissues and its function is to decompose superoxide as soon as it is formed and thus protects the tissues against the harmful action of superoxide. The H_2O_2 formed is decomposed by catalase.

Electron transport system (Respiratory chain)

Hydrogen removed from the substrates is oxidised to water through the electron transport system. The system consists of the following carriers: (1) Nicotinamide adenine dinucleotide (NAD) and Nicotinamide adenine dinucleotide phosphate (NADP); (2) Flavin adenine nucleotides (FMN, FAD); (3) Ubiquinone (CoQ) and (4) Cytochromes (Cyt) (Fig.21.2 and 21.3).

Nicotinamide Adenine Nucleotides (NAD and NADP): These act as coenzymes for several enzymes in the TCA cycle. They exist both in the oxidised and reduced forms as indicated below:

$$NAD^+ \longleftrightarrow NADH$$
$$NADP^+ \longleftrightarrow NADPH$$

Flavin Adenine Nucleotides (FMN, FAD): They are present as part of a group of enzymes known as flavoproteins. The flavoprotein enzymes accept hydrogen atoms from reduced nicotinamide nucleotides as indicated below. The enzyme NADH dehydrogenase is a flavoprotein containing FMN.

$$NADH + FMN + H^+ \longleftrightarrow FMNH_2 + NAD$$
$$NADPH + FMN + H^+ \longleftrightarrow FMNH_2 + NADP$$

The enzyme succinic dehydrogenase contains FAD as the prosthetic group and catalyses oxidation of succinate to fumarate. This enzyme does not require NAD and the hydrogen taken up by FAD is passed on to CoQ (Fig 21.2 and 21.3).

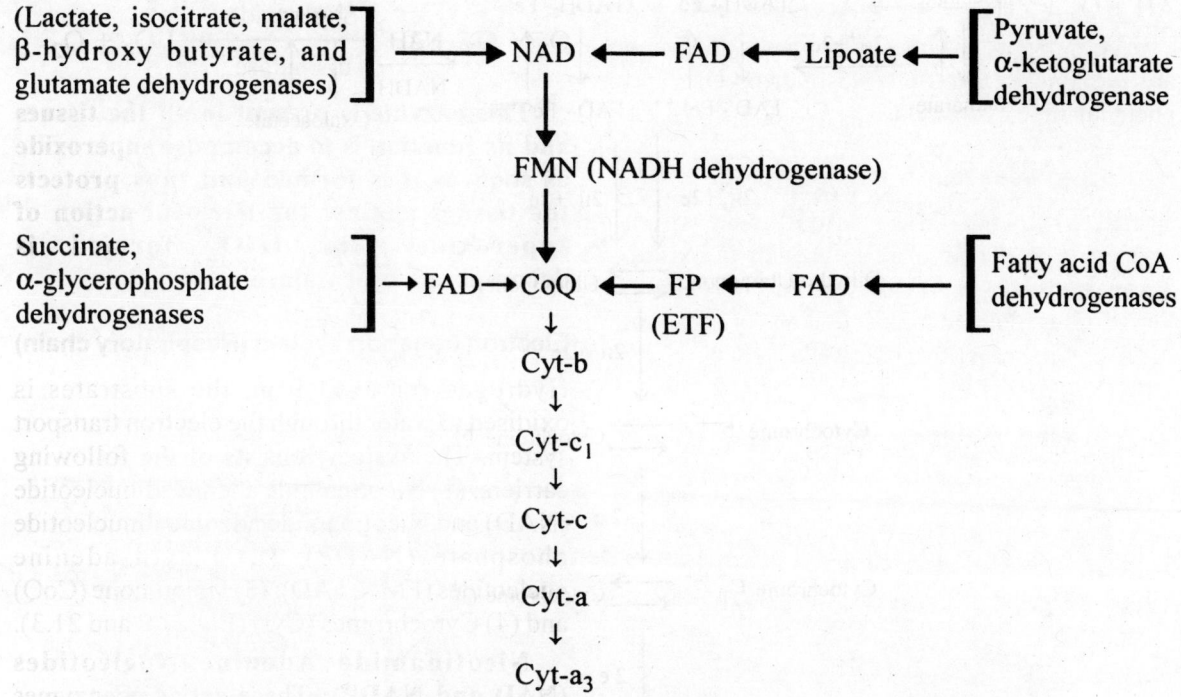

Fig. 21.2 : Electron transport chain (respiratory chain) carriers and metabolites oxidised

Ubiquinone (CoQ): There is good evidence that ubiquinone serves as a carrier between flavoproteins and cytochromes. It exists in reduced and oxidised forms as indicated below:

$$CoQ + 2H^+ + 2e \rightleftharpoons CoQH_2$$

Cytochromes: These were among the earliest components of the electron transport chain to be studied. The studies of Warburg and co-workers and Keilin and co-workers have revealed the presence of five cytochromes (a, a_3, b, c and c_1). All these cytochromes a, b, c and c_1 contain iron prophyrin as the prosthetic group. Cytochromes b, c and c_1 function as anaerobic dehydrogenases and carry electrons from the substrate (Fig. 21.3). Cytochrome oxidase (a_3) is the terminal member of the chain and is capable of oxidasing hydrogen removed from the substrates to water. It contains copper and iron. Recent studies indicate that cytochromes a and a_3 together constitute

cytochrome oxidase. The reduced form of cytochrome oxidase reduces molecular O_2, a process requiring four electrons for each mol of O_2 reduced.

Cytochrome b: It is a haem protein. The purified protein has a molecular weight of 28,000. In the absence of cation detergent, this protein aggregates readily to a larger polymer. The reduced form does not autooxidise nor does the oxidised form react with cyanide. Cytochrome b takes up electrons from reduced ubiquinone (Fig.21.3).

Cytochrome c_1: This is one of the recently recognised members of this group. It is a haem protein. The molecular weight is 38,000. It is rapidly converted into a polymer. It takes up electrons from reduced cytochrome b (Fig. 21.3).

Cytochrome c: It is the oldest member of the group. It has been isolated in the crystalline form. It is a haem protein and has a molecular

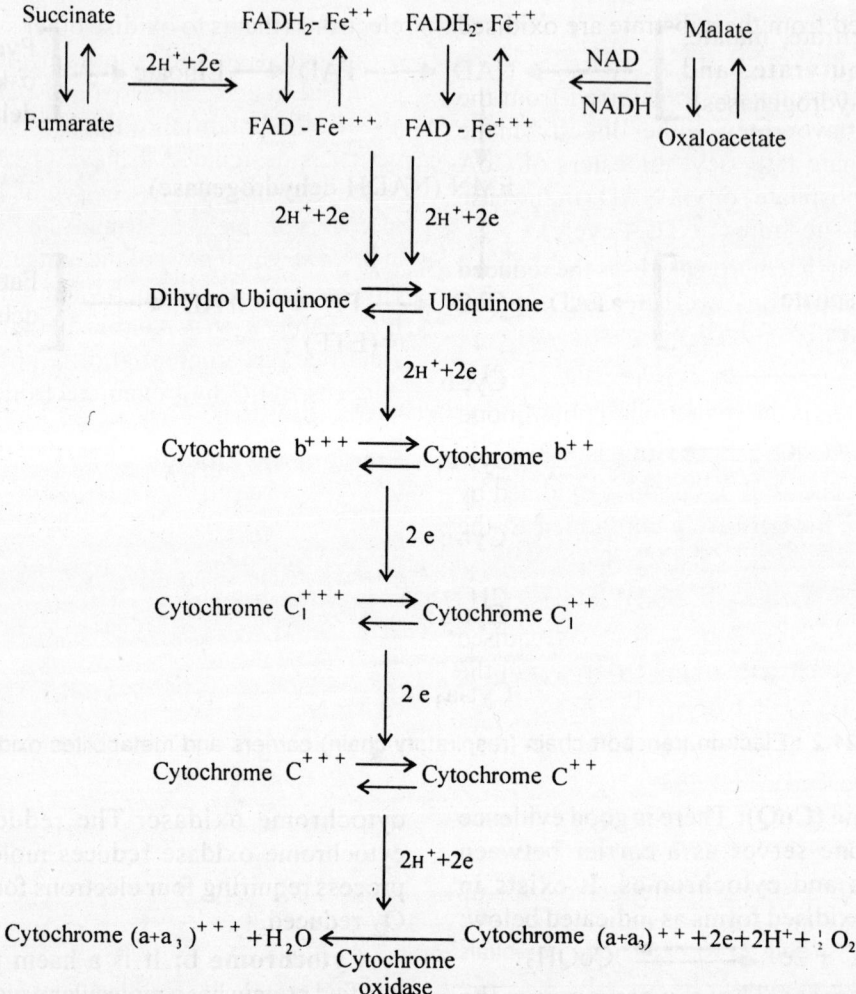

Fig. 21.3 : Electron transport chain i.e. Respiratory chain (Oxidation of hydrogen removed from substrate to water).

weight of 12,400 to 13,000. At neutral pH, ferrocytochrome c does not react with Co or O_2 nor does the ferric form react with cyanide. It only serves to transport electrons. It takes up electrons from cytochrome c_1 (Fig. 21.3). The reduced cytochrome c acts as a substrate for cytochrome oxidase.

Cytochrome Oxidase (a + a$_3$) : It is the terminal member of the cytochrome group. Recent studies indicate that it is a mixture of cytochrome a and a$_3$. Cytochrome oxidase is a

polymer of sub units of molecular weight about 72,000; each of which contains one haem as well as one atom of copper. Cytochrome oxidase is capable of oxidising hydrogen and electrons carried from the substrates by cytochrome c by molecular oxygen (Fig. 21.3). It combines with CO and CN and is thereby inactivated.

The electron transport system indicating the manner of transport of electrons and hydrogen from the substrate through different carriers is indicated in Fig. 21.2 and 21.3. The hydrogen atoms removed from the substrate are oxidised to water.

1.Hydrogen atoms are transferred from the substrate to a flavoprotein, either directly (in the case of succinate fatty acyl thioesters of CoA and glycerophosphate) or via NAD (in the case of lactate and substrates of TCA cycle).

2.As the non- haem iron oxidises the reduced flavoproteins, protons are released into the medium.

$$FADH_2 + 2Fe^{+++} \longrightarrow FAD + 2Fe^{++} + 2H^+$$

The next step is the reduction of ubiquinone

$$2Fe^{++} + 2H^+ + CoQ \rightleftharpoons CoQH_2 + 2Fe^{+++}$$

3.As the reduced ubiquinone is oxidised by cytochrome b, protons are again added to the medium.

$$CoQH_2 + Cyt\ c^{+++} \longrightarrow CoQ + Cyt\ c^{++} + 2H^+$$

4.At the end of the chain, hydrogen is oxidised to water by cytochrome oxidise (a + a_3) in the presence of oxygen as follows:

$$\frac{1}{2}O_2 + H^+ + 2e \longrightarrow OH^-$$
$$OH^- + H^+ \longrightarrow H_2O$$

Oxidation-reduction or redox potential

A system with a strong tendency to take up electrons (that is to oxidise other systems) has a large negative redox potential. The redox potential of a system (Eo) is usually compared against the potential of the hydrogen electrode which is designated to have O volts at pH-O. Since enzymes are not active at low pH, it is more reasonable to determine the redox potential at pH 7 in which most of the oxidation- reduction enzymes are active. Such values are designated E'o (Table 21.6). At this pH, the hydrogen electrode has a potential difference of -0.42 V with respect to hydrogen electrode at pH-O.

Free energy change

When two oxidation reduction systems react with one another, the difference in redox potential between the two systems ΔE'o is related to the free energy change of the reaction (ΔG or ΔF) by the following equation:

$$\Delta G = -nF\Delta E'o \quad \text{Coulomb joules}$$

Where n is the number of electrons transferred and F is the Faraday constant (96,500 coulomb per one gram equivalent). The value of ΔG thus obtained may be converted into calories by dividing by the factor 4.18.

Table 21.6 : Electrode potentials of some oxidation - reduction systems

System				E'o volts
$\frac{1}{2}O_2/H_2O$	..	..	..	0.82
$\frac{1}{2}O_2 + H_2O/H_2O_2$	..	..	..	0.30
Fe^{+++}/Cytochrome a Fe^{++}	..	..	..	0.29
Fe^{+++}/Cytochrome c Fe^{++}	..	..	..	0.22
Fe^{+++}/Cytochrome b_2 Fe^{++}	..	..	..	0.12
Dehydroascorbic acid/ascorbic acid	..	..	..	0.08
$FMN/FMNH_2$	..	..	..	-0.12
Oxaloacetic acid/malic acid	..	..	..	-0.17
Pyruvic acid/lactic acid	..	..	..	-0.19
$NAD/NADH + H^+$	..	..	..	-0.32
Pyruvic acid + CO_2/malic acid	..	..	..	-0.33
Uric acid/xanthine	..	..	..	-0.36

$$\Delta G = \frac{nF \times \Delta E'o}{4.18} \text{ calories}$$

FREE ENERGY CHANGES AND OXIDATION-REDUCTION POTENTIAL

Relation between Eo and Free energy

Since the oxidation reactions produce energy, it will be of interest to calculate the free energy of different oxidation-reduction reactions. This can be calculated by the following formula.

$$- \Delta F^o = nF\Delta Eo$$

where ΔF^o = Standard free energy of reaction

n = number of electrons (or hydrogen atoms)

and ΔF^o = Coulomb volts of joules which can be converted into units of free energy since 4.18 joules = 1 g Cal. The value obtained for ΔF^o is for the oxidation of one molecule of reactant.

Example: For example, the free energy of the reaction involving oxidation of malic acid to oxaloacetic acid by cytochrome c under

circumstance such that equimolar concentrations always exist of each of the reactants of the two systems. Since the Eo value are -0.17 volts and 0.2 volt (Table 21.7), the free energy can be calculated from the equation.

$$- \Delta F^o = nF\Delta Eo$$

$$- \Delta F^o = \frac{-2 \times 96,500 \times \{0.2 - (-0.17)\}}{4.18}$$

$$= - 18,246 \text{ cal or } 18.2 \text{ kcal.}$$

The oxidation of one molecule of malic acid by cytochrome c results in the release of 18,246 cal or 18.2 kcal.

Free energy changes in various steps in the Electron Transport Chain

Free energy changes calculated from the oxidation potential difference of the various oxidation-reduction systems involved in the respiratory chain are given in Table 21.7.

The energy released at each step is directly proportional to the difference in redox potentials

Table 21.7 : Free energy changes in the various oxidation-reduction system of the respiratory Chain

Step of transference of H or $\bar{e}$	Difference in redox potential (E)	Free energy changes Kcals
NADH $\xrightarrow{2H}$ FP	0.26 volts	- 12.0
FP $\xrightarrow{2\bar{e}}$ 2 cyt b	0.10 volts	4.6
2cyt b $\xrightarrow{2\bar{e}}$ 2 cyt c	0.23 volts	- 10.6
2cyt c $\xrightarrow{2\bar{e}}$ 2cyt a	0.02 volts	- 0.9
2cyt a $\xrightarrow{2\bar{e}}$ 2cyt a_3	0.21 volts	- 9.6
2cyt a_3 $\xrightarrow{2\bar{e}}$ O_2	0.32 volts	14.7
Total	1.14 volts	52.4 Kcal

of the two consecutive systems operating in the step (Table 21.8). Thus it is evident that when 1 molecule of NADH is oxidised by $\frac{1}{2}O_2$, about 52 Kcal of free energy are set free. Assuming the free energy required for the conversion of one mol. of ADP to ATP is 7-8 Kcal, the free energy conserved in the formation of 3 mol. of ATP from ADP per mol. of NADH oxidised will be from 21 to 24 KCal. Thus the efficiency of conservation of energy is 21 x 100/52 = 40% or 24 x 100/52 = 46%.

BIOENERGETICS (High Energy Compounds)

In the oxidation of glucose, fatty acids and amino acids in the tissues, certain energy- rich phosphate compounds are formed or hydrolysed, leading to the conservation or release of free energy. The most important of these include phosphate esters of adenine (ATP, ADP, AMP), acyl phosphates, enol phosphates, guanidine phosphates, and thiol esters. When these compounds are hydrolysed, free energy is released (Table 21.8).

Oxidative Phosphorylation: The term oxidative phosphorylation refers to the formation of ATP from ADP during the oxidation of metabolites through the electron transport system. The oxidation of NADH leads to the formation of 3 mols of ATP and of $FADH_2$ to the formation of 2 mols of ATP. Since the formation of ATP from ADP requires about 7 kcals of energy, ATP formation is possible at the sites where the free energy released is more than 8 kcals. (Table 21.8) i.e. between (1) NAD and FP (2) cyt. b and cyt. c (3) cyt. a and cyt. a_3 and (4) cyt. a_3 and O_2.

Substrate level phosphorylation: Substrate level phosphorylation also leads to the production of ATP but the reactions are not dependent on electron transport system. Some examples of this type of phosphorylation are: (1) the reactions of glycolysis in which phosphoenolpyruvic acid and 1:3 diphosphoglyceric acids are first formed and react later with ADP to form ATP and (2) the reaction catalysed by succinic thiokinase in TCA cycle which leads to the formation of GTP which in turn reacts with ADP forming ATP.

Conservation of Energy as ATP during Oxidation of Glucose and Fatty Acids: As explained above, the electron transport system and the oxidative phosphorylation mechanism

Table 21.8 : Free energy of hydrolysis of some important **energy- rich (high energy)** compounds

High energy compound	Δ G (Cal)
Phosphoenolpyruvate	14,800
1:3 Diphosphoglycerate	11,800
Phosphocreatine	10,300
Acetyl-CoA	7,500
ATP to ADP	7,300
ATP-AMP and Pyrophosphate	8,600
ADP-AMP	6,500
Glucose-1-phosphate	5,000
Fructose-1-phosphate	3,800
Glucose-6-phosphate	3,300
Phosphocreatine+ADP $\longrightarrow$ Creatine + ATP	33,000

help to form ATP. Substrate level phosphorylation also leads to the formation of ATP. It is evident that the cell has the mechanism to conserve part of the energy obtained in the oxidation to glucose, fatty acids and amino acids in the form of ATP which can be used for several biochemical reactions requiring ATP such as the synthesis of fatty acids, phosphorylation reactions, etc.

ATP formed during Glucose Oxidation: If there was no mechanism in the cell for trapping energy, all the energy will be released as heat. The cell has, however, the mechanism for conserving part of the energy as newly formed ATP. During the complete oxidation of 1 mol. of glucose in the cell, it has been estimated (Table 21.9) that 38 mols of ATP are synthesised

from ADP. The free energy conserved in 38 mols. of ATP will be 38 x 7,300 or 277,400 cal. When 1 mol. of glucose is oxidised, the total energy output will be 686,000 cal. Out of this, 277,400 cal. are conserved as ATP, i.e., the efficiency of energy conservation is about 40 percent.

ATP formed during oxidation of Fatty Acids: The complete oxidation of 1 mol. of palmitic acid will yield 2,440,000 cal. The number of mols of ATP formed (Table 21.10) during the oxidation of 1 mol. of palmitic acid is 131. The energy conserved in 131 mols. of ATP will be 131 x 7,300 or 956,300 calories, i.e., about 40 percent of the total energy. In the case of fat oxidation also, 40 percent of the energy is conserved as ATP.

Table 21.9 : ATP formed during oxidation of glucose

Reaction	ATP (Mols)
Glucose $\longrightarrow$ Fructose 1, 6- diphosphate	-2
2 mols of triophosphate $\longrightarrow$ 2 mols of 3-phospho glyceric acid	2
2 NADP $\longrightarrow$ 2NADPH $\longrightarrow$ 2NADP	6
2 mols of phosphoenol pyruvic acid $\longrightarrow$ 2 mols of pyruvic acid	2
2 mols of pyruvic acid $\longrightarrow$ 2mols of acetyl CoA	6
2 mols of acetyl CoA $\longrightarrow$ 4 CO_2 + 4H_2O	24
Total	38

Table 21.10: ATP formed in the oxidation of palmitic acid

Reaction	ATP (Mols)
Palmityl CoA + 7O_2 $\longrightarrow$ 8 Acetyl CoA	35
8 Acetyl CoA + 16 O_2 $\longrightarrow$ 16 H_2O + 16 CO_2	96
(8 revolutions of TCA cycle yielding 12 ATP per revolution)	
Total	131

CHAPTER 22

RADIOISOTOPES

Thanks to H. Bacqueral, Curie and Curie and others for the discovery of us. We are of great use to the Biologists/Biochemists/ Chemists/ Physicians etc. as we are extensibly used in the studies of intermediary metabolism i.e., in the follow up of metabolic pathways, etc. and in medicine as we can cure the most fierceful disease of the day i.e. cancer. We are used in the treatment of hyperthyroidism, certain types of cancers of the thyroid, leukaemias, etc.

Side by side, ours wrongful handling and exposure is very dangerous as we may cause genetic defects. Teratogenic effects are those that may be observed in children who were exposed during the fetal and embryonic stages of development. Teratogenic effects, such as cancer, congenital malformation and reduced intelligence have been observed in certain irradiated groups (for example, Japanese atomic bomb survivors) but only at relatively high doses (20 rem or more acute exposure).

USE OF RADIOACTIVE AND STABLE ISOTOPES IN STUDIES IN INTERMEDIARY METABOLISM AND MEDICINE

Isotopes of elements have the same atomic number but different atomic weights. Isotopes may be broadly divided into two groups: (i) Radioactive isotopes; and (ii) Stable isotopes. Both the types of isotopes have been used in studies in the metabolism of carbohydrates, proteins, fats, nucleic acids and minerals.

Radioactive isotopes

Radioactivity (emitted by the element uranium) was first discovered by H. Becqueral in 1895.

Soon after, Curie and Curie discovered radium (another radioactive element) in 1902. The radioactive elements emit radiations. The radiations have been classified as follows: (i) Emission of alpha particle; (ii) Emission of beta particle; (iii) Emission of positron (positively charged electron of nuclear origin); and (iv) Emission of gamma rays.

α-Particle: The α- particle consists of two protons and two neutrons i.e., a helium nucleus.

β-Particle: The β- particle is an electron of nuclear origin. During its emission, a neutron is transformed into a proton.

Positron: Positron is a positively charged

electron of nuclear origin. During the emission of positron, a proton is changed into a neutron. The positron is "short" lived. After ejection , it loses its kinetic energy and combines with an electron. This results in the annihilation of both the particles and liberation of two gamma rays.

Gamma Rays: Gamma rays are electro-magnetic radiations and have no mass or charge. They are more penetrating than $\alpha-$ or $\beta-$ rays.

The half lives of some radioactive isotopes used in the studies of intermediary metabolism or in clinical medicine are given in Table 22.1

Measurement of' Radioactivity

Two types of instruments are commonly used: (i) Scintillation counters; and (ii) Geiger-Muller counter.

Scintillation Counters: The sample containing the radioactive isotope is mixed with certain type of phosphor. The radiation emitted by the sample is converted into light radiations which are picked up by a photomultiplier tube and measured using a counter.

Geiger-Muller Counter: Rays from the radioactive isotope enters an ionization chamber which contains gas. The rays interact with the gas and produce ions which in turn causes discharge of current. The current is amplified and recorded in a counter.

Stable Isotopes

The stable isotopes which have found use in studies in intermediary metabolism are H^2 (Deuterium), N^{15} and O^{18}. They do not emit any radiations. They can be measured by the use of **Mass Spectrophotometer.**

USE OF ISOTOPES IN BIOCHEMICAL STUDIES AND MEDICINE

Biochemical and Physiological Studies

The different type of studies may be discussed under the following heads: (i) Distribution studies; (ii) Dilution studies; (iii) Membrane transfer studies; (iv) Studies on life span and fate of cells; and (v) Metabolic studies.

Distribution Studies: Distribution studies have been widely used in biochemical research in medicine. For example, in study of thyroid physiology, the distribution of I^{131} administered

Table 22.1: Half lives of some Radioactive Isotopes used in the studies of Intermediary Metabolism and Medicine

Element	Half life	Radiation with energy in Mev
H^3	12.5 years	$(0.0185)\,\beta$
C^{14}	5760 years	$(0.156)\,\beta$
P^{32}	14.3 days	$(1.712)\,\beta$
S^{35}	87.1 days	$(0.169)\,\beta$
Fe^{59}	45.1 days	$\beta\,(0.46),\ \gamma\,(1.3)$
I^{131}	8.1 days	$\beta\,(0.69),\ \gamma\,(0.72)$
Ca^{45}	152 days	$\beta\,(0.26)$
Na^{24}	15.1 hours	$\beta\,(1.59),\ \gamma\,(2.89)$
K^{42}	12.4 hours	$\beta\,(3.85)$
Cl^{36}	4.4×10^5 years	$\beta\,(0.71)$
Co^{60}	5.2 years	$\gamma\,(1.33),\ \beta\,(0.306)$

as Na^{131} has provided much information. About one third the iodine ingested was taken up by the thyroid and about two thirds was excreted by the kidney in normal human adults.

Dilution Studies: Some of the dilution studies carried out with radioactive isotopes are: (i) measurement of plasma volume using I^{131} labelled serum albumin; (ii) measurement of erythrocyte volume using Cr^{51} labelled erythrocytes; and (iii) measurement of total body water using I^{131} labelled iodoantipyrin or tritiated water.

Membrane Transfer Studies- Absorption and Excretion Studies: Radioactive isotopes have been used in several absorption-excretion studies. These include: , (i) absorption of fat containing I^{131} using I^{131} triolein or I^{131} oleic acid; (ii) absorption of iron using Fe^{59} ferrous salts; and (iii) measurement of intestinal protein loss by intravenous injection of I^{131} or Cr^{51} labelled protein.

Live Span of R.B.C.: The life span of RBC has been determined by tagging Cr^{51} to RBC.

Metabolic Studies: The greatest area of application of radioactive isotopes has been in the study of the intermediary metabolism. Almost every phase of metabolism viz., photosynthesis, carbohydrate degradation, the tricarboxylic acid cycle, amino acid metabolism, protein biosynthesis, nucleic acid synthesis, biosynthesis of haem and cholesterol, fatty acid synthesis and oxidation and steroid metabolism have been studied using compounds containing C^{14}, N^{15}, H^2, H^3, P^{32}, S^{35}, etc. Several aspects of mineral metabolism have been studied using Ca^{45}, Fe^{54}, I^{131}, Na^{24}, K^{42} and Cl^{36}.

As Radiation Sources in Clinical Medicine

Radioactive isotopes are used as a radiation source in medicine for the treatment of certain disorders. Examples of such clinical use are: (i) the use of radioactive iodine in the treatment of hyperthyroidism and some types of cancer of the thyroid, (ii) the use of P^{32} labelled sodium phosphate in the treatment of polycythemia vera or leukaemias. Radioactive isotopes are used clinically in the form of sealed needles for insertion directly into tumours. More recently $Cobalt^{60}$ is used to deliver radiations (α- rays) to tumours.

PRECAUTIONS IN HANDLING RADIOISOTOPES

Ionizing radiation can be hazardous to the healthy body and unnecessary exposure should be avoided. It appears that the human body can receive 5 rem per year after the age of 18 years without any apparent harmful effect. The hands and forearms can receive 75 rem per year without harmful effect. In most laboratories using isotopes mainly as tracers, personnel receive only a small fraction of the recommended limits. In order to keep the exposure to a minimum, certain precautions should be observed :

(i) Radioactive isotopes should be stored in a special area, properly marked by signs, and properly shielded. The plastic or glass container or containers made up of several centimetres of **lucite** are adequate. (ii) The handling of radioactive isotope should be carried out in such a way that the hands and body should receive less than the recommended limit. (iii) As far as possible, remote control handling equipment should be used and if possible unbreakable containers should be employed. In case of breakage or spillage, the containers or absorbent material should be placed appropriately. (iv) **Pipetting should always be done with the automatic or remote devices and never by mouth.** (v) **Rubber gloves should be worn whenever there is a danger or skin contact with a radioactive isotope. (vi) Eating, drinking and smoking should be prohibited in the laboratory. (vii) Whenever work with volatile radioisotopes is necessary, it should be carried out in a closed system or in a fume - hood with proper ventilation as prescribed by the Atomic Energy Commission.**

CHAPTER 23

PHYSICOCHEMISTRY PHENOMENA (BIOPHYSICS)

(HYDROGEN ION CONCENTRATION, pH, BUFFERS, COLLOIDS, OSMOSIS, VISCOSITY, SURFACE TENSION, DIALYSIS, ETC.

We are of extreme importance in many ways as we make the '*logic*' of physiology/biochemistry phenomena of human chemistry and give the answers of how, why and when of entire physiology/biochemistry. That who understands us seriously, can go to the height of searching answers of numerous unsolved problems of disorders/diseases. We are also of immense significance to pharmacologists and physicians.

HYDROGEN ION CONCENTRATION, pH AND BUFFERS

One of the important factors governing biochemical and biophysical changes is the concentration of various ions present in the blood, body fluids and glandular secretions. The important cations that are present are H^+, Ca^{++}, Na^+, K^+ etc. and the important anions are bicarbonate (HCO_3^-), chloride (Cl^-), phosphate (HPO_4^{--} and $H_2PO_4^-$) etc.

The origin of H^+ in living tissues is water as all forms of life contain water and as water feebly ionises to liberate H^+ in addition to OH^-. Water contains 10^{-7} g of H^+/litre and as it is the source for H^+ in the body, the concentration of H^+ in biological fluids will be in the neighbourhood of 10^{-7} g of H^+/litre.

As a result of ionisation of water for each H^+ there should be equivalent amount of OH^-

according to the following equation:

$$H_2O \rightleftharpoons H^+ + OH^-$$

(It has to be remembered that the degree of ionisation is very slight and it could be shown as if just one molecule out of nearly 550 million molecules of water undergoes complete ionisation. Also, the H^+ ion gets hydrated and is present as hydroxonium ion, H_3O^+.) In water which is neutral, the H^+ concentration is 10^{-7} g ions/litre (equal to 10^{-7} g/litre). As there should be an equivalent number of OH^-, the concentration of OH^- also is 10^{-7} g ions/litre. But each g ion of OH^- is equal to 17 g. So 10^{-7} g ions of OH^- will be equal to 17×10^{-7} g.

H^+ concentration is responsible for acidity while it is OH^- for alkalinity. If in any system H^+ and OH^- are of equal concentration, the solution is neutral, e.g. water. If H^+ concentration exceeds that of OH^-, the solution will become acidic. For example if the concentration of H^+ in an aqueous medium is 10^{-2} it is acidic. Alternately if the H^+ is less than 10^{-7}, the solution will be basic (for example a solution with a concentration of 10^{-10} of H^+). In any aqueous solution the ionic product ($H^+ \times OH^-$) should not exceed 10^{-14} g ions/litre which is arrived at by experimental finding that there are 10^{-7} g ions of H^+ and 10^{-7} g ions of OH^- ($10^{-7} \times 10^{-7} = 10^{-14}$) per litre of water.

In order to do away with the negative powers as 10^{-7} or 10^{-x} in representing H^+ concentration especially of biological fluids, S.P.L. Sorensen suggested a convenient notation known as pH notation (**pH meaning Puissance Hydrogen,** Potenz Hydrogen or Hydrogen power). In this, the negative powers vanish and positive numbers result and at the same time one is able to appreciate the concentration of Hydrogen ions:

pH is defined as the negative logarithm to the base 10 of H^+ concentration (or better H^+ activity).

pH = $-\log_{10} H^+$

pH of water: The H^+ of water is 10^{-7} g/litre

$H^+ = 10^{-7}$ g

$\log_{10} H^+ = \log_{10} 10^{-7} = -7$

Negative $\log_{10} H^+ = 7$

$(-\log_{10} H^+)$

Therefore, the pH of water is 7

Thus the H^+ concentration of 10^{-7} involving negative power (-7) becomes a positive number 7 in pH notation. The different H^+ concentrations and their corresponding pH values are given below:

As already indicated, the product of ionic concentrations or H^+ and OH^- should be only 10^{-14} in any aqueous solution, the highest pH could be only 14. The pH of a solution containing 1 g of H^+ (say 1 N HCl on complete ionisation) is 0 and that of 1 N alkali (on complete ionisation) is 14. The pH scale is thus between 0 and 14, pH 0 indicating almost pure acid solution and pH 14 almost pure alkali solution. pH 7 is that of water which is neutral as it contains equal number of H^+ and OH^-. An increase of H^+ concentration will mean decrease of negative power, the pH of acid solutions will be less than 7. If the pH is above 7, the solution is alkaline.

Neutral pH 7

Acid pH 0 upto 7

Alkaline pH above 7 to 14

The pH of blood is 7.35 to 7.45 i.e. slightly on the alkaline side. The pH of urine is on the acid side, i.e. less than 7.

DEFINITIONS OF BUFFERS, ACIDS AND BASES

Buffers

A buffer solution is one which resists or minimizes change of pH when acid or base is added. Thus the buffers in the body fluid act as a physicochemical defence against pH change; other mechanisms such as the physiological control mechanisms of the kidneys and lungs also operate to minimize changes in pH and also to restore the composition of the body fluids to a normal state following a disturbance.

A buffer always consists of a mixture of a

H^+	1	10^{-1}	10^{-2}	10^{-3}	10^{-4}	10^{-5}	10^{-6}	10^{-7}	10^{-8}	10^{-9}	10^{-10}	10^{-11}
pH	0	1	2	3	4	5	6	7	8	9	10	11

acidic   neutral   basic

	10^{-12}	10^{-13}	10^{-14}
	12	13	14

basic

weak acid (or base) and its conjugate base (or acid) respectively.

Acid

An acid is a proton donor, that is anything which dissociates into one or more protons, i.e. a hydrogen ion, plus a conjugate base.

e.g. $HA \rightleftharpoons H^+ + A^-$
        acid   proton   conjugate base

example : carbonic acid $H_2CO_3 \rightleftharpoons H^+ + HCO_3^-$

Base

A base is a proton acceptor, i.e. anything which can combine with a proton to form a conjugate acid.

e.g. $B + H^+ \rightleftharpoons BH^+$
       base   conjugate acid

or $BH + H^+ \rightleftharpoons BH_2^+$
     base   conjugate acid

example : ammonia $NH_3 + H^+ \rightleftharpoons NH_4^+$

bicarbonate $HCO_3^- + H^+ \rightleftharpoons H_2CO_3$

Note that some biological substances (e.g. phosphates and amino acids, see below) can behave as both bases and acids, i.e. they can both accept and donate protons respectively. Such substances are described as being amphiprotic or amphoteric.

e.g. $H_2PO_4^- \rightleftharpoons H^+ + HPO_4^{--}$
       acid

$H_2PO_4^- + H^+ \rightleftharpoons H_3PO_4$
base

Water is also an example of an amphoteric molecule since it can both donate and accept protons:

$H_2O \rightleftharpoons H^+ + OH^-$
acid

and $H_2O + H^+ \rightleftharpoons H_3O^+$
     base

The Henderson-Hasselbalch Equation

From the definitions

$Acid \rightleftharpoons H^+ + base^-$

$pH = -\log [H^+]$

$pK = -\log K$

$K = [H+] \dfrac{[base^-]}{[acid]}$

one can simply derive the Henderson equation:

$$[H+] = \frac{[K . \{acid\}]}{[base^-]}$$

or the more useful logarithmic version, the Henderson-Hasselbalch equation which is:

$$pH = pK + \log \frac{[base^-]}{[acid]}$$

This equation is fundamental to the consideration of all acid- base equilibria.

Obviously, according to the law of mass action, addition of H^+ ions to a mixture containing acid and base.

acid $\rightleftharpoons H^+ + base$

will displace the equilibrium towards the left as written above; thus the concentration of the base component will fall, while the concentration of the acid component must rise by an exactly corresponding amount. The Henderson-Hasselbalch equation enables one to relate quantitatively the change in [base], [acid] and pH. One therefore can see that the pH of a solution depends on the logarithm of the ratio of base to acid concentration;* and not on the ratio

---

* In turn, the hydrogen ion concentration itself depends upon the ratio of base to acid concentration (not logarithm) according to the Henderson equation:

$$[H^+] = K \times \frac{[base^-]}{[acid]}$$

itself or on one or other concentration by itself.

Consider the equilibrium:

$$\text{acid} \rightleftharpoons H^+ + \text{base}^-$$

$$pH = pK + \log \frac{[\text{base}^-]}{[\text{acid}]}$$

Addition of x mole of H^+ ions per litre will reduce [base] by an amount x, and will increase [acid] by an equal amount x, so that the pH becomes

$$pH = pK + \log \left\{ \frac{[\text{base}] - x}{[\text{acid}] + x} \right\}$$

It can be shown that the smallest change in the ratio will be produced (for a given value of x) if initially [acid] = [base]. This means that a buffer is best, i.e. it minimizes pH change most effectively, when it consists or an equimolar mixture of its acid and base forms. Therefore, a buffer mixture is best when:

$$pH = pK + \log \frac{[\text{base}^-]}{[\text{acid}]}$$

$$= pK + \log (1)$$

$$= pK$$

Hence, a buffer function is best when the pH is close to the buffer's pK value; roughly speaking it is only useful as a buffer if the pH is within 1 pH unit of the pK value. Hence, acids with pK values in the vicinity of 2 to 3, such as α-COOH groups in amino acids and proteins are of no value as buffers around physiological pH (7.4).

Buffer solutions

A buffer solution is one which is resistant to changes in pH on the addition of small amounts of acid or alkali: Such solutions usually consist of a mixture of a weak acid and its salt (e.g. acetic acid and sodium acetate), a weak base and its salt (ammonium hydroxide and

ammonium chloride). A salt of a weak acid and a weak base (e.g. ammonium acetate) also has buffer action.

Buffers of the Body Fluids

Here, we will consider various buffer systems in blood and other extracellular fluids. The two principal buffers in blood are the bicarbonate / CO_2 system and the haemoglobin system. Plasma proteins and phosphate make minor but sometimes significant contributions. Except for haemoglobin, the same substances are important buffers in the other extracellular tissue fluids, including cerebrospinal fluid (CSF). Proteins and phosphates (organic and inorganic) are probably the principal intracellular buffers, but since one cannot measure readily the composition of intracellular fluids in practice, therefore, they will not be considered further. However, these buffers are summarized below in Table 23.1.

Table 23.1: Principal buffer systems in body fluids

1.	Blood	CO_2/HCO_3^-
		HHb/Hb^- and $HHbO_2/HbO_2^-$
		i.e. haemoglobin
		H. Protein/Protein$^-$
		$(H_2PO_4^-/HPO_4^{--})$
2.	CSF, ECF	CO_2/HCO_3^-
		(H. Protein/Protein$^-$)
		$(H_2PO_4^-/HPO_4^{--})$
3.	Intracellular fluids	H.Protein/Protein$^-$
		$H_2PO_4^-/HPO_4^{--}$
		P organic/P $^-$organic
		CO_2/HCO_3^-
4.	Urine	$H_2PO_4^-/HPO_4^{--}$
		NH_4^+/NH_3

It is important to bear in mind that measurements in specific extracellular fluids such as blood and CSF do not necessarily give a true picture of the acid-base status of the intracellular fluids or of the body fluids as a whole.

Bicarbonate/carbondioxide system

This is of major importance, especially because the acid component (or, strictly, the acid anhydride), carbon dioxide is volatile and its concentration can be regulated physiologically by the respiratory system, that is by pulmonary ventilation together with control from the chemoreceptors and respiratory centre. Additionally the conjugate base, bicarbonate, can be independently regulated to a certain extent by the kidneys although this is not very rapid. There is fairly large quantity of this buffer present owing to large carbon dioxide production during even basal oxidative metabolism since CO_2 is the principal end product of normal carbohydrate and fat oxidation. **A sedentary adult produces about 13,000 m mol CO_2 per day and an active person may produce over twice this amount.**

Consider the equilibrium
$$CO_2 + H_2O \rightleftharpoons H_2CO_3 \rightleftharpoons H^+ + HCO_3^-$$

In the presence of the enzyme carbonic anhydrase which is found in red-blood cells, the formation of carbonic acid by the hydration of CO_2 is rapid:
$$CO_2 + H_2O \rightleftharpoons H_2CO_3$$

Since carbonic acid cannot be easily measured, and since it is CO_2 (the acid anhydride) rather than the H_2CO_3 (the acid itself) which is regulated by ventilation, it is convenient to ignore the 'true' acid base equilibrium
$$H_2CO_3 \rightleftharpoons H^+ + HCO_3^-$$
which gives
$$pK = -\log \frac{[H+].[HCO_3^-]}{[H_2CO_3]}$$
and to consider the overall equilibrium:
$$CO_2 + H_2O \rightleftharpoons H_2CO_3 \rightleftharpoons H^+ + HCO_3^-$$

Regulation of bicarbonate concentration

In addition to the lungs regulating the Pco_2 in blood, the kidneys can regulate the bicarbonate concentration to some extent, although this regulatory mechanism acts more slowly than does the respiratory one. The kidneys can regulate the plasma bicarbonate concentration by controlling the rate of tubular reabsorption of bicarbonate and the rate at which bicarbonate is regenerated in the renal tubule cells via the rate of H^+ secretion into the urine.

The HCO_3^-/CO_2 system can be regarded as the main buffer system in extracellular fluids.

Haemoglobin

Proteins and amino acids as buffers

All proteins are, to some extent, buffers by virtue of the acid-base dissociations or associations of their component amino acids. However, the equilibrium of the α-amino and α-carboxyl groups, viz.

$$\underset{\text{base}}{\underset{\text{COOH}}{\overset{R}{|}}\overset{|}{CH}-NH_2} + H^+ \rightleftharpoons \underset{\text{acid}}{\underset{\text{COOH}}{\overset{R}{|}}\overset{|}{CH}^- -NH_3^+} \quad \text{(association of the α-amino group)}$$

and

$$\underset{\text{acid}}{\underset{\text{COOH}}{\overset{R}{|}}\overset{|}{CH}-NH_2} \rightleftharpoons \underset{\text{base}}{\underset{\text{COO}^-+H^+}{\overset{R}{|}}\overset{|}{CH}-NH_2} \quad \text{(dissociation of the α-carboxyl group)}$$

are not important since these two groups are involved in the formation of the peptide linkage between amino acids.

In addition, haemoglobin is present in blood at a remarkably high concentration of around 15g/100ml and since the buffering capacity of any buffer depends upon its concentration, therefore, it's a very powerful buffer system.

Plasma proteins

All proteins contain dissociating and associating side-chain groups in their constituent amino acids and hence they are capable of acting as buffers. While proteins are likely to be of major importance for intracellular buffering but they have limited capability of buffering in blood because most of the plasma proteins are present only in quite small concentrations. Albumin (3-4.5 g/100 ml) is the most abundant plasma protein and does contribute significantly to blood buffering.

Phosphate

Phosphoric acid is a tribasic acid which can be dissociated, thus:

$$H_3PO_4 \rightleftharpoons H^+ + H_2PO_4^- \quad pK_1 = 2.0$$
$$H_2PO_4^- \rightleftharpoons H^+ + HPO_4^{--} \quad pK_2 = 6.8$$
$$HPO_4^{--} \rightleftharpoons H^+ + PO_4^{---} \quad pK_3 = 11.7$$

At physiological pH values, virtually all the phosphate is in the $H_2PO_4^-$ and the HPO_4^{--} forms, and therefore only the second equation above need be considered.

Since pK = 6.8 is so close to pH 7.4, one can see that this is potentially a good buffer at blood pH on physicochemical grounds. However, the phosphate concentration in plasma is so low (0.8-1.4 m mol/litre in fasting) that this system is normally of trivial importance.

However, phosphate is the principal buffer of normal urine, the concentration in urine obviously can vary over a wide range, depending mainly on phosphate and fluid intake, but a figure of 50 m mol/litre may be typical.

Bone buffering

In prolonged acidosis, phosphate buffering can become important, although it is often loosely stated that under these conditions bone acts as a buffer. Calcium phosphate, which is present in hydroxyapatite form in the inorganic part of bone, is relatively insoluble; however the solubility is greater at lower pH. Hence, if the pH falls below normal, some calcium phosphate in bone goes into solution and the plasma levels of both calcium and phosphate rise. The increased phosphate is

thus able to buffer H^+ ions. Thus, calcium phosphate in bone can be regarded as an **'alkali reserve'**, which is mobilized in response to reduced pH.

Ammonia

Ammonia is excreted by the renal tubule cells into the urine where it acts as a buffer (or, strictly, on a proton 'sink') by combining with H^+ ions to form ammonium ions:

$$NH_3 + H^+ \rightleftharpoons NH_4^+$$

Ammonium buffering in urine becomes increasingly important as the amount of acid to be excreted increases such as in metabolic acidosis. Ammonia, being a toxic molecule, is not found in appreciable concentration in the blood of a normal individual except perhaps in portal venous blood.

Mechanism of buffer action

The mechanism of buffer action can well be explained by taking the buffer pair of acetic acid and sodium acetate.

Acetic acid feebly ionises to give acetate ion and hydrogen ion.

$$CH_3COOH \rightleftharpoons (CH_3COO)^- + H^+$$

Sodium acetate being a salt ionises considerably and gives a high concentration of acetate ions.

$$CH_3COO\,Na \longrightarrow (CH_3COO)^- + Na^+$$

If a strongly ionising acid like HCl tending to decrease the pH is now added to the above buffer, the acetate ions available combine with the H^+ entering the buffer and convert it into the weakly ionising acetic acid. Thus, the influence of added H^+ in decreasing pH is overcome by the salt of the buffer.

$$H^+ + (CH_3 - COO)^- \longrightarrow CH_3 - COOH$$
(of the acid   weakly ionising
added)   acid

On the other hand, if a strongly ionising base like NaOH tending to increase the pH enters the buffer, the H+ of the acid combines with the hydroxyl ion and converts it into undissociated molecules of water. Thus, the influence of added OH- ion in increasing the pH is overcome by the acid part of the buffer.

$$OH^- + H^+ \longrightarrow H_2O$$

(from alkali   (of the acid
added)   of buffer)

Thus a buffer solution resists any alteration in pH by the addition of small amounts of acid or alkali.

Indicators

Indicators are substances which change colour with change of pH of the solution. They are organic substances and are either weak acids or weak bases. They partially ionise. The undissociated molecules have one colour and the dissociated ions another colour.

Indicator molecules $\longrightarrow$ $H^+ + (Ind)^-$ ions
(one colour) $\longleftarrow$ (different colour)

Just as acids have dissociation constant, dissociation of indicator also has indicator constant K. Henderson-Hasselbalch equation could be used for dissociation of indicator.

$$pH = pK + \log_{10} \frac{\text{(indicator ions)}}{\text{(undissociated molecules)}}$$

Range of an indicator is that part of the pH scale (0-14) over which the eye can appreciate a change in colour of the indicator.

It is roughly 2 units in the pH scale.

For example Methyl orange 3.1 to 4.4

Phenolphthalein 8.3 to 10

In addition to individual indicators, mixtures of indicators known as universal indicators have been found useful for covering the entire pH range and determining the approximate pH of experimental solution.

A convenient and simple form of universal indicator covering a range of pH from 4 to 11 is made from methyl red, alpha naphtholphthalein, phenolphthalein and bromophenol blue. The colours and corresponding pH values for the

above universal indicators are

colour	red	orange red	yellow	greenish-yellow
pH	4	5	6	7
	green	blue green	blue	violet
	8	9	10	11

Determination of pH

pH can be determined either by colorimetric methods or EMF methods.

All colorimetric methods use indicators in one form or the other. Hence they are also called indicator methods.

a) using buffer solutions

The pH of the experimental solution is first determined approximately by means of universal indicator by matching the colour developed with the colour chart given for the various pH units. If the colour developed when a drop of universal indicator is added to about 2 ml of experimental solution is, say, red, the approximate pH is 4. Knowing the approximate pH, the individual indicator working at that range is chosen. In this case it is methyl orange whose indicator range covers the pH of 4.

A fixed quantity of the individual indicator (methyl orange) is added to a certain volume of the experimental solution. The same quantity of the indicator is added to equal volumes of various buffer standards differing in pH by say 0.1 unit in the neighbourhood of 4: (say 3, 3.1, 3.2, 3.3...3.9,4, 4.1, 4.2...5). In the buffer standards colours of different intensities will be produced. The experimental solution also would have developed a colour with the indicator. This colour obtained in the test solution is matched with the colours in the buffer standards. The pH of the buffer standard whose colour matches with the colour developed in the test solution is the pH of the test solution. If, for instance, the colour developed in the test solution matches with that in the buffer standard with pH 3.6, the pH of the test solution is 3.6.

b) without using buffer solutions

i) by using universal indicator papers or individual indicator papers.

The papers are supplied by companies. A drop of the solution is placed on the indicator paper. The colour developed is compared with the colour chart given for different pH units.

ii) by using comparators

Various comparators like Lovibond comparator, Hellige comparator are available. Discs with different shades of colours for different pH values are supplied. The test solution is treated with the prescribed quantity of indicator specified or supplied. The colour developed is matched with the colours in the disc. The pH for the colour in the disc matching with the colour of the experimental solution is the pH of the test solution.

iii) pH can also be determined without using buffer standards from a knowledge of the dissociation constant of the acid of the buffer and the concentrations of salt and acid in the buffer. For this the Henderson-Hasselbalch equation should be used.

2) In EMF methods, difrerent electrodes like the hydrogen electrode, quinhydrone electrode or the glass electrode can be used. Direct reading pH meters are available working on this principle and using the glass electrode.

Determination of pH by glass electrode

When a glass surface is in contact with a solution, it acquires a potential difference which has been found by experiment to be dependent upon the pH of the solution.

The glass electrode (Fig. 23.1) consists of a glass tube terminating in a thin-walled bulb. A special glass of relatively low melting point and high electrical conductivity is used. The bulb contains a solution of constant pH and an electrode of definite potential. A platinum wire inserted in pH 4 buffer solution containing a small quantity of quinhydrone is usually employed. The glass bulb containing the above is inserted in the experimental solution whose pH is to be determined. This constitutes the glass electrode which is a half cell.

In actual determination of pH, the glass electrode is coupled with calomel electrode and the EMF of the cell is determined experimentally.

$$E_{cell} = E_{glass} + E_{calomel}$$
$$E_{glass} = E_{cell} - E_{calomel}$$

Assuming $E_{calomel}$ to be 0 .3333, E_{glass} can be determined.

pH of the solution is related to the E_{glass} by the equation

$$pH = \frac{E_{glass} - K}{0.0002\ T}$$

where T is the absolute temperature and K is a constant for the glass electrode. (K for any glass electrode can be determined in a separate experiment using a solution of known pH).

The glass electrode can be used for almost any solution except that which is very acidic or very alkaline.

Direct reading pH meters incorporating the glass and calomel electrodes are available.

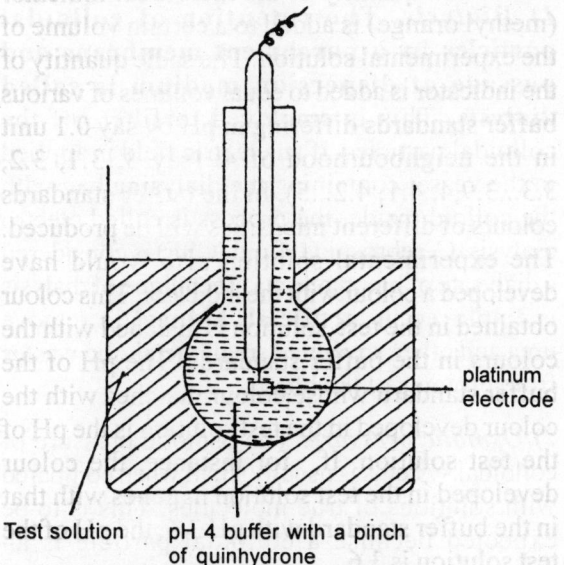

platinum electrode

Test solution   pH 4 buffer with a pinch of quinhydrone

Fig. 23.1 : Glass electrode

Beckmann's pH meter, Cambridge pH meter are such instruments which are routinely used in biochemical laboratories.

COLLOIDAL STATE

Graham, the father of colloid chemistry, classified substances into crystalloids and colloids. Substances like sodium chloride, sugar, etc. which while present in solution pass through parchment membrane were called crystalloids where substances like albumin, gelatin etc. which were retained by parchment membrane were called colloids (glue-like). This classification was later found to be unacceptable as one and the same substance could be a crystalloid or a colloid depending on the experimental conditions. Thus, sodium chloride which is a crystalloid according to Graham can be obtained as a colloid in benzene or alcohol. Soap behaves as a colloid in water but crystalloid in alcohol. Thus any substance can be obtained in colloidal form by employing suitable methods. The term 'colloid' therefore does not concern the nature of the substance but only the state of subdivision of matter. Any substance is said to be in colloidal state if the diameter of its particles ranges from $1m\mu$ to 200 $m\mu$ [$1 m\mu$ (millimicron) $= 10^{-3}$ of μ (micron) or 10^{-6} mm]. Colloidal state of matter is intermediate between molecules and suspensions; molecules having a diameter below $1 m\mu$ and hence could not be seen at all with the help of a microscope and suspensions having a diameter above $200 m\mu$ and can be seen even with the naked eye. Colloidal particles can be seen with the aid of ultramicroscope, each particle appearing as a small disc of light. Because of the very small size, the colloidal particles pass through ordinary filter paper, the pores of which are too big to retain the particles. However, colloidal particles are retained by parchment, collodion or animal membranes.

A colloidal system is a heterogeneous diphase system. The phase which constitutes the bulk is called the dispersion medium (external medium) which contains the dispersed or internal phase. Combination of any two phases can form a colloid of any of the following types-gas/liquid; gas/solid; liquid/gas; liquid/liquid; liquid/solid; solid/gas; solid/liquid and solid/solid. The phase written first forms the dispersed phase.

Solid/liquid colloid is termed a **'sol'** while liquid/liquid colloid is called an **'emulsion'** which contains two immiscible liquids-the one in smaller amounts forming the dispersed phase.

Sols in which water is the dispersion medium are called hydrosols. If alcohol is the medium, sols are called alcohols. Sols are divided into lyophobic (liquid-hating) and. lyophilic (liquid-loving) types depending on the affinity between the solid and the liquid. If it is hydrosol, the terms hydrophobic (water hating) and hydrophilic (water-loving) are employed. The terms **'suspensoid'** for lyophobic sols and **'emulsoid'** for lyophilic sols are used by biochemists while they are not used by physical chemists.

Good examples of hydrophilic sols are those of proteins, gum, gelatin, starch, agar in water.

Properties of colloidal solutions

1) Dialysis. **The retention of colloidal particles by a parchment membrane and passage of dispersion medium is called dialysis.** This is employed to filter off the colloidal particles. If an electric field is applied in the vessel containing the dialysing bag with the colloid inside, the process is called electro dialysis. Cerebrospinal fluid (CSF) is considered a dialysate of blood plasma. Technique of dialysis is employed in **'artificial kidney'** to remove urea and other unwanted small metabolic wastes from proteins of the blood.

2) Osmotic pressure. The osmotic pressure of colloidal systems is usually small when compared with solutions of true molecules. This is to be expected because a colloidal particle is an aggregate of thousands of molecules. Osmotic pressure being a colligative. Property depends on the number of particles. The osmotic pressure of proteins of plasma is called **'oncotic'** pressure which has a significant role in maintaining blood volume.

3) Optical properties. Colloidal particles scatter light. This property is called **Tyndall effect**. It is Tyndall effect which is applied in ultra microscope in which the light scattered by the particles is seen.

4) Brownian movement. The colloidal particles are in continual haphazard motion. This is called Brownian movement which is due to the bombardment of the colloidal particles by molecules of dispersion medium.

5) Electrical properties of colloids. Colloidal state of matter possesses great surface area per unit weight in view of the presence of a large number of particles in it. Every particle possesses, around it, certain fields of force which are probably largely electromagnetic. Such fields of force which are on the surface of each particle are relatively free when compared with those inside the particle. Inside the particles the forces are internally neutralised by the atoms present, while forces on the surface are only partially neutralised. Hence the surface of colloidal particle has free fields of force or attraction, which impart to it peculiar properties. One very important property arising out of surface forces is adsorption. Traces of ions are adsorbed on to the surface of colloidal particles. This adsorption together with primary ionisation of ionisable groups in the colloidal substance is responsible for the electrical properties of colloids.

Emulsions

Emulsions are liquid/liquid colloids. The two liquids should be immiscible. Either liquid can be dispersed in the other. That which is in smaller amounts forms the disperse phase, the droplets of which have a diameter of 0.1 to 1 mμ. In general two types of emulsions are recognised:

(1) Oil in water emulsions and (2) water in oil emulsions, depending upon whether water is excess or the other liquid.

Emulsions are generally unstable unless a third substance known as an emulsifying agent is present. The emulsifier reduces the interfacial tension between the oil (or organic liquid) and water and this imparts stability to the liquid/liquid colloid. Soaps, gelatin, gum, proteins and bile salts are good examples of emulsifying substances.

Milk is a common example of an emulsion and contains droplets of liquid fat dispersed in an aqueous medium. The emulsifier is the protein casein.

Emulsions also can be separated by electrophoresis and can be coagulated, broken or de-emulsified by the addition of material which destroys the emulsifier and neutralises the electric charge. Boiling and freezing also cause de-emulsification.

Membrane phenomena

The living cell membrane is quite different from artificial membranes made of non-living matter in composition, electrical properties and permeability. The surface tension lowering substances which concentrate at the interface according to Gibbs Thomson effect are found to predominate in the living membrane. Membrane is thus made up of phospholipids, cholesterol, fatty acids, soap and protein; most of which are surface tension lowering substances. Electron microscopy, x-ray diffraction and histochemical studies have shown the living membrane to be composed of two long thin monolayers of protein between which occurs a layer of lipid, chiefly phospholipid and cholesterol.

Resting membrane has an electrical potential which is about - 70 mv. The electrical charge of the membrane is due to different factors like ionisation of the protein of the membrane, adsorption of ions and Helmholtz double layer and to a considerable extent diffusion potential due to concentration cells of Na^+, K^+ and Cl^-. The value of electrical potential appears to depend on K^+ ion diffusion potential as a first approximation. The inside of a membrane is negative and outside positive while the pore walls also are negatively charged. The electrical nature of membrane influences the permeability of substances across the membrane.

Many biochemical reactions take place inside the cells. Hence entry of substances across the cell membrane decides metabolic reactions. Various factors operate in the transport of substances across the membrane. For small molecules and ions, it is simple diffusion. Urea and sugar are equally distributed between the cells and plasma. The differential distribution of Na^+ and K^+ between cells and extracellular fluid and chiefly the accumulation of K^+ inside the cells is explained by relative decrease in the size of hydrated K^+ when compared with hydrated Na^+ (1: 1.47), increased motility of K^+ (1×10^{-6} moles/sq cm/see of membrane while for Na^+ it is less, i.e. 2×10^{-8} moles only) and Donnan effect.

Sieve effects due to cell membrane mosaic and pinocytosis also account for selective membrane permeabilitles. Lipid soluble substances are easily transported as they get dissolved in lipids of the cell membrane.

Permeability is also concerned in some cases with the nature of the substances, structure and their configuration. Iron passes through the membrane of intestinal cells only if it is in ferrous form Fe^{++} and not Fe^{+++} while in rats it is shown that Fe^{+++} also can be absorbed. Glucose is transported more easily than galactose and cholic acid with greater ease than fatty acids. Even the configuration of a substance in certain regions of the molecule is a factor in absorption. D-glucose, D-galactose and L-arabinose have similar configuration around the 3 carbon atoms, as shown over here:

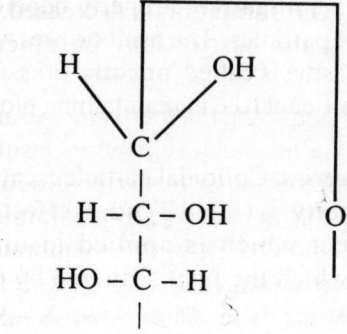

D-arabinose which has a different configuration is not transported easily as L-arabinose.

In some cases when the substance crosses the membrane, chemical reaction can take place and this might hasten absorbtion. Sucrose when it passes through the membrane is hydrolysed to glucose and fructose by enzyme effect. Galactose is epimerised to glucose. Cholesterol which does not pass through the membrane easily passes through when it is as a complex in bile. The permeability of membrane is considerably influenced by membrane-bound cyclic AMP.

Carrier systems bring about efficient transport in certain cases. For K^+ and Na^+ the same carrier is considered to be involved. For sodium pump mechanism, a carrier (p) is said to be involved and forms with Na^+ the complex pNa^+ which is more soluble in lipid membrane than either p or Na^+. This pNa^+ moves out, dissociates, p gets destroyed or inactivated, and Na^+ is thus channelled out. The carrier p is speculated to be histamine pyridoxal phosphate or phosphatidyl serine. Even for the mode of action of insulin, according to Randall and Smith, a carrier is implied. The carrier is said to combine with glucose and the complex moves easily across the membrane. They suggest that the carrier is more active when it is in dephosphorylated form. Thus the carrier is active in anoxia when ATP formation is decreased. It is predicted that the carrier may be glucan peptide.

Recently it is suggested that both glucose and Na^+ have carrier for intestinal absorption. Insulin increases the movement of carrier-glucose complex across the membrane by combining with **'receptor'** molecules in the membrane. Insulin can also change the cyto-skeletal structure of membrane when its $-S-S-$ interacts with -SH of protein of the cell wall reversibly. This affects the coiling of the membrane and facilitates free entry of glucose in muscle cells. More significantly insulin is said to convert the laminar form of the membrane to micellar form and thus increases the permeability for glucose. However, insulin is not required for transport of glucose across liver cells as also fructose for any cell.

Membrane phenomenon is of utmost importance in nerve induction. Acetyl choline causes an efflux of potassium and influx of sodium leading to a reversal of polarisation. A wave of negative electricity passes through the membrane until choline esterase hydrolyses acetyl choline and this restores the original condition in respect of potassium and sodium ions and the negative charge on the internal side of the membrane is restored.

Donnan membrane equilibrium

Colloidal state is responsible for the so-called selective absorptions or selective membrane permeability of certain ions. This role of colloids is explained by the Donnan membrane equilibrium. If a membrane is freely permeable and if on either side of the membrane there are electrolytes (e.g. NaCl and KNO_3), at equilibrium all the four ions Na^+, Cl^-, K^+ and NO_3^- will be equally distributed on each side of the membrane. On the other hand if the membrane is not permeable to all the ions, then there will be an unequal distribution of ions on either side of the membrane. **According to Donnan, the non-diffusible ion or ions on one side of the membrane influences the diffusion of the diffusible ion or ions.** Both the quality and quantity of diffusible ions will be influenced.

Sodium salt of protein (sodium proteinate) is a colloidal electrolyte as it ionises to give sodium ion and proteinate (Pr^-) ion. The proteinate ion is colloidal and is not diffusible through a membrane. Its nature and concentration will influence the diffusion of electrolytes across the membrane and cause accumulation of certain ions on one side.

Let it be assumed that sodium proteinate is separated from NaCl by a membrane.

Na^+		Na^+
Pr^-		Cl^-
	membrane	
(A)		(B)

Diffusion occurs across the membrane of the easily diffusible ions; Na^+ and Cl^-. After equilibrium is attained, the following will be the state of affairs.

Na^+		Na^+
Pr^-		Cl^-
Cl^-		
(A)		(B)

In the side (A), the Na^+ ion has to balance the two negative ions Pr^- and Cl^- while in the side (B) it has to balance only the Cl^- ion. So the concentration of Na^+ in the side (A) will be greater than that at side (B)

$$Na^+ (A) > Na^+ (B)$$

The total ionic concentration in side (A) will be greater than in side (B).

From thermodynamical consideration, after equilibrium is established, the concentrations (more, correctly **'activity'**) of NaCl on both the sides should be the same.

$$Na^+ Cl^- (A) = Na^+ Cl^- (B)$$

But $Na^+ (A) > Na^+ (B)$

It follows therefore that concentration of chloride ions in (A) should be less than in side (B)

$$C^- (A) < Cl^- (B)$$

or chloride concentration in (B) should be greater than that in (A).

Thus Donnan equilibrium has brought the following effects on the distribution of Na+ and Cl⁻.

1) On the side in which the non-diffusible ion is present, there is accumulation of oppositely charged diffusible ion. (In the present case Pr^- ion has resulted in accumulation of Na^+ on the same side).

2) On the other side of the membrane, the non-diffusible ion pauses the accumulation of diffusible ion of the same charge. It is as if the diffusible ion of the same charge is excreted out from its side by the non-diffusible ion (Pr^- ion causes the accumulation of Cl^- ion on the opposite side).

3) The total concentration of all the ions will be greater on the side in which the non-diffusible ion is present. This will lead to an osmotic imbalance between the two sides.

The amount of sodium chloride diffusing across the membrane can be related mathematically as fallows with the initial concentration of sodium chloride.

Let the initial concentration of sodium proteinate ($Na^+ Pr^-$) be 'a' moles on the side I and that of sodium chloride on the other side (side II) be 'b' moles and both of them are separated by a membrane.

Na^+ (a)		Na^+ (b)
Pr^- (a)		Cl^- (b)
I		II

'a' moles of Na^+ Pr– would mean 'a' moles of each ion while 'b' moles of sodium chloride would mean 'b' moles of each ion. If it is assumed that 'x' moles of sodium chloride diffuse through the membrane from side II to side I, then after equilibrium the concentrations of sodium ions and chloride ions on either side would be as follows:

Na^+ (a + x)		Na^+ (b - x))
Pr^-		
Cl^- (x)		Cl^- (b - x)
I		II

(After equilibrium also there will be diffusion of sodium chloride both ways but the rates of diffusion from II to 1 and I to II will be equal. Such a dynamic equilibrium will not affect the distribution of ions after equilibrium is established).

The amount of sodium chloride diffusing from either side is proportional to the products of their concentrations (more correctly their activities). So at equilibrium, amount diffusing from II to I is proportional to $(b - x)(b - x)$; amount diffusing from I to II is proportional to $(a + x)(x)$.

As the rates of diffusion at equilibrium are equal

$$(a + x)(x) = (b - x)(b - x)$$
$$ax + x^2 = b^2 - 2bx + x^2$$
$$ax + 2bx = b^2$$
$$x(a + 2b) = b^2$$
$$x = \frac{b^2}{(a + 2b)}$$

The above equation shows that the amount of sodium chloride diffusing, i.e. x is dependent on not only the concentration of sodium chloride (b) but on the concentration of non-diffusible ion, i.e. 'a'. Thus the quality and quantity of non-diffusible ion influences the extent of diffusion of easily diffusible ion across a membrane. As an example, inside the red blood cells, the pH is relatively less than that of plasma. This could be because the negatively charged protein haemoglobin of the RBC abstracts the oppositely charged H^+ ion by the Donnan effect tending to cause a decrease of pH inside the RBC.

By Donnan effect, there will he unequal distribution of ions on either side of the membrane and this will create a difference in **Osmotic Pressure.** The total number of ions on one side is greater than that on the other side. This can be shown qualitatively that in the side containing the non-diffusible ion (Pr^-) in the above example, in addition to the existing Na^+ Pr^-, sodium chloride (Na^+ & Cl^-) enters. Hence the ionic concentration on such a side could increase. Secondly from the equation:

$$(a + x) x = (b - x) (b - x)$$
$$\text{I} \qquad\qquad \text{II}$$

On side II it is a square say 8 X 8. To get the product 64, for side I, if $(a + x)$ could be greater than 8, x will be less than 8. But the total of $(a + x)$ and x will always be mathematically greater than 16 (than on the right side i.e. 8 + 8). Thus mathematically also the ionic concentration could be shown to be greater on the side having the non-diffusible ion. As osmotic pressure depends upon the number of ions, the side having nondiffusible ion will exert greater osmotic pressure than the other side. For example if a = 1 mole and b = 2 moles, x the

amount diffused will be $\dfrac{b^2}{a + 2b} = \dfrac{4}{1 + 4} = 0.8$

Side I will have 1.8 $(a + x)$ of Na^+; 1 of Pr^- (a) and 0.8 (x) of Cl^- with a total of 3.6 moles while side II will have 1.2 (b-x) of Na+ and 1.2 (b - x) of Cl^- making a total of 2.4 moles. Thus side I has (3.6 - 2.4) = 1.2 moles excess leading to greater osmotic pressure at that side. Imbibition of gels is said to be due to this type of osmotic imbalance. Inside the gel are large non-diffusible protein ions. At equilibrium the total ionic concentration will be greater within the gel than in the solution in which it is placed. Osmotic flow of water will therefore occur and thus the gel imbibes.

Membrane hydrolysis

Donnan effect causes membrane hydrolysis and makes one side relatively acidic or alkaline depending on the charge of the non-diffusible ions. As in this system one side is concerned with H^+ and OH^- of water this shift of ions is called membrane hydrolysis.

The interaction between sodium proteinate and water (H^+ and H^-) through a membrane results in accumulation of H^+ (oppositely charged to Pr^-) on the side containing sodium proteinate. Hence pH of that side drops down and it becomes acidic.

1) Initial state

Na^+		H+
Pr^-		OH^-
		(Neutral)

2) At equilibrium

Na^+		H^+ (less)
Pr^-		OH^- (more)
H^+(more)		Na^+
OH^-(less)		
acidic		basic

On the other hand, if protein salts as Pr^+ Cl^- are separated from water by a membrane, the protein ion with positive charge will cause accumulation of OH^- of water making the pH of the side containing water acidic.

1) Initial

Pr^+		H^+
Cl^-		OH^-
		(Neutral)

2) At equilibrium

Pr^+		H^+ (more)
Cl^-		
H^+ (less)		OH^- (less)
OH^-(more)		Cl^-
		acidic

Thus it could be stated that acid is excreted by Pr^+Cl^- across the membrane. Donnan points out that it is possible to attain in this way a concentration of H^+ ions as great as is present in gastric juice.

If a number of ions are separated by a membrane, a relationship could be arrived for their relative concentrations. It is known that

$$Na^+_{(1)} \times Cl^-_{(1)} = Na^+_{(2)} \times Cl^-_{(2)}$$

or

$$\frac{Na^+_{(1)}}{Na^+_{(2)}} = \frac{Cl^-_{(2)}}{Cl^-_{(1)}}$$

If a system contains a number of diffusible ions like Na^+, K^+, Ca^{++}, Cl^-, SO_4^{2-} distributing on either side of a membrane then

$$\frac{Na^+_{(1)}}{Na^+_{(2)}} = \frac{K^+_{(1)}}{K^+_{(2)}} = \frac{Ca^{++}_{(1)}}{Ca^{++}_{(2)}} = \frac{Cl^-_{(2)}}{Cl^-_{(1)}} = \frac{SO_4^{2-}_{(2)}}{SO_4^{2-}_{(1)}}$$

This can be applied to distribution of ions between cells and plasma

$$\frac{HCO_3^-_{(plasma)}}{HCO_3^-_{(cell)}} = \frac{Cl^-_{(plasma)}}{Cl^-_{(cell)}}$$

or between plasma and lymph

$$\frac{Plasma\ Na^+}{Lymph\ Na^+} = \frac{Plasma\ K^+}{Lymph\ K^+} = \frac{Lymph\ Cl^-}{Plasma\ Cl^-}$$

As plasma contains more of negatively charged proteins it has more of positively charged ions Na^+, K^+ etc. and less or negatively charged ion i.e. Cl^-. However, concentration of HCO^-_4 is greater in plasma than in lymph and this is an exception. This is required for the transport of CO_2 produced by the cells during metabolism.

Physiological importance of colloids

1) Enzyme action due to large surface area of colloids and adsorption.

The small size of the colloidal particles gives them a great specific surface. The enzymes which are colloidal have thus a great specific surface. Because of great specific surface there is efficient adsorption which leads to efficient enzyme catalysis.

Adsorption is also important in drug action, detoxification, orientation of protoplasmic constituents etc. Thus colloidal state leads to good adsorption in the above cases.

2) Maintenance of blood pH due to electro-kinetic potential.

Because of the electro-kinetic potential, proteins, phospholipids, etc. serve as amphoteric colloids reacting either with acids or alkalies. Because of the amphoteric nature, they help in maintaining the pH of blood.

3) Fat absorption and protection of bile contents. Colloidal proteins and phospholipids hold the fatty substances of living cells in an invisible colloidal form and protect them; again, colloidal lyophilic proteins keep the difficult soluble substances like cholesterol, calcium bilirubinate etc. in dissolved state in bile and protect them from precipitation by electrolytes.

4) Water transport and formation of urine due to colloidal osmotic pressure.

The colloidal systems exert osmotic pressure which is very important in water transport in the body and in the formation of urine.

5) Glandular secretions by imbibition and syneresis. Tissue fluid is imbibed by the colloids in glandular cells. The imbibed fluid is squeezed out as glandular secretions by syneresis.

6) Donnan membrane equilibrium. Colloidal state is responsible for the so-called selective absorptions or selective membrane permeabilities of certain ions. This application of colloids is explained by Donnan's membrane equilibrium, and membrane hydrolysis.

OSMOSIS

Osmosis is an important property of solutions. **It is the spontaneous flow of a solvent into a solution when the two are separated by a semi-permeable membrane. It is also the flow of a solvent from a more dilute solution to a relatively concentrated solution through a semi-permeable membrane.** Osmosis strictly, refers to the flow of the solvent only. It is a colligative property depending upon the number of the particles of the solute.

Osmotic pressure

Osmotic pressure is defined as the equivalent of excess pressure which must be applied to the solution to prevent the passage the solvent into it through a semi-permeable membrane separating the two. Osmotic pressure can also be defined as the excess pressure which must be applied to it in order to increase the vapour pressure of the solution until it becomes equal to that of the solvent.

Strictly speaking even a semi-permeable membrane is not required for osmotic flow of a solvent. If a solvent and solution are kept side by side in a closed chamber (Fig. 23.2) there will be osmosis of the solvent to the solution though there is no semi-permeable membrane between the two. The osmosis of the solvent is due to the fact that the chemical potential or activity or partial free energy of solvent is less on the solution side than on the solvent side. Hence the movement of the solvent to the solution is accompanied by a decrease of free energy and is, therefore, spontaneous.

In the body there is no membrane which is typically semipermeable, i.e. permeable to solvent and impermeable to the solute. Hence the term 'osmotic potency' is preferred to actual osmotic pressure by some authors.

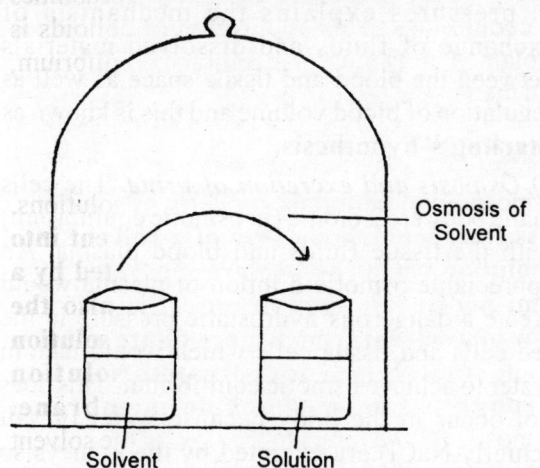

Osmosis of Solvent

Solvent   Solution

Fig. 23.2 : To show osmosis

The osmotic pressure of a solution is directly proportional to the concentration of the solute and in turn depends on the number of molecules or ions contained in the solution. Though dependent on the number of molecules of the solute, osmotic pressure is independent of the nature of the solute; hence it is a colligative property. A substance of lower molecular weight will have more molecules per unit volume than a substance of higher molecular weight and will therefore exert a greater osmotic pressure. Albumin which has a lower molecular weight than globulin exerts a greater osmotic pressure than globulin on a weight to weight basis.

If two solutions have the same osmotic pressure, these are described as iso-osmotic solutions. Iso-osmotic solutions will have the same vapour pressure. When the osmotic pressure of one is greater than that of the other it is called **hypertonic**. If it is less than that of the other, it is called **hypotonic**.

Abnormal osmotic pressures

The osmotic pressure of electrolytes gives results considerably higher than those calculated from their formulae. This is due to ionisation of the electrolytes in solution. The number of particles will increase due to ionisations of electrolytes in aqueous medium. Therefore, the osmotic pressure of electrolytes determined experimentally is greater than the theoretically calculated value (not assuming ionisation). **This greater osmotic pressure is referred to as the abnormal osmotic pressure of electrolytes.**

Role of osmosis in physiological processes

Osmosis has an important role in (1) the regulation of blood and volume, (2) in the excretion of urine, (3) in absorption etc. Osmosis also explains the haemolysis of red cells which is applied in the fragility test.

1) Regulation of blood volume. The concentration of electrolytes and of organic solutes in plasma and tissue fluids is substantially

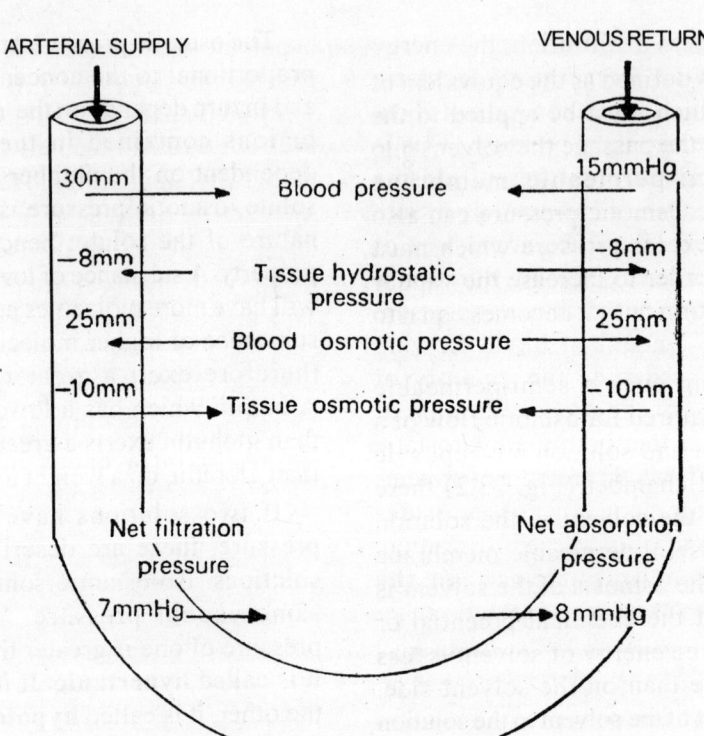

Fig. 23.3 : To Show the phenomenon of osmotic pressure

the same. So the osmotic pressure due to these substances is practically identical. (see figure 23.3).

The blood proteins are responsible for about 25 mm of total osmotic pressure of plasma (about 4940 mm of Hg). Osmotic pressure of proteins is referred to oncotic pressure. This oncotic pressure is opposed by the oncotic pressure of tissue fluid protein which is about 10 mm. Hence the effective osmotic pressure of blood over that of tissue fluid is (25-10) = 15 mm; the net hydrostatic pressure on the arterial side is (30 - 8) = 22 mm. Hence there is excess hydrostatic pressure over osmotic pressure by (22-15) =7 mm at the arterial end and this favours forcing out of fluid outward from the capillary to the tissue spaces. On the other hand, the net hydrostatic pressure at venous end (15-8) = 7 mm while the effective osmotic pressure is

15 mm. Hence the excess osmotic pressure over hydrostatic pressure by (15-7) = 8 mm is in favour of reabsorption of water as intravascular osmotic pressure predominates. The difference in pressures explains the mechanism of exchange of fluids and dissolved materials between the blood and tissue space as well as regulation of blood volume and this is known as **Starling's hypothesis.**

2) Osmosis and excretion of urine. The cells in the body are isotonic (in osmotic equilibrium) with the tissue fluids and blood plasma. An appreciable osmotic dilution of plasma would create a dangerous hydrostatic pressure in the red cells and tissue cells which would take in water to achieve osmotic equilibrium. This does not occur in the body because water or salt (chiefly NaCl) are excreted by the kidneys so as to keep the blood isotonic with the cells. Urine is formed by a process of filtration, the energy for which is derived from the hydrostatic pressure of blood. A gross filtration force of about 75 mm of Hg is the capillary pressure. This is opposed by the oncotic pressures of plasma proteins (about 30 mm), renal interstitial pressure of 10 mm Hg and renal intratubular pressure of 10 mm Hg. The total force opposing filtration is 50 mm (30 + 10 + 10). The net filtration pressure of 25 mm and the amount of blood flowing through the kidneys decide the quantity of glomerular filtrate. For the proper filtration of urine; it is thus clear that both the hydrostatic pressure of blood and oncotic pressure of proteins have a part to play and changes in their pressures will affect the exctent of glomerular filtration. **Osmosis is of great importance in the process of urine excretion.**

3) Absorption.

Intestinal contents (Lumen)	Blood plasma (Capillaries of the villi)

Mucosa

In absorption, the processes of osmosis and diffusion work hand in hand. Hence, whatever may be the osmotic pressure of the intestinal contents, hypotonic or hypertonic with blood plasma, water of course moves osmotically depending on the osmotic pressure but salts or sugars move by diffusion. (Mucosal membrane is permeable to salts or sugar in either direction). This may be illustrated in the case of the absorption of say isotonic glucose which is easily absorbed into blood. First, the sugar diffuses into the blood and makes the isotonic solution hypotonic. Now, osmotic flow of water occurs into blood and makes the sugar solution isotonic again. Thus by diffusion and osmosis, absorption of sugar and salt solutions takes place.

4) Destruction of red cells by haemolysis occurs both in vivo and in vitro.

Since the red cell membrane is permeable to water, the volume of the cell changes according to its osmotic environment. When placed in a hypotonic solution, red cells swell owing to water passing in osmotically **(endosmosis)**. If the solution is sufficiently hypotonic, the cells may even rupture and the cell contents diffuse into the surrounding fluid. This is called **haemolysis.**

5) If RBCs are placed in hypertonic solution, water passes out of the cells **(exosmosis)** and the red cells shrink due to diminution in volume. This process is called crenation.

Clinical applications

1) The practice of giving 5% glucose or 0.9% saline for intravenous infusions has also a tremendous bearing on osmotic pressure considerations and Vant Hoff's factor, 'i'.

The osmotic pressure of plasma is about 280 to 300 milli osmols/litre. Any intravenous infusion should have iso osmolality. 5% glucose (50 g/litre) solution will give rise to $(50/180 \times 1000) =$ about 280 milli osmols/litre. In case of 0.9% saline (9 g/litre), this amount equals to $9/58.5 \times 1000 =$ about 150 milli moles/litre. But as NaCl (of saline) is an electrolyte unlike glucose, it undergoes ionisation. Each molecule of NaCl will give rise to 2 osmotically active ions (Vant Hoff's factor is 2). Hence, 150 milli moles/litre of NaCl will be equal to $150 \times 2 = 300$ milli osmols/litre. Thus 5% glucose and 0.9% saline are iso-osmotic with plasma and hence used for intravenous infusions.

2) *Fragility Test.* The extent of haemolysis of RBCs is observed in a series of tubes with hypotonic NaCl solutions adding a drop of blood in each and observing after about two hours. If there is no haemolysis, there will be a colourless supernatant layer over an opaque red suspension of cells. If haemolysis is complete, a transparent red solution is seen. In normal human blood, complete haemolysis occurs only below about 0.35% NaCl; the cells resist haemolysis above about 0.45%. In between, there is partial haemolysis. Diminished resistance (increased fragility) is seen in haemolytic jaundice (upto 0.7

to 0.8 %) and increased resistance in certain anaemias.

3) *Cause of oedema in cases of albuminuria.* **In albuminuria, plasma proteins, mainly albumin, are excreted.** When the concentration of plasma proteins is thus reduced, the oncotic pressure of plasma is lowered. This would naturally mean increase of hydrostatic pressure which causes oedema which is accumulation or excess fluid in tissue space.

4) Another clinical application of osmotic pressure is the injection of hypertonic solutions of salts such as sodium chloride to reduce cerebral oedema. Water is withdrawn from the brain osmotically.

ADSORPTION

Adsorption is an important property of surfaces. It describes the existence of a higher concentration of any particular substance at the surface of a liquid or solid than is present in the bulk.

Adsorption of gases by solids

Adsorption of gases by solids refers to an excess concentration of gases at the surface and is different from **'absorption'** which means uniform penetration of solid by the gas. Best known adsorbents are charcoal (by burning coconut shells in a limited supply of air), silica gel, alumina, metals like platinum, palladium etc. Increase of pressure and decrease of temperature increase the extent of the adsorption of a gas by a solid.

Adsorption isotherm

The term isotherm or isothermal is used to describe a curve which gives the variation of volume with pressure of a gas at constant temperature.

The variation of gas adsorption with pressure at constant temperature can be represented by the equation $a = kp^n$ where 'a' is the amount of gas adsorbed by unit mass, e.g. 1 g of adsorbing

material at the pressure p; k and n are constants for the given gas and adsorbent at the particular temperature. An equation of this type is known as an adsorption isotherm since it is applicable at constant temperature.

Gibbs adsorption equation

Gibbs adsorption equation is a significant equation in connection with adsorption at the surface of a solution. For a dilute solution of concentration 'c' and surface tension 'r', the equation is $S = -c/RT \cdot dr/dc$ where S is the excess concentration of solute per sq. cm. of surface, as compared with that in the bulk of the solution; dr/dc is the rate of increase of surface tension of the solution with the concentration of the solute, R is the gas constant and T the absolute temperature.

According to the equation, if the solute causes the surface tension of the solvent to decrease, dr/dc will become negative and S positive indicating that the solute will have a higher concentration in the surface than in the bulk of the solution. Thus, according to Gibbs adsorption equation a substance which decreases the surface tension (or interfacial tension) will be adsorbed at that interface. On the other hand if any substance increases the surface tension of the solvent, dr/dc will be positive and S will be negative, that is, the concentration of the solute will be lower in the surface than in the bulk of the solution. In other words surface tension increasing substances like some electrolytes are not adsorbed at the interface.

SURFACE TENSION

A molecule in the interior of a liquid is completely surrounded by other molecules and so, on an average, it is attracted equally on all directions and hence can move with equal freedom in any direction. On a molecule in the surface, however, there is a resultant attraction inwards because the number of molecules per unit volume is greater in the bulk of the liquid than in the vapour (which would be always present above the liquid column). Hence, the freedom of movement of the molecule at the surface is restricted. As a consequence, the surface of a liquid pulls itself-together tending to occupy the least possible area. Because, of this tendency to contract, a surface behaves as if it were in a state of tension. The surface film of a liquid has thus the properties of an elastic skin and is resistant to rupture as can be seen by the experiment of floating a needle on water.

The force with which the surface molecules are held is called **'The Surface Tension'** of the liquid. **It is defined as the force in dynes acting at right angles to any imaginary line of 1 cm.** length on the surface.

Other manifestations of Surface Tension are formation of drops of liquids falling through air, the rise of liquid in a capillary tube and formation of a miuiscus at the surface of liquids.

The surface tension occurring at the surface of separation of two immiscible phases (e.g. liquid-liquid, or liquid-solid) is called interfacial tension.

Role of Surface Tension in physiological processes

Gibbs- Thomson principle: Substances which lower the Surface Tension become concentrated in the surface layer whereas substances which increase surface tension are distributed in the interior of the liquid. Soaps, oils, proteins and bile salts reduce the Surface Tension of water while sodium chloride and most inorganic salts increase the Surface Tension. Substances which reduce the Surface Tension are used for emulsification.

1) Bile salts which reduce Surface Tension bring about a stable emulsion of fats and help in fat absorption.

2) Lipids and proteins which are both Surface Tension lowering substances are found concentrated in the cell wall. This facilitates adsorption of these substances (taking up of substances from solutions by surfaces).

Surface Tension leads to efficient Adsorption. This is applied in :

a) Enzymatic reactions

b) formation of complex compounds of proteins and lipids, of proteins and salts etc. in protoplasm.

c) in the action of drugs and poisons.

A practical application of lowering of Surface Tension is Hay's test for bile salts in urine. The surface skin of normal urine is sufficiently dense to prevent fine particles of sulphur sprinkled on the surface from penetrating the skin and sinking to the bottom. The presence of bile salts as in the urine of certain types of jaundice so lowers the Surface Tension that the surface-skin can no longer support the sulphur particles which sink to the bottom of the tube. Thus bile salts are detected in urine.

VISCOSITY

Viscosity of a liquid is the resistance to flow. It is the manifestation of the frictional effect due to the passage of one layer of liquid over another.

Coefficient of viscosity of a fluid is defined as the force required per unit area to maintain unit difference of velocity between two parallel planes in the fluid 1 cm apart. The smaller the coefficient of viscosity the more rapidly the liquid flows. Oils, liquids like glycerine have a high coefficient of viscosity while ether and so-called mobile liquids possess a low coefficient of viscosity.

The unit of viscosity is a poise.

Determination of coefficient of viscosity

When a liquid flows through a capillary tube of length 'l' and radius 'r' for a time 't', under a constant pressure head 'p' and if the volume of the liquid flowing out from the tube is v, then the coefficient of viscosity η is given by the equation

$$\eta = \frac{P \, \pi r^4}{8 \, l \, v} \times t$$

Instead of finding the absolute coefficient of viscosity, it is easy to determine the relative coefficient of viscosity of liquids with respect to water. Ostwalds's viscometer (Fig. 23.4) is used for this purpose.

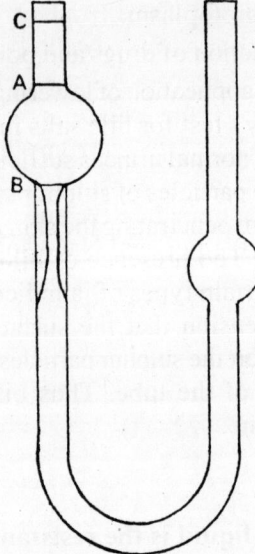

Fig. 23.4 : Ostwald's viscometer to determine coefficient of viscosity of liquids

First water is taken in the viscometer and is sucked to the level C. Time taken for the flow of water from the mark A to B is noted using a stopwatch. The experiment is repeated with the liquid whose coefficient of viscosity is to be known. If the densities of water and the liquid are d_1 and d_2, their coefficient of viscosities η_1 and η_2, the times taken being t_1 and, t_2 then

$$\frac{\eta_1}{\eta_2} = \frac{d_1 \, t_1}{d_2 \, t_2}$$

If η_1 is assumed η_2 can be known

Applications of viscosity

a) In determining the approximate molecular weight of certain liquids and to know whether the liquids are normal or associated.

According to Dunstan $\dfrac{d}{M} \times \eta \times 10^6 = 40$ to 60

where d is the density of the liquid, η the coefficient of viscosity and M the molecular weight. If d and η are known, approximate value of M can be calculated.

This relation holds good for non-associated liquids only. For associated liquids the value is considerably greater than 60. Benzene has the value of 73 while water 559.

b) *Viscosity and chemical constitution.*

In the homologous series of organic compounds, increase of viscosity per CH_2 group is approximately constant.

From a knowledge of viscosity and molecular weight and the density, the molecular viscosity of a liquid can be determined.

$$\text{Mol. viscosity} = \left(\frac{M^{\frac{2}{3}}}{d} \right) \times \eta$$

Thorpe and Rodger found that molecular viscosity is an additive property at the boiling point. For H it is 80, 0 in OH 196. Like Parachor, Mol. viscosity can be employed to solve structural problems.

Viscosity of protoplasm

This is determined by gravity or centrifugation methods. In this, granules or inclusions are moved through the protoplasm by gravity or centrifugal force. By applying Stokes's law (F = 6 $\pi \eta$ a.v where F is the force pushing a sphere through the liquid, a the radius of the sphere and v its velocity) η can be determined.

In another method, the speed of Brownian movement is used as a measure of viscosity.

Heilbrunn has shown that the viscosity of protoplasm depends on the nature and concentration of granular suspension. The value is roughly 3-5 centi poises. It is affected during cell division, or when a muscle or nerve is thrown into activity or when a cell is subjected to the influence of an anaesthetic like ether. Usually the viscosity of protoplasm at the cortical region is higher than that of the interior. The high protoplasmic viscosity in the cortical region seems to be due to the presence of increased amounts of calcium at the cortex and the influence of calcium in clotting. This is the case with amoeba. When the organism is exposed to stimulus as mechanical agitation, electric shock or ultra violet irradiation, calcium ions move to the interior. This results in a sharp increase of viscosity of the protoplasm of the interior.

Change of protoplasmic viscosity in the cells under stimulus is thus primarily due to the movement of calcium ions.

Anaesthetics prevent the clotting reaction of protoplasm. They cause a 'liquefaction' of cortex, tend to prevent the gelatin of the interior and bring about alterations in viscosity.

Viscosity of blood

This is determined by Hess viscometer. This consists of essentially two capillaries of equal bore and equal length and connected by T tube with suction bulb. Simultaneously blood is sucked through one capillary and water through the other. The relative viscosity of blood as compared with that of water is determined from the volumes of water and blood that have flowed through the capillaries, the viscosities being inversely proportional to the volume of flow for a given time.

Blood is nearly 4.5 times as viscous as water. **Viscosity of blood is lowered in anaemia, nephritis, leukemia, malaria, diabetes mellitus, jaundice and pneumonia.** Excessive sweating and traumatic shock lead to increase

Hypotonic, Hypertonic and Isotonic Solutions

The maintenance of normal water content of animal cells is largely controlled by osmotic pressure relationship between the cell contents and the surrounding tissue fluid. If, for example, red blood cells are placed in 0.1 percent NaCl solution, water enters the cells and the cells break and haemolysis takes place. If on the other hand, RBC is placed in 10 percent NaCl solution, water is drawn from the RBC and it shrinks. It is evident, 0.1 per cent NaCl solution is hypotonic and 10 per cent NaCl is hypertonic with respect to the osmotic pressure of the RBC contents. If RBC is placed in 0.9 per cent NaCl, it retains its shape and size. Hence 0.9 per cent NaCl solution is isotonic with RBC contents, i.e., it has the same osmotic pressure as RBC contents. An isotonic solution of glucose contains 5 per cent glucose (Table 23.2).

of blood viscosity. **High viscosity of blood is encountered in the congenital disease Waldenstrom's macroglobulinemia.**

Hydrogen Ion Concentration of HCl of Varying Normality

The hydrogen ion concentrations of a strong acid like HCl of varying normality are given in Table 23.3. In dilute solutions HCl is completely ionised.

It is evident that H ion concentration of HCl decreases with increasing dilution of the acid

Table 23.2 : Isotonic solutions of sodium chloride, sodium bicarbonate, sodium lactate and glucose

Substance	Mol wt. (g)	Isotonic solution	
		g/100 ml	Molarity
Glucose	180	5	M/3.6
NaCl	58.5	0.9	M/6.5
NaHCO$_3$	84	1.4	M/6.0
Sodium Lactate	112.2	1.87	M/6.0

Table 23.3: Hydrogen Ion concentration of HCl of varying normality

Normality of HCl	Hydrogen ion g/litre	Concentration of H ion	pH value
N/10	0.1	1/10 or 10^{-1}	1
N/100	0.01	$1/10^2$ or 10^{-2}	2
N/1000	0.001	$1/10^3$ or 10^{-3}	3
N/10000	0.0001	$1/10^4$ or 10^{-4}	4
N/100000	0.00001	$1/10^5$ or 10^{-5}	5
N/1000000	0.000001	$1/10^6$ or 10^{-6}	6

Table23.4 : H and OH Ion concentration of dilute sodium hydroxide

Strength of NaOH	OH ion	H ion	pH
N/10	10^{-1}	10^{-13}	13
N/100	10^{-2}	10^{-12}	12
N/1000	10^{-3}	10^{-11}	11
N/10000	10^{-4}	10^{-10}	10
N/100000	10^{-5}	10^{-9}	9
N/1000000	10^{-6}	10^{-8}	8

starting from N/10 HCl.

H and OH Ion Concentration of Dilute Sodium Hydroxide

Alkalinity of dilute sodium hydroxide is due to the OH ions. When sodium hydroxide is dissolved in water, there is preponderance of OH ions and this suppresses the hydrogen ion concentration as indicated in Table 23.4.

It is evident that as the concentration of OH ion increases, the H ion decreases. The product of H and OH ions in an aqueous solution of very dilute acid or alkali is always 10^{-14}.

TRANSFER OF SUBSTANCES ACROSS MEMBRANES

Food after digestion is absorbed from the small intestines into the circulation. The different nutrients absorbed are glucose, amino acids, vitamins, minerals and emulsified and finely divided lipids as chylomicrons and lipoproteins. The cells of different tissues obtain their nutrient requirements in the form of glucose, amino acids, vitamins, minerals and lipids (free fatty acids and lipoproteins). The passage of water and nutrients across the intestinal membranes, blood capillaries and cell membranes is a highly complex physico-chemical process. The following aspects of the problem are discussed (1) Intestinal mucosal structure; (2) Nature of tissue cell membranes; (3) Permeability of cell membranes; and (4) Mechanism of transfer of nutrients and excretory products across the membrane.

Intestinal Mucosal Structure

The small intestine in the adult is about 380 cm long. The entire epithelial lining has its surface extended by villi. This enormous surface area is further increased by brush borders (micro villi). The rate of renewal of intestinal mucosal cells has been found to be extremely rapid, a greater part of the intestinal lining being replaced in 3-6 days as compared with 120 days for RBC.

There are specific sites in the small intestine for the absorption of various nutrients (Fig. 23.5).

The intestinal mucosa contains a large group of enzymes (i) Disaccharidases to hydrolyse disaccharides; (2) Peptidases to hydrolyse

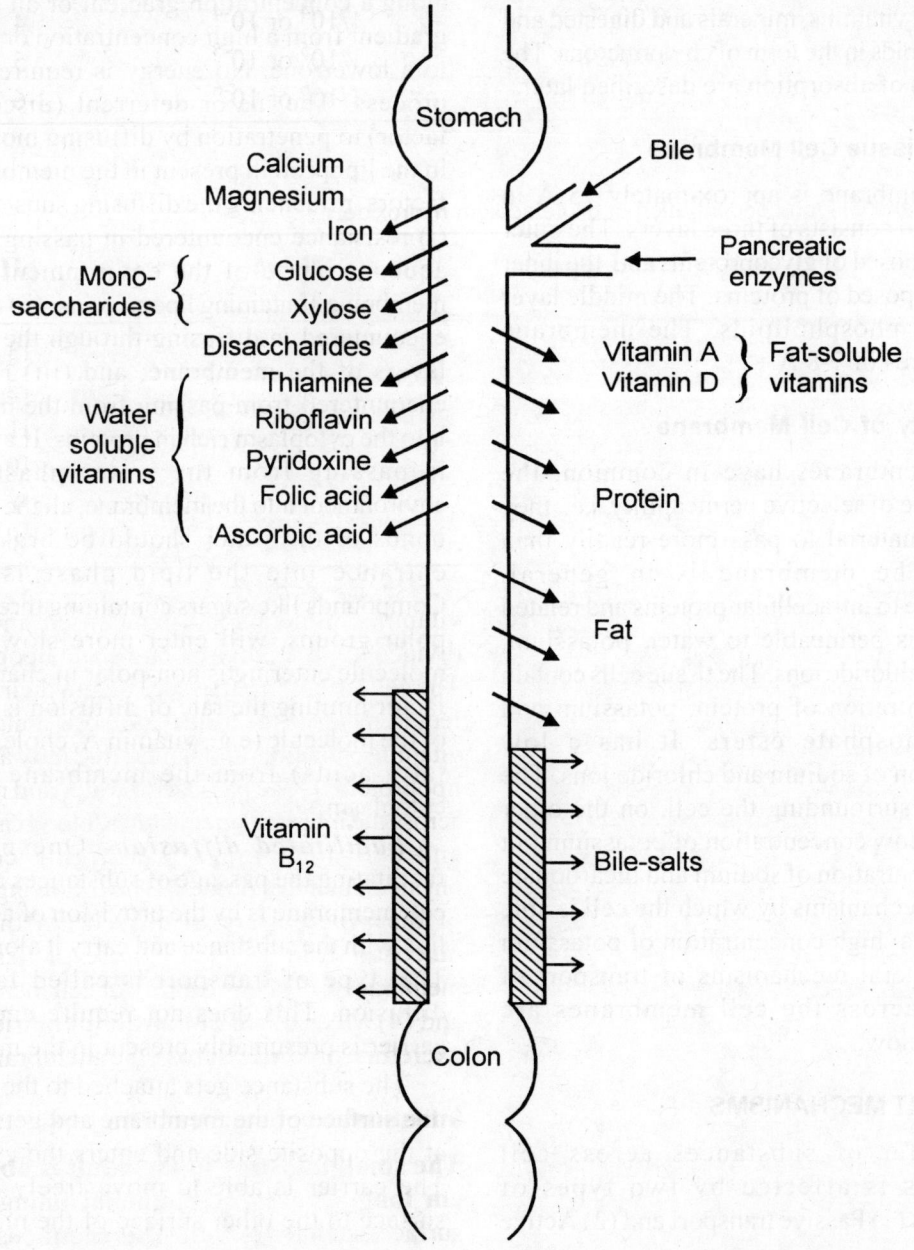

Fig. 23.5 : Specific sites for the absorption of nutrients in the small intestine

peptides; and (3) Lipid synthesising enzymes to synthesise neutral lipids and phosphoipids from the hydrolytic products of lipids. The main function of small intestines is the absorption of nutrients into the systematic circulation in the form of glucose and other monosaccharides, amino acids, vitamins, minerals and digested and emulsified lipids in the form of chylomicrons. The mechanisms of absorption are described later.

Nature of Tissue Cell Membrane

The cell membrane is approximately 75 Å in thickness and consists of three layers. The outer layer is composed of glycoproteins and the inner layer is composed of proteins. The middle layer consists of phospholipids. The membrane contains pores of 7-8 Å.

Permeability of Cell Membrane

All cell membranes have in common, the characteristic of selective permeability, i.e., they allow one material to pass more readily than another. The membrane is in general, impermeable to intracellular proteins and related anions but is permeable to water, potassium, sodium and chloride ions. The tissue cells contain high concentration of protein, potassium and organic phosphate esters. It has a low concentration of sodium and chloride ions. The tissue fluid surrounding the cell, on the other hand, has a low concentration of potassium but a high concentration of sodium and bicarbonate ions. The mechanisms by which the cell is able to maintain a high concentration of potassium and the general mechanisms of transport of materials across the cell membranes are discussed below:

TRANSPORT MECHANISMS

The transfer of substances across cell membranes is affected by two types of mechanisms (1) Passive transport and (2) Active transport.

Passive Transport

There are three major types of passive transport (i) Simple diffusion; (ii) Facilitated diffusion; and (iii) Exchange diffusion.

Simple Diffusion: Simple diffusion occurs along a concentration gradient or an electrical gradient from a high concentration or potential to a lower one. No energy is required for the process. The major deterrent (discouraging factor) to penetration by diffusing molecules is in the lipoprotein present in the membrane. The factors influencing the diffusing substances are: (i) resistance encountered in passing from the aqueous phase of the environment into the membrane containing lipoproteins; (ii) resistance encountered in diffusing through the different layers of the membrane; and (iii) resistance encountered from passing from the membrane into the cytoplasm rich in proteins. If a molecule is passing from the water phase of the environment into the membrane, all the hydrogen bonds of the water should be broken when entrance into the lipid phase is gained. Compounds like sugars containing three or more polar groups, will enter more slowly. If the molecule entering is non-polar in character, the factor limiting the rate of diffusion is the entry of the molecule (e.g., vitamin A, cholesterol and fatty acids) from the membrane into the cytoplasm.

Facilitated diffusion: One means of facilitating the passage of substances across the cell membrane is by the provision of a carrier to link with the substance and carry it along with it. This type of transport is called facilitated diffusion. This does not require energy. The carrier is presumably present in the membrane.

The substance gets attached to the carrier at one surface of the membrane and gets released at the opposite side and enters the cytoplasm. The carrier is able to move freely from one surface to the other surface of the membrane.

Exchange Diffusion: Another type of carrier dependent transport has been shown to operate in the passage of certain ions and amino acids. This is called exchange diffusion. For each molecule or ion transported into the cell, a similar molecule is transported out of the cell on the return trip of the carrier. This type of diffusion is responsible for the major exchange of labelled ions and molecules for non labelled ones.

Active Transport

A greater part of the transport of nutrients across the intestinal mucosa and cell membranes takes place by **'active transport'**. The term **'Active Transport'** means the movement of substances across the cell membrane against a concentration or electrochemical gradient. Energy is required for active transport. Further, active transport is carrier mediated and the carrier is a specific transport protein that is present in the membrane. ATP provides the energy required for the active transport. 'Active Transport' is essential for the transport of Na ion out of the cell and K ion into the cell, and for the absorption of glucose and amino acids across the intestinal mucosa. The transport of glucose and amino acids into the cell by active transport mechanisms is accompanied by the simultaneous movement of sodium ion along with them and it is carrier dependent. The movement of Na ion out of the cell and the K ion into the cell is constantly going on by active transport mechanism and the concentration of these ions in the cell is thus maintained at constant level. The active transport mechanism functions in the (i) maintenance of high K content in RBC and other cells; (ii) movement of Na, K and Ca ions in nerve cells; (iii) secretion of digestive juices; (iv) absorption and secretion by kidney tubules; and (v) secretion of hormones by endocrine glands.

Endocytosis: The term **'Endocytosis'** was suggested by De Duve for the gulping (swallow hastily) one intact cell by another cell1. The important examples of mammalian cells involved in endocytosis are: (i) the granular leucocytes; (ii) the macrophages of the reticulo endothelial system; and (iii) the endothelial lining of the sinusoids of the liver. **The gorging (devouring i.e., to eat greedily) of solids is called phagocytosis and of liquids pinocytosis.**

Secretion: The term **'secretion'** is used to include two consecutive processes: (i) the formation of specific constituents; (ii) their transfer across a membrane in the form of a liquid. Examples are : (i) secretion of saliva and other digestive juices; (ii) secretion of hormones by various ductless glands; and (iii) secretion by kidney tubules, etc.

Filtration: The term **'filtration'** refers to the passage of fluid through a membrane owing to difference of hydrostatic pressure on the two sides of the membrane. The fluid passes from the high pressure side to the low pressure side. It will contain all dissolved substances to which the membrane is permeable. The passage of water and electrolytes from the arterial end of the capillaries to the tissue space is due to the fact that the arterial capillary blood pressure (22 mm Hg) is higher than the colloidal osmotic pressure (15 mm Hg) of plasma while the passage of fluid and electrolytes from tissue space into the capillaries at the venous end of the capillaries is due to the fact that the colloidal osmotic pressure of plasma (15 mm. Hg) is greater than the capillary blood pressure at the venous end (7 mm Hg). The formation of filtrate from blood by the capillaries of the glomeruli of the kidney is due to the high capillary blood pressure (70 mm Hg) exerted in these capillaries as compared with (30 mm Hg) in the arterial end of capillaries elsewhere.

CHAPTER 24

COMMON PROCEDURES (TECHNIQUES) USED IN BIOCHEMISTRY

The common procedures (techniques) of importance in biochemistry are: (1) Colorimetry (2) Electrophoresis; (3) Chromatography (4) Flame photometry (5) Spectrophotometry (6) Elisa (7) Atomic absorption spectrophotometry (8) Autoanalysers, etc. Out of these, we shall discuss over here colorimetry, electrophoresis and chromatography only. These techniques may be legitimately and safely compared with the tools of a *carpenter*. As the value of a carpenter is zero without his tools; likewise a *biochemist/pathologist / molecular biologist* is nothing without such techniques as mentioned above.

Principle

Many biochemical analytical methods produce solutions of coloured compounds. Colorimetry is the technique for determining the concentration of these solutions by measuring the amount of absorption of light which occurs when light rays are passed through them. The more concentrated a solution, the more light is absorbed, and hence the less light it transmits; that is, dilute solutions permit the passage of more light than do concentrated solutions of the same substance.

The law which expresses the relationship between the intensity of light entering and leaving a solution is the Beer-Lambert law.

For a solution of an absorbing solute in a colourless solvent, the fraction of the incident light absorbed is proportional to the number of solute molecules in the light path. That is:

$\text{Log}_{10}\left(\dfrac{I_o}{I}\right) = \varepsilon tc$, where

$I_o =$ the incident light intensity

$I =$ the transmitted light intensity

$t =$ the thickness of solution (in cm.)

$c =$ concentration in moles / l

$\varepsilon =$ a constant called the molar extinction coefficient which depends upon temperature, wavelength and solvent.

Figure 24.1 shows the decrease in intensity of light from $I_o \rightarrow I$ after passing through absorbing material. The wavelength of light is not affected.

Other terms

$\text{Log}_{10}\left(\dfrac{I_o}{I}\right)$ called the optical density, D (or

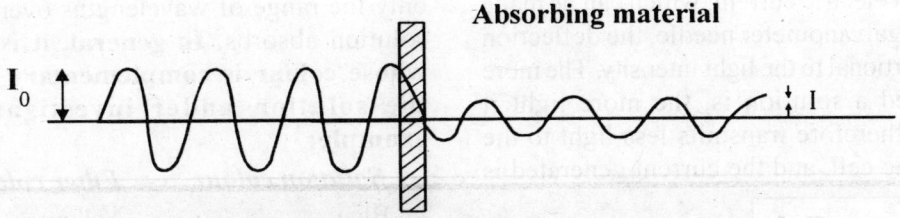

I_0 Absorbing material I

Fig. 24.1 : Showing decrease in the intensity of light

absorbance or extinction of the solution).

$\dfrac{I \times 100}{I_0}$ is called the percentage transmission.

According to the **Beer-Lambert law,** the optical density is constant provided the product of path length and concentration is constant, that is, the density of a solution of concentration 0.1 mole / l, and path length 1 cm is the same as for a solution of 0.01 mole / l and path length 10 cm.

The Beer-Lambert law is obeyed by most solutions provided they are dilute. In a more concentrated solution there may be deviations from the law caused by the association of molecules and so forth. Also, the law only applies to monochromatic light, that is, light of a narrow band of wavelengths.

COLORIMETERS

Colorimeters are instruments used for measuring light intensity. They may either be calibrated in terms of optical density ($D = \log I_0/I$)

or percentage transmission ($\times\ 100\ \dfrac{I}{I_0}$)

Provided the thickness of solution is constant, that is a standard cuvette is used throughout, then D is directly proportional to concentration. If D is plotted against the concentration, straight line is obtained. If the instrument is calibrated as percentage transmission, and a graph is plotted against concentration of solutions, then a logarithmic curve is obtained as shown below in figures.

There are two types of instruments for measuring light intensity, photoelectric absorptiometers which employ photocells as light detectors, and visual instruments which are much less accurate as they depend on the naked eye to detect differences in light intensity.

PHOTOELECTRIC ABSORPTIOMETERS

Photoelectric absorptiometers use photoelectric cells, either of the barrier layer type, or the emissive type. Light falling on these cells

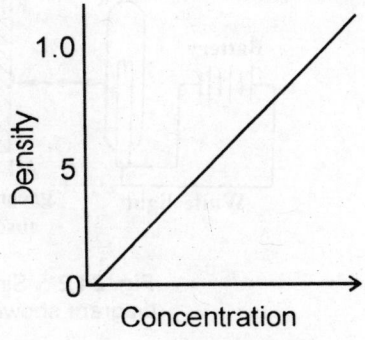

generates an electric current, which can be made to deflect a galvanometer needle, the deflection being proportional to the light intensity. The more concentrated a solution is, the more light it absorbs; it therefore transmits less light to the photoelectric cell, and the current generated is smaller.

Absorptiometers using barrier layer (selenium) self generating photocells may either be direct reading, single photocell instruments, or be 'null-point' reading double cell instruments. In the latter, filtered light from a single source reaches both photocells. Some light will be absorbed by a coloured solution inserted in front of one of the cells, and this will be reflected by the galvanometer reading. By varying a resistance in the circuit, or by closing a diaphragm, the two currents may be balanced, the galvanometer acting as a **null-point** indicator.

THE USE OF COLOUR FILTERS

To increase the sensitivity of readings, that is to give the greatest difference in photocell response between two concentrations of a solution, a suitable colour filter is placed between the test solution and the photoelectric cell. These filters are made up of coloured gelatin, mounted between two pieces of glass. Usually these filters have narrow transmission bands, so they transmit monochromatic light. The filter is chosen so that the range of wavelengths it transmits, includes only the range of wavelengths over which the solution absorbs. **In general, it is the filter whose colour is complementary to that of the solution under investigation. For example:**

Solution colour	Filter colour
Blue	Yellow
Bluish-green	Red
Purple	Green
Red	Bluish-green
Yellow	Blue
Yellow-green	Violet

To understand the use of light filters, consider a solution which absorbs light in the red part of the spectrum. Such a solution, when illuminated by white light, absorbs red colour wavelengths and emits bluish-green light, together with a small amount of red. The greater the concentration of the solution, the smaller the amount of red light transmitted.

The most sensitive readings of the galvanometer will be obtained, therefore, by allowing only the transmitted red light to activate the cell. A red filter achieves this by being opaque to bluish-green light, and allowing only the red to pass through as shown in Figure 24.2.

When colorimetric determinations are being made (analyses resulting in coloured solutions which are proportional to the concentration of the original substance), it is essential to ensure

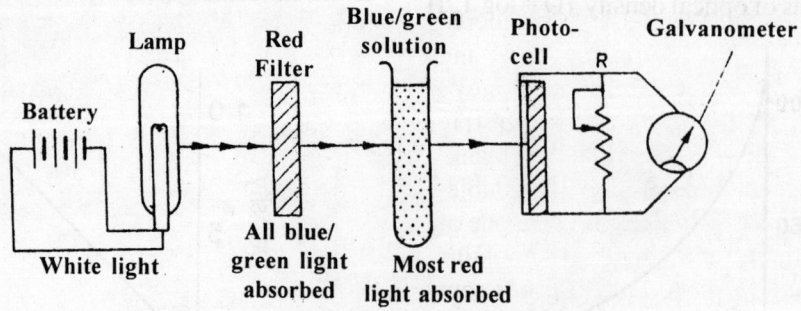

Fig. 24.2 : Single cell photoelectric absorptiometer (diagram showing light path, and use of colour filter)

that the colour being measured is only due to the substance under test, and is not due to any of the reagents used. Whenever such determinations are being made, therefore, it is essential to include the following:

(a) The *Test* solution. This contains the unknown concentration of substance under test, together with the reagents used in that test.

(b) The *Blank* solution. This solution is identical to that of the test solution in that it has been carried through the test procedure and contains all the reagents used, but without the test substance. Any colour given by the reagents used in the analysis can be detected and eliminated.

(c) The *Standard* solution. This is identical with the test solution, except that it contains a known amount of the substance being determined, and is approximately equal in concentration to that expected in the test solution.

It is also essential to avoid any errors due to dirty glassware, turbidity of solutions or air bubbles, as all these factors will seriously interfere with light transmission. It is especially important to remember not to handle the cuvette by its optical surfaces, which must be clean and dry.

In order to be sure that the optical density is due solely to the substance under test, the reading given by the 'blank' solution must be considered with the reading obtained from the 'test' and 'standard' solutions. This can be done in one of two ways. If a single-cell photoelectric absorptiometer is used, it is set so that the ' blank' solution is 100 percent transmission. If a double-cell photoelectric absorptiometer is used, one of the cells, called the reference, always contains distilled water, and is set to read 100 per cent transmission. The blank, test and standard

solutions are then placed one after another in the second cuvette, and a series of readings obtained. The blank reading must then be subtracted from the test and the standard reading, i.e.,

$$\frac{\text{Test - Blank}}{\text{Standard - Blank}} \text{ X Concentration of standard}$$

It is possible to check that the instrument is still at 100 per cent transmission between each set of readings. The actual details of use vary with each instrument.

GENERAL PROCEDURE FOR USING A SINGLE CELL PHOTOELECTRIC ABSORPTIOMETER

(1) Choose a suitable filter and place this in the light path.

(2) Switch on the lamp, and allow 5 minutes for the instrument to stabilize.

(3) Using the special tube or glass cell (cuvette) provided with the instrument, insert a 'blank' solution in the path of filtered light. Be careful not to touch the optical surfaces of the glass as this will interfere with light transmission. The glass must be chemically clean.

(4) Adjust the scale reading until it reads full scale. This is now 100 percent transmission with the particular reference solution used, or zero optical density.

(5) Without altering anything else, remove the tube and replace it with a similar tube containing the 'unknown' solution.

(6) Note the meter reading for this test solution.

(7) Immediately remove the test solution, and replace it with a 'standard' solution of known concentration.

(8) Note the meter reading for the

standard solution.

General calculation

T = Reading of test solution

S = Reading of standard solution

$$\frac{T}{S} \times \text{Concentration of standard} = \text{Concentration of test}$$

When a number of determinations are being made using a photoelectric absorptiometer, it is not necessary to read a standard with each unknown but to make use of a calibration curve. The instrument may be calibrated as follows.

A series of solutions is prepared, in dilutions ranging from the lowest expected concentration to the highest. The optical density of each solution is very carefully measured, using the standard technique for the instrument. From the figures obtained, a calibration curve is drawn by plotting optical densities (meter readings) directly against the concentrations.

ELECTROPHORESIS OF PROTEINS

The movement of ions or charged particle in solution to the anode or cathode under the influence of an electric current is called **'Electrophoresis'**. Protein molecules contain some basic groups and carboxyl groups. The basic groups are provided by the epsilon amino groups of lysine, guanido group of arginine and imidazole group of histidine while the acidic groups are provided by the free carboxyl groups of dicarboxylic acids, the phenolic group of tyrosine and SH group of cysteine. Since the number of acidic and basic groups present varies from one protein to another, the net positive or

As the name implies, colorimetry involves the quantitative estimation of colour. So the substance, to be estimated colorimetrically, must be either coloured by itself or capable of forming coloured complex through chemical reactions. Furthermore the intensity of the colour must be dependent upon the concentration. Colorimetry basically is of two types:

1. Visual Colorimetry. This is in which we compare the light intensities transmitted out of the solutions.

2. Photometry. This is in which we compare the absorption of the light by the solutions.

When absorption measurements are done by photoelectric colorimeters in visible range of the spectrum (i.e., between 400-760 mμ of wavelength), the device is termed as photoelectric colorimetry. On the other hand, if these absorption measurements are done in invisible region of spectrum (i.e., in ultraviolet and infrared regions), the technique is termed as spectrophotometry, in which we make use of spectrophotometers.

Absorption maxima. At a particular wavelength, any light absorbing material (colour) absorbs maximum light, which is termed as **absorption maxima.**

Approximate wavelength of colours

(a)	Ultra Violet	< 400 mμ
(b)	Violet	400 - 450 mμ
(c)	Blue	450 - 500 mμ
(d)	Green	500 - 570 mμ
(e)	Yellow	570 - 590 mμ
(f)	Orange	590 - 620 mμ
(g)	Red	620 - 760 mμ
(h)	Infrared	>760 mμ

negative charge in the protein differs from one protein to another. **At iso-electric point, proteins carry equal number of positive and negative charges and do not move in an electric field.** The iso-electric points of some proteins are given in Table 24.1.

Table 24.1 : Iso-electric point of some proteins

Proteins	Iso-electric point (pH)
Serum albumin (human)	4.7
γ-globulin (human)	6.4
Haemoglobin (human)	6.7

On the acid side of the iso-electric point, the proteins in solution carry net positive charge due to the basic groups and move to the cathode or negative pole while on the alkaline side of the iso-electric point, the protein carries a net negative charge due to the carboxyl groups and migrate to the positive pole or anode. Tiselius (1937) developed an elegant method of separating proteins by electrophoresis using a 'U' tube. The solution of the proteins (at suitable alkaline pH) e.g., plasma is placed in the 'U' tube

and electric current is passed at the end of the 'U' tube. The charged protein particles migrate to the anode. The rate at which the proteins migrate will depend on the net negative charge on the protein and the molecular weight of the proteins.

Electrophoresis using filter paper and gels as medium

Several improvements and simplification have been made in the electrophoretic technique using filter paper, starch gel, agar gel, acrylamide gel. The technique of paper electrophoresis of plasma proteins is described below and shown in Fig. 24.3. A small quantity of bromophenol blue is added to plasma. A drop of the plasma is spotted at the centre of a strip of special paper, saturated with barbitone buffer (pH 8.6). The centre of the paper is supported over a glass rod. The ends of the paper dip in the same buffer solution kept in two troughs on either side of the glass rod. The entire system is covered with a glass sheet. An electric current of suitable amperage and voltage (2 to 8v) is passed across

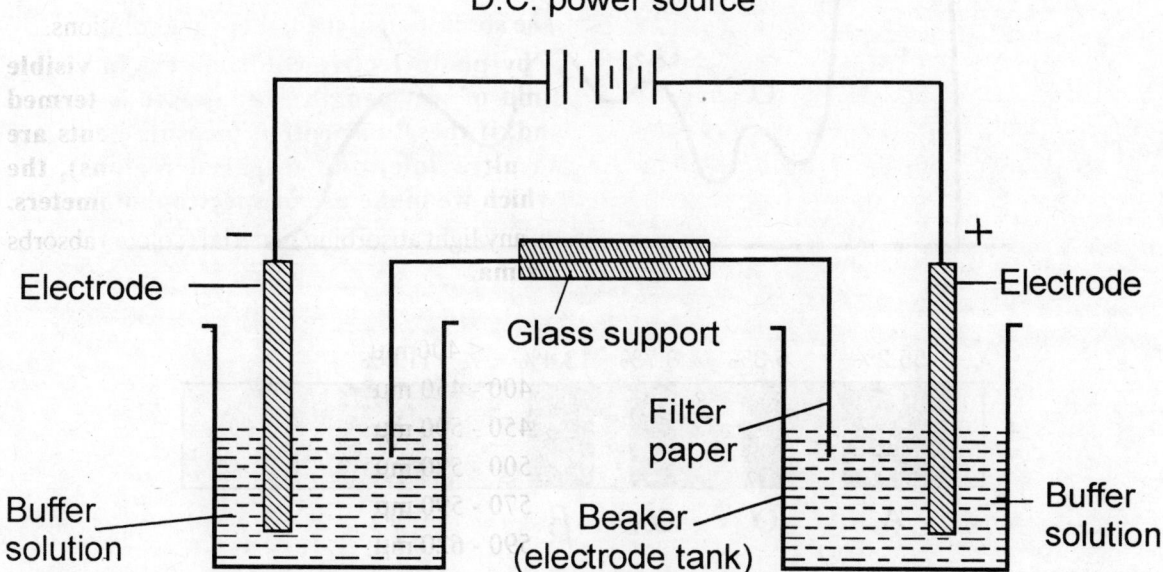

Fig : 24.3 : Diagram of Electrophoresis apparatus

the paper, when the proteins carrying different electric charges migrate at different rates. The proteins stained blue by bromophenol blue will be found migrating to the anode at different rates. After a run of about 6 hours, the paper is removed and dried in an oven at 100°C for 30 minutes. The paper is again stained with a solution containing bromophenol blue. The different protein fractions appear as blue coloured bands in the following order: (1) albumin; (2) α_1-globulin; (3) α_2-globulin; (4) β-globulin; and (5) mixture of γ-globulins and fibrinogen. Albumin, being the fastest moving fraction, moves to the farthest end of the paper towards anode while γ-globulin and fibrinogen

being the slowest moving proteins form a band towards the other end. If a quantitative estimation is required, the intensity of blue colour in each band can be scanned using an optical densitometer. Alternately, the bands may be cut and the colour eluded in barbitone buffer and measured in a photoelectric colorimeter. The concentration of different proteins in plasma expressed as percentage of total proteins is as follows: (1) albumin, 55.2 percent; (2) α_1-globulin, 5.3 percent; (3) α_2-globulin, 8.7 percent; (4) β-globulin, 13.4 percent; (5) γ-globulin, 11.0 percent; and (6) fibrinogen, 6.5 percent. Graphic representation of concentrations of serum proteins as obtained by scanning in a densitometer is shown in Fig. 24.4.

Immuno Electrophoresis

This technique offers a very sensitive method for the separation and identification of the different proteins present in the γ-globulin fraction. It is a modified agar-gel electrophoresis technique. The procedure combines electrophoresis with specific antigen-antibody precipitin

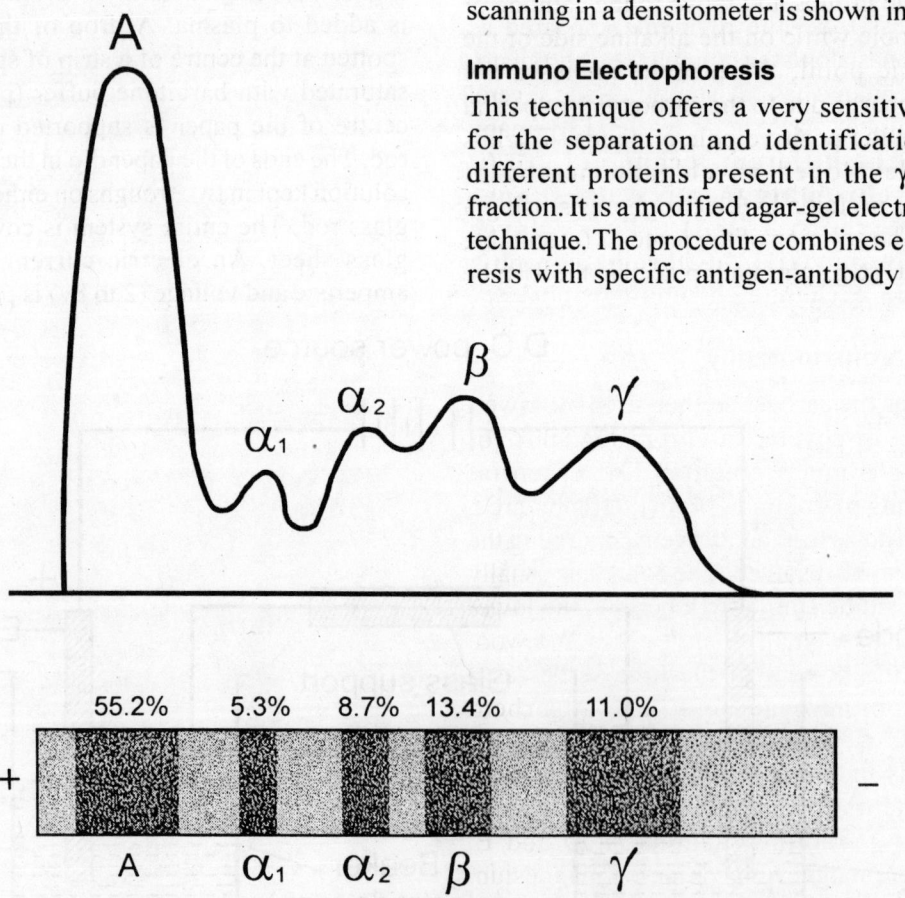

Fig : 24.4 : Graphic representation of concentration of serum protein fractions as obtained by scanning in a Densitometer.

reactions. The separated proteins are allowed to react with specific immune serum placed in a groove prepared in the gel. The immune serum diffuses into the gel and reacts with tho immunoglobulin forming precipitation lines.

CHROMATOGRAPHY

The term 'Chromatography' was used originally by the Polish Botanist, Tswett (1906) to a procedure evolved by him for separating a mixture of plant pigments using a column of calcium carbonate. He made the important discovery that when solution of plant pigments in ether was allowed to drip through a column of calcium carbonate powder packed in a long narrow glass tube, the pigments appeared as separate zones along the column. The chromato-graphic-technique has been modified and several new techniques have been evolved by many workers. **The different techniques are (i) Column chromatography; (ii) Paper chromatography; (iii) Thin layer chromatography; (iv) Gas chromatography; and (v) Ion exchange chromatography.**

Column chromatography

This was the earliest method used by Tswett (1906), the discoverer of chromatography for separating plant pigments. The essential requirements of column chromatography are a column, an adsorbent and solvent containing the substances to be resolved. The column is usually a long glass tube similar to a burette, the lower end tapering. A small quantity of cottonwool placed at the bottom of the tube serves as a support for the adsorbent. The adsorbent commonly used are alumina or $CaCO_3$ (for carotenoids and other plant pigments), celite or supercel (for proteins), cellulose (organic compounds), kaolin (vitamins A, D and E, porphyrins), magnesium oxide or magnesium silicate (for steroids), silicic acid (hydrocarbons, amino acids). The solvents used commonly are acetone, petroleum ether, ether, alcohol, etc. The

solution is allowed to drip through the column. The substances undergo separation into separate zones. These can be identified by reacting with specific reagents or spectrophotometrically.

Paper chromatography (Partition chromatography)

Partition chromatography is based on the distribution of a mixture between two immiscible liquids. Filter paper is commonly used as the supporting medium for this technique. Solvents commonly used are mixtures of water and butanol or phenol. **This method is used widely for the separation of amino acids or sugars.**

Rf Values: The movement of a particular solute is measure in terms of Rf values. Rf value is the ratio between the distance travelled by the substance from the starting point to the distance travelled by the solvent from the starting point.

$$Rf = \frac{\text{Distance travelled by the solute}}{\text{Distance travelled by the solvent}}$$

The Rf value is less than one. The value is constant for a particular solute with the same solvent system.

Chromatographic technique

Two types of techniques are commonly used: (1) Single dimensional chromatography; and (2) Two dimensional chromatography.

Single dimensional paper chromatography: Two types of techniques are used: (1) Ascending paper chromatography (Fig. 24.5); (2) Descending paper chromatography (Fig. 24.5). The principle of both the methods is the same. A small volume (about 0.005 ml) of the amino acid mixture solution containing about 100 μg of amino acids is applied with a syringe needle at a pencil mark point 5 cm from one end (A) of the filter paper strip and allowed to dry. The filter paper strip is suspended in a jar or glass cabinet so that the end (A) of the paper dips into a solution of butanol-acetic acid-water

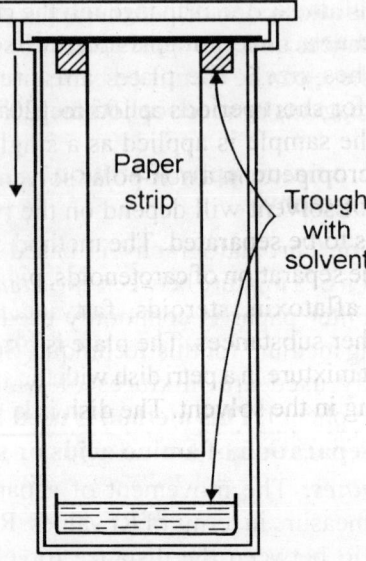

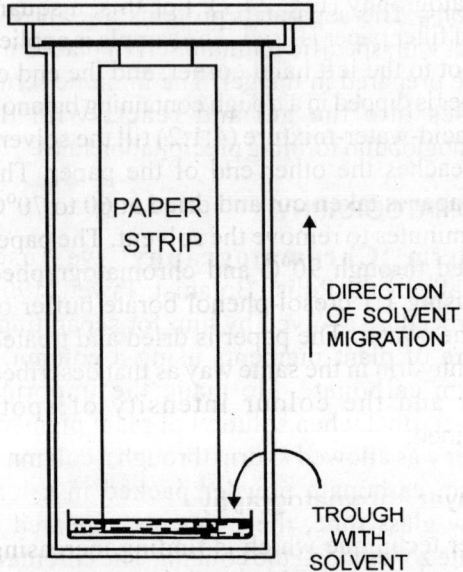

Fig : 24.5 : Apparatus for **Descending** (left) and **Ascending** (right) **Paper Chromatography**

kept in a trough at the bottom of the cylinder or chamber (ascending paper chromatography) or at the top of the cylinder or chamber (descending paper chromatography). The chromatogram is allowed to develop till the solvent front has reached the other end of the filter paper. The filter paper is removed, dried in an oven at 70 to 80°C for 15 minutes. The paper is sprayed with 0.5 percent ninhydrin in acetone and dried for 3 minutes at 90 to 100°C. Purple coloured spots appear with all amino acids except proline which gives an yellow spot and hydroxyproline, a brown spot (Fig. 24.6). The spots can be cut, eluded with acetone and the intensity of colour determined against standard amino acid spots obtained under similar conditions. Alternately, the colour intensities of the spots on the paper can be determined by means of a scanner (recording transmittance or reflectance photometer device).

Two dimensional paper chromatography: In the single dimensional paper chromatography, the Rf values of some amino acids are so close that they overlap each other. All the amino acids occurring in a protein hydrolysate can be separated on a two dimensional paper

chromatogram may be run. In this method, a sheet of filter paper is dotted with the sample as a spot to dry. Keeping the sample end of the paper dipped in a suitable chromatography solvent (e.g. n-butanol – acetic acid – water mixture (4:1:5) till the solvent front reaches the other end of the sheet. The filter paper is taken out and dried at 70°C for 30 minutes to remove the solvent. The paper is turned through 90° and chromatographed again using another sheet of butanol butter or chloroform. The spots detected earlier with ninhydrin in the same way as the earlier center and the colour intensity of the spot determined.

This layer chromatography can be used as another technique of chromatography using use in place of paper is thin layer chromatography. In this method, a layer of suitable adsorbent. The developing solvents are the same as in paper chromatography.

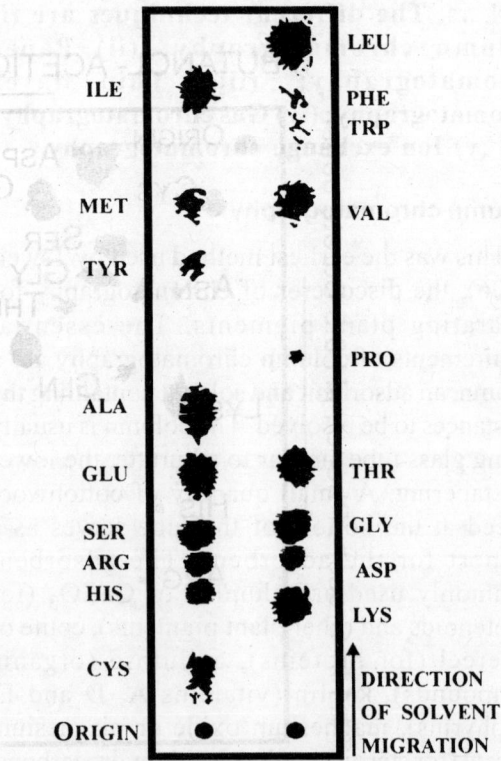

Fig : 24.6 : Chromatogram showing the separation of Amino acids by **Ascending Paper Chromatography**

chromatography (Fig. 24.7). For this, a square sheet of filter paper is used. The sample is applied as a spot to the left hand corner, and the end of the paper is dipped in a trough containing butanol-acetic acid-water-mixture (4:1:2) till the solvent front reaches the other end of the paper. The filter paper is taken out and dried at 60 to 70°C for 30 minutes to remove the solvent. The paper is turned through 90°C and chromatographed again using 1:1 cresol-phenol borate buffer or collidine- water. The paper is dried and treated with ninhydrin in the same way as that described earlier and the colour intensity of spots determined.

Thin layer chromatography

Another technique which is finding increasing use in biochemistry is thin layer chromatography. In this method, thin layer of adsorbents such as

silica gel, alumina, ion exchange resin, sephadex are spread as a slurry on glass plates (6 x 6 or 8 x 8 inches size). The plates are dried and activated for short periods at 105 to 120°C and cooled. The sample is applied as a single spot with a micropipette in a non-polar solvent. The selection of solvent will depend on the type of substances to be separated. The method can be used for the separation of carotenoids, pigments, vitamins, aflatoxin, steroids, fatty acids and several other substances. The plate is placed in the solvent mixture in a petri dish with the spotted end dipping in the solvent. The dish is kept in a glass chamber which is closed tightly with a glass sheet. The solvent rises rapidly through the plate and the separation of the substances takes place in a short time (30 min to 3 hours). The plates are removed, dried at low temperature (50 to 60°C). The spots are detected by spraying the

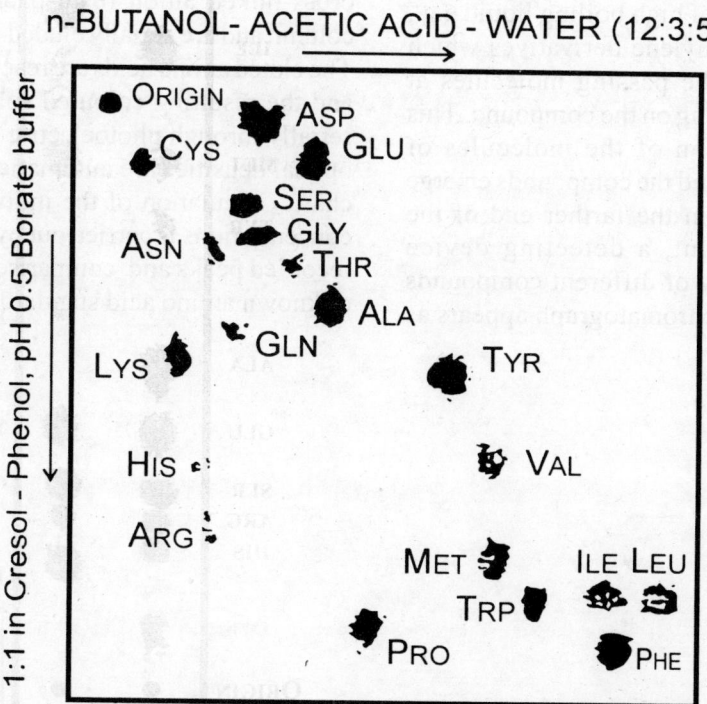

Fig : 24.7 : Chromatogram showing the separation of Amino acids by **Two Dimensional Paper Chromatography**

plate with a suitable reagent. The intensity of colour is evaluated in the same way as in paper chromatography. The advantages of TLC are: (1) lesser time (as separation can be completed in about 30 minutes to 3 hours as compared to paper chromatography which takes 16 to 24-hours); (2) better separation; and (3) sensitivity. Its disadvantages are poor reproducibility of Rf values.

Gas chromatography

Gas chromatography was discovered by James and Martin in 1952. In gas chromatography, a mixture of compounds to be separated is injected into one end of a long heated column through which passes an inert gas carrier. The material should vapourise at high temperature without decomposing. The columns are several feet in length and one quarter inch or less in diameter are packed with microglass beads coated with a variety of high boiling liquid e.g., silicones polyoxy ethylene derivatives which absorb and release the passing molecules at different rates depending on the compound. This results in a separation of the molecules of different compounds and the compounds emerge one after another from the farther end of the column. At this point, a detecting device measures the quantity of different compounds emerging out. A gas chromatograph appears as a series of peaks on a graphical chart where each peak position is characteristic of a specific material and each peak area is directly related to its relative concentration. By the application of gas chromatography to the analysis of expired air, the presence of 15 short chain volatile organic molecules has been detected.

Ion exchange chromatography-automatic amino acid analyser

Moore and Stein utilised an ion exchange resin (Dowex) and various buffers to accomplish separation on a chromato-graphic column of all the amino acids present in a protein hydrolysate. Modifications in this procedure introduced by Moore, Spackman and Stein led to the development of an automatic amino acid analyser for the separation and estimation of amino acids. The principle of the method is as follows: Amino acids are absorbed on a highly cross-linked anion resin packed in a suitable column and are serially eluded in a specific order. The eluted amino acids are reacted with ninhydrin and the resulting coloured solutions are passed serially through photoelectric colorimeters. The optical densities are automatically recorded in a chart. Calculation of the individual amino acid concentrations is carried out by integration of the recorded peaks and comparison with peak areas of known amino acid standards.

CHAPTER 25

LIVER AND KIDNEY FUNCTION TESTS

LIVER: As you know, me is the evermost important organ of the body where metabolism of all the compounds takes place. If somehow, I get sick then whole body gets disturbed. Surgeons have so far tried unsuccessfully for my transplantation. As I am very complex in structure and functioning, therefore, in my case, adaptability of transplantation had not been a success so far.

I have several very important functions to perform in the body like I am responsible for (i) making proteins, (ii) making bile for digestion of food, (iii) breaking down fats and amino acids, (iv) filtering poisonous chemicals from the blood and then breaking them down, etc.

KIDNEYS: We are small in size and ours shape is very beautiful, just like that of the seed of a bean. Ours function is of very high order as we are *'excretory organs'* (scavangers/sweepers) and excrete all the toxins/wastage/garbage, etc. out of the body and make it clean.

Liver is the most important tissue of our body, the importance of which can be evaluated from the fact that the metabolism of all the main substances viz. carbohydrates, lipids, proteins, nucleic acids, etc. takes place in this very tissue. By chance, if it is out of order, now, one can very well imagine the harm one is bound to face in one or the other way. **Its functions are innumerable, its reserve capacity is enormous and its ability to recover is also enormous.** For the assessment of liver functioning one has, therefore, to be aware with both i.e. its reserve capacity and the battery of functions it performs. It, therefore, becomes more rationale to have some knowledge of its anatomy.

A. ANATOMY - SALIENT FEATURES

Liver (Fig. 25.1) of a healthy adult weighs between 0.85-2.6 kg with an average of about 1.6 kg. Grossly, it is constituted of lobes of various size which differ to some extent in the sources of afferent blood supplies. Each lobe has a tree

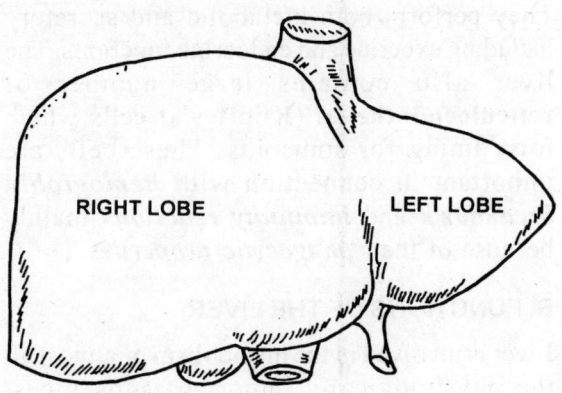

Fig. 25.1 : Diagram of liver

Metabolic functions of the liver

* Conversion of absorbed monosacc-harides i.e. galactose and fructose into glucose.
* Biosynthesis of cholesterol and its esterification and excretion.
* Conversion of NH_3 into urea.
* Biosynthesis of proteins.
* Biosynthesis of nucleic acids.
* Metabolism of vitamins and minerals to some extent.
* Synthesis of blood coagulation factors.
* Secretory and excretory functions.
* Detoxication and protective functions.
* Storage functions, etc.
* Formation of blood in embryo and some abnormal states in adults.

Functions of the liver

1. Metabolic functions
2. Secretory function
3. Detoxication and protective functions
4. Storage functions
5. Synthesis of blood coagulation factors
6. Excretory functions
7. Handling of enzymes
8. Miscellaneous functions

like framework of connective tissue supporting parenchymal cells, blood vessels and the bile ducts. Blood reaches the lobules from the portal vein and the hepatic artery. The blood enters into spaces between cords or sheets of hepatic cells, sinusoids, and after passing through them is drained into central vein of the lobule.

The most abundant and the characteristic cells of the liver are the parenchymal cells which are arranged in such a manner that each cell faces both a duct and a sinusoid containing blood. They perform both metabolic and secretory including exocrine and endocrine functions. The liver also contains large number of **reticuloendothelial (Kupffer's) cells** which form lining for sinusoids. These cells are important in connection with *hemoglobin breakdown* and *immunity reactions* mainly because of their *phagocytic properties.*

B. FUNCTIONS OF THE LIVER

Liver is involved in the metabolism of almost all the physiologically important substances/

compounds and is also independently involved in many other important biochemical functions. Various function tests are categorised on the basis of following diverse functions of the liver.

Basic functions of liver are divided into:

(a) Storage and filtration of blood attrib-uted to its vascular functions.

(b) Secretion of bile into gastrointestinal tract (GIT) attributed to its secretory functions.

(c) Anabolism and catabolism of physiologi cally important compounds attributed to its metabolic functions.

1. Metabolic functions

Liver is a key organ and hence believed to be the principal site for the following reactions:

(a) Conversion of absorbed monosaccharides e.g. galactose and fructose into glucose.

(b) Cholesterol biosynthesis, its esterification and excretion.

(c) Biosynthesis of plasma proteins e.g. albumin and globulins.

(d) Conversion of ammonia into urea.

2. Secretory functions

Liver is largely responsible for bile pigment metabolism by converting bilirubin, formed from heme catabolism, into bilirubin diglucuronides and secreting them through bile.

3. Detoxication and protective functions

Liver **(Kupffer cells)** can remove foreign bodies from blood by phagocytosis. It can detoxify various drugs and hormones by converting them into less toxic substances which are excreted.

4. Storage functions

Liver stores glucose in the form of **glycogen.** It is also responsible to some extent for the storage of some vitamins e.g. **vitamin A and B$_{12}$.**

5. Synthesis of blood coagulation factors

Preprothrombin (inactive form) is converted into prothrombin in liver in the presence of vitamin K. Other coagulation factors e.g. factor V, VII and X are also synthesised in the liver.

6. Excretory functions

Bromosulphthalein(BSP) and Rose Bengal dye are exclusively found to be excreted through liver cells.

7. Handling of enzymes

Much significance is attributed to liver for handling of enzymes like alkaline phosphatase (ALP) and release of transaminases e.g. aspartate transaminase (GOT) and alanine transaminase (GPT).

8. Miscellaneous functions

    (a) Blood formation in embryo
    (b) Blood formation in adults in some abnormal states

C. DISEASES OF THE LIVER AND BILIARY TRACT

Disturbances of metabolism occurring in liver diseases are mainly due to failure of parenchymal cells to carry out vital functions. Various reasons attributed to these disturbances include infections, decreased mass of functioning cells, decreased blood supply, impaired nutrition and reactions of other organs e.g. brain, kidney, pancreas, adrenal, gonads and spleen etc.

Viral hepatitis, infectious diseases of the liver, are mainly due to degeneration and necrosis of parenchymal cells followed by their complete disappearance causing destruction of normal lobule architecture. Recovery, however, may occur within 24-48 hours due to astonishing regenerating capability of these cells. In earlier time viral hepatitis has been often mistaken as **"Catarrhal Jaundice"** a disease of bile duct.

Overnutrition, dietary deficiencies of betaine, choline, methionine or other extrinsic sources of methyl groups and the action of toxic substances may contribute to the occurrence of fatty liver. Liver diseases of purely nutritional origin are more prevalent in those parts of the world where consumption of low nutritional quality protein is more common. Other diseases such as infectious mononucleosis, malaria, lobar pneumonia, typhoid fever, anaemias, syphilis, cholera, diabetes mellitus and thyrotoxicosis too contribute to liver damage by causing strain on various metabolism.

Proliferation of connective tissues of the liver may also occur spontaneously due to diminished blood supply resulting from circulatory and other factors. Disorganisation of liver structure and further interference with blood supply may also arise due to overgrowth of connective tissue. This finally may produce shrunken liver with markedly reduced mass of parenchymal, reticuloendothelial and vascular tissue. Such **"scarred livers"** are usually witnessed in portal, atrophic and **Laennec's Cirrhosis.** Profound biliary obstruction may also be manifested as biliary cirrhosis.

Obstruction of bile duct often causes jaundice as witnessed in liver damage. Therefore, it becomes rather more judicious to distinguish between jaundices due to obstruction, hepatic or excessive destruction of blood (hemolytic).

Other causes include neoplastic disease of the ducts and carcinoma of head of pancreas. Gall stones entering common bile duct are mainly responsible for biliary obstruction. Damage of parenchymal cells with widespread necrosis, which may be fatal are not as a result of liver damage caused either by drugs or chemicals. Excessive destruction of blood due to increased hemolysis is as a result of incompatible blood transfusion; hemolytic poisons are largely responsible for hemolytic jaundice.

Metabolism and functions of other organs e.g. brain and kidney are also impaired due to liver disease. Impairment of renal function commonly accompanies liver disease and hence jointly referred to as hepatorenal syndrome.

LIVER FUNCTION TESTS (Table 25.1)

The choice of tests for the study of the diseases of the liver or biliary tract varies with the type of information sought. A decision about the number of tests to be got done requires experience and judgement. Various tests according to the functions of liver involved may be listed as follows:

1. **Tests based on the abnormalities of bile pigment metabolism:**
   (a) Serum bilirubin and Van den Bergh reaction. Icteric index.
   (b) Urinary and fecal urobilinogen.
   (c) Urinary coproporphyrin.

2. **Tests based on the role of liver in carbohydrate metabolism:**
   (a) Galactose tolerance test.
   (b) Fructose tolerance test.

3. **Tests based on the changes in plasma proteins (disturbances in protein metabolism) :**
   (a) Determination of total serum proteins and A/G ratio.
   (b) Flocculation tests.
   (c) Amino acids in blood and urine.

Icteric Index

It measures the degree of jaundice by measuring the intensity of the yellow colour of the serum. Serum or plasma is diluted with physiological saline until it matches in colour to a 1 in 10,000 solution of potassium dichromate. **The dilution factor is termed as the Icteric index.**

The normal range is from 4 to 6 whereas, in latent jaundice it is from 7 to 15. With an index over 15 clinically obvious jaundice should be present. In jaundice the icteric index parallels the serum bilirubin but below 1 mg%, it is roughly 5 times the serum bilirubin. **The Icteric index is not specific for bilirubin but influenced by the carotenes present in the serum.**

4. **Tests based on the abnormalities of lipids (disturbances in lipid metabolism) :**
   (a) Determination of serum cholesterol and the ratio of free and esterified cholesterol.
   (b) Determination of fecal fats.

5. **Tests based on the detoxicating function of the liver**
   (a) Hippuric acid synthesis test.

6. **Tests based on the excretion of injected substances by the liver:**
   (a) Bromsulphthalein test.

7. **Determination of serum enzymes:**
   Common (Routine Enzymic Investigations)
   (a) Aspartate transaminase (GOT).
   (b) Alanine transaminase (GPT), and
   (c) Alkaline phosphatase.
   Investigations Rarely Recommended:
   (a) γ-glytamyl transpeptidase.
   (b) Isocitrate dehydrogenase.
   (c) Choline esterase.
   (d) Lactate dehydrogenase.

8. **Formation of prothrombin**

Table 25.1 : Liver Function Tests

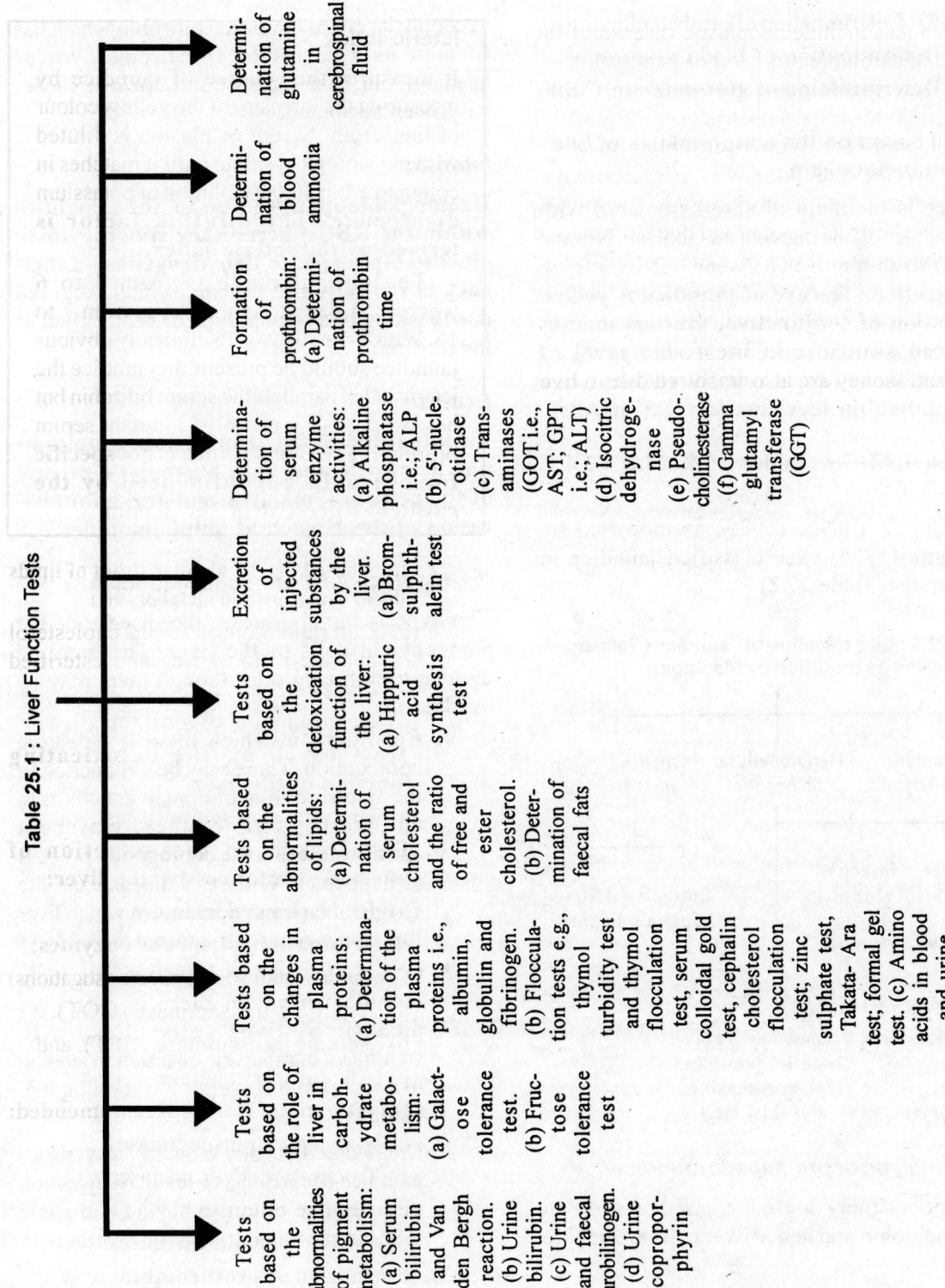

| Tests based on the abnormalities of pigment metabolism:
(a) Serum bilirubin and Van den Bergh reaction.
(b) Urine bilirubin.
(c) Urine and faecal urobilinogen.
(d) Urine coproporphyrin | Tests based on the role of liver in carbohydrate metabolism:
(a) Galactose tolerance test.
(b) Fructose tolerance test | Tests based on the changes in plasma proteins:
(a) Determination of the plasma proteins i.e., albumin, globulin and fibrinogen.
(b) Flocculation tests e.g., thymol turbidity test and thymol flocculation test, serum colloidal gold test, cephalin cholesterol flocculation test; zinc sulphate test, Takata- Ara test; formal gel test. (c) Amino acids in blood and urine | Tests based on the abnormalities of lipids:
(a) Determination of serum cholesterol and the ratio of free and ester cholesterol.
(b) Determination of faecal fats | Tests based on the detoxication function of the liver:
(a) Hippuric acid synthesis test | Excretion of injected substances by the liver.
(a) Brom-sulphthalein test | Determination of serum enzyme activities:
(a) Alkaline phosphatase i.e.; ALP
(b) 5'-nucleotidase
(c) Transaminases (GOT i.e., AST; GPT i.e.; ALT)
(d) Isocitric dehydrogenase
(e) Pseudocholinesterase
(f) Gamma glutamyl transferase (GGT) | Formation of prothrombin:
(a) Determination of prothrombin time | Determination of blood ammonia | Determination of glutamine in cerebrospinal fluid |

(a) Determination of prothrombin time.

9. **Determination of blood ammonia**

10. **Determination of glutamine in C.S.F.**

1. Tests based on the abnormalities of bile pigment metabolism

Jaundice is the main disease associated with abnormalities of bile pigment metabolism. Normal serum bilirubin ranges between 0.2-1.0 mg/dl. **Characteristic feature of jaundice is yellow colouration of conjunctiva, mucous membrane and skin due to increased level of bilirubin. Jaundice is usually visible when serum bilirubin level exceeds 2.5 mg/dl.**

CLASSIFICATION (Tables 25.2, 25.3, 25.4 & 25.5)

Rolleston & McNee (1929) as modified by **Maclagan** (1964) have classified jaundice in three groups (Table 25.2) :

Table 25.2 : Classification of Jaundice (Rolleston and McNee as modified by Maclagan)

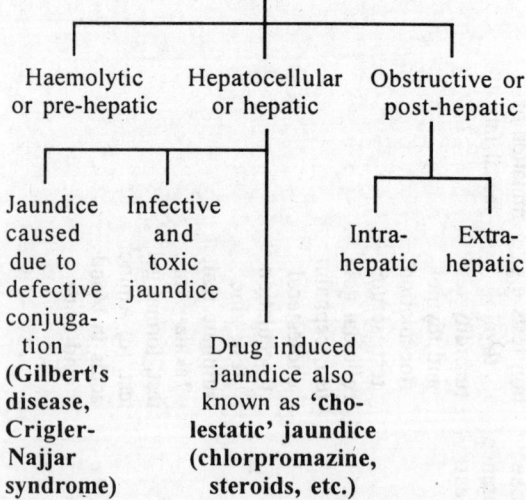

(a) Haemolytic or pre-hepatic jaundice

This type is largely due to increased breakdown of haemoglobin and hence liver cells are unable to conjugate entire increased bilirubin which has formed as a result of the breakdown of haemoglobin. Both intrinsic and extrinsic causes have been attributed.

Intrinsic

Haemoglobinopathies due to abnormalities within the RBCs, hereditary spherocytosis, glucose-6-phosphate dehydrogenase deficiency in red cells and favism (which is caused due to eating of a special type of bean called as fava beans).

Extrinsic

Incompatible blood transfusion, autoimmune hemolytic anaemia, haemolytic disease of the newborn, malaria, and oral administration of drugs such as sulphonamides.

(b) Hepatocellular or hepatic jaundice

This type is largely due to the disease of the parenchymal cells of the liver. This may be divided into three groups though there may be overlapping:

1. Conditions in which there is defective conjugation. There may be a reduction in the number of functioning liver cells as in chronic hepatitis or there may be a specific defect in the conjugation process as happens in **Gilbert's disease** and the **Crigler-Najjar syndrome,** in which liver function is otherwise normal.

2. Conditions such as infective and toxic jaundice in which there is extensive damage of liver cells along with significant intrahepatic obstruction leading to appreciable absorption of conjugated bilirubin.

3. Drug induced jaundice known as "cholestatic" jaundice occurring as a result of ingestion of drugs e.g. chlorpromazine and some steroids causing intrahepatic obstruction.

Table 25.3: Classification, causes and clinical findings of 'Jaundice'

	Hemolytic or prehepatic jaundice	Hepatic or parenchymatous jaundice	Obstructive or post-hepatic jaundice
1. Causes	Due to excessive haemolysis 1. Defects in red blood cells 2. External causes Incompatible blood transfusion/ hemolytic poison/drug reaction	Occlusion of biliary passage (a) Intrahepatic cholestasis (b) Extrahepatic gall stones, tumours, lymphnodes.	1. Parenchymal cell destruction 2. Viral hepatitis/toxic jaundice 3. Cirrhosis of liver-fibrosis
2. Clinical findings			
(a) Extent of jaundice	Low	Very high	Very high
(b) Faecal matter	Dark brown	Clay coloured	Variable pale

Table 25.4: Biochemical findings for differential diagnosis of 'Jaundice'

Parameter	Hemolytic or pre-hepatic	Hepatic	Obstructive or post-hepatic
1. Serum bilirubin	Slightly high < 5 mg/dl	High > 20 mg/dl	Very high >50 mg/dl
2. Van den Bergh reaction	Indirect	Mixed biphasic	Direct
3. Bile pigments in urine			
(a) Bilirubin	Absent	Present	Present
(b) Urobilinogen	High	Normal or high	Decreased/Absent
4. SGPT (ALT)	Normal	Very high	High
5. ALP (alkaline phosphatase)	Normal	High upto 30 KA units	Very high > 35 KA units
6. 5′ Nucleotidase	Normal	Slightly high	Very high
7. Prothrombin time	Normal	Increased	Increased but returns back to normal after vitamin K administration
8. Flocculation test: Thymol turbidity	Negative	Raised	Negative

In this type also, liver functions are otherwise normal.

(c) Obstructive or post-hepatic jaundice (Fig. 25.3)7

This type is mainly due to obstruction in the flow of bile in the extrahepatic ducts. It is found to be associated with patients having gall stones, carcinoma of the head of the pancreas or enlarged lymph glands pressing bile duct. Obstruction may be either intra-hepatic in nature or extra-hepatic.

Rich's classification of jaundice

1. Retention Jaundice

It includes hemolytic jaundice and conditions causing impaired removal of bilirubin from the blood. **In this type, there is an increase in indirect reacting bilirubin.** This is characterised by impaired conjugation of bilirubin.

2. Regurgitation Jaundice

It includes obstructive jaundice and cholestasis. In this type, there is reabsorption of bilirubin into the blood which has been excreted by the liver cells. **In this type, there is an increase in the direct reacting conjugated bilirubin.**

Interpretation

It helps in the assessment of the intensity of jaundice. Serum bilirubin level is found to be much higher in obstructive jaundice as compared to hemolytic jaundice. Quantitative estimation of serum bilirubin is useful in :

1. Sub clinical jaundice: In this type, there are small increases in serum bilirubin ranging between 1.0 and 3.0 mg%.
2. Clinical jaundice: Where it is used to follow the development and course of the jaundice.

BILIRUBIN METABOLISM {Fig 25.2 (a) and (b)}

Differential diagnosis of jaundice is based on **Van den Bergh reaction** which is based on the reaction of bilirubin differently with Diazo reagent e.g. conjugated and unconjugated bilirubin. **Bilirubin derived from haemoglobin which does not pass through liver cells is called unconjugated bilirubin, soluble in methanol and gives indirect reaction.**

Biliverdin, $C_{33}H_{34}O_6N_4$

Bilirubin, $C_{33}H_{36}O_6N_4$

Where : M = $- CH_3$ (methyl group)
P = $- CH_2CH_2COOH$ (propionic acid)
V = $- CH = CH_2$ (vinyl group)
E = $- CH_2CH_3$ (ethyl group)

Table 25.5: Pathophysiologic Classification of Jaundice

1. Predominantly Unconjugated Hyperbilirubinemia

A. Overproduction

* Intravascular hemolysis - hemolytic anemias
* Extravascular hemolysis - resorption of blood from large hematomas, large internal hemorrhages (e.g., gastrointestinal bleeds), hemorrhagic infarcts (e.g., lungs), etc.
* Ineffective erythropoiesis

B. Decreased hepatocellular uptake
* Drugs
* Sepsis
* Markedly reduced caloric intake (near-starvation)

C. Decreased hepatocellular conjugation
(hereditary lack or impaired function of enzyme glucuronyl transferase)

* Gilbert's syndrome
* Crigler-Najjar syndrome
* Neonatal jaundice
* Drug inhibition, e.g., chloramphenicol
* Diffuse hepatocellular diseases e.g., hepatitis, cirrhosis, etc.

2. Predominantly Conjugated Hyperbilirubinemia (Cholestasis)

A. Impaired hepatocellular secretion

(i) "Pure" cholestasis
* **Dubin-Johnson and Rotor syndromes**
* Congenital atesia or strictures in the intrahepatic ducts
* "Early" biliary cirrhosis
* Fibrocystic disease of the pancreas
* Drugs, e.g., oral contraceptives, estrogens, methyl testosterone; Benign familial recurrent cholestasis, and recurrent jaundice of pregnancy

(ii) Hepatocellular cholestasis
* Some cases of viral hepatitis ("cholangiolitic" viral hepatitis)
* Some cases of alcohol-induced fatty liver or hepatitis
* Some forms of chemical or drug-induced injury

B. Extrahepatic obstruction to biliary apparatus
* Obstructive gallstones
* Carcinoma of the head of the pancreas
* Obstructive carcinoma of extrahepatic ducts or papilla of Vater
* Inflammatory stenosis strictures usually related to previous biliary surgery
* Congenital atresia of the extrahepatic ducts

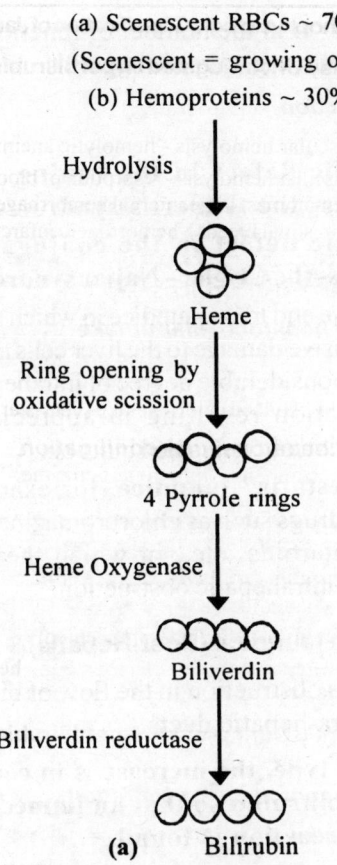

(a) Scenescent RBCs ~ 70%

(Scenescent = growing old)

(b) Hemoproteins ~ 30%

Hydrolysis

Heme

Ring opening by
oxidative scission

4 Pyrrole rings

Heme Oxygenase

Biliverdin

Billverdin reductase

(a) Bilirubin

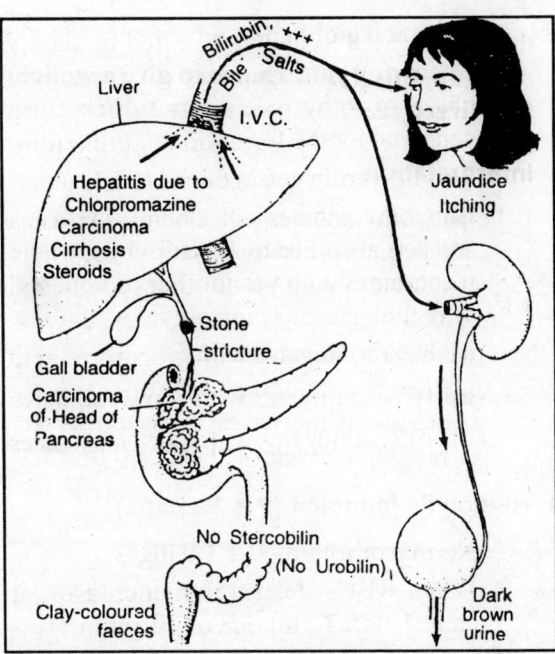

Fig. 25.3 : Main causes and features of obstructive jaundice

Bilirubin {Fig. 25.2 (a) and (b)} is formed from haemoglobin in the RES i.e., reticuloendothelial system (spleen, bone marrow and Kupffer's cells of the liver) and then circulates attached to the plasma albumin, in low concentration in the blood. This bilirubin is insoluble in water but dissolves in chloroform. Recent work has shown that the bilirubin gets conjugated with glucuronic acid in the liver cells and is excreted in the bile mainly as the diglucuronide.

On the other hand, bilirubin passing through liver cells undergoes conjugation and hence termed as conjugated bilirubin. It is water soluble and hence gives direct reaction.

Formation (Biosynthesis) of bilirubin

* When RBCs complete their life span of 120 days, then they get phagocytized in reticuloendothelial system (R.E.S.).

* Haemoglobin is also phagocytized to give

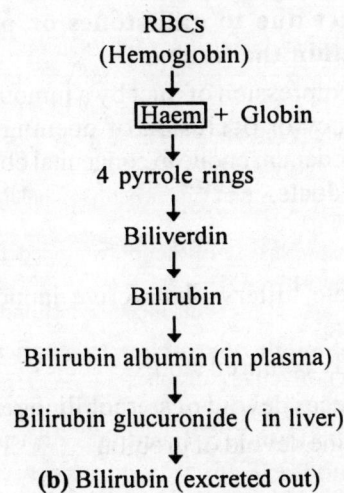

RBCs
(Hemoglobin)

Haem + Globin

4 pyrrole rings

Biliverdin

Bilirubin

Bilirubin albumin (in plasma)

Bilirubin glucuronide (in liver)

(b) Bilirubin (excreted out)

Fig. 25.2 : (a) and (b) Bilirubin metabolism

haem and globin protein.

* Haem ring gets opened to give a straight chain of 4 pyrrole rings which form substrate for the formation of biliverdin.
* This biliverdin gets reduced to bilirubin.
* Bilirubin combines with albumin in plasma and gets absorbed by hepatic cells, where it combines with yet another protein and after that gets conjugated:
    (a) 80% conjugates with glucuronic acid
    (b) 10% conjugates with some sulphates
    (c) 10% conjugates with other substances

1. Hemolytic jaundice (Pre-Hepatic)

* Normal bilirubin - 0.2-1.0 mg%
* When RBCs destruction increases, it causes more formation of bilirubin.
* **A normal liver can excrete 2000 mg to 3000 mg bilirubin during hemolysis and patient may exhibit little icterus (yellow pigmentation) (Hemolytic Jaundice).**

Causes

* Liver cells are unable to conjugate all the increased bilirubin formed.
* Excessive breakdown of red cells may be due to abnormalities within the cells, e.g., hemoglobinopathies, and hereditary spherocytosis or due to the factors external to the cells as happens in the transfusion of incompatible blood and hemolytic disease of the newborn, malaria, drugs such as sulphonamides.
* Other causes are congenital defects and enzyme defects such as glucose-6-phosphate dehydrogenase which is responsible for hemolysis of RBCs.

2. Hepatocellular jaundice (Hepatic)

* It is a disease of the parenchymal cells.
* There is found defective conjugation.

* Reduction in the number of functioning liver cells, e.g. chronic hepatitis.

Causes

1. **Specific defect in the conjugation process- the Gilbert's syndrome.**
2. **Specific defect in the conjugation process- the Crigler - Najjar syndrome.**
3. Infective and toxic jaundice in which there is extensive damage to the liver cells along with a considerable degree of intrahepatic obstruction resulting in appreciable absorption of conjugated bilirubin.
4. **"Cholestatic" jaundice,** for example due to drugs such as chlorpromazine and some steroids, etc., in which there is mainly intrahepatic obstruction.

3. Obstructive jaundice (Post-Hepatic)

* There is obstruction in the flow of bile in the extra-hepatic ducts.
* **In this type, the increase is in conjugated bilirubin so that an immediate direct reaction is found.**

Causes

* **Blockage of hepatic and common bile duct due to gall-stones or parasites within the lumen.**
* Compression of duct by a tumour/ malignancy or occlusion of opening into the duodenum or due to congenital obliteration of ducts.

Findings

In complete biliary obstructive jaundice, the findings are:

* Clay coloured stools
* Faeces devoid of stercobilinogen
* Urine devoid of urobilin

Physiological jaundice

* It develops mostly in full term infants

between 2nd and 7the day of life.

* There is found no evidence of hemolysis in such type of jaundice and the cause has been ascertained which is the deficiency of enzyme glucuronyl transferase.

* In intrauterine life bilirubin formed is eliminated via placenta.

* **Immediately after birth, liver has to eliminate all the bilirubin formed, it is seen that in some cases liver is unable to deal adequately with the task, that is why, during the first 10 days of life, jaundice develops-known as physiological jaundice.** In such cases as soon as the concerned enzyme is adequately synthesised, such type of jaundice disappears.

* **Normal level of serum bilirubin is from 0.2 - 1.0 mg%.**

* Bilirubin is the major end product of hemoglobin breakdown.

* If its concentration reaches 3-4 times of the normal level, the excess amount of it starts diffusing from capillaries as a result of which the skin, conjunctiva, mucous membrane and even the deep tissues assume a pale yellow tint.

* The pigment is not merely dissolved in the tissues but appears to be bound in some way to the tissues. Such kind of yellowness is called "Jaundice" **(Jaune = Yellow).**

* **Jaundice = yellow pigmentation + hyperbilirubinemia of the connective tissue.**

* **Sometimes concentration of bilirubin may rise upto 40 mg/dl, which is a most severe condition.**

Vanden Bergh Reaction

Results of **Van den Bergh direct and indirect reactions** are interpreted as follows:

1. Haemolytic jaundice

It is associated with increase in unconjugated bilirubin, hence indirect reaction is obtained. Only unconjugated bilirubin can cross blood brain barrier.

2. Obstructive jaundice

It is associated with increased conjugated bilirubin giving immediate direct reaction.

3. Hepatocellular jaundice

It gives mixed results. In viral hepatitis, direct reaction is rule.

An immediate direct reaction is also witnessed in cholestatic jaundice. Same results are also obtained irrespective of obstruction being intrahepatic or extrahepatic. Hence, direct Van den Bergh reaction is only of limited value.

(b) Urinary and faecal urobilinogen : Urinary Urobilinogen

Urobilinogen, maximum normal range is upto 4 mg/24 hrs. It is a normal constituent of urine.

1. In complete obstruction, no urobilinogen is found in urine as a rule because bilirubin is unable to get into intestine to form urobilinogen. Hence presence of bilirubin in urine without urobilinogen is strongly suggestive of obstructive jaundice.

2. On the other hand increased urobilinogen in urine and absence of bilirubin are strongly conclusive evidence of hemolytic jaundice.

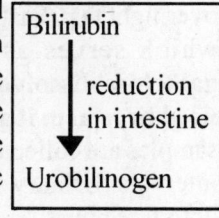

3. Increased urinary urobilinogen is also observed in cirrhosis of liver.

Fecal urobilinogen

1. It is increased, normal range is 50-250 mg per day, in hemolytic jaundice associated with dark coloured fecal matter.

2. Fecal urobilinogen is decreased or absent

in obstructive jaundice or in extreme cases of hepatic parenchymal damage. A complete absence of fecal urobilinogen is strongly conclusive evidence for malignant obstruction.

2. Tests based on the role of liver in carbohydrate metabolism

Several tests of liver (hepatic) function based upon the role played by the liver in carbohydrate metabolism have been used. When the liver cells are damaged, a decreased rate of glycogen formation is there as a result of which more of the sugar absorbed from the alimentary tract into the portal circulation passes into the peripheral circulation. To test this function of the liver, monosaccharides have been mainly employed.

Glucose tolerance test is not, however, of much diagnostic value in liver diseases. Normal liver is able to convert galactose and fructose into glucose. This function is, however, impaired in liver dysfunction and hence used for the assessment of liver function.

Oral galactose tolerance test

Procedure

The test is performed in the morning after overnight fast. Fasting blood sample is collected which serves as a control. **40 grams of galactose dissolved in a cup full of water (if need be, warm it a little) is given orally.** Blood samples are collected for two hours at 1/2 hourly intervals. Urinary specimens are also collected upto five hours.

Interpretation

1. In normal persons or in patients suffering from obstructive jaundice, blood galactose level returns back to normal within one hour with the excretion of upto 3 gm of galactose in urine between 3-5 hours.

2. Intra-hepatic (Parenchymatous) jaundice is associated with excretion of more galactose (4-5 gms) during the first five hours.

Galactose index

It is obtained by adding the four blood galactose values.

Interpretation

1. Upper normal limit is taken as 160
2. In liver diseases, very high values are obtained

Intravenous (I. V.) galactose tolerance test

procedure

Same as oral test except that I.V. injection of galactose equivalent to 0.5 gm/kg body weight is given as sterile 50% solution. Blood galactose is estimated after 5 minutes, half, one, one and a half and two hours.

Interpretation

1. In normal persons, curve begins with average value of 200 mg galactose/dl, falling-steeply during the first hour and reaching a figure between 0 and 10 mg% by the end of two hours.

2. In obstructive jaundice, the pattern is similar as witnessed in normal persons, there being little or no galactose in the blood at the end of the two hours.

3. In persons with liver cell damage, the fall in blood galactose is much slower.

Though this intravenous test avoids errors due to impaired absorption of galactose from the intestine but the oral galactose tolerance test is the method of choice because of its simplicity. It is even more useful than the fructose tolerance test because of the fact of very slow absorption of fructose from the intestine if compared to galactose.

Fructose tolerance test

50 gms of fructose is given to the fasting subject as for glucose tolerance test (GTT).Fasting blood sample and other blood samples are collected at 12 hour intervals upto 2½ hours after taking fructose. Useful methods for the estimation of blood sugar measure both glucose and fructose present.

Interpretation

In the normal person, one finds little or no rise in the blood sugar level in column I of the following table. The highest blood sugar reached during the test should not exceed the fasting level by more than 30 mg per 100 ml. The rise in blood sugar is greater than this when there is **liver cell damage** but the increases met with are never great. In column II of the table there is shown an abnormal response from a case of **infective hepatitis.**

3. Tests based on the changes in plasma proteins

These tests reveal useful information in chronic liver diseases because liver is the main site of albumin and fibrinogen synthesis and possibly of some of the α and β-globulins also. Determination

Sample No.	I (Normal person)	II (Case of infective hepatitis)
1. Fasting blood sugar	95 mg%	85 mg%
2. Blood sugar ½ hour after 50 g. fructose	100 mg%	130 mg%
3. Blood sugar 1 hour after 50 g fructose	105 mg%	145 mg%
4. Blood sugar 1½ hours after 50 g fructose	100 mg%	150 mg%
5. Blood sugar 2 hours after 50 g fructose	95 mg%	135 mg%
6. Blood sugar 2½ hours after 50 g fructose	90 mg%	120 mg%

of A/G ratio provides much significant information.

Interpretation

1. Infective hepatitis

Quantitative estimation of albumin and globulin may give normal results in the early stages and sometimes a small increase in γ-globulin develops so that for a short time, the albumin globulin ratio may fall below one.

2. Obstructive jaundice

It also reveals normal levels of albumin and globulins in blood unless there is considerable liver cell damage.

3. Parenchymal liver disease

In advanced liver diseases, albumin gets decreased and the globulin often increased, therefore, the albumin - globulin ratio may be reversed. The albumin may fall below 2.5 per cent and is a contributory factor in causing edema present in such cases. The globulin, on the other hand, may be found to be increased so much so that it may even sometimes exceed 7 per cent, a finding which is said to indicate a bad prognosis. Fractionation of the globulins reveals that the increase is usually in the γ-globulin fraction, but in some cases, there is also found a smaller increase in β-globulins.

4. Fibrinogen

It is normal (200 to 400 mg per cent) unless considerable liver damage has taken place. Then values below 100 mg per 100 ml have been reported. These are found in severe acute liver insufficiency for e.g. acute hepatic necrosis, poisoning by carbontetrachloride, advanced stages of liver cirrhosis, etc.

Flocculation tests

These tests are independent on alteration in the type of proteins present in plasma. These changes may be both quantitative as well as qualitative.

(a) Thymol turbidity

The degree of turbidity produced when serum. is treated with a buffered solution of thymol is measured; it is compared with a set of protein standards containing 10, 20, 30, 40, 50, 60, 70, 80, 90 and 100 mg per 100 ml. A greater turbidity is given at lower temperatures (optimum temperature being 25°C).

Interpretation

Normal range is 0-4 units (each unit corresponds to 10 mg/100 ml protein standard). **It is found to be highest in infective hepatitis.**

(b) Thymol flocculation

It was observed that when the thymol turbidity test was allowed to stand overnight, flocculation sometimes occurred. This was made the basis of a thymol flocculation test. After the turbidity has been measured, leave the tube to stand in the dark overnight (that is for 18 hours) and then read the degree of flocculation which may be graded: negative (no flocculation); 1+, 2+, 3+, and 4+.

The flocculation test proves to be positive in some cases in which the turbidity test is found to be negative. It has been claimed that the sensitivity of the thymol turbidity test gets increased by this additional 'flocculation' observation.

Other turbidity and flocculation tests e.g. **cephalin cholesterol flocculation test, Takata-Ara test, Jirgl's flocculation test, formal gel test have become obsolete in reference to liver diseases.**

(c) The serum colloidal gold test

Results obtained in liver diseases by this method are almost the same as given by thymol turbidity test. Scientist Maclagan (1944) obtained 92 percent positive tests in infective hepatitis; 47 percent in post-arsphenamine jaundice; 87 percent in hepatic cirrhosis, but only 8 percent in obstructive jaundice.

(d) Cephalin cholesterol flocculation test

This test also gives almost similar results as obtained by the thymol turbidity test. It is positive in the early stages of infective hepatitis before the jaundice develops.

(e) Zinc sulphate test

In this test, serum is mixed with a buffered zinc sulphate solution and the turbidity produced is read in the same way as in case of thymol turbidity test. This test gives an index of the amount of γ-globulin present. The test is best done using fresh serum and more consistent results are obtained if the same temperature i.e., 25°C is used.

Interpretation

The normal range lies between 2 to 8 units with results upto 80 units in disease. It gives a positive test in cases of cirrhosis of the liver.

(f) Formal gel test

This is another test for detecting increase in globulin.

In this test formalin is used. When positive, the serum solidifies within a few minutes, sometimes becoming opaque. A positive test is mainly found in conditions in which there is increased serum globulin. **Although this is found to be positive in chronic liver diseases, it has been mainly used in other conditions, such as kala-azar, whilst positive findings have been reported in a number of diseases such as multiple myeloma, sarcoidosis, severe malarial infections, trypanosomiasis, and in many other chronic infections.**

Summary

Flocculation tests have aroused considerable interest in recent years. In liver diseases and particularly in acute hepatitis, cephalin cholesterol, colloidal gold and thymol turbidity tests are most useful. The tests are found to be positive in about 90 percent cases of infective hepatitis and cirrhosis. In obstructive jaundice, thymol and colloidal gold tests give more consistently negative results than the cephalic test. The cephalic cholesterol test has the advantage of being positive earlier in infective hepatitis, whilst the thymol turbidity remains positive longer.

If only one test is used, the thymol turbidity test is the best, since the thymol buffer is readily reproducible and the test is most easily read. Some workers have preferred to use two and select the thymol turbidity test and the colloidal gold test.

In interpreting these tests, it should be borne in mind that all tests give positive results in a number of diseases other than those involving the liver, and some, for example the formal gel test, have been mainly used in such conditions. Positive results in non-hepatic diseases are less frequent in the colloidal gold, cephalic cholesterol and thymol turbidity tests.

Scientists **Carter** and **Maclagan**, using the thymol turbidity test have reported 80 per cent positive results in malaria, 38 percent in rheumatoid arthritis, 36 percent in heart failure, 58 percent in glandular fever and 86 percent in subacute bacterial endocarditis.

4. Tests based on the abnormalities of Lipids (Lipid Metabolism Disturbances)

Liver is an important site for cholesterol biosynthesis, its esterification, oxidation and excretion. Normal total cholesterol level ranges between 150-200 mg% of which approximately 70-75% remains in esterified form. There occurs almost a little change in the ratio of free and esterified cholesterol in the cases of obstructive jaundice which is associated with elevation of both the fractions. The degree of reduction in both these fractions roughly parallels the degree of liver damage in parenchymatous liver diseases. In liver diseases, the percentage of ester cholesterol decreases for e.g. in infective hepatitis during the earlier phases whilst the jaundice is developing, the tendency is that the total cholesterol either remains normal or falls a little whereas the ratio of ester cholesterol falls appreciably low. In severe acute hepatic necrosis, the total serum cholesterol is usually low and may fall below 100 mg per 100 ml, whereas there is a marked reduction in the percentage of esterified cholesterol fraction. **In xanthomatous biliary cirrhosis the increase is almost entirely in the free cholesterol fraction.**

Tests based on the abnormalities of lipids are the following:

(a) determination of serum cholesterol and of the proportion of free and ester cholesterol.

(b) determination of faecal fats.

5. Tests based on the Detoxicating Function of the Liver

Hippuric Acid synthesis test of **'Quick'** is the best known test for the assessment of detoxicating function of the liver.

Liver is responsible for the removal of benzoic acid, by combining it with glycine to form hippuric acid which is excreted via urine.

Test

Dissolve 6.0 gms of sodium benzoate in about 200 ml of water and give it orally or 1.77 gms of sodium benzoate dissolved in 20 ml of distilled water is given intravenously.

Oral test is preferred unless there is possibility of impaired absorption of the benzoate or nausea. For reliable results renal functions should be normal. Oral test starts after 3 hours of light breakfast. Food should not be given until the test is over. Urine sample immediately before ingestion of sodium benzoate is discarded. Urine samples at 4 hours after the ingestion and in between are collected and pooled. Hippuric acid is estimated in pooled sample. Normal response includes excretion of at least 3.0 gms of hippuric acid expressed as benzoic acid or 3.5 gms of sodium benzoate. Both acute or chronic liver damage result in lesser excretion. In infective hepatitis, patients excrete less than 1.0 gm.

6. Tests based on the excretion of injected substances by the Liver

Bromsulphthalein (BSP) test

The ability of the liver to excrete certain dyes is utilised for this test. Fasting patient is given 5 mg BSP/kg body weight as 5% BSP solution intravenously. Blood is withdrawn at the end of 25 and 45 minutes after the injection and then allowed the specimens to clot. Quantity of dye is estimated in each sample. In normal healthy individuals not more than 5% of the dye should be retained in the blood at the end of 45 minutes. Bulk of the dye should be removed in 25 minutes with only 15% remaining at the end of 25 minutes. Removal proceeds more slowly, if liver functioning is impaired. Approximately 50% of the dye is¹retained after **45 minutes in advanced cases of liver cirrhosis. This test is contra-indicated in obstructive jaundice.** This test is mostly useful in liver cell damage without jaundice, in cirrhosis and chronic hepatitis. In these conditions, it may be the most sensitive of the liver function tests. Rose Bengal dye can also be used alternatively. p31 labelled Rose Bengal dye has been used where isotope laboratory is available. After the administration of this isotope intravenously, count is taken over the neck and abdomen. As the dye is excreted through liver, in normal persons, neck count goes

down and abdomen count increases. Due to retention of dye in parenchymal liver diseases, neck count is always higher with hardly any rise in abdomen count.

7. Tests based on the determination of the activity of liver enzymes

(a) SGOT (AST) and SGPT (ALT)

Increases in both transaminases are found in liver diseases. Determination of the activities of these enzymes are although of limited value in differential diagnosis of jaundice but of extreme use in assessment of severity and prognosis of parenchymal liver diseases specially acute infective and serum hepatitis. Normal ranges for these enzymes are as follows:

SGOT (AST) - 4-17 IU/L or 8-40 units/ml

SGPT (ALT) - 3-15 IU/L or 5-35 units/ml

In liver diseases the ratio of ALT/ AST is always more than unity. Both enzymes increase to much lesser extent in obstructive jaundice. Very high enzyme activities are obtained in toxic hepatitis due to carbon tetrachloride poisoning but the elevation is much less in **drug (chlorpromazine) induced hepatitis.**

(b) Serum alkaline phosphatase

It is widely distributed but most plentiful in bone and liver. Normal range is 3-13 King Armstrong units/100 ml. It gets increased in both i.e. infective hepatitis and post hepatic jaundice. However, the rise is usually much greater in cases of obstructive jaundice than in jaundice due to hepatitis. Using King-Armstrong units, the dividing line which has been suggested is 35 KA units/100 ml. **A value higher than this suggests obstructive jaundice, in which very high figures upto 200 units and over may be encountered.** On the other hands, results below 35 units suggest conditions such as infective hepatitis. Sometimes, then there is observed overlapping, mostly in the range of 30-45 units per 100 ml. Serum alkaline phosphatase is found within its normal range in the cases of haemolytic jaundice.

Quite a large number of enzyme estimations for example isocitrate dehydrogenase, 5 '-nucleotidase, pseudo-cholinesterase, etc are of diagnostic value in liver cell damage but the above three have been most commonly and routinely employed in laboratories.

8. Determination of prothrombin time

Prothrombin is formed from inactive preprothrombin in liver cells; vitamin K being required for this formation. Prothrombin activity is assessed as 'Pro-thrombin Time' (PT) which has been defined as the time required for clotting to take place in citrated plasma to which optimum amounts of thromboplastin and Ca^{++} have been added. Normal range has been reported between 10-16 seconds with an average of 14 seconds. Results are always expressed as prothrombin time of patients (in seconds) to normal control value.

Interpretation

Although determination of prothrombin time is mostly used in controlling anticoagulant therapy, it has also been used n liver diseases and jaundice. Determination of prothrombin time is also used to decide whether there is danger of bleeding during operation in biliary tract diseases or not.

9. Determination of ammonia

Ammonia is mostly formed in the body from nitrogenous material by the bacterial action in the intestine, and is also produced in the kidneys in which an enzyme **glutaminase** can split glutamine to give ammonia and glutamic acid and in the muscles from adenine. Metabolism of ammonia takes place mainly in the liver where it is converted to urea. In liver diseases, the ability to remove ammonia coming to it from the intestine may be impaired. Considerable increase in the level of ammonia may be found for instance over 250 µg per 100 ml in cases of advanced cirrhosis and hepatic coma. Normal range is 40-75 µg ammonia nitrogen per 100 ml blood.

An ammonia tolerance test has been used to test the ability of the liver to deal with ammonia coming to it from the intestine.

10. Determination of glutamine in C.S.F. (Indirect method of liver function test)

Normal range of glutamine in cerebrospinal fluid varies between 6 to 14 mg per 100 ml. It is found to be raised both in cases of cirrhosis of liver and hepatic coma. Prognosis is usually fatal if level increases beyond 40 mg/dl.

Conclusion

To apply simultaneously the entire group of tests described above would seldom be justified. Selection of tests relating to cause can, however, be made on the following outlines.

1. Detection of liver damage in the absence of jaundice e.g. early or subclinical hepatitis

B.S.P. retention, direct and indirect bilirubin, SGOT and urine urobilinogen.

2. Detection of residual liver damage e.g. chronic hepatitis, recovery stages of hepatitis

B.S.P. retention, total proteins, A/G ratio, direct and indirect bilirubin, prothrombin time, SGOT and urine urobilinogen.

3. Detection of jaundiced patient with parenchymatous disease

Direct and total serum bilirubin, SGOT, SGPT, serum proteins, A/G ratio, and prothrombin time.

4. Differentiation of hemolytic jaundice

Direct and indirect serum bilirubin, erythrocyte fragility and reticulocyte count.

5. Differentiation of parenchymatous disease from biliary disease

Serum alkaline phosphatase, SGOT, galactose tolerance test, and prothrombin time.

6. Differentiation of extrahepatic biliary obstruction due to gall stone from neoplasm, stricture etc.

Faecal urobilinogen.

7. Following course of biliary tract surgery

Prothrombin time, serum alkaline phosphatase, SGOT, direct and total bilirubin, electrolytes, creatinine, blood NPN, and serum lipids.

Functions of the liver

The liver performs many vital functions. It stores chemicals and carries out many different chemical processes. **It is the site of metabolism of all the substances/compounds.**

* Makes bile for digesting food
* Breaks down fats and amino acids
* Helps maintain blood sugar level
* Store fat- soluble vitamins and some minerals

* Makes proteins
* Helps clot blood
* Controls blood cells formation and their destruction.
* Filters poisonous chemicals from the blood and breaks them down

---

Liver

The liver in a normal, 70-kg human adult weighs approximately 1.5 kg, or about 2% of body weight. Its major cell type, the hepatocyte, is of epithelial origin. Interposed between the intestinal tract and the general circulation, the **liver is uniquely related to the endocrine pancreas which plays a prominent role in metabolic homeostasis.** The liver receives a large volume of blood from the intestinal tract via the portal vein and a small volume of blood via the hepatic artery, and it drains via the hepatic veins into the inferior vena cava. **It is the first organ to meet nutrients delivered from the intestine, with the exception of lipid, and to meet the secreted insulin and glucagon. By delivering bile (which contains bile acids and cholesterol) into the intestine, the liver predominates in cholesterol homeostasis.** It has the greatest metabolic flexibility of any organ and shows tremendous adaptability to fluxes of metabolites and nutrients. It rapidly undergoes changes in size and glycogen and protein content. In the fed state, 5-10% of its wet weight consists of glycogen but after a 24-hours fast the glycogen disappears almost entirely. **After a day or two on a high-protein diet, the liver shows a large increase in activity of enzymes involved in amino acid metabolism and in gluconeogenesis.** A high-carbohydrate diet produces the opposite effect. The liver is the primary site of glycogen deposition and blood glucose maintenance. It also plays a central role in lipid, protein, and nitrogen homeostasis. **In the typical adult, the liver exports daily 180 g of glucose, 100 g of triacylglycerol, and 14 g of albumin. Its metabolic energy is derived primarily from fatty acid oxidation.**

RENAL (KIDNEY) FUNCTION TESTS

The kidneys, each of which weighs **between 120 and 170 g,** lie behind the peritoneum on either side of the vertebral column extending from the 12th thoracic to the 3rd lumbar vertebrae. Their position in relation to the vertebral column, however, varies with the posture and respiration. In healthy persons, **the kidneys measure from 11 to 13 cm in length, the left being larger.** Their shape is just like that of a seed of a bean and these are two in number and **their main function is excretory,** that is to say that these are **excretory organs.** One can visualise the role of a scavenger/sweeper who if, somehow one day does not turn up, then the wastage/ garbage/ dust pile up. In the same way, if these organs stop their functioning partially or fully then the wastage piles up in blood hampering various normal biochemical functions of the body; meaning to say that the **'biochemistry'** of the body gets disturbed. Therefore, in order to know whether these excretory organs i.e., kidneys are working properly or not, there are certain tests to evaluate their functioning as given in Table 25.6. **Out of these tests, determination of urea and creatinine in blood are of paramount importance while the rest are routinely not used and of less importance at a glance (Table 25.6).**

RENAL FAILURE

Acute renal failure may be caused by rapidly progressive irreversible disease processes but more commonly it is the result of some acute disturbance to renal blood flow (as in shock) and from this the patient may recover. The production of urine falls below 400 ml per day **(oliguria)** and the quality of the urine is also impaired. The urine volume may be as low as 20 to 30 ml per day and rarely, there may be no urine at all **(anuria). The concentration of nitrogenous products such as urea and creatinine in the blood rapidly increases, the plasma potassium rises and acidaemia develops. Death is likely to occur in a week or two if** these biochemical abnormalities are not corrected.

Chronic renal failure develops more gradually over a number of months or years as a result of progressive destruction of nephrons. Here again acidaemia and a gradually increasing blood urea and creatinine are the result. The increase in blood urea and of other nitrogeneous substance in the blood is proportional to the loss of nephrons, usually, measured in terms of creatinine clearance but it should be appreciated that the kidney has a very considerable reserve of function and the blood urea, for example, seldom shows any increase until the creatinine clearance is less than half the normal value. Thereafter the rise is progressively steeper but life is still possible even with a creatinine clearance as low as 2 ml per minute. Once the creatinine clearance has fallen significantly, the surviving nephrons subjected to a greater load of material to be excreted (filtered load), are in a state of persistent **osmotic diuresis** so that the patient passes relatively large amounts of dilute urine **(polyuria).** The fractional excretion of electrolytes as well as of water is increased and at a GFR of 3.0 ml per minute, some 80 percent of the fluid filtered and 50 to 60 percent of the filtered load of sodium and chloride may be excreted. Finally, of course, as the number of functioning nephrons falls still further, the volume of urine falls and death occurs from **'uraemia'. The main features of uraemia are nausea and vomiting, pigmentation of the skin (urochrome), drowsiness, stupor (unconciousness) and coma.**

Patients with severe renal failure may now be treated by dialysis, a procedure which seeks to replace temporarily some of the functions of the patients' kidneys. This may be done outside the body by connecting one of the patients' arteries to a cellophane tube lying in a bath of dialysing solution, isotonic with blood, containing physiological concentrations of electrolytes but no urea or other nitrogenous substance.

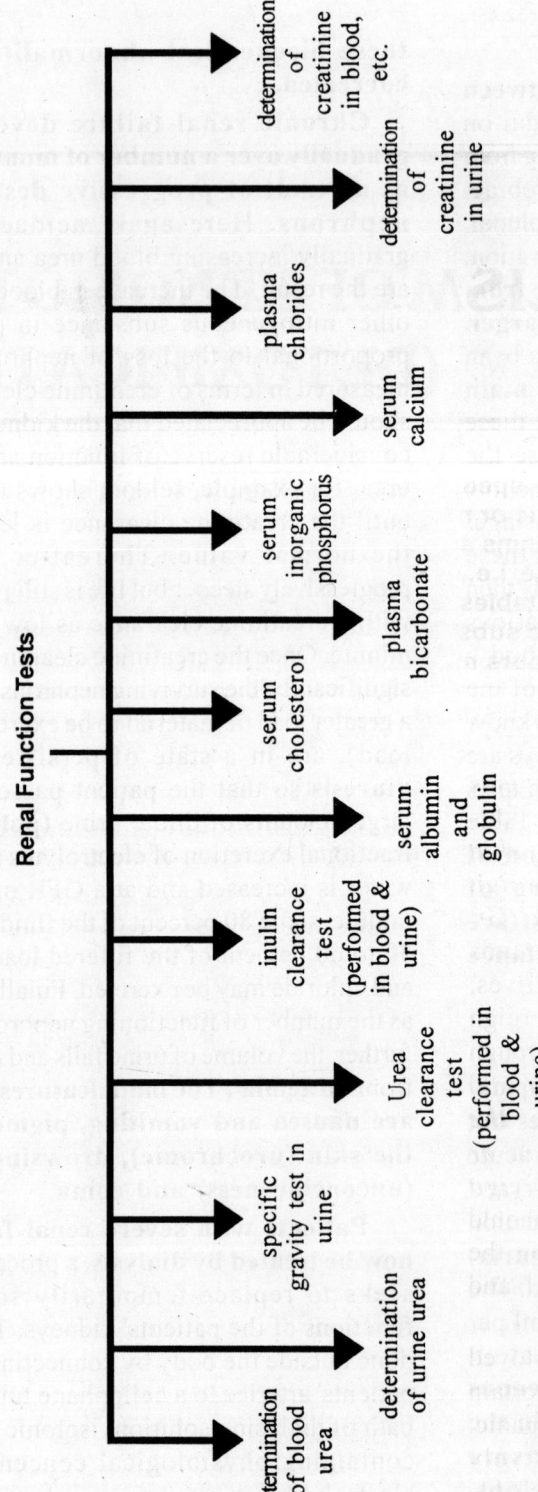

Renal Function Tests

- determination of blood urea
- determination of urine urea
- specific gravity test in urine
- Urea clearance test (performed in blood & urine)
- inulin clearance test (performed in blood & urine)
- serum albumin and globulin
- serum cholesterol
- plasma bicarbonate
- serum inorganic phosphorus
- serum calcium
- plasma chlorides
- determination of creatinine in urine
- determination of creatinine in blood, etc.

Table 25.6 : To show various tests for knowing the functioning of kidneys

CHAPTER 26

METABOLISM OF XENOBIOTICS (DETOXIFICATION)

Ours mechanisms have got a special favour for the body as they convert toxic substances into less toxic or non - harmful substances and ultimately eliminate them. Ours mechanisms are so strong that they can even convert the most dreadful substance i.e., potassium cyanide (if consumed in micrograms or via natural eatables as it remains present in them in very minute quantity) to a less toxic substance. Now, you can very well imagine, how much well - wishers are ours mechanisms to the human body.

INTRODUCTION

Certain unwanted and harmful chemical agents may enter the human body through various routes such as *inhalation, ingestion,. skin contact* and *injections,* etc. These foreign compounds are known as *Xenobiotics (Gr. Xenos=Strange).* These foreign compounds may be in the form of food, drugs, additives, preservatives or pollutants etc. Besides, foreign molecules are also produced in intestine through bacterial enzymatic actions upon normal digestion products. *The metabolism of the Xenobiotics is known as 'detoxication or detoxification or the metabolism of foreign compounds'.* It is an important aspect and should be studied properly before understanding the pharmacology, toxicology, cancer research and drug addiction.

The term **'detoxication'** has been employed to denote biochemical transformation of certain foreign compounds, both organic and inorganic, which makes these compounds relatively harmless to animals by making them more soluble

(so, more readily they are excreted).

Site and importance

Most of the detoxication reactions take place in the liver, but kidney and other tissues may also contribute. Toxic substances should be removed immediately from the body otherwise, they may cause certain undesired and harmful effects and sometimes they may even be fatal. Occasionally a xenobiotic may be excreted unchanged. A potentially toxic xenobiotic in free form may combine with DNA and RNA or cell protein to cause serious damage to the cell.

Mechanism of detoxication

After entering the blood stream through various routes, foreign chemicals may either:

(i) bind to plasma protein (partial or complete)

(ii) pass into ECF, CSF

(iii) permeate into tissue cell or

(iv) be excreted through kidney, bile, feces and milk etc. Inside the cell, metabolism of these foreign chemicals takes place. In most of the cases metabolism of foreign compounds takes place in two stages:

Liver is the main site for the detoxication. Compounds that are produced within the body, such as ammonia, as well as compounds that enter the body from outside, such as alcohol, drugs, and other substances, are detoxified.

By this process, such harmful substances become more *water soluble,* as a result of which they are in a position to be excreted promptly by the kidneys.

The cells in which detoxication takes place are the hepatocytes; a large number of detoxifying enzymes are located on the endoplasmic reticulum. The reactions are oxidation (largely hydroxylation), reduction (via NADPH), hydrolysis, and conjugation (including methylation).

— *Preliminary stage or initial alteration:* In preliminary stage, either of these three reactions takes place- **(i) Oxidation (ii) Reduction (iii) Hydrolysis. Out of these three, oxidation is the main reaction.**

— *Final alteration : Products* which are formed by preliminary changes are, in all cases, ready for excretion but in most instances further alterations are required. These changes are classed as conjugation or synthesis reactions.

The overall purpose of the two stages (or phases) of metabolism of xenobiotics is to increase their solubility and thus, to facilitate their excretion. A brief description of the above mentioned changes is as follows:

Detoxication by Oxidation

Oxidation is the most general reaction in the biochemical disposal of normal or foreign compounds by the body. Reactions of this type include hydroxylation of ring systems, oxidation of alcohol and aldehydes to acids, oxidation of sulfur compounds to sulfoxides and sulfones, oxidative splitting of rings, oxidative dealkylation and deamination and the oxidation of alkyl groups and side chains to alcohols and acids. Oxidative reactions are mostly carried out by a group of *"mixed-function oxidases"* in the liver which in the final step involve a cytochrome P-450 haemoprotein, NADPH and O_2

(i) *Aromatic hydrocarbons-These* on oxidation are converted into phenol e.g.

$C_6H_6 \longrightarrow C_6H_5OH \longrightarrow$ Conjugation later on
Benzene   Phenol

(ii) *Alcohols and aldehydes* -These are converted into acids.

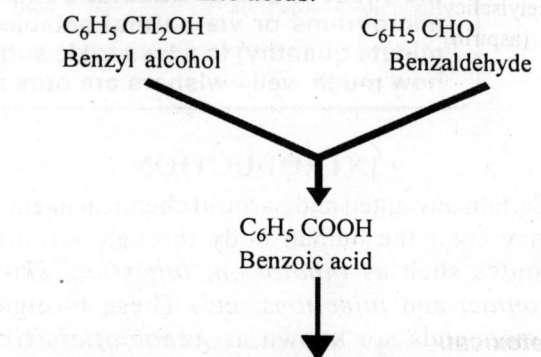

$C_6H_5 CH_2OH$ $C_6H_5 CHO$
Benzyl alcohol   Benzaldehyde

$C_6H_5 COOH$
Benzoic acid

Conjugation later on

(iii) *Amines-Many* primary aliphatic amines undergo oxidation to the corresponding acids as a result of which nitrogen is converted to urea according to the general reaction-

$R - CH_2NH_2 \longrightarrow R - COOH + NH_2CONH_2$
$C_6H_5CH_2NH_2 \longrightarrow C_6H_5COOH \longrightarrow$ Conjugation
benzylamine   benzoic acid   later on

(iv) *Drugs-Meprobamate* (tranquilizer drug used for the control of anxiety, tension and muscle spasm) is hydroxylated during its metabolism.

           Hydroxylation
Meprobamate $\longrightarrow$ Hydroxymeprobamate

Detoxication by Reduction

In human beings this mechanism is less common than the oxidation. Many nitrocompounds are reduced in the body to amino compounds e.g.,

Picric acid $\longrightarrow$ Picramic acid

p-Nitrobenzene $\longrightarrow$ p-Nitrophenol

Dibenzyldisulfides $\longrightarrow$ Sulphhydryl derivatives (2-benzylthiol)

Detoxication by Hydrolysis

The hydrolytic cleavage of ester, amide, glucoside and other linkages causes molecular alteration of foreign molecules, e.g.

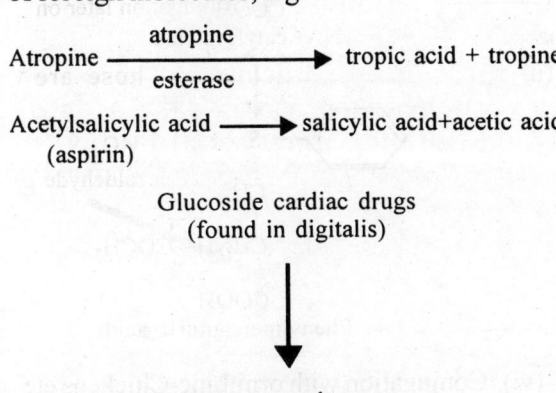

Atropine $\xrightarrow[\text{esterase}]{\text{atropine}}$ tropic acid + tropine

Acetylsalicylic acid $\longrightarrow$ salicylic acid+acetic acid
(aspirin)

Glucoside cardiac drugs
(found in digitalis)

$\downarrow$

sugars + aglucone

Detoxication by Conjugation or Synthesis

As already mentioned, conjugation reactions follow oxidation, reduction or hydrolysis which cause foreign compounds to become more soluble as a result of which they are more readily excretable. Many conjugating agents are known, most of these are derived from carbohydrate and amino acid metabolisms e.g., glucuronic acid, glycine, sulfuric acid, acetic acid, glutamine, ornithine, cysteine and the methyl group. Most of the conjugation reactions take place in the liver but kidney and other tissues may also participate.

(i) *Conjugation with glucuronic acid-This* is the most common type of conjugation reaction which is carried out by *glucuronyl transferase enzyme.* In this reaction formation of an ester or an ether type of linkage with glucuronic acid with a carboxyl or a hydroxyl group of the foreign compound takes place. Various substances like phenol, benzoic acid, chloramphenicol, bilirubin, etc. are excreted as glucuronides, e.g.,

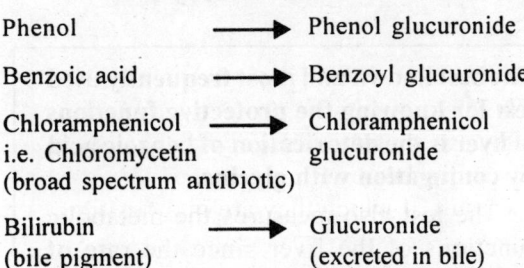

Phenol $\longrightarrow$ Phenol glucuronide

Benzoic acid $\longrightarrow$ Benzoyl glucuronide

Chloramphenicol $\longrightarrow$ Chloramphenicol
i.e. Chloromycetin   glucuronide
(broad spectrum antibiotic)

Bilirubin $\longrightarrow$ Glucuronide
(bile pigment)   (excreted in bile)

(ii) *Conjugation with glycine-Glycine,* the simplest amino acid, also acts as a conjugating agent for the removal of toxic metabolites or foreign chemicals. Benzoic acid may again be detoxified by conjugation with glycine and as a result of which hippuric acid is formed, which is excreted in the urine. In this reaction benzoic acid is first activated by conversion to benzoyl CoA

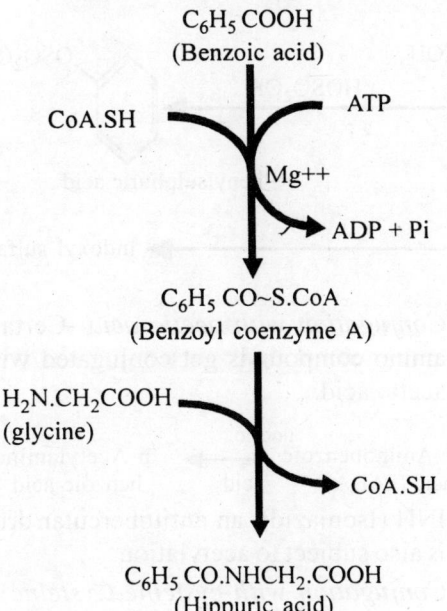

$C_6H_5\,COOH$
(Benzoic acid)

CoA.SH $\qquad$ ATP

Mg^{++}

ADP + Pi

$C_6H_5\,CO{\sim}S.CoA$
(Benzoyl coenzyme A)

$H_2N.CH_2COOH$
(glycine)

CoA.SH

$C_6H_5\,CO.NHCH_2.COOH$
(Hippuric acid)

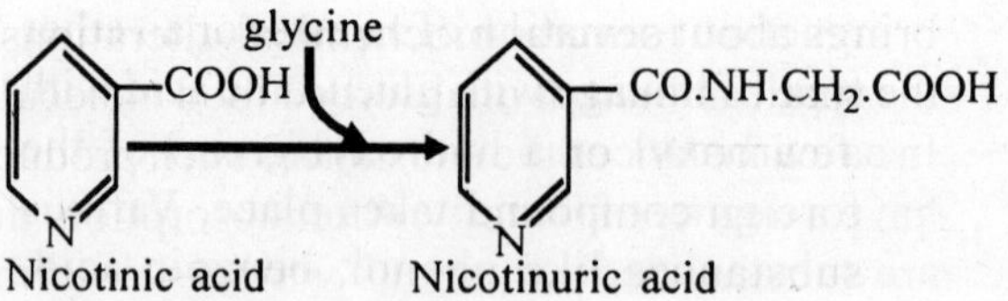

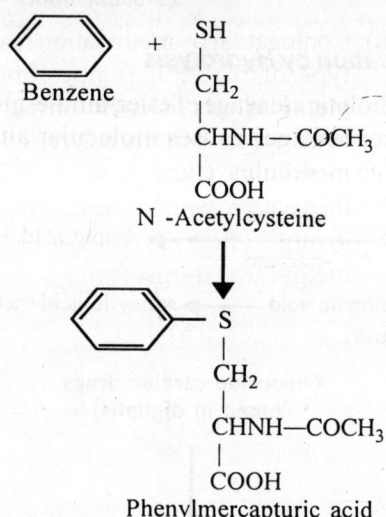

glycine

Nicotinic acid → Nicotinuric acid

Salicylic acid ──────────→ Salicyluric acid

> **The best known and most frequently used test for knowing the protective functions of liver is the detoxication of benzoic acid by conjugation with glycine.**
>
> The test also measures the metabolic functions of the liver since the rate of formation of hippuric acid also depends upon the concentration and the amount of glycine available.

(iii) *Conjugation with sulfuric* acid-Sulfuric acid is used by the body for detoxication of various compounds with phenolic hydroxyl groups. Sulfate donors are glycolipids, glycoproteins, glycoaminoglycans, etc.

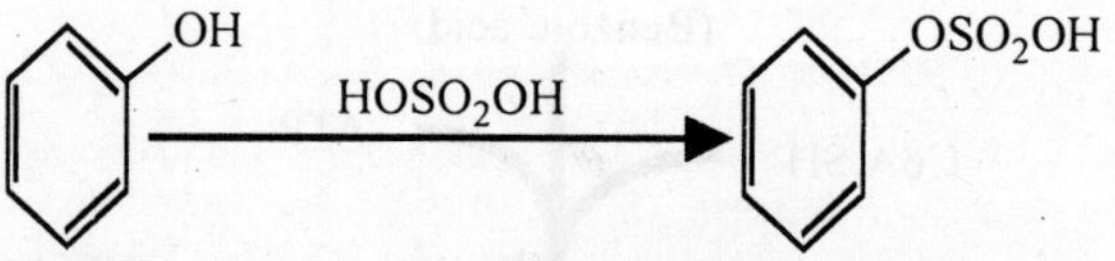

Phenol

$HOSO_2OH$

Phenylsulphuric acid

Indole ──────────→ Indoxyl sulfate

(iv) *Conjugation with acetic acid* -Certain amino compounds get conjugated with acetic acid.

p-Aminobenzoic acid (PABA) ──acetic acid──→ p-Acetylamino-benzoic acid

INH (Isoniazid), an antitubercular drug is also subject to acetylation.

(v) *Conjugation with cysteine-Cysteine* is

also involved in the detoxication of aromatic compounds such as benzene.Cysteine is first acetylated to form N-acetyl cysteine which then reacts with benzene to give phenylmercapturic acid which is excreted in urine. Similar reactions are used for the disposal of other aromatic compounds.

Benzene +

SH
|
CH_2
|
$CHNH—COCH_3$
|
COOH
N -Acetylcysteine

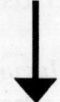

S
|
CH_2
|
$CHNH—COCH_3$
|
COOH
Phenylmercapturic acid

(vi) Conjugation with ornithine-Chickens etc. detoxify phenylacetic acid by conjugation with ornithine.

Penylacetic acid

↓

Diphenylacetylornithine

(vii) Conjugation with glutamine—phenylacetic acid is conjugated with glutamine.

Phenylacetic acid + glutamine

↓

Phenylacetyl glutamine

Detoxication of phenylacetic acid is an interesting example of species difference in detoxication mechanisms. In human body, it is detoxified by conjugation with glutamine; in chickens by conjugation with ornithine and in dogs or some other species by conjugation with glycine.

(viii) Conjugation by methylation reaction -This type of reaction is not common. The methyl donor is methionine; an amino acid, which is firstly converted into active methionine (S-adenosyl methionine) and then active methionine donates its methyl group. The reaction is catalysed by methyl transferase, e.g.,

Pyridine

$+CH_3$

N-Methylpyridinium hydroxide

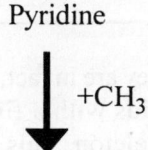

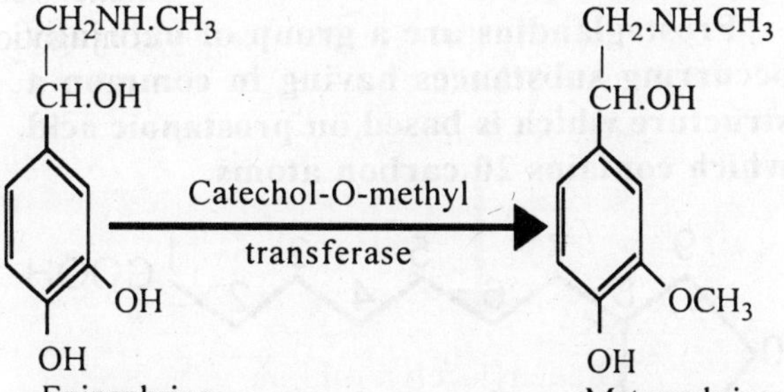

CH$_2$NH.CH$_3$		CH$_2$.NH.CH$_3$
CH.OH	Catechol-O-methyl transferase →	CH.OH

OH
OH
Epinephrine

OCH$_3$
OH
Metanephrine

Production and metabolism of foreign compounds in large intestine

Bacterial enzyme system in the large intestine brings about several biochemical alterations of the small amount of unabsorbed food molecules. In a few instances the substances such produced have a degree of toxicity. After absorption, they are metabolized in various ways as described earlier so that their elimination occurs afterwards, for instance, neutral fats are hydrolyzed by bacterial action and the products so formed are normal to gut, however, the choline fraction of phospholipids may yield an abnormal amine neurine which has a low older of toxicity.

Choline $\longrightarrow$ Neurine

Many amino acids undergo decarboxylation as a result of the action of intestinal bacteria to produce toxic amines (ptomaines).

Amino acid $\longrightarrow$ Ptomaine

CO_2

Detoxication of cyanides

Although the cyanide radical (CN$^-$) is very poisonous to the body, even then, very small quantities of it may be harmless. The CN$^-$ radical is converted to relatively nontoxic thiocyanate radical—SCN$^-$, and excreted as salts of this acid radical; **this reaction is catalysed by an enzyme known as rhodanese (thiosulfate sulfur transferase) in the presence of thiosulfate or colloidal sulfur as shown below:**

$$HCN+Na_2S_2O_3 \xrightarrow{\text{rhodanese}} NaHSO_3+NaCNS$$

Enzyme 'rhodanese' is of considerable significance in the animals that eat foods containing cyanogenic substances.

CHAPTER 27

EICOSANOIDS
(PROSTAGLANDINS, THROMBOXANES AND LEUKOTRIENES)

> We are C_{20} fatty acids derivatives having complicated structures and play numerous very important roles in the body like we help in controlling (i) blood pressure (ii) secretion of gastric HCl, (iii) inflammation (anti inflammatory agents), etc.

Arachidonic acid and some other C_{20} fatty acids with methylene-interrupted bonds give rise to eicosanoids which are physiologically and pharmacologically very active compounds and are known as **prostaglandins (PG)**, **thromboxanes (TX)**, and **leukotrienes (LT)**.

Arachidonic acid which is usually derived from the 2nd position of phospholipids in the plasma membrane, as a result of phospholipase A_2 activity, is the substrate for the biosynthesis of the PG_2, TX_2, and LT_4 compounds. The pathway for the synthesis of prostaglandins and thromboxanes is known as a **'cyclooxygenase pathway'** whereas the pathway for the synthesis of leukotrienes is known as a **'Lipooxygenase pathway'** as shown in Figure 27.1.

The figure indicates various stimulants as well as inhibitors. **It also indicates as to why steroids, which inhibit total eicosanoids production, are better anti-inflammatory agents than aspirin like drugs which inhibit only the cyclooxygenase pathway.**

PROSTAGLANDINS (PG)
Prostaglandins may be defined as the compounds which are fatty acid derivatives with hormones

like activities. They are in fact, unsaturated cyclic hydroxy fatty acids with a five membered ring in a 20 carbon skeleton. This group of hormone like substances was first of all detected in seminal fluid of man and other species, hence the name given as prostaglandins.

Prostaglandins are a group of naturally occurring substances having in common a structure which is based on prostanoic acid which contains 20 carbon atoms.

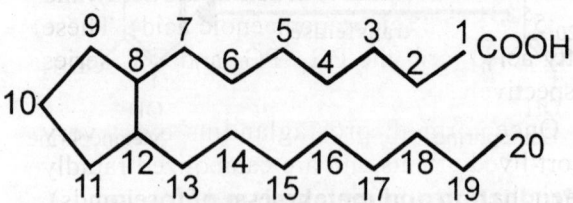

Prostanoic acid

Sixteen naturally occurring prostaglandins have been described (Table 27.1), but only seven along with two thromboxanes are found commonly throughout the body. These are termed as the **primary prostaglandins.**

Although PGs appear **hormone like in action** but they are different from hormones in

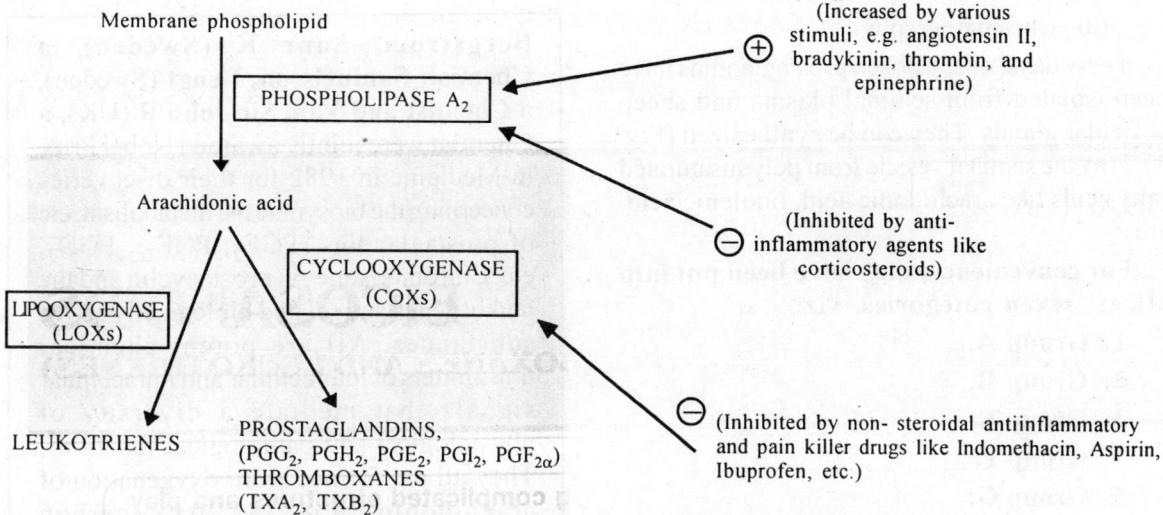

Fig. 27.1 : Conversion of archidonic acid to prostaglandins and thromboxanes via cyclooxygenase pathway and leukotrienes via lipooxygenase pathway

atleast two respects; they are synthesized at the site of action and made in almost all the tissues. **Linoleic acid** ($C_{18}:2^{9,12}$) is the precursor of two of the three 20- carbon fatty acids that form PGs; **linolenic acid** ($C_{18}:3^{9,12,15}$) is the other precursor. **Both these fatty acids are considered essential because they can not be synthesized in the body and therefore must be taken through diet.** The three C_{20} fatty acids subsequently formed are $C_{20}:3^{5,8,11}$ (eicosatrienoic acid), $C_{20}:4^{5,8,11,14}$ (eicosatetraenoic acid or **arachidonic acid),** and $C_{20}:5^{5,8,11,14,17}$ (eicosapentaenoic acid). These fatty acids form the PG_1, PG_2 and PG_3 series respectively.

Once formed, prostaglandins exert very short-lived effects and are catabolized rapidly (their half-life being expressed in seconds). Inactivation of prostaglandin appears to be mediated by two enzymes, 15α-hydroxy-prostaglandin dehydrogenase and Δ^{13}-prostaglandin reductase. **Prostaglandins are not stored; instead the precursor C_{20} fatty acids are present in tissues attached to the C-2 of phosphoglycerides. When needed, the C_{20} precursor is hydrolyzed by**

Table 27.1: Naturally occurring Prostaglandins

Primary PG	Other PG
PGE_1	PGA_1
$PGF_{1\alpha}$	PGA_2
PGE_2	19 α- OH PGA_1*
$PGF_{2\alpha}$	19 α- OH PGA_2**
PGG_2	PGB_1
PGH_2	PGB_2
PGI_2	19 α- OH PGB_2
Thromboxane A_2	PGE_3
Thromboxane B_2	$PGF_{3\alpha}$

* hydroxy-prostaglandin A,** hydroxy-prostaglandin B

phospholipase A_2, which is specific for the C-2 atom of the phosphoglyceride. The release of the C_{20} fatty acid appears to be the rate-limiting step in prostaglandin synthesis and is stimulated by the effect of bradykinin, thrombins, or angiotensin II.

Besides seminal fluid, these have also been found in various other tissues like lung, brain, pancreas etc. These are lipid soluble and may be isolated by any of the following techniques:

    (i)   Counter-current extraction technique, and

(ii) Chromatography

These days, over a dozen prostaglandins have been isolated from seminal plasma and sheep vesicular glands. They can be synthesized (Fig. 27.2) by the seminal vesicle from polyunsaturated fatty acids like arachidonic acid, linolenic acid, etc.

For convenience, they have been put into atleast seven categories, viz:

1. **Group A,**
2. **Group B,**
3. **Group E,**
4. **Group F,**
5. **Group G,**
6. **Group H and**
7. **Group I**

This classification is based upon the difference in the structure of the 5-carbon ring.

A, B and E have an oxo-grouping at position 9, whereas F, has a hydroxyl group in this position. 'A' has a double bond between positions 10 and 11 whereas 'B' has a double bond between positions 8 and 12. 'E' and 'F' do not have a double bond in the ring but possess a

Bergstrom, Sune K (Sweden), a **Chemist; Samuelsson, Bengt** (Sweden), a **Chemist and Van, Sir John R** (UK), a **Chemist** were jointly awarded Nobel Prize in Medicine in 1982 for their discoveries concerning the biosynthesis, metabolism, etc of prostaglandins (PGF$_2$, PGF$_{2a}$, PGD$_2$, etc.), thromboxane A$_2$ prostacyclin and the leukotrienes and related biologically active substances. All are potent chemical transmitters of intercellular and intracellular signals that mediate a diversity of physiological and pathological functions. They all are formed from oxygenation of arachidonic acid, a 20 - carbon polyunsaturated fatty acid.

hydroxyl group at position 11. It has been studied that all the active prostaglandins have got at least one double bond between positions 13 and 14; even some have two double bonds, the second being between positions 5 and 6 and finally some are found to have three double bonds; the additional bond being between positions 17 and 18. The structures of some of the more important

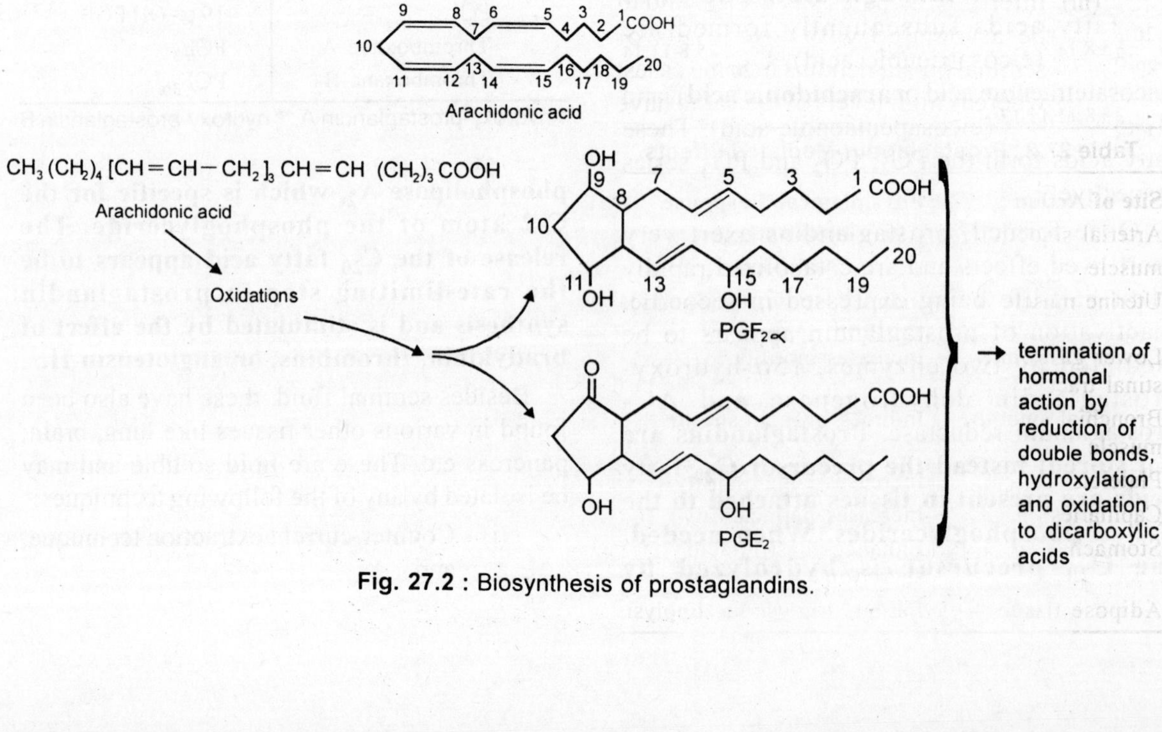

Fig. 27.2 : Biosynthesis of prostaglandins.

prostaglandins ($PGF_{2\alpha}$ and PGE_2) and that of arachidonic acid are given in Fig 27.3.

Some of the important prostaglandins include PGE_1, PGE_2, PGE_3, $PGF_{1\alpha}$, $PGF_{2\alpha}$, $PGF_{3\alpha}$ PGG_2, PGH_2, PGI_2, etc. There may be some 10 or 15 intermediate forms. Other prostaglandins are derivatives of PGE_1, varying in structural details, including the number of double bonds and hydroxyl groups and the stereo configuration of the hydroxyl groups.

Physiological functions/biochemical roles

Prostaglandins have been found to play following important roles in the human body (Table 27.2):

(i) They exert profound effects in facilitating fertilization of the ovum by causing uterine and cervical movements that help in the movement of the spermatozoa from the vagina into the cervix and uterus. In this way, they are believed to stimulate the smooth muscle of the uterus, particularly at the time of ovulation.

(ii) They help in controlling blood pressure.

(iii) Infertility in males has been found to be associated with low levels of seminal prostaglandins in some cases; whereas high levels of the same have been noticed in the amniotic fluid of those women who have a tendency of premature abortion.

(iv) Prostaglandins are believed to inhibit lipolysis in adipose tissue, possibly by inhibiting the conversion of ATP to cyclic AMP. Prostaglandins, thus, have the opposite effect of epinephrine, norepinephrine, glucagon and ACTH on the release of fatty acids from adipose tissue.

(v) **They also appear to control the secretion of gastric hydrochloric acid, the excess of which may otherwise cause gastric ulcers.**

(vi) They antagonize the action of catecholamines, in general.

(vii) They are also being extensively used as **abortificants** in some countries as they have got a tendency to induce abortions. The use of PGE_2 and $PGE_{2\alpha}$ are under extensive clinical trials in countries like Sweden, U.K., U.S., Uganda, etc., that is to say they help preventing conceptions.

(viii) Their exact role · in human reproduction is still uncertain.

(ix) They give relief in **asthma** and **nasal congestion.**

(ix) **They help in controlling inflammation.**

THROMBOXANES

These are synthesized in platelets and when released are responsible for vasoconstriction and platelet aggregation. They are of different types like TXA and TXB etc. Structures of some important thromboxanes are as given in Fig. 27.3.

LEUKOTRIENES

These are arachidonic acid metabolites. When these are conjugated to glutathione, then they are termed as peptidoleukotrienes. These are

Table 27.2 : Prostaglandin-Mediated Effects	
Site of Action	**Physiological Response**
Arterial smooth muscle	Alters blood pressure
Uterine muscle	Induces labour, therapeutic abortion
Lower gastrointestinal tract	Increases motility
Bronchial smooth muscle	Induces bronchospasm
Platelets	Increases coagulability
Capillaries	Increases permeability
Stomach	Enhances gastric-acid secretion
Adipose tissue	Inhibits triglyceride lipolysis

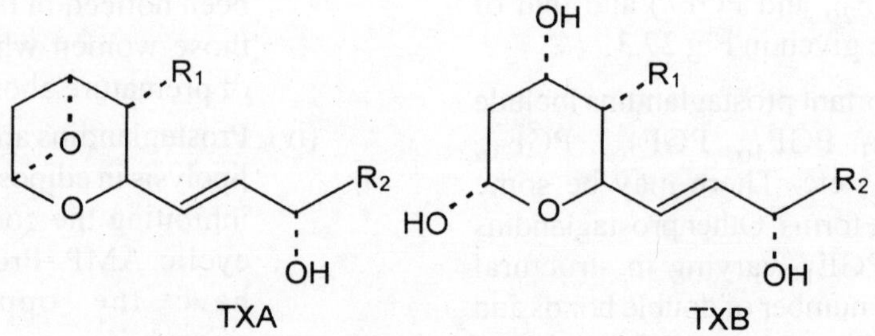

Fig 27.3: Structures of thromboxanes (TXA & TXB)

abbreviated as LT, thus LTC_3 denotes leukotriene C_3. These are of various types like LTA, LTB, LTC, LTD etc. Structure of LTB_4 is as shown in Fig. 27.4.

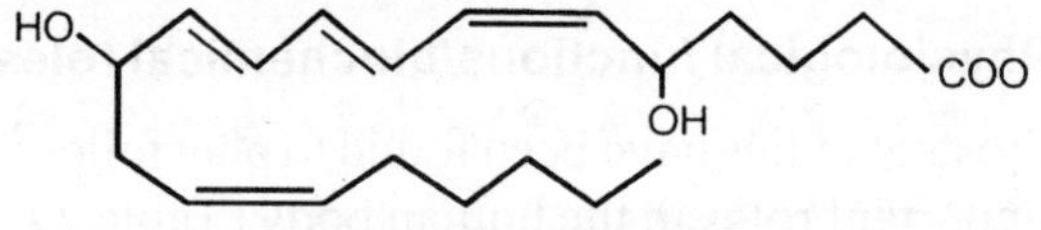

Fig 27.4: Leukotriene B_4

Functions/Importance

(i) They are responsible for the causation of **vascular permeability.**

(ii) They are also responsible for the attraction and activation of leukocytes.

(iii) They appear to be important regulators in many diseases which involve inflammation or immediate hypersensitivity reactions, such as asthma.

Nonsteroidal anti-inflammatory drugs (NSAIDs), such as aspirin, ibuprofen, and indomethacin, inhibit the COXs, thereby decreasing prostaglandins synthesis. **Two isoforms of COX are known- COX-1 and COX-2. COX-1 level is in general rather constant in cells, whereas COX-2 is synthesized in response of inflammation. Certain drugs that inhibit both COXs have nephrotoxic and ulcerogenic side effects.** Therefore, new NSAIDs are being tested to inhibit preferentially COX-2 to reduce side effects while maintaining the desirable anti-inflammatory therapy.

Prostaglandin I_2, or prostacyclin, is derived from arachidonic acid in the vascular endothelium. It has a powerful vasodilatory action, especially on the coronary arteries, and also is responsible for inhibiting platelet aggregation. Thromboxane A_2 is synthesized from arachidonic acid but also is produced by platelets. It has the opposite effect of prostacylin; that is, it stimulates the contraction of arterial smooth muscle and enhances platelet aggregation. It has a very short half-life, about 30 seconds, and is converted rapidly to its inactive metabolite thromboxane B_2. The thromboxanes are slightly different from the other prostaglandins in that they contain six sided rings of five carbon atoms and one oxygen atom (Figure 7.4). Table 7.2 lists some of the reported functions of the various prostaglandins. With the increasing knowledge of the physiological role of the prostaglandins, discrete disorders of prostaglandin metabolism are likely to be discovered, and prostaglandins, prostaglandin analogues, or prostaglandin antagonists are likely to be used in clinical practice.

BIOCHEMICAL VALUES

Biochemical Values

Table - I Normal Human Biochemical Values in Blood / Plasma / Serum

S.No.	Constituent	Normal range	High in	Low in
	DIABETES MELLITUS			
1.	Blood Sugar (Fasting)	70 - 100 mg%	Diabetes mellitus	Hyperinsulinism
2.	Blood Sugar (PP)	Less than 140 mg%	Diabetes mellitus	—
3.	Renal Threshold Value	160 - 180 mg%	Diabetes mellitus	—
4.	Blood Sugar Level, (Random)	80 - 120 mg%	Diabetes mellitus	—
	RENAL FUNCTION TESTS			
1.	Blood Urea	14 - 43 mg%	Nephritis, Renal Failure	Nephrosis
2.	Serum Creatinine	0.1 - 1.2 mg%	Nephritis, Renal Failure	Nephrosis
	LIVER FUNCTION TESTS			
1.	Serum Bilirubin	0.2 - 1.0 mg%	Obstructive Jaundice, Haemolytic Jaundice, Neonatal Jaundice and Hepatitis	—
2.	SGOT (AST)	4 - 17 IU/l (8 - 40 units/ml)	Myocardial Infarction, Infective Hepatitis etc.	—
3.	SGPT (ALT)	3 - 15 IU/l	Liver Disorders	—
4.	Serum Alkaline Phosphatase	4 - 11 KA Units	Obstructive Jaundice, Biliary Cirrhosis, Rickets, Osteomalacia etc.	Scurvy, Severe Anaemia, Mal-nutrition, Hypo-phosphatasia
5.	Serum Proteins, Total	6.0 - 8.0 g%	Multiple Myeloma, Anhydraemia, etc.	Nephrotic Syndromes, Neoplastic Disease, Malnutrition, Kwashiorkor Syndrome, Cirrhosis of Liver.

S.No.	Constituent	Normal range	High in	Low in
6.	Serum Albumin	3.5 - 5.0 g%	—	Cirrhosis of Liver, Nephrotic Syndromes, Malnutrition, Malignancies, etc.
7.	Serum Globulins,	2.3 - 3.6 g%	Anhydraemia, Nephrosis, Infections, Advanced Liver Diseases, etc.	—
8.	Albumin / Globulins Ratio	1.2 - 1.5	—	Less than 1 in Infective Hepatitis
9.	Fibrinogen (Plasma)	0.3 - 0.6 g%	Infections	Cirrhosis of Liver
	CARDIAC ENZYMES			
1.	SGOT (AST)	4 - 17 IU / l (8 - 40 units / ml)	Myocardial Infarction, Infective Hepatitis, etc.	—
2.	Lactic Dehydrogenase (LDH)	230 - 460 IU / l	Myocardial Infarction, Infective Hepatitis, Toxic Jaundice, etc.	—
3.	Creatine Phosphokinase (CPK or CK)	20 - 50 IU / l (men) 10-37 IU / l (Women)	Myocardial Infarction, Hypothyroidism, Progressive Muscular Atrophy, etc	—
	CARDIAC MARKERS			
1.	Troponin - T		Myocardial Infarction	—
2.	Homocysteine		Myocardial Infarction	Pregnancy
	THYROID FUNCTION TESTS			
1.	Triiodothyronine (T_3)	60 - 190 ng/dl (RIA mehtod)	Pregnancy, Hyperthyroidism	Hypothyroidism
2.	Thyroxine (T_4)	1.5 - 4.0 ng/dl (RIA mehtod)	Hyperthyroidism	Hypothyroidism
3.	TSH	0.3 - 6.0 μIU / ml	Hypothyroidism	Hyperthyroidism
4.	Thyroid Binding Globulin (TBG)	2.0 - 4.8 ng/dl	Pregnancy, Acute Liver Disease	Major illness, Nephrosis, Thyrotoxicosis
5.	Protein Bound Iodine (PBI)	4 - 8 μg/dl	Hyperthyroidism	Hypothyroidism, Nephrosis, etc.

S.No.	Constituent	Normal range	High in	Low in
	PANCREATIC FUNCTION TESTS			
1.	Serum Amylase	80 - 180 Somogyi Units	Pancreatitis, Stone and Cancer in Biliary Duct, Perforated Peptic Ulcer	Liver diseases
2.	Serum Lipase	Less than 150 U / l	Pancreatitis, Cancer in Pancreas, Cirrhosis of Liver, Hepatitis, Duodenal ulcer, Disease of the biliary tract, etc.	—
	LIPID PROFILE			
1.	Serum Cholesterol	150 - 200 mg %	Diabetes, Nephritis, etc	Hyperthyroidism, Severe liver damage
2.	HDL - Cholesterol	30 - 63 mg %, (men) 35 - 75 mg % (women)	The Combined Risk Factor of Coronary Heart Disease (CHD) can be determined following the estimations of Serum Cholesterol and HDL - Cholesterol.	
3.	LDL - Cholesterol	up to 150 mg /dl	**The Ratio of Cholesterol to HDL - Cholesterol has Predictive Value in Determining the Risk of CHD more accurately. For normal males the ratio of 5:1 and for normal females the ratio of 4.5:1 are considered as average risk.** Lower ratios significantly reduce the risk, whereas ratios **9.5:1 and 7:1** for males and females respectively, are believed to double the risk of CHD. An inverse relationship has been observed between the risk of CHD and the concentration of HDL-cholesterol. HDL - cholesterol represents approximately 20-25% of the total cholesterol in serum.	

S.No.	Constituent	Normal range	High in	Low in
4.	VLDL	up to 28 mg / dl	Hyperlipidaemia	—
5.	Serum Triglycerides	30 - 140 mg%	Hyperlipidaemia, Atherosclerosis, Nephrosis	—
6.	Lipids, Total	360 - 820 mg%	Diabetes Mellitus	—
	STOMACH FUNCTION TEST			
1.	Fractional Test Meals (FTM) i.e., Gastric Analysis	Free Acidity 0.0 - 40 meq / l ; Total Acidity 20 - 55 meq / l	Duodenal Ulcer and Gastric Ulcer	Hypochlorhydria (Hypoacidity)
	HORMONES			
1.	Insulin	5 - 20 µU / ml (Adult Fasting)	Hypoglycaemia, Insulinoma	Diabetes Mellitus
2.	Testosterone	350 - 1000 ng /dl , (Males)	-	Hypogonadism (Males)
		20 - 70 ng /dl, (Females)	Elevated (females)-Adrenal or Ovarian Tumors	—
3.	Thyrocalcitonin	20 - 400 pg / ml	Medullary Carcinoma of the Thyroid	—
4.	Human Chorionic Gonadotropin (HCG)	2,000 - 40,000 IU/l	Detectable level confirms Pregnancy	Threatened Pregnancy
5.	Gastrin	< 300 pg/ml	Stomach or Duodenal Ulcer, Zollinger Ellison Syndrome	—
	ANAEMIA			
1.	Haemoglobin (males)	14 - 18 g%	Polycythemia	Anemias
2.	Haemoglobin (females)	11 - 16 g%	Polycythemia	Anemias

S.No.	Constituent	Normal range	High in	Low in
	MISCELLANEOUS			
1.	Serum Acid Phosphatase	1 - 4 KA Units	Carcinoma of Prostate Gland, Paget's Disease, Hyperparathyroidism	—
2.	Serum Uric Acid	2 - 7 mg %	Gout, Nephritis, Arthritis, Eclampsia	Wilson's Disease, Fanconi Syndrome
3.	Serum Calcium	9-11 mg%	Hyperparathyroidism	Infantile Tetany, Rickets
4.	Serum Inorganic Phosphorus	2.5-4.5 mg%	Nephritis, Renal Failure	Rickets, Fanconi Syndrome
5.	Serum Sodium Serum Potassium	137-148 meq/l 3.6-5.4 meq/l	— Pneumonia, Acute Infections and Uremia	Diabetic Acidosis 6. —
7.	Serum Magnesium	1-3 mg%	—	Vomiting and Diarrhoea
8.	Serum Lithium	Absent or in Traces	—	—
9.	Lipoprotein (a)	0 - 30 mg/ dl		

DESIRED LIPID PROFILE

Risk Category	Total Cholesterol mg / dl	HDL Cholesterol mg /dl	LDL Cholesterol mg / dl	Triglycerides mg / dl
DESIRABLE	<200	>=35	<130	<200
BORDERLINE HIGH	200 - 239	...	130 - 159	200 - 400
WORRISOME	>=240	<35	>=160	401 - 1000

IMPORTANT TUMOR MARKERS

Sl. No	TUMOR MARKERS	ASSOCIATED CANCER
1.	Carcino Embryonic Antigen (CEA)	Colon, Lung, Breast, Pancreas
2.	Alpha Fetoprotein (AFP)	Liver, Gonadal Germ Cell Tumor
3.	Prostate - Specific Antigen (PSA)	Prostate Cancer
4.	Prostatic - Acid Phosphatase (PAP)	Prostate Cancer
5.	Lactic Dehydrogenase (LDH)	Lymphoma, Ewing's Syndrome
6.	Calcitonin (CT)	Medullary Cancer of the Thyroid
7.	Human Chorionic Gonadotropin (HCG)	Trophoblast, Gonadal Germ Cell Tumor

Table - II : Commonly used Anticoagulants

S.No.	Anticoagulant	mg/ml Blood	Use	Mode of Action
1.	Heparin	0.2	Procedures requiring whole blood or plasma especially useful when intact erythrocytes are desired	Inhibits conversion of prothrombin to thrombin
2.	Ethylenediamine - Tetraacetic Acid (EDTA)	1	Procedures requiring whole blood or plasma	Chelates ionic calcium
3.	Oxalates (a) Lithium (b) Sodium (c) Potassium (d) Ammonium	1 - 2	Procedures requiring whole blood or plasma. Causes shrinkage of cell volume, should not be used in haematological procedures.	Forms unionized calcium oxalate complex; reduces level of ionized calcium below that required for clotting
4.	Sodium Citrate	5	As for oxalates	Forms unionized complex with calcium
5.	Sodium Fluoride	10	**Combination anticoagulant and preservative for blood glucose determination by inhibiting blood enzymes causing glycolysis;** causes erythrocyte shrinkage. Combined with thymol (1mg +10 mg NaF) for effective control of microbial growth in stored blood samples.	Forms unionized calcium fluoride complex

APPENDIX - I

CSF in Differential Diagnosis

Disease	Appearance	Cells/cmm	Protein (mg%)	Glucose (mg%)
Normal pH (7.35-7.4)	-	-	-	-
Normal level	Crystal clear	< 5 cells, all lymphocytes	15 - 45	50 - 80
Acute purulent meningitis	opalescent to purulent clot	500-20,000 mostly poly's	45 - 100 +	0 - 45
Tuberculous meningitis	opalescent fibrin web, pellicle	10 - 500 mostly lympho's	45 - 500 +	0 - 45
Early, acute syphilitic meningitis	clear to turbid, occasional clot	25 - 2,000 mostly lympho's	45 - 400 +	15-75
Late CNS syphilis	Normal	Normal or ↑	Normal or ↑	Normal
Viral encephalitis (arthropod borne)	Normal	0 - 100 mostly lympho's	Normal or increased	45-100
Viral meningoencephalitis	Normal	0 - 2000+	Normal or ↑	Normal

APPENDIX - II

Typical composition of human blood in health and certain disorders

Constituent	Normal level (mg per 100 ml)	Nephritis (mg per 100 ml)	Diabetes mellitus mg per 100 ml
Calcium (serum)	8.5 - 10.5	5 - 7	-
Chlorides as NaCl	580 - 630	to 700	to 400
Cholesterol (serum)	150 - 200	to 900	to 800
Creatinine	0.1 - 1.2	to 28	to 4
Glucose	70 - 120	to 300	to 1,200
Inorganic phosphorus (serum) (higher in children)	2.5 - 4.8	to 20	-
Blood/Plasma Urea	14 - 43	to 400	-
Plasma carbondioxide (vol%)	55 - 75	to 45	10 - 50
Blood/Plasma Urea nitrogen (BUN)	6 - 20	to 300	to 30
Uric acid	2.5 - 7.0 (men) 1.5 - 6.0 (women)	to 27	to 10

APPENDIX - III

Variations in activities of intracellular enzymes in Myocardial Infarction

Enzyme	Earliest significant increase (hours)	Time of maximum (hours)	Time of return to normal (days)
CPK	2 - 4	24 - 36	3
GOT	4 - 6	24 - 48	5
LDH	8 - 10	48 - 72	14

APPENDIX - IV

Qualitative Analysis of a Normal Urine

Total 24 hours volume	1-2litres
Colour	pale to deep amber
Transparancy	clear
Sediments	Nil
Odour	characteristic and faintly aromatic
Reaction	acidic (about pH 6.0)
Specific gravity	1.008-1.030
Albumin	Nil
Sugar	Nil
Ketone bodies	Nil
Bile pigments	Nil
Bile salts	Nil
Urobilinogen	Nil
Crystals	may or may not be present
Pus cells	Nil
RBCs	Nil
Casts	Nil
Microorganisms	Nil

APPENDIX - V

Urine, Quantitative analysis of a normal urine

Sl. No.	Constituent	Normal range (per 24 hours)
1.	Acetone	5-7.5 mg
2.	Acidity, titratable	20-50 meq/litre
3.	Aldosterone	2-23 mcg
4.	Allantoin	25-35 mg
5.	Amino acids, total	500-1000 mg
6.	Ammonia	500-1200 mg
7.	Amylase	5-20 Somogyi units
8.	Androgens	6-20 mg
9.	Ascorbic acid	6-18 mg
10.	Calcium (as Ca)	100-300 mg
	meq/litre	5-15
11.	Chlorides (as Nacl)	10-15 g
	meq/litre	170-250
12.	Cholesterol, total	0.3-1 mg
13.	Citric acid	210-470 mg
14.	Copper	< 30 mg
15.	Coproporphyrins	60-280 mcg
16.	Creatine	< 200 mg
17.	Creatinine	100-1800 mg
18.	Glucose	15-130 mg
19.	Hexosamines	80-110 mg
20.	Hippuric acid	100-1000 mg
21.	17-Hydroxycorticosteroids	6-20 mg
22.	5-Hydroxy-3-indoleacetic acid	<10 mg
23.	Indican	40-150 mg
24.	Iodine	10-200 mcg
25.	Iron	< 1 mg
26.	17-ketogenic steroids (men)	2-7 mg
	(women)	1-5.5 mg
27.	Ketone bodies	< 50 mg
	acetone	0-7.5 mg
	β-hydroxybutyric acid	30mg
28.	17-ketosteroids (neutral) men	9-24 mg
	(women)	5-17 mg

Contd

Sl. No.	Constituent	Normal range (per 24 hours)
29.	Lactic acid	100-300 mg
30.	Lead	0.03-0.08 mg
31.	Leucine aminopeptidase (men)	50-175 G-R units
	(women)	20-70 G-R units
32.	Magnesium (as Mg)	50-200 mg
	meq/litre	4-20
33.	Nicotinic acid	0.1-1 mg
34.	Nitrogen, total	12-18 g
35.	Oxalic acid	15-50 mg
36.	pH	5.0-8.0
37.	Pentoses	< 500 mg
38.	Phenols, total	< 71 mg
	conjugated	20- 70 mg
	free	0.2 - 0.4 mg
39.	Phosphatase, acid	80-300 King-Armstrong units
40.	Phosphorus (as P)	1-1.2 g
41.	Potassium	1-3 g
	meq/litre	40-65
42.	Proteins, total	< 150 mg
43.	Purine bases	16-60 mg
44.	Reducing substances, total (as glucose)	0-200 mg
45.	Sodium	3-5 g
	meq/litre	130-200
46.	Sulfates (total), (as S)	0.6-2 g
47.	Thiocyanate	5-8 mg
48.	Total solids	70g
49.	Urea	20-35 g
50.	Urea N	10-15 g
51.	Uric acid	580-1000 mg
52.	Urobilinogen, Ehrlich units	< 2
53.	Uroporphyrins	10-50 mcg
54.	Zinc	0.3-0.4 mg

INDEX